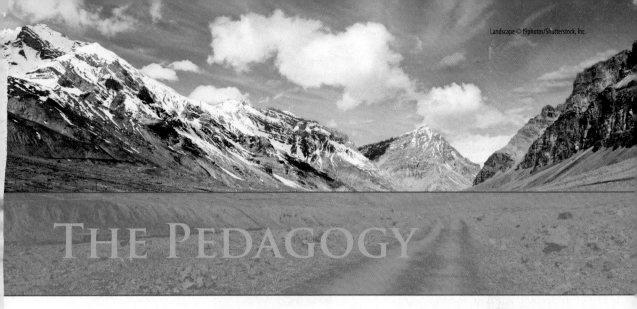

THE PEDAGOGY

Professional Nursing Concepts: Competencies for Quality Leadership, Third Edition drives comprehension through various strategies that meet the learning needs of students, while also generating enthusiasm about the topic. This interactive approach addresses different learning styles, making this the ideal text to ensure mastery of key concepts. The pedagogical aids that appear in most chapters include the following:

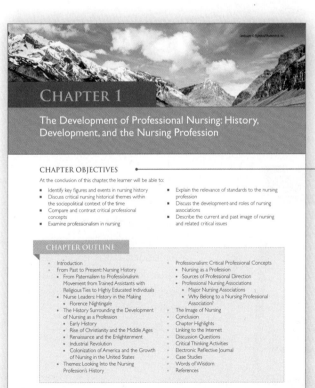

Chapter Objectives
These objectives provide instructors and students with a snapshot of the key information they will encounter in each chapter. They serve as a checklist to help guide and focus study.

Key Terms

Found in a list at the beginning of each chapter, these terms will create an expanded vocabulary in professional nursing concepts.

Introduction

Important concepts and topics are highlighted at the beginning of each chapter to focus students' attention on the essential material.

Linking to the Internet

Links to supplemental material are included at the end of each chapter for students interested in exploring topics of interest in greater depth.

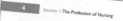

4   Section I: The Profession of Nursing

KEY TERMS

Accountability
Autonomy
Code of ethics

Nursing
Professionalism
Responsibility

Scope of practice
Social policy statement
Standards

INTRODUCTION

This text presents an introduction to the nursing profession and critical aspects of nursing care and the delivery of health care. To begin the journey to graduation and licensure, it is important to understand several aspects of the nursing profession. What is professional nursing? How did it develop? Which factors influence the view of the profession? This chapter addresses these questions.

FROM PAST TO PRESENT
Nursing History

It is important for nursing students to learn about nursing history. Nursing's history provides a framework for understanding how nursing is practiced today and which societal trends are shaping the profession. The characteristics of nursing as a profession and what nurses do today have their roots in the past, not only in the history of nursing but also in the history of health care and society in general. Today, health care is highly complex; diagnostic methods and therapies have been developed that offer many opportunities for prevention, treatment, and cures that did not exist even a few years ago. Understanding the health process is part of this discussion to appreciate where nursing is today as a stimulus for changes in the future. Nursing is "realized as a practice discipline to serve the needs of society to enhance the health of the community" (Shaw, 1993, p. 1654).

The past portrayal of nurses as handmaidens and assistants to physicians has its roots in the profession's religious beginnings. The following sections examine the story of nursing and explore how it developed.

From Paternalism to Professionalism: Movement from Trained Assistants with Religious Ties to Highly Educated Individuals

The discipline of nursing slowly evolved from the traditional role of women, apprenticeship, humanitarian aims, religious ideals, intuition, common sense, trial and error, theories, and research, as well as the multiple influences of medicine, technology, politics, war, economics, and feminism (Brooks & Kleine-Kracht, 1983; Gorenberg, 1983; Jacobs & Huether, 1978; Keller, 1979; Kidd & Morrison, 1988; Lynaugh & Fagin, 1988; Perry, 1985). It is impossible to provide a detailed history of nursing's evolution in one chapter, so only critical historical events will be discussed here.

Writing about nursing history itself has its own interesting history (Connolly, 2004). Historians who wrote about nursing prior to the 1950s tended to be nurses, and they wrote for nurses. Although nursing, throughout its history, has been intertwined with social issues of the day, the early publications about nursing history did not link nursing to "the broader social, economic, and cultural context in which events unfolded" (Connolly, 2004, p. 10). There was greater emphasis on the "profession's purity, discipline, and faith" (p. 10). Part of the reason for this narrow view of nursing history

---

Chapter 1: The Development of Professional Nursing   35

LINKING TO THE INTERNET

- American Association for the History of Nursing: http://www.aahn.org
- Directory of Links: http://dmoz.org/health/nursing/history
- Barbara Bates Center for the Study of the History of Nursing, University of Pennsylvania: http://www.nursing.upenn.edu/history/Pages/default.aspx
- Experiencing War: Women at War (Includes nurses): http://www.loc.gov/vets/stories/ex-war-womenatwar.html
- National Student Nurses Association: http://www.nsna.org
- American Assembly of Men in Nursing: http://aamn.org
- Nursing: The Ultimate Adventure pamphlet (NSNA): http://www.nsna.org/Publications/Ultimate_Adventure.aspx

CASE STUDIES

Case Study 1

You and your friends in the nursing program are having lunch after a class that covered content found in this chapter. One of your friends says, "I was bored when we got to all that information on professionalism and nursing organizations. What a waste of time. I just want to be a nurse." All of you are struggling to figure out what you have gotten yourself into. You turn to your friends and suggest it might be helpful to have an open discussion on the comment just made. So over lunch you all talk about the comment made by one of your friends. It was clear that the students who had read the chapter were better able to discuss the issue, but everyone had an opinion.

Case Questions

Here are some questions to consider:
1. What is the purpose of nursing organizations?
2. What role should professional organizations assume to increase nursing status in the healthcare system?
3. What are some of the advantages and disadvantages to joining a professional organization?
4. What do you know about your school's NSNA chapter? How would you join your school's student nursing association?
5. Which nursing organization mentioned in this chapter interests you and why? Compare your response with those of your other classmates.
6. Search on the Internet for a specialty nursing organization and pick one that interests you. What can you find out about the organization?

(continues)

Chapter Highlights
Chapter highlights summarize the most important material for quick review.

Discussion Questions
Each chapter includes discussion questions students should be able to answer after reading through the chapter.

Critical Thinking Activities
Each chapter includes critical thinking activities that students can work through individually or in a group.

Electronic Reflection Journal
At the end of each chapter, the electronic reflection journal activity prompts students to think about how content will affect and apply to them.

Chapter 1: The Development of Professional Nursing   33

Landscape © flphoto/Shutterstock, Inc.

CONCLUSION

This chapter has highlighted the history of nursing, societal trends, image of nursing, and other influences that shape nursing as a profession. It presented an overview of the remainder of this text. Professional nursing includes many key aspects that will be discussed in more detail: art and science of nursing; education; critical issues related to health care, such as those involving consumers; the continuum of care; the healthcare delivery system; policy, and legal and ethical concerns; the five core competencies; and current issues regarding the practice of nursing.

Landscape © flphoto/Shutterstock, Inc.

CHAPTER HIGHLIGHTS

1. Nursing history provides a framework for understanding how nursing is practiced today.
2. The history of nursing is complex and has been influenced by social, economic, and political factors.
3. Florence Nightingale was instrumental in changing the view of nursing and education to improve care delivery.
4. Nursing meets the critical requirements for a profession.
5. The sources of professional direction include ANA documents that describe the scope of practice, accountability, and an ethical code.
6. Professional organizations play a key role in shaping nursing as a profession.
7. The image of nursing is formulated in many ways by the public, the media, interprofessional colleagues, and nurses. Nursing's image as a profession has both positive and negative aspects.

Landscape © flphoto/Shutterstock, Inc.

DISCUSSION QUESTIONS

1. How might knowing more about nursing history affect your personal view of nursing?
2. How did the image of nursing in Nightingale's time influence nursing from the 1860s through the 1940s?
3. How would you compare and contrast accountability, autonomy, and responsibility?
4. Based on content in this chapter, how would you define professionalism in your own words?
5. Why are standards important to the nursing profession and to healthcare deli
6. Review the ANA standards of professional performance. Are by any of the standards? If so, w
7. How would you explain to so not in health care the reason phasizes its social policy statem

---

34   Section 1: The Profession of Nursing

Landscape © flphoto/Shutterstock, Inc.

CRITICAL THINKING ACTIVITIES

1. Describe how the Nightingale Pledge has relevance today and how it might be altered to be more relevant. Work with a team of students to accomplish this activity and arrive at a consensus statement.
2. Interview two nurses and ask them if they think nursing is a profession, and determine the rationale for their viewpoint. How does what they say compare with what you have learned about professionalism in this chapter?
3. Attend a National Student Nurses Association meeting at your school. What did you learn about the organization? What did you observe in the meeting about leadership and nursing? Do you have any criticisms of the organization and how might it be improved?
4. Complete a mini-survey of six people (non-nurses), asking them to describe their image of nursing and nurses. Try to pick a variety of people. Summarize and analyze your data to identify any themes and unusual views. How does what you learned relate to the content in this chapter? List the similarities and differences, and then discuss your findings with a group of your classmates and compare with their findings.
5. Analyze a television program that focuses on a healthcare situation/story line. How are nurses depicted compared with other healthcare professionals? Compose a letter to the program describing your analysis, and document your arguments to support your viewpoint. This could be done with a team of students: watch the same program and then discuss opinions and observations.

Circuit Board: © Photos.com

ELECTRONIC Reflection Journal

You are asked to develop an Electronic Reflection Journal that you will use after you complete each chapter. This is the place for you to comment on some aspect identified at the end of the chapter. You may also keep notes about issues that you want to expand on—reflect on—as you progress through your nursing education. If you are using technology that allows you to make visuals, use drawings and graphics to expand your journal thoughts.

In your first entry in your Electronic Reflection Journal, consider the following questions related to the image of nursing. Connect your responses so that you can better understand the importance of image to the profession and the meaning of profession.

1. Why is the image of nursing important to the profession?
2. What role do you think you might have as a nurse in influencing the image of nursing? Provide specific examples.
3. What is your opinion about nursing uniforms, and how do you think they influence the image of nursing?
4. What stimulated your interest in nursing as a profession? Was the image of nursing in any way related to your decision, and in what way did it impact your decision?

Special assignment for this chapter: Write your own definition of nursing and include it in your Electronic Reflection Journal. Work on this definition throughout this course as you learn more about nursing. Save the final draft, and at the end of each semester or quarter, go back to your definition and make any changes you feel are necessary. Keep a draft of each definition so that you can see your changes. When you graduate, review all your definitions; see how you have developed your view of professional nursing. Ideally, you would then review your definition again one year post graduation.

Case Studies

Case studies encourage active learning and promote critical thinking skills. Students can analyze the situation they are presented with and solve problems, learning to apply the information in the text to everyday practice.

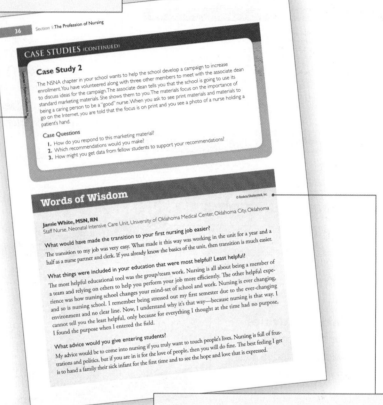

CASE STUDIES (CONTINUED)

Case Study 2

The NSNA chapter in your school wants to help the school develop a campaign to increase enrollment. You have volunteered along with three other members to meet with the associate dean to discuss ideas for the campaign. The associate dean tells you that the school is going to use its standard marketing materials. She shows them to you. The materials focus on the importance of being a caring person to be a "good" nurse. When you ask to see print materials and materials to go on the Internet, you are told that the focus is on print and you see a photo of a nurse holding a patient's hand.

Case Questions
1. How do you respond to this marketing material?
2. Which recommendations would you make?
3. How might you get data from fellow students to support your recommendations?

Words of Wisdom

© Rodola/Shutterstock, Inc

Jamie White, MSN, RN
Staff Nurse, Neonatal Intensive Care Unit, University of Oklahoma Medical Center, Oklahoma City, Oklahoma

What would have made the transition to your first nursing job easier?
The transition to my job was very easy. What made it this way was working in the unit for a year and a half as a nurse partner and clerk. If you already know the basics of the unit, then transition is much easier.

What things were included in your education that were most helpful? Least helpful?
The most helpful educational tool was the group/team work. Nursing is all about being a member of a team and relying on others to help you perform your job more efficiently. The other helpful experience was how nursing school changes your mind-set of school and work. Nursing is ever changing, and so is nursing school. I remember being stressed out my first semester due to the ever-changing environment and no clear line. Now, I understand why it's that way—because nursing is that way. I cannot tell you the least helpful, only because for everything I thought at the time had no purpose, I found the purpose when I entered the field.

What advice would you give entering students?
My advice would be to come into nursing if you truly want to touch people's lives. Nursing is full of frustrations and politics, but if you are in it for the love of people, then you will do fine. The best feeling I get is to hand a family their sick infant for the first time and to see the hope and love that is expressed.

Words of Wisdom

Words of wisdom from practicing nurses help students better understand how their education and training will prepare them for their work as a nurse. These features highlight advice from practicing nurses about their experience as a student and their transition to the field.

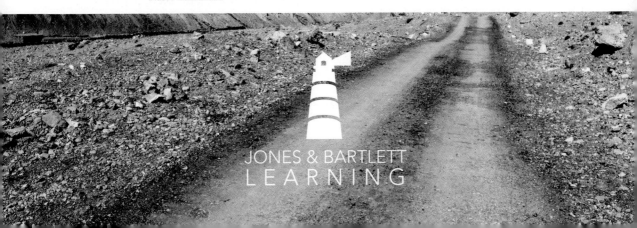

PROFESSIONAL NURSING CONCEPTS

Competencies for Quality Leadership

THIRD EDITION

ANITA FINKELMAN, MSN, RN
Visiting Faculty
Northeastern University
Bouvé College of Health Sciences
School of Nursing
Boston, Massachusetts
Nurse Consultant

CAROLE KENNER, RN, FAAN
Dean and Professor
School of Nursing
Health and Exercise Science
The College of New Jersey
Ewing, New Jersey

JONES & BARTLETT
LEARNING

World Headquarters
Jones & Bartlett Learning
5 Wall Street
Burlington, MA 01803
978-443-5000
info@jblearning.com
www.jblearning.com

Jones & Bartlett Learning books and products are available through most bookstores and online booksellers. To contact Jones & Bartlett Learning directly, call 800-832-0034, fax 978-443-8000, or visit our website, www.jblearning.com.

Substantial discounts on bulk quantities of Jones & Bartlett Learning publications are available to corporations, professional associations, and other qualified organizations. For details and specific discount information, contact the special sales department at Jones & Bartlett Learning via the above contact information or send an email to specialsales@jblearning.com.

04888-9

Production Credits
VP, Executive Publisher: David Cella
Executive Editor: Amanda Martin
Associate Acquisitions Editor: Rebecca Myrick
Production Editor: Sarah Bayle
Marketing Communications Manager: Katie Hennessy
Art Development Editor: Joanna Lundeen
VP, Manufacturing and Inventory Control: Therese Connell
Composition: Cenveo Publisher Services
Cover and Text Design: Kristin E. Parker
Manager of Photo Research, Rights & Permissions: Lauren Miller
Cover Image: © f9photos/Shutterstock, Inc.
Printing and Binding: Manufactured in the United States by RR Donnelley
Cover Printing: Manufactured in the United States by RR Donnelley

Library of Congress Cataloging-in-Publication Data
Finkelman, Anita Ward, author.
 Professional nursing concepts : competencies for quality leadership / Anita Finkelman, Carole Kenner. — Third edition.
  p. ; cm.
 Includes bibliographical references and index.
 ISBN 978-1-284-06776-7
 I. Kenner, Carole, author. II. Title.
 [DNLM: 1. Nursing—United States. 2. Leadership—United States. 3. Nurse's Role—United States. 4. Nursing Care—United States. WY 100 AA1]
 RT82
 610.7306'9—dc23
                    2014024735

6048

Printed in the United States of America
18 17 16 15   10 9 8 7 6 5 4 3

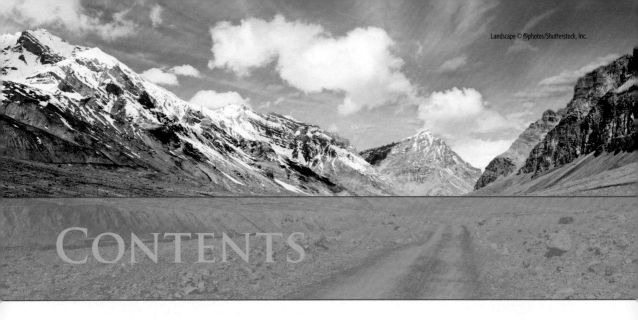

Landscape © f9photos/Shutterstock, Inc.

CONTENTS

SECTION II: THE HEALTHCARE CONTEXT

Chapter 5 Health Policy and Political Action: Critical Actions for Nurses 149

Chapter 6 Ethics and Legal Issues 173

Chapter 7 Health Promotion, Disease Prevention, and Illness: A Community Perspective 197

Chapter 8 The Healthcare Delivery System: Focus on Acute Care 233

SECTION III: CORE HEALTHCARE PROFESSIONAL COMPETENCIES

SECTION IV: THE PRACTICE OF NURSING TODAY AND IN THE FUTURE

Chapter 14 The Future: Transformation of Nursing Practice Through Leadership ... 451

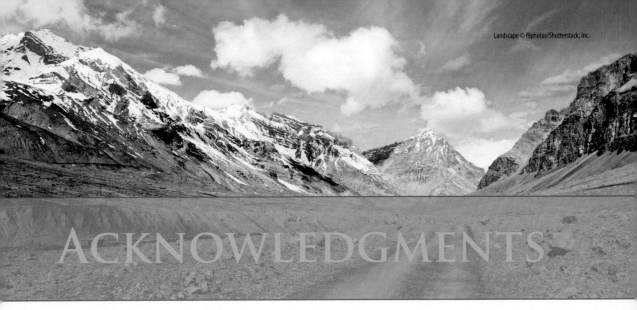

ACKNOWLEDGMENTS

We would like to thank our families: Fred, Shoshannah, and Deborah Finkelman, and Lester Kenner. Thank you to Elizabeth Karle for providing administrative assistance with research and the manuscript, to Amanda Martin for her guidance in the development of this book, and to Sarah Bayle and the Jones & Bartlett Learning editorial staff for their expertise. We also want to recognize all the students we have worked with who have taught us so much about what students need to know to practice competently.

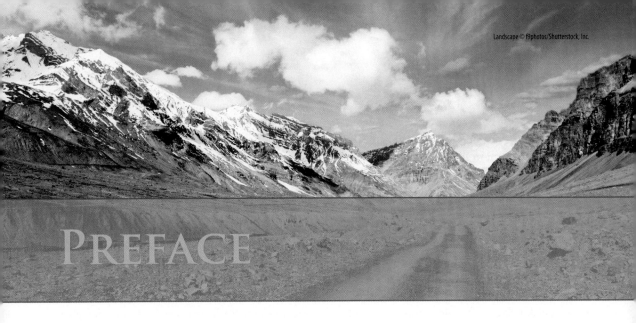

Landscape © f9photos/Shutterstock, Inc.

PREFACE

This text was motivated by the need to include more information in nursing education about the Institute of Medicine (IOM) reports on quality health care, with a focus on the five core competencies identified by the IOM for all healthcare professions. This goal is even more imperative today for the *Third Edition* given the strong emphasis on improving health care in the United States and concern that the quality of care continues to need improvement. The IOM core competencies provide the framework for this text, which introduces nursing students to the nursing profession and healthcare delivery (IOM, 2003). The five competencies are:

1. Provide patient-centered care
2. Work in interprofessional teams
3. Employ evidence-based practice
4. Apply quality improvement
5. Utilize informatics

Nursing students today are asked to cover much information in their courses and to develop clinical competencies in a short period of time. It is critical that each student recognize that nursing does not happen in isolation, but rather it is part of the entire healthcare experience. Nurses need to assume critical roles in this experience through their unique professional expertise and leadership.

They are also members of the healthcare team; they must work with others to provide and improve care.

This text consists of 14 chapters and is divided into 4 sections. Section I focuses on the profession of nursing. In these chapters, students will learn about the dynamic history of nursing and how the profession developed; the complex essence of nursing (knowledge and caring); nursing education, accreditation, and regulation; and how to succeed as nursing students.

Section II explores the healthcare context in which nursing is practiced. Health policy and political action are very important today in health care and in nursing. Students need to know about ethical and legal issues that apply to their practice now and that will also apply in their future as registered nurses. Students typically think most about caring for the acutely ill, but the health context is broader than this and includes health promotion, disease prevention, and illness across the continuum of care in the community. Though nursing is practiced in many different settings and healthcare organizations, the final chapter in this section focuses on acute care organizations, providing students with an in-depth exploration of one type of healthcare organization.

Section III moves the discussion to the core healthcare competencies. Each chapter focuses on one of the five IOM core competencies. Though this section covers these competencies in depth, the competencies are relevant to all the content in this text.

Section IV brings us to the end of this text, although not to the end of learning. The chapter in this section focuses on the transformation of nursing practice through leadership, connecting the key concepts in the text.

This edition also includes three new appendices. The first focuses on quality improvement measurement and analysis methods, providing students with a quick reference for information about quality improvement that can be used throughout the nursing program and to develop their expertise in quality improvement. The other appendices provide students with important employment information related to staffing and healthy work environments, as well as finding the right job.

Each chapter includes objectives, an outline of the chapter to help organize students' reading, key terms that are found in the chapter and are defined in the glossary, content with headers that apply to the chapter outline, and references. The end-of-chapter content includes Internet links, expanded discussion questions and critical thinking activities, and two case studies with questions. The Electronic Reflection Journal is new to this edition. This activity has students develop a log or diary over the course of using the text. The journal can be maintained in students' computers or tablets and updated as students progress in this course; it can also be expanded as students progress in their nursing program. It provides students with opportunities to reflect on content, supporting the development of professional self-awareness. Chapters also include "Words of Wisdom"—stories and conversations with nurses who practice, teach, manage, lead, and do much more to improve health care and ensure that patients get what they need. Above all, this text is patient centered. Nurses care for and about patients.

REFERENCE

Institute of Medicine (IOM). (2003). *Health professions education: A bridge to quality.* Retrieved from http://www.iom.edu/Reports/2003/Health-Professions-Education-A-Bridge-to-Quality.aspx

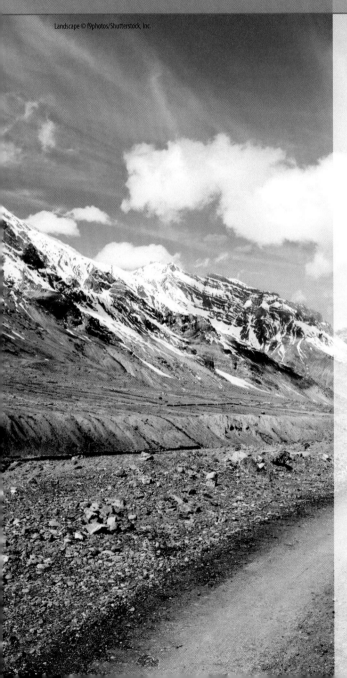

SECTION 1

The Profession of Nursing

The first section of this text introduces the nursing student to the profession of nursing. The framework for content in this text is the Institute of Medicine (IOM) core competencies for healthcare professions. The Development of Professional Nursing: History, Development, and the Nursing Profession chapter discusses the history and development of the nursing profession and what it means for nursing to be a profession. The Essence of Nursing: Knowledge and Caring chapter discusses the essence of nursing, focusing on the need for knowledge and caring and how nursing students develop throughout the nursing education program to be knowledgeable, competent, and caring. The Nursing Education, Accreditation, and Regulation chapter examines nursing education, accreditation of nursing education programs, and regulation of the practice of nursing. The Success in Your Nursing Education Program chapter provides information about the nursing student experience.

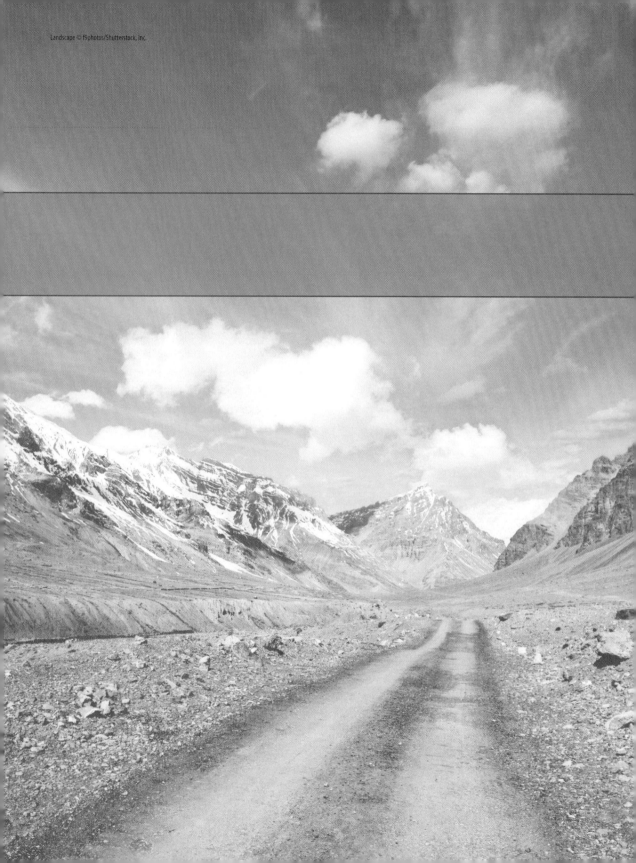

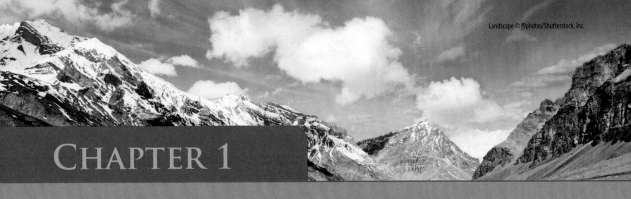

CHAPTER 1

The Development of Professional Nursing: History, Development, and the Nursing Profession

CHAPTER OBJECTIVES

At the conclusion of this chapter, the learner will be able to:

- Identify key figures and events in nursing history
- Discuss critical nursing historical themes within the sociopolitical context of the time
- Compare and contrast critical professional concepts
- Examine professionalism in nursing
- Explain the relevance of standards to the nursing profession
- Discuss the development and roles of nursing associations
- Describe the current and past image of nursing and related critical issues

CHAPTER OUTLINE

KEY TERMS

Accountability	Nursing	Scope of practice
Autonomy	Professionalism	Social policy statement
Code of ethics	Responsibility	Standards

INTRODUCTION

This text presents an introduction to the nursing profession and critical aspects of nursing care and the delivery of health care. To begin the journey to graduation and licensure, it is important to understand several aspects of the nursing profession. What is professional nursing? How did it develop? Which factors influence the view of the profession? This chapter addresses these questions.

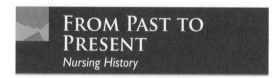

FROM PAST TO PRESENT
Nursing History

It is important for nursing students to learn about nursing history. Nursing's history provides a framework for understanding how nursing is practiced today and which societal trends are shaping the profession. The characteristics of nursing as a profession and what nurses do today have their roots in the past, not only in the history of nursing but also in the history of health care and society in general. Today, health care is highly complex; diagnostic methods and therapies have been developed that offer many opportunities for prevention, treatment, and cures that did not exist even a few years ago. Understanding this growth process is part of this discussion; it helps us to appreciate where nursing is today and may provide stimulus for changes in the future. "Nursing is conceptualized as a practice discipline with a mandate from society to enhance the health and well-being of humanity" (Shaw, 1993, p. 1654).

The past portrayal of nurses as handmaidens and assistants to physicians has its roots in the profession's religious beginnings. The following sections examine the story of nursing and explore how it developed.

From Paternalism to Professionalism: Movement from Trained Assistants with Religious Ties to Highly Educated Individuals

The discipline of nursing slowly evolved from the traditional role of women, apprenticeship, humanitarian aims, religious ideals, intuition, common sense, trial and error, theories, and research, as well as the multiple influences of medicine, technology, politics, war, economics, and feminism (Brooks & Kleine-Kracht, 1983; Gorenberg, 1983; Jacobs & Huether, 1978; Keller, 1979; Kidd & Morrison, 1988; Lynaugh & Fagin, 1988; Perry, 1985). It is impossible to provide a detailed history of nursing's evolution in one chapter, so only critical historical events will be discussed here.

Writing about nursing history itself has its own interesting history (Connolly, 2004). Historians who wrote about nursing prior to the 1950s tended to be nurses, and they wrote for nurses. Although nursing, throughout its history, has been intertwined with social issues of the day, the early publications about nursing history did not link nursing to "the broader social, economic, and cultural context in which events unfolded" (Connolly, 2004, p. 10). There was greater emphasis on the "profession's purity, discipline, and faith" (p. 10). Part of the reason for this narrow view of nursing history is that the discipline of history had limited, if any, contact with the nursing profession. This began to change in the 1950s and 1960s, when the scholarship of nursing history began to expand, albeit very slowly. In the 1970s, one landmark publication, *Hospitals, Paternalism, and the Role of the Nurse* (Ashley, 1976), addressed social issues as an important aspect of nursing history. The key issue considered in this document was feminism in the society at large and its impact on nursing. As social history became more important, increased examination of nursing, its history, and influences on that history took place. In addition, nursing is tied to political history today. For example, it is very difficult to understand current healthcare delivery concerns without including nursing (such as the impact of the nursing shortage). All of these considerations have an impact on health policy, including legislation at the state and national levels.

Schools of nursing often highlight their own history for students, faculty, and visitors. This might be done through exhibits about the school's history and, in some cases, a mini-museum. Such materials provide an opportunity to identify how the school's history has developed and how its graduates have affected the community and the profession. The purpose of this chapter is to explore some of the broad issues of nursing history, but this discussion should not replace the history of each school of nursing as the profession developed.

Nurse Leaders: History in the Making

The best place to begin to gain a better understanding of nursing history is with a description of its leaders—that is, the nurses who made a difference to the development of the profession. The vignettes in **Exhibit 1-1** describe the contributions of some nursing leaders. People do not operate in a vacuum, of course, and neither did the nurses highlighted in this exhibit. Many factors influenced nurse leaders, such as their communities, the society, and the time in which they practiced.

Exhibit 1-1   A Glimpse into the Contributions of Nurses

This list does not represent all the important nursing leaders but does provide examples of the broad range of their contributions and highlights specific achievements. These glimpses are written in the first person, but they are not direct quotes.

Dorothea Dix (1840–1841)

I traveled the state of Massachusetts to call attention to the present state of insane persons confined within this Commonwealth, in cages, stalls, pens! Chained, naked, beaten with rods, and lashed into obedience. Just by bettering the conditions for these persons, I showed that mental illnesses aren't all incurable.

Linda Richards (1869)

I was the first of five students to enroll in the New England Hospital for Women and Children and the first to graduate. Upon graduation, I was fortunate to obtain employment at the Bellevue Hospital in New York City. Here I created the first written reporting system, charting and maintaining individual patient records.

Clara Barton (1881)

The need in America for an institution that is not selfish must originate in the recognition of some evil that is adding to the sum of human suffering, or diminishing the sum of happiness. Today my efforts to organize such an institution have been successful: the National Society of the Red Cross.

Isabel Hampton Robb (1896)

As the first president for the American Nurses Association, I became active in organizing the

(continues)

Exhibit 1-1 (continued)

nursing profession at the national level. In 1896, I organized the Nurses' Associated Alumnae of the United States and Canada, which later became the American Nurses Association. I also founded the American Society of Superintendents of Training Schools for Nurses, which later became the National League of Nursing Education (NLNE; later changed to the National League for Nursing [NLN]). Through these professional organizations, I was able to initiate many improvements in nursing education.

Sophia Palmer (1900)

I launched *American Journal of Nursing* and served as editor-in-chief of the journal for 20 years. I believe my forceful editorials helped guide nursing thought and shape nursing practice and events.

Lavinia L. Dock (1907)

I became a staunch advocate of legislation to control nursing practice. Realizing the problems that students faced in studying drugs and solutions, I wrote one of the first nursing textbooks, *Materia Medica for Nurses*. I served as foreign editor of *American Journal of Nursing* and coauthored the book, *The History of Nursing*.

Martha Minerva Franklin (1908)

I actively campaigned for racial equality in nursing and guided 52 nurses to form the National Association of Colored Graduate Nurses.

Mary Mahoney (1909)

In 1908, the National Association of Colored Graduate Nurses was formed. As the first professional Black nurse, I gave the welcome address at the organization's first conference.

Mary Adelaide Nutting (1910)

I advocated for university education for nurses and developed the first program of this type. Upon accepting the chairmanship at the Department of Nursing Education at Teachers College, Columbia University, I became the first nurse to be appointed to a university professorship.

Lillian Wald (1918)

My goal was to ensure that women and children, immigrants and the poor, and members of all ethnic and religious groups would realize America's promise of life, liberty, and the pursuit of happiness. The Henry Street Settlement and the Visiting Nurse Service in New York City championed public health nursing, housing reform, suffrage, world peace, and the rights of women, children, immigrants, and working people.

Mary Breckenridge (1920)

Through my own personal tragedies, I realized that medical care for mothers and babies in rural America was needed. I started the Frontier Nursing Service in Kentucky.

Elizabeth Russell Belford, Mary Tolle Wright, Edith Moore Copeland, Dorothy Garrigus Adams, Ethel Palmer Clarke, Elizabeth McWilliams Miller, and Marie Hippensteel Lingeman (1922)

We are the founders of the Sigma Theta Tau International Honor Society of Nursing. Each of us provided insights that advanced scholarship, leadership, research, and practice.

Susie Walking Bear Yellowtail (1930–1960)

I traveled for 30 years throughout North America, walking to reservations to improve health care and Indian health services. I established the Native American Nurses Association and received the President's Award for Outstanding Nursing Healthcare.

Virginia Avenel Henderson (1939)

I am referred to as the first lady of nursing. I think of myself as an author, an avid researcher, and a visionary. One of my greatest contributions to the nursing profession was revising Harmer's *Textbook of the Principles and Practice of Nursing*, which has been widely adopted by schools of nursing.

Lucile Petry Leone (1943)

As the founder of the U.S. Cadet Nurse Corps, I believe we succeeded because we had a saleable

Exhibit 1-1 (continued)

package from the beginning. The women immediately liked the idea of being able to combine war service with professional education for the future.

Esther Lucille Brown (1946)

I issued a report titled *Nursing for the Future*. This report severely criticized the overall quality of nursing education. Thus, with the Brown report, nursing education finally began the long-discussed move to accreditation of nursing education programs.

Lydia Hall (1963–1969)

I established and directed the Loeb Center for Nursing and Rehabilitation at Montefiore Hospital in the Bronx, New York. Through my research in nursing and long-term care, I developed a theory (core, care, and cure) that the direct professional nurse-to-patient relationship is itself therapeutic and nursing care is the chief therapy for the chronically ill patient.

Martha Rogers (1963–1965)

I served as editor of *Journal of Nursing Science*, focusing my attention on improving and expanding nursing education, developing the scientific basis of nursing practice through professional education, and differentiating between professional and technical careers in nursing. My book, *An Introduction to the Theoretical Basis of Nursing* (1970), marked the beginning of nursing's search for a theoretical base. Later, my work led to a greater emphasis on research and evidence-based practice.

Loretta Ford (1965)

I co-developed the first nurse practitioner program in 1965 by integrating the traditional roles of the nurse with advanced medical training and the community outreach mission of a public health official.

Madeleine Leininger (1974)

I began, and continued to guide, nursing in the recognition that the culture care needs of people

in the world will be met by nurses prepared in transcultural nursing.

Florence Wald (1975)

I devoted my life to the compassionate care for the dying. I founded Hospice Incorporated in Connecticut, which is the model for hospice care in the United States and abroad.

Joann Ashley (1976)

I wrote *Hospitals, Paternalism, and the Role of the Nurse* during the height of the women's movement. My book created controversy with its pointed condemnation of sexism toward, and exploitation of, nurses by hospital administrators and physicians.

Luther Christman (1980)

As founder and dean of the Rush University College of Nursing, I have been linked to the "Rush Model," a unified approach to nursing education and practice that continues to set new standards of excellence. As dean of Vanderbilt University's School of Nursing, I was the first to employ African American women as faculty at Vanderbilt and became one of the founders of the National Male Nurses Association, now known as the American Assembly for Men in Nursing.

Hildegard E. Peplau (1997)

I became known as the "Nurse of the Century." I was the only nurse to serve the American Nurses Association as executive director and later as president, and I served two terms on the Board of the International Council of Nurses. My work in psychiatric–mental health nursing emphasized the nurse–patient relationship.

Linda Aiken (2007)

My policy research agenda is motivated by a commitment to improving healthcare outcomes by building an evidence base for health services management and providing direction for national policy makers, resulting in greater recognition of the role that nursing care has on patient outcomes.

Florence Nightingale

Florence Nightingale is viewed as the "mother" of modern nursing throughout the world. Most nursing students at some point say the Nightingale Pledge, which helps all new nurses connect the past with the present. The Nightingale Pledge is found in **Box 1-1**. It was composed to provide nurses with an oath similar to the physician's Hippocratic Oath. The oath was not written by Nightingale but was supposed to represent her view of nursing.

Volumes have been written about Nightingale. She has become almost the perfect vision of a nurse. However, although Nightingale did much for nursing, many who came after her provided even greater direction for the profession. A focus on Nightingale helps to better understand the major changes that occurred. In 1859, Florence Nightingale wrote, "No man, not even a doctor, ever gives any other definition of what a nurse should be than this— 'devoted and obedient.' This definition would do just as well for a porter. It might even do for a horse. It would not do for a policeman" (Nightingale, 1992,

---

Box 1-1	The Original Nightingale Pledge

I solemnly pledge myself before God and in the presence of this assembly, to pass my life in purity and to practice my profession faithfully. I will abstain from whatever is deleterious and mischievous, and will not take or knowingly administer any harmful drug. I will do all in my power to maintain and elevate the standard of my profession, and will hold in confidence all personal matters committed to my keeping and all family affairs coming to my knowledge in the practice of my calling. With loyalty will I endeavor to aid the physician, in his work, and devote myself to the welfare of those committed to my care.

Source: Composed by Lystra Gretter in 1893 for the class graduating from Harper Hospital, Detroit, Michigan.

---

p. 20). This quote clearly demonstrates that she was outspoken and held strong beliefs, though she lived during a time when this type of forthrightness from a woman was extraordinary.

Florence Nightingale was British and lived and worked in the Victorian era during the Industrial Revolution. During this time, the role of women— especially women of the upper classes—was clearly defined and controlled. These women did not work outside the home and maintained a monitored social existence. Their purpose was to be a wife and a mother, two roles that Nightingale never assumed. Education of women was also limited. With the support of her father, Nightingale did obtain some classical education, but there was never any expectation that she would "use" the education (Slater, 1994). Nightingale grew up knowing what was expected of her life: Women of her class ran the home and supervised the servants. Although this was not her goal, the household management skills that she learned from her mother were put to good use when she entered the hospital environment. Because of her social standing, she was in the company of educated and influential men, and she learned the "art of influencing powerful men" (Slater, 1994, p. 143). This skill was used a great deal by Nightingale as she fought for reforms.

Nightingale held different views about the women of her time. She had "a strong conviction that women have the mental abilities to achieve whatever they wish to achieve: compose music, solve scientific problems, create social projects of great importance" (Chinn, 2001, p. 441). She felt that women should question their assigned roles, and she herself wanted to serve people. When she reached her 20s, Nightingale felt an increasing desire to help others and decided that she wanted to become a nurse. Nurses at that time came from the lower classes, and, of course, any training for this type of role was out of the question. Her parents refused to support her goal, and because women were not free to make this type of decision by themselves, she was blocked. Nightingale became angry and then depressed. When her depression worsened, her parents finally relented and allowed her to attend nurse's training in Germany. This venture was kept a secret, and people she knew were told that she was away at a spa for 3 months' rest (Slater, 1994). Nightingale was also educated in math and science, which would lead her to use statistics to demonstrate the nurse's impact on health outcomes. Had it not been for her social standing and her ability to obtain some education, coupled with her friendship with Dr. Elizabeth Blackwell, nurses might well have remained uneducated assistants to doctors, at least for a longer period of time than they did.

An important fact about Nightingale is that she was very religious—to the point that she felt God had called on her to help others (Woodham-Smith, 1951). She also felt that the body and mind were separate entities, but both needed to be considered from a health standpoint. This view later served as the basis of nursing's holistic view of health. Nightingale's convictions also influenced her views of nurses and nursing practice. She viewed patients as persons who were unable to help themselves or who were dying. She is quoted as saying, "What nursing has to do ... is to put the patient in the best condition for nature to act upon him" (Seymer, 1954, p. 13). Nightingale also recognized that a patient's health depends on environmental impacts such as light, noise, smells or effluvia, and heat—something that we examine more closely today in nursing and in health care. In her work during the Crimean War, she applied her beliefs about the body and mind by arranging activities for the soldiers, providing them with classes and books, and supporting their connection with home—an early version of what is now often called holistic care. Later, this type of focus on the total patient became an integral part of psychiatric mental health nursing. Nightingale's other interest—in sanitary reform—grew from her experience in the Crimean War, and she worked with influential men to make changes on this front. Although she did not agree with the new theories about contagion, she did support the value

of education in improving social problems and believed that education included moral, physical, and practical aspects (Widerquist, 1997). Later nurses based more of their interventions on science and evidence-based practice.

Nightingale wrote four small books—or treatises, as they were called—thus starting the idea that nurses need to publish about their work. The titles of the books were *Notes on Matters Affecting the Health, Efficiency, and Hospital Administration of the British Army* (1858a), *Subsidiary Notes as to the Introduction of Female Nursing into Military Hospitals* (1858b), *Notes on Hospitals* (1859), and *Notes on Nursing* (1860, republished in 1992). The first three focused on hospitals that she visited, including military hospitals (Slater, 1994). Nightingale collected a lot of data. Her interest in healthcare data analysis helped to lay the groundwork for epidemiology, highlighting the importance of data in nursing, particularly in a public health context, and also established the foundation for nursing research and evidence-based practice. An interesting fact is that *Notes on Nursing* was not written for nurses, but rather for women who cared for ill family members. As late as 1860, Nightingale had not completely given up on the idea of care provided by women as a form of service to family and friends. This book was popular when it was published because at the time, family members provided most of the nursing care.

Nightingale's religious and upper-class background had a major impact on her important efforts to improve both nursing education and nursing practice in the hospital setting. Nurses were of the lower class, usually had no education, and were often alcoholics, prostitutes, and women who were down on their luck. Nightingale changed all that. She believed that patients needed educated nurses to care for them, and she founded the first organized school of nursing. Nightingale's school, which opened in London in 1860, accepted women of a higher class—not alcoholics and former prostitutes, as had been the case with previous generations of nurses. The students were not viewed as servants, and their loyalty was to the school, not to the hospital. This point is somewhat confusing and must be viewed from the perspective that important changes were made; however, these were not monumental changes but a beginning. For example, even in Nightingale's school, students were very much a part of the hospital; they staffed the hospital, representing free labor, and they worked long hours. This approach developed into the diploma school model, considered an apprenticeship model. Today, diploma schools have less direct relationships with the hospitals, and in some cases, they offer associate degrees; some offer baccalaureate degrees. There are also few schools of nursing today that are diploma schools (see the *Nursing Education, Accreditation, and Regulation* chapter).

Nightingale's students did receive some training, which had not been provided in an organized manner prior to her efforts. Nightingale's religious views also had an impact on her rigid educational system, and she expected students to have high moral values. Training was still based on an apprenticeship model and continued to be for some time in Britain, Europe, and later the United States. The structure of hospital nursing was also very rigid, with a matron in charge. This rigidity persisted for decades, and in some cases may still be present in hospital nursing organizations.

Nurses in Britain began to recognize the need to band together, and they eventually formed the British Nurses Association. This organization took on the issue of regulating nursing practice. Nightingale did not approve of efforts by the British Nurses Association toward state registration of nurses, mostly because she did not trust the leaders' goals regarding registration (Freeman, 2007). There were no known standards for nursing, so how one became a registered nurse was unclear. Many questions were raised regarding the definition of nursing, who should be registered, and who controlled nursing. Some critics suggest that Nightingale did make changes, but the way she made the changes also had negative effects, including delaying the

development of the profession (particularly regarding nurses' subordinate position to physicians), failing to encourage nursing education offered at a university level, and delaying licensure (Freeman, 2007). Despite this criticism, Nightingale still holds an important place in nursing history.

The History Surrounding the Development of Nursing as a Profession

When nursing history is described, distinct historical periods typically are discussed: early history (AD 1–500), rise of Christianity and the Middle Ages (500–1500), Renaissance (mid-1300s–1600s), and the Industrial Revolution (mid-1700s–mid-1800s). In addition, the historical perspective must include the different regions and environments in which the historical events took place. Early history focuses on Africa, the Mediterranean, Asia, and the Middle East. The focus then turns to Europe, with the rise of Christianity and subsequent major changes that span several centuries. Nursing history expands as colonists arrive in America and a new environment helps to further the development of the nursing profession. Throughout all these periods and locations, wars have had an impact on nursing. As a consequence of the varied places and times in which nursing has existed, major historical events, different cultures and languages, varying views on what constitutes disease and illness, roles of women, political issues, and location and environment have influenced the profession. Nursing has probably existed for as long as humans have been ill; someone always took care of the sick. This does not mean that there was a formal nursing position; rather, in most early cases, the nurse was a woman who cared for ill family members. This discussion begins with this group and then expands.

Early History

Early history of nursing focused on the Ancient Egyptians and Hebrews, Greeks, and Romans.

During this time, communities often had women who assisted with childbearing as a form of nursing care, and some physicians had assistants. The Egyptians had physicians, and sick persons looking for magical answers would go to them or to priests or sorcerers.

Hebrew (Jewish) physicians kept records and developed a hygiene code that examined issues such as personal and community hygiene, contagion, disinfection, and preparation of food and water (Masters, 2005). This occurred at a time when hygiene was very poor—a condition that continued for several centuries. Disease and disability were viewed as curses and related to sins, which meant that afflicted persons had to change or follow the religious statutes (Bullough & Bullough, 1978).

Greek mythology recognized health issues and physicians in its gods. Hippocrates, a Greek physician, is known as the father of medicine. He contributed to health care by writing a medical textbook that was used for centuries, and he developed an approach to disease that would later be referred to as epidemiology. Hippocrates also developed the Hippocratic Oath (Bullough & Bullough, 1978), which is still said by new physicians today and also influenced the writing of the Nightingale Pledge. The Greeks viewed health as a balance between body and mind—a different perspective from earlier views related to curses and sins.

Throughout this entire period, the wounded and ill in the armies required care. Generally, in this period—which represents thousands of years and involved several major cultures that rose and fell—nursing care was provided, but not nursing as it is thought of today. People took care of those who were sick and those going through childbirth, representing an early nursing role.

Rise of Christianity and the Middle Ages

The rise of Christianity led to more structured nursing care, but still it was far from professional nursing. Women continued to carry most of the burden of caring for the poor and the sick. The church set up a system for care that included the role of the deaconess, who provided care in homes. Women who served in these roles had to follow strict rules set by the church. This role eventually evolved into that of nuns, who began to live and work in convents. The convent was considered a safe place for women. The sick came to the convents for nursing care and also received spiritual care (Wall, 2003). The establishment of convents and the nursing care provided there formed the seed for what, hundreds of years later, would become the Catholic system of hospitals that still exists today.

Men were also involved in nursing at this time. For example men in the Crusades cared for the sick and injured. These men wore large red crosses on their uniforms to distinguish them from the fighting soldiers.

Altruism and connecting care to religion were major themes during this period. Even Nightingale continued with these themes in developing her view of nursing. Disease was common and spread quickly, and medical care had little to offer in the way of prevention or cure. Institutions that were called hospitals were not like modern hospitals; they primarily served travelers and sometimes the sick (Kalisch & Kalisch, 1986, 2005).

The Protestant Reformation had a major impact on some of the care given to the sick and injured. The Catholic Church's loss of power in some areas resulted in the closing of hospitals, and some convents closed or moved. The hospitals that remained were no longer staffed by nuns, but rather by women from the lower classes who often had major problems, such as alcoholism, or were former prostitutes. This is what Florence Nightingale found when she entered nursing.

Renaissance and the Enlightenment

The Renaissance had a major impact on health and the view of illness. This period was one of significant advancement in science, though by today's standards, it might be viewed as limited. These early discoveries led to advancements that had never been imagined before.

This is the period, spanning many years, of Columbus and the American and French Revolutions. Education became more important. Leonardo da Vinci's drawings of the human anatomy, which were done to help him understand the human body for his sculptures, provided details that had not been recognized before (Donahue, 1985). The 18th century was a period of many discoveries and changes (Dietz & Lehozky, 1963; Masters, 2005; Rosen, 1958), including the following:

- Jenner's smallpox vaccination method was developed during a time of high death rates from smallpox.
- Psychiatry became a medical specialty area, through the influence of Freud and others.
- The pulse watch and the stethoscope were developed, changing how physical assessment was conducted.
- Pasteur discovered the process of pasteurization, which had an impact on food and milk contamination.
- Lister used some of Pasteur's research and developed approaches to antiseptic surgery; as a result of work, he became known as the father of surgery.
- Koch studied anthrax and cholera, both major diseases of the time, demonstrating that they were transmitted by water, food, and clothing. As a result of this work, he became known as the father of microbiology.
- Klebs, Pasteur, Lister, and Koch all contributed to the development of the germ theory.

All of these discoveries and changes had an impact on nursing over the long term and changed the sociopolitical climate of health care. Nightingale did not agree with the new theory of contagion, but over time the nursing profession accepted these new theories, which remain critical components of patient care today. Nightingale stressed, however, that the mind–body connection—putting patients in

the best light for healing—ultimately made the difference. Discovering methods for preventing disease and using this information in disease prevention is an important part of nursing today. Public and community health are certainly concerned with many of the same issues that led to critical new discoveries so many years ago, such as contamination of food and water and preventing disease worldwide.

Industrial Revolution

The Industrial Revolution brought changes in the workplace, but many were not positive from a health perspective. The crowded factories of this era were hazardous and served as breeding grounds for disease. People worked long hours and often under harsh conditions. This was a period of great exploitation of children, particularly those of the lower classes, who were forced to work at very young ages (Masters, 2005). No child labor laws existed, so preteen children often worked in factories alongside adults. Some children were forced to quit school to earn wages to help support their families. Cities were crowded and very dirty, with epidemics erupting about which little could be done. There were few public health laws to alleviate the causes.

Nightingale and enlightened citizens tried to reform some of these conditions. Indeed, as Nightingale stated in *Notes on Nursing* (1992), "there are five essential points in securing the health of houses: pure air, pure water, efficient drainage, cleanliness, and light." Nightingale strongly supported more efforts to promote health and felt that this was more cost-effective than treating illness—important healthcare principles today—but she did not support progressive thought at the time regarding contagion and germs. These ideas are good examples reflecting the influence of the environment and culture in which a person lives and works on personal views and problems. If one did not know anything about the history of the time, one might wonder why Nightingale held these ideas to be important.

Colonization of America and the Growth of Nursing in the United States

The initial experiences of nursing in the United States were not much different from those described for Britain and Europe. Nurses were of the lower class and had limited or no training; hospitals were not used by the upper classes, but rather by the lower classes and the poor. Hospitals were dirty and lacked formal care services.

Nursing in the United States did move forward, as described in Exhibit 1-1 demonstrating the nursing activity and change that occurred over time. Significant steps were taken to improve nursing education and the profession of nursing. The first nursing schools—or, as they were called, training schools—were modeled after Nightingale's school. Some of the earlier schools were in Boston, New York, and Connecticut. The same approach was taken in these schools as in Britain: Stress was placed on moral character and subservience, with efforts to move away from using lower-class women with dubious histories, as was done in the early days of nursing even in the United States (Masters, 2005). Limitations regarding what women could do on their own still constituted a major problem. Women could not vote and had limited rights. This situation did begin to change in the early 1900s when women obtained the right to vote, but only with great effort. The Nurses' Associated Alumnae, established in 1896, was renamed the American Nurses Association (ANA) in 1911. Isabel Robb and Lavinia Dock led this effort. At the same time, the first nursing journal, *American Journal of Nursing* (*AJN*), was created through the ANA. The *AJN* was published until early 2006, when the ANA replaced it with *American Nurse Today* as its official journal. The *AJN*, the oldest U.S. nursing journal, still exists today, but is published by a company not associated with ANA. Its content has always focused on the issues facing nurses and their patients.

Although some nurse leaders such as Dock were ardent suffragists, Nightingale was not interested in these ideas, even though women in Britain did not have the right to vote. Nightingale felt that the focus should be on allowing (a permissive statement indicative of women's status) women to own property and then linking voting rights to this ownership right (Masters, 2005). There was, however, communication across the ocean between U.S. and British nurses. They did not always agree on the approach to take on the road to professionalism; in fact, nurses did not always agree on this issue within the United States. Nurse leaders and practicing nurses helped nursing to grow into a profession during times of war (the American Revolution, the Civil War, the Spanish–American War, World War I, World War II, the Korean War, the Vietnam War, and modern wars today). The website *Experiencing War: Women at War*, which is mentioned in the "Linking to the Internet" section of this chapter, offers information about nurses who served in these wars, providing leadership and further developing the nursing profession.

In the 1930s, the Great Depression also had an impact on the nursing field, "resulting in widespread unemployment of private duty nurses and the closing of nursing schools, while simultaneously creating the increasing need for charity health services for the population" (Masters, 2005, p. 28). This meant that there were fewer student nurses to staff the hospitals. As a consequence, nurses were hired, albeit at very low pay, to replace them. Until that time, hospitals had depended on student nurses to staff the hospitals, and graduate nurses served as private-duty nurses in homes. Using students to staff hospitals continued until the university-based nursing effort grew; however, during the Depression, there was a greater need to replace nursing students with nurses when schools closed. On one level, this could be seen as an improvement in care, but the low pay obstacle was difficult to overcome, resulting in a long history of low pay scales for nurses.

In 1922, the Goldmark report, *Nursing and Nursing Education in the United States*, had a major impact on nursing education; this report recommended that university schools of nursing should be established. In 1948, the Brown report was also critical of the quality of nursing education. This led to the implementation of an accreditation program for nursing schools, which was conducted by the National League for Nursing (NLN). Accreditation is a process of reviewing what a school is doing and its curriculum based on established standards. (See the *Nursing Education, Accreditation, and Regulation* chapter.) Movement toward the university setting and away from hospital-based schools of nursing and establishment of standards with an accreditation process were major changes for the nursing profession. The ANA and the NLN continue to establish standards for practice and education and to support implementation of those standards. In addition, the American Association of Colleges of Nursing (AACN) developed a nursing education accreditation process (discussed in the *Nursing Education, Accreditation, and Regulation* chapter).

The Carnegie report, *Educating Nurses: A Call for Radical Transformation*, describes the current status of nursing education. Patricia Benner led this study of current nursing education (Benner, Sutphen, Leonard, & Day, 2010). It is the most significant review of nursing education since the Goldmark and Brown reports. This report is discussed in the *Nursing Education, Accreditation, and Regulation* chapter.

In the 1940s and 1950s, other changes occurred in the healthcare system that had a direct impact on nursing. Certainly, scientific discoveries were changing care, but important health policy changes occurred as well. The Hill-Burton Act (1946) established federal funds to build more hospitals; as a result of this building boom, at one point in the 1980s, there were too many hospital beds. In turn, many nurses lost their jobs in hospitals because their salaries represented the largest operating expense and there were not enough patients to fill the beds.

There is some belief that this decision still impacts the current nursing shortage, though its scope has varied over the last few years. When more nurses are needed, some of the nurses who are laid off move into new jobs or careers or leave the workforce so they are not available when the need for nurses increases again. The latter half of the 20th century represented a period of rapid change in reimbursement for health care, owing to the growth of health insurance and the establishment of Medicare and Medicaid; such rapid changes are now being seen again in the 21st century with the passage of the Affordable Care Act of 2010. During these times, typically more nurses and other healthcare providers are needed. The *Healthcare Delivery System: Focus on Acute Care* chapter discusses some of these issues in more detail. The *Health Policy and Political Action: Critical Actions for Nurses* chapter examines the most significant issue in current healthcare delivery—namely, the healthcare reform of 2010 (Patient Protection and Affordable Care Act of 2010).

Little has been said in this description of nursing history about the role of men and minorities in nursing; these groups had little involvement in the profession's early history. This lack of diversity plagues nursing even today, though certainly there has been improvement. Segregation and discrimination also existed in nursing, just as they did in the society at large. The National Association of Colored Graduate Nurses closed in 1951 when the ANA began to accept African American nurses as members. Nevertheless, concern remains about the limited number of minorities in health care. The Sullivan Commission's report on health profession diversity, *Missing Persons: Minorities in the Health Professions* (Sullivan & Sullivan Commission, 2004), is an important document offering recommendations to improve diversity in the health professions. The American Association of Colleges of Nursing responded to this critical report by recommending the following actions (AACN, 2004):

- Health profession schools should hire diversity program managers and develop strategic plans that outline specific goals, standards, policies, and accountability mechanisms to ensure institutional diversity and cultural competence.

- Colleges and universities should provide an array of support services to minority students, including mentoring, resources for developing test-taking skills, and application counseling.
- Schools granting baccalaureate nursing degrees should provide and support bridging programs that enable graduates of 2-year colleges to succeed in the transition to 4-year institutions. Graduates of associate degree (AD) nursing programs should be encouraged to enroll in baccalaureate nursing programs and supported after they enroll.
- AACN and other health profession organizations should work with schools to promote enhanced admissions policies, cultural competence training, and minority student recruitment.
- To remove financial barriers to nursing education, public and private funding organizations should provide scholarships, loan forgiveness programs, and tuition reimbursement to students and institutions.
- Congress should substantially increase funding for diversity programs within the National Health Service Corps and Titles VII and VIII of the Public Health Service Act.

These recommendations and efforts to improve the number of minorities in all health professions have had some impact as will be discussed in the *Nursing Education, Accreditation, and Regulation* chapter, but more improvement is required. This topic also relates to the problem of healthcare disparities, as noted in other chapters.

The number of men in nursing has increased over the years but still is not where it should be. Men served as nurses in the early history period, such as in the Crusades, and monks provided care in convents. However, after this period, men were not accepted as nurses because nursing was viewed as a woman's role. The poet Walt Whitman was a nurse in the Civil War. Thus, there were men in nursing, though few, and some were well known—but perhaps not for their nursing (Kalisch & Kalisch, 1986). Early in the history of nursing schools in the United States, men were not accepted, and this may have been influenced by the gender-segregated housing for nursing students and the model of apprenticeship that focused on women (Bullough, 2006). In part, this female dominance was also the result of nursing's religious roots, which promoted sisters as nurses. This made it difficult for men to come into the system and the culture—it was a women's profession.

After the major wars—such as World Wars I and II, the Korean War, and the Vietnam War—medics came home and entered nursing programs, and they continue to do so. In 1940, the ANA did recognize men by having a session on men in nursing at its convention. With the return of medics from the wars, many of whom were men, and the movement of schools of nursing into more academic settings, more men began to apply to nursing programs. Men in nursing have to contend with male-dominated medicine, which has had an influence on the practice. Male nurses were also able to get commissions in the military (Bullough, 2006). The changes did have an impact, but the increase in salaries and improvement in work conditions had the strongest effect on increasing the number of men in nursing.

In 2001, Boughn conducted a study to explore why women and men choose nursing. The results of this study indicated that female and male participants did not differ in their desire to care for others. Both groups had a strong interest in power and empowerment, but female students were more interested in using their power to empower others, whereas male students were more interested in empowering the profession. The most significant difference was found in the expectations of salary and working conditions, with men expecting more. Why would not both males and females expect higher salaries and better working conditions? Is this still part of the view of nursing and nurses from nursing's past?

Luther Christman was a well-known nurse leader who served as a nurse for many years, retiring at the age of 87, and after retirement he continued to be an active voice for the profession and for men in nursing until his death in 2011. According to Sullivan (2002), Christman stated that "men in medicine were reluctant to give up power to women and, by the same token, women in nursing have fought to retain their power. Medicine, however, was forced to admit women after affirmative action legislation was enacted" (2002, p. 10). "Sadly," Christman reported, "nursing, with a majority of women, was not required to adhere to affirmative action policies" (Sullivan, 2002, p. 12). Today, more men and minorities enter baccalaureate degree programs than any other level of nursing education, as supported by national workforce data from the NLN and the AACN on an annual basis (Cleary, 2007; Sochalski, 2002). There is an organization for men in nursing, the American Assembly for Men in Nursing (http://www.aamn.org), and men are also members of other nursing organizations.

There is no question that the majority of nurses are White females, and this needs to change. There has been an increase in the number of male and minority nurses, but not enough. There is a greater need to actively seek out more male and minority students (Cohen, 2007). Men and minorities in nursing should reach out and mentor student nurses and new nurses to provide them with the support they require as they enter a profession predominantly composed of White women. More media coverage would also be helpful in publicizing the role of men and minorities in nursing; for example, when photos are distributed to local media, and to media in general, they should emphasize the diversity of the profession. Men still constitute a very small percentage of the total number of registered nurses (RNs) living and working in the United States, although their numbers continue to grow (U.S. Department of Health and Human Services, 2010). Before 2000, 6.2% of RNs were men; by 2008, this percentage had increased to 9.6%. Male and female RNs are equally likely to have a baccalaureate degree, but male RNs are more likely to also have a non-nursing degree.

Themes: Looking into the Nursing Profession's History

Nursing's past represents a movement from a role based on family and religious ties and the need to provide comfort and care (because that was perceived as a woman's lot in life) to educated professionals serving as the "glue" that holds the healthcare system together. From medieval times through Nightingale's time, nursing represented a role that women played in families to provide care. This care extended to anyone in need, but after Nightingale highlighted what a woman could do with some degree of education, physicians/doctors recognized that women needed to have some degree of training. Education was introduced, but mainly to serve the need of hospitals to have a labor force. Thus, the apprenticeship model of nursing was born. Why would nursing perceive a need for greater education? Primarily because of advances in science, increased knowledge of germs and diseases, and increased training of doctors, nurses needed to understand basic anatomy, physiology, pathophysiology, and epidemiology to provide better care. To carry out a doctor's orders efficiently, nurses must have some degree of understanding of causes and effects of environmental exposures and of disease causation. Thus, the move from hospital nursing schools to university training occurred.

Critics of Nightingale suggest that although the "lady with the lamp" image—that is, a nurse with a light moving among the wounded in the Crimea—is laudable, it presented the nurse as a caring, take-charge person who would go to great lengths and even sacrifice her own safety and health to provide care (Shames, 1993). The message sent to the public was that nurses were not powerful. They were caring, but they would not fight to change the conditions of hospitals and patient care. They instead acted, as many do today, as victims. Hospitals "owned" nurses and considered them cheap labor. Today, many hospitals still hold the same view, though they would never admit it publicly. This view of health suggests that doctors are defined by their scope of practice in treating diseases, whereas nurses are seen as promoting health, adding to the view of the lesser status of nursing (Shames, 1993). This view also has led to problems between the two professions, as they argue over which profession is better at caring for patients. The view that nurses are angels of mercy rather than well-educated professionals reinforces the idea that nurses care but really do not have to think; this view is perpetuated by advertisements that depict nurses as angels or caring ethereal humans (Gordon, 2005). Most patients—especially at 3 a.m., when few other professionals are available—hope that the nurse not just caring, but a critical thinker who uses clinical reasoning and judgment and knows when to call the rest of the team.

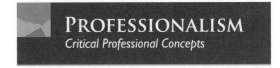

PROFESSIONALISM
Critical Professional Concepts

Today, nursing is an applied science, a practice profession. To appreciate the relevance of this statement requires an understanding of **professionalism** and how it applies to nursing. Nursing is more than just a job; it is a professional career requiring commitment. **Table 1-1** describes some differences in attitudes related to an occupation/job and a career/profession.

But what does this really mean, and why does it matter? As described previously in this chapter, getting to where nursing is today was not easy, nor did it happen overnight. Many nurses contributed to the development of nursing as a profession; it mattered to them that nurses be recognized as professionals.

Nursing as a Profession

The current definition of **nursing**, as established by the ANA (2010c), is "the protection, promotion,

Table 1-1	Comparison of Attitudes: Occupation Versus Career	
	Occupation	**Career**
Longevity	Temporary, a means to an end	Lifelong vocation
Educational preparation	Minimal training required, usually associate degree	University professional degree program based on foundation of core liberal arts
Continuing education	Only what is required for the job or to get a raise/promotion	Lifelong learning, continual effort to gain new knowledge, skills, and abilities
Level of commitment	Short-term, as long as job meets personal needs	Long-term commitment to organization and profession
Expectations	Reasonable work for reasonable pay; responsibility ends with shift	Will assume additional responsibilities and volunteer for organizational activities and community-based events

Source: From Wilfong, D., Szolis, C., & Haus, C. (2007). *Nursing school success: Tools for constructing your future.* Sudbury, MA: Jones and Bartlett.

and optimization of health and abilities, prevention of illness and injury, alleviation of suffering through the diagnosis and treatment of human response, and advocacy in the care of individuals, families, communities, and populations" (p. 10). **Box 1-2** provides several definitions of nursing that provide a historical perspective on the development of a definition for nursing.

The Essence of Nursing: Knowledge and Caring chapter contains a more in-depth discussion of the nature of nursing, but a definition is needed here to gain further understanding of nursing as a profession. Is nursing a profession? What is a profession? Why is it important that nursing be recognized as a profession? Some nurses may not think that nursing is a profession, but this is not the position taken by recognized nursing organizations, nursing education, and boards of nursing that are involved in licensure of nurses. Each state has its own definition of nursing that is found in the state's nurse practice

---

Box 1-2   Definitions of Nursing: Historical Perspective

The following list provides a timeline of some of the definitions of nursing.

Florence Nightingale

Having "charge of the personal health of somebody ... and what nursing has to do ... is to put the patient in the best possible condition for nature to act upon him." (Nightingale, 1859, p. 79)

Virginia Henderson

"The unique function of the nurse is to assist the individual, sick or well, in the performance of those activities contributing to health or its recovery (or to peaceful death) and that he would perform unaided if he had the necessary strength, will or knowledge. And to do this in such a way as to help him gain independence as rapidly as possible." (Henderson, 1966, p. 21)

Martha Rogers

"The process by which this body of knowledge, nursing science, is used for the purpose of assisting human beings to achieve maximum health within the potential of each person." (Rogers, 1988, p. 100)

American Nurses Association

"Nursing is the protection, promotion, and optimization of health and abilities, prevention of illness and injury, alleviation of suffering through the diagnosis and treatment of human response, and advocacy in the care of individuals, families, communities, and populations." (ANA, 2004, p. 4)

International Council of Nursing

"Nursing encompasses autonomous and collaborative care of individuals of all ages, families, groups and communities, sick or well and in all settings. Nursing includes the promotion of health, prevention of illness and the care of ill, disabled and dying people. Advocacy, promotion of a safe environment, research, participation in shaping health policy and in patient and health systems management, and education are also key nursing roles." (International Council of Nursing, n.d.)

Sources: Nightingale, F. (1859). *Notes on nursing: What it is and what it is not* (commemorative ed.). Philadelphia, PA: Lippincott; Henderson, V. (1966). *The nature of nursing: A definition and its implications for practice, research, and education.* New York, NY: Macmillan; Rogers, M. (1988). Nursing science and art: A prospective. *Nursing Science Quarterly, 1,* 99; American Nurses Association. (2004). *Nursing scope and standards of practice.* Silver Spring, MD: Author; International Council of Nursing. (n.d.). Retrieved from http://www.icn.ch/

act, but the ANA definition noted here encompasses the common characteristics of nursing practice.

In general, a profession—whether nursing or another profession, such as medicine, teaching, or law—has certain characteristics (Bixler & Bixler, 1959; Finkelman, 2012; Huber, 2014; Lindberg, Hunter, & Kruszewski, 1998; Quinn & Smith, 1987; Schein & Kommers, 1972):

- A systematic body of knowledge that provides the framework for the profession's practice
- Standardized, formal higher education
- Commitment to providing a service that benefits individuals and the community
- Maintenance of a unique role that recognizes autonomy, responsibility, and accountability
- Control of practice responsibility of the profession through **standards** and a **code of ethics**
- Commitment to members of the profession through professional organizations and activities

Does nursing demonstrate these professional characteristics? Nursing has a standardized content, although schools of nursing may configure the content in different ways; there is consistency in content areas such as adult health, maternal–child health, behavioral or mental health, pharmacology, assessment, and so on. The National Council Licensure Examination (NCLEX) covers standardized content areas. This content is based on systematic, recognized knowledge as the profession's knowledge base for practice (ANA, 2010a), and it is expected to be offered in higher education programs. The *Nursing Education, Accreditation, and Regulation* chapter discusses nursing education in more detail. It is clear, though, that the focus of nursing is practice—care provided to assist individuals, families, communities, and populations.

Nursing as a profession has a social contract with society, as described in *Nursing's Social Policy Statement*: "The authority for the practice of professional nursing is based on a social contract that acknowledges professional rights and responsibilities

as well as mechanisms for accountability. Nurses make contributions to society (the community in which nurses practice), and because of this, nurses have a relationship to the society and its culture and institutions. Nurses do not operate in a vacuum, without concern for what the individuals in a community and the community need. Understanding needs and providing care to meet those needs are directly connected to the social context of nursing. There are critical value assumptions related to the contract between nursing and society that provide an explanation of the importance of this contractual relationship" (ANA, 2010a, pp. 6–7). These assumptions include the following:

- Humans manifest an essential unity of mind, body, and spirit.
- Human experience is contextually and culturally defined.
- Health and illness are human experiences. The presence of illness does not preclude health, nor does optimal health preclude illness.
- The relationship between the nurse and the patient occurs within the context of the values and beliefs of the patient and the nurse.
- Public policy and the healthcare delivery system influence the health and well-being of society and professional nursing.
- Individual responsibility and interprofessional involvement are essential.

Autonomy, responsibility, and **accountability** are intertwined with the practice of nursing and are critical components of a profession. Autonomy is the "capacity of a nurse to determine his/her own actions through independent choice, including demonstration of competence, within the full scope of nursing practice" (ANA, 2010a, p. 39). It is the right to make a decision and take control. Nurses have a distinct body of knowledge and develop competencies in nursing care that should be based on this nursing knowledge. When this is accomplished, nurses can then practice nursing. "Responsibility refers to being entrusted with a particular function" (Ritter-Teitel, 2002, p. 34). "Accountability means being responsible and accountable to self and others for behaviors and outcomes included in one's professional role. A professional nurse is accountable for embracing professional values, maintaining professional values, maintaining competence, and maintenance and improvement of professional practice environments" (Kupperschmidt, 2004, p. 114). A nurse is also accountable for the outcomes of the nursing care that the nurse provides; what nurses do must mean something (Finkelman, 2012). The nurse is answerable for the actions that the nurse takes. Accountability and responsibility are not the same thing, however. A nurse often delegates tasks to other staff members, telling staff what to do and when. The staff member who is assigned a task is *responsible* both for performing that task and for the performance itself. The nurse who delegated the task to the staff person is *accountable* for the decision to delegate the task. Delegation is discussed in more detail in the *Work in Interprofessional Teams* chapter.

Sources of Professional Direction

Professions develop documents or statements about what the members feel is important to guide their practice, to establish control over practice, and to influence the quality of that practice. Some of the important sources of professional direction for nurses follow:

1. *Nursing's Social Policy Statement* (ANA, 2010c) is an important document that is mentioned elsewhere in this chapter. This **social policy statement** describes the profession of nursing and its professional framework and obligations to society. The original 1980 statement has been revised three times—in 1995, 2003, and 2010. This document informs consumers, government officials, other healthcare professionals, and other important stakeholders about nursing and its definition, knowledge base, scope of practice, and regulation.

2. *Nursing: Scope and Standards of Practice* (ANA, 2010b) was developed by the ANA and its members. Nursing standards, which are "authoritative statements defined and promoted by the profession by which the quality of practice, service, or education can be evaluated" (ANA, 2010b, p. 67), are critical to guiding safe, quality patient care. Standards describe minimal expectations. "We must always remember that as a profession the members are granted the privilege of self-regulation because they purport to use standards to monitor and evaluate the actions of its members to ensure a positive impact on the public it serves" (O'Rourke, 2003, p. 97).

Standards include a **scope of practice** statement that describes the "who, what, where, when, why, and how" of nursing practice. The ANA definition of nursing is the critical foundation. As noted in Box 1-2, the definition of nursing evolved and will most likely continue to evolve over time as needs change and healthcare delivery and practice evolve. Nursing knowledge and the integration of science and art, which are discussed in more detail in *The Essence of Nursing: Knowledge and Caring* chapter, are part of the scope of practice, along with the definition of the "what and why" of nursing. Nursing care is provided in a variety of settings by the professional registered nurse, who may have an advanced degree and specialty training and expertise. Additional information about the standards, as well as the nurse's roles and functions, is found throughout this text. Part of being a professional is having a commitment to the profession—a commitment to lifelong learning, adhering to standards, maintaining membership in professional organizations, publishing, and ensuring that nursing care is of the highest quality possible.

To go full circle and return to the social contract, nursing care must be provided and should include consideration of health, social, cultural, economic, legislative, and ethical factors. Content related to these issues is discussed in other chapters in this text. Nursing is not just about making someone better; it is about providing health education, assisting patients and families in making health decisions, providing direct care and supervising others who provide care, assessing care and applying the best evidence in making care decisions, communicating and working with the treatment team, developing a plan of care with a team that includes the patient and family when the patient agrees to family participation, evaluating patient outcomes, advocating for patients, and much more.

The *Apply Quality Improvement* chapter discusses safe, quality care in more detail, but as the student becomes more oriented to nursing education and nursing as a profession, it is important to recognize that establishing standards is part of being in a profession. The generic standards and their measurement criteria, which apply to all nurses, are divided into two types of standards: standards of practice and standards of professional performance. The major content areas of the standards follow (ANA, 2010b, pp. 9–11).

Standards of Practice (competent level of practice based on the nursing process)

1. Assessment
2. Diagnosis
3. Outcomes identification
4. Planning
5. Implementation (coordination of care, health teaching and health promotion, consultation, and prescriptive authority)
6. Evaluation

Standards of Professional Performance (competent level of behavior in the professional role)

1. Ethics
2. Education
3. Evidence-based practice and research
4. Quality of practice
5. Communication
6. Leadership
7. Collaboration
8. Professional practice evaluation
9. Resource utilization

Nursing specialty groups—in some cases, in partnership with the ANA—have developed specialty standards, such as those for cardiovascular nursing, neonatal nursing, and nursing informatics. However, all nurses must meet the generic standards regardless of their specialty.

The *Code of Ethics for Nurses* (ANA, 2010a) describes nursing's central beliefs and assists the profession in controlling its practice. This code is "the profession's public expression of those values, duties, and commitments" (ANA, 2010a, p. xi). Implementation of this code is an important part of nursing's contract with society. As nurses practice, they need to reflect these values. The *Ethics and Legal Issues* chapter focuses on ethical and legal issues related to nursing practice and describes the code in more detail.

State boards of nursing also assume an important role in guiding and in some cases determining professional direction through legislation. Each state board operates under a state practice act, which allows the state government to meet its responsibility to protect the public—in this case, the health of the public—through nursing licensure requirements. Each nurse must practice, or meet the description of, nursing as identified in the state in which the nurse practices. Regulation is discussed in more detail in the *Nursing Education, Accreditation, and Regulation* chapter.

Professional Nursing Associations

Nurses have a history of involvement in organizations that foster the goals of the profession. The existence of professional associations and organizations is one of the characteristics of a profession. A professional organization is a group that has specific goals, objectives, and functions that relate to the mission of a specific profession. Typically, membership is open to members of that profession and requires payment of dues. Some organizations have more specific membership requirements or may be by invitation only. Nursing has many organizations at the local, state, national, and international levels, and some organizations function on all of these levels.

Professional organizations often publish journals and other information related to the profession and offer continuing education opportunities through meetings, conferences, and other formats. As discussed previously, many of the organizations, particularly ANA, have been involved in developing professional standards. Professional education is a key function of many organizations. Some organizations are very active in policy decisions at the government levels and in taking political action to ensure that the profession's goals are addressed. This activity is generally done through lobbying and advocacy. Some of the organizations are involved in advocacy in the work environment, with the aim of making the work environment better for nurses.

Major Nursing Associations

The following description highlights some of the major nursing organizations (keep in mind that many other professional organizations exist). Organizations that focus on nursing specialties have expanded. Other organizations related to nursing education are described in the *Nursing Education, Accreditation, and Regulation* chapter. **Exhibit 1-2** lists some of these organizations and their websites.

American Nurses Association.   The ANA is the organization that represents all RNs in the United States, but not all RNs belong to the ANA. The ANA also represents nurses who are not members because many in government and business view the ANA as the voice of nursing. When the ANA lobbies for nursing, it is lobbying for *all* nurses, not just its membership. This organization represents more than 3.1 million RNs through its 54 constituent member associations and state and territorial associations, although the actual membership is only approximately 180,000 (ANA, 2013). This shift in membership must be considered in light of generational issues. New nurses typically do not join organizations, and there is continual unrest regarding

the perception by some nurses of the ANA's lack of response to vital nursing issues. In addition to being a professional organization, the ANA is a labor union, which is not true for most nursing professional organizations. Participation in the labor union is optional for members, and each state organization's stance on unions has an impact on membership. The ANA's major publication is *American Nurse Today*.

The organization's 2012 annual report identifies the eight pillars on which the organization bases its programs, products, and services (ANA, 2012):

- *Leadership*: We prepare and support nurses to advocate and lead in a full range of practice and policy settings. In fall 2012, ANA launched its Leadership Institute with programs focused on addressing the needs of developing leaders. In 2013, programs are planned for emerging and advanced leaders.
- *Cornerstone Documents*: These documents articulate the views of ANA on ethical, professional and policy issues that impact contemporary nursing practice and nursing's unique contributions to patients, health care and society. Examples include the *Code of Ethics for Nurses* and *Scope and Standards of Practice*.
- *Scope of Practice*: We promote and support the ability of RNs and APRNs to practice to the full extent of their knowledge and professional scope through multiple strategies. This pillar also encompasses ANA's recognition of specialty scope and standards.
- *Care Innovation*: We influence national policy to advance nursing service delivery models to enhance patient-centricity and to expand economic opportunities for nurses.
- *Quality*: This work encompasses ANA's commitment to advocate and promote nursing quality and patient safety outcomes through research and measurement, collaborative learning, consultative services, and advocacy.

Exhibit 1-2	Specialty Nursing Organizations

Academy of Medical–Surgical Nurses: http://www.medsurgnurse.org

Academy of Neonatal Nursing: http://www.academyonline.org

American Academy of Ambulatory Care Nursing, http://www.aaacn.org

American Academy of Nurse Practitioners: http://www.aanp.org

American Academy of Nursing: http://www.aannet.org

American Assembly for Men in Nursing: http://aamn.org

American Association for the History of Nursing: http://www.aahn.org

American Association of Colleges of Nursing: http://www.aacn.nche.edu

American Association of Critical-Care Nurses: http://www.aacn.org

American Association of Diabetes Educators: http://www.diabeteseducator.org

American Association of Legal Nurse Consultants: http://www.aalnc.org

American Association of Managed Care Nurses: http://www.aamcn.org

American Association of Neuroscience Nurses: http://www.aann.org

American Association of Nurse Anesthetists: http://www.aana.com

American Association of Nurse Attorneys: http://www.taana.org

American Association of Occupational Health Nurses: http://www.aaohn.org

American College of Nurse–Midwives: http://www.midwife.org

American College of Nurse Practitioners: http://www.acnpweb.org

American Holistic Nurses' Association: http://www.ahna.org

American Nephrology Nurses' Association: http://www.annanurse.org

American Nurses Association: http://www.nursingworld.org

American Nurses Foundation: http://www.nursingworld.org/anf

American Nursing Informatics Association: http://www.ania.org

American Organization of Nurse Executives: http://www.aone.org

American Psychiatric Nurses Association: http://www.apna.org

American Public Health Association–Public Health Nursing: http://www.apha.org

American Radiological Nurses Association: http://www.arinursing.org

American Society of PeriAnesthesia Nurses: http://www.aspan.org

American Society of Plastic Surgical Nurses: http://www.aspsn.org

Association for Nursing Professional Development: http://anpd.org

Association of Camp Nurses: http://www.campnurse.org

Association of Nurses in AIDS Care: http://www.anacnet.org

Association of Pediatric Hematology/Oncology Nurses: http://www.apon.org

Association of PeriOperative Registered Nurses: http://www.aorn.org

Association of Rehabilitation Nurses: http://www.rehabnurse.org

(continues)

Exhibit 1-2 (*continued*)

Association of Women's Health, Obstetric and Neonatal Nurses: http://www.awhonn.org

Commission on Graduates of Foreign Nursing Schools: http://www.cgfns.org

Council of International Neonatal Nurses: http://www.coinnurses.org

Developmental Disabilities Nurses Association: http://www.ddna.org

Emergency Nurses Association: http://www.ena.org

Home Healthcare Nurses Association: http://www.hhna.org

Hospice and Palliative Nurses Association: http://www.hpna.org

Infusion Nurses Society: http://www.ins1.org

International Association of Forensic Nurses: http://www.iafn.org

International Council of Nurses: http://www.icn.ch

International Homecare Nurses Association: http://ihcno.org

International Society for Psychiatric–Mental Health Nurses: http://www.ispn-psych.org

International Transplant Nurses Society: http://itns.org

National Alaskan Native American Indian Nurses Association: http://www.nanainanurses.org

National Association of Clinical Nurse Specialists: http://www.nacns.org

National Association of Neonatal Nurses: http://www.nann.org

National Association of Orthopaedic Nurses: http://www.orthonurse.org

National Association of Pediatric Nurse Practitioners: http://www.napnap.org

National Association of School Nurses: http://www.nasn.org

National Black Nurses Association: http://www.nbna.org

National Council of State Boards of Nursing: https://www.ncsbn.org

National Gerontological Nursing Association: http://www.ngna.org/

National League for Nursing: http://www.nln.org

National Nursing Staff Development Organization: http://www.nnsdo.org

National Student Nurses Association: http://www.nsna.org

Oncology Nursing Society: http://www.ons.org

Pediatric Endocrinology Nursing Society: http://www.pens.org

Society of Gastroenterology Nurses and Associates: http://www.sgna.org

Society of Pediatric Nurses: http://www.pedsnurses.org

Society of Trauma Nurses: http://www.traumanurses.org

Society of Urologic Nurses and Associates: http://www.suna.org

Society for Vascular Nursing: http://www.svnnet.org

State Nurses Associations: http://www.nursingworld.org/functionalmenucategories/aboutana/whoweare/cma.aspx

Transcultural Nursing Society: http://www.tcns.org

Wound, Ostomy and Continence Nurses Society: http://www.wocn.org

- *Work Environment*: ANA advocates a culture of safety. These programs promote a healthy and safe environment for patients and nurses.
- *Safe Staffing*: These programs, products, and services assist nurses in promoting safe staffing at every practice level and in all settings.
- *Healthy Nurse*: We champion the health, safety and wellness of the nurse through programs, products and services with your health in mind.

Content on all of these pillars is included in this text, as they are critical elements of health care today.

The ANA has three affiliated organizations: the American Nurses Foundation (ANF), the American Academy of Nursing (AAN), and the American Nurses Credentialing Center (ANCC).

American Nurses Foundation. "The American Nurses Foundation is the only philanthropic organization with a mission to transform the nation's health through the power of nursing. We help nurses step into leadership roles in their communities and workplaces to ensure that they can play a meaningful role in shaping decisions on the quality and capacity of health care" (ANF, 2012). In 2012, ANF awarded $1.16 million in grants.

American Academy of Nursing. The AAN was established in 1973, and it serves the public and the nursing profession through its activities to advance health policy and practice (AAN, 2013b). The academy is considered the "think tank" for nursing. Membership as an academy fellow is by invitation; fellows may then list "FAAN" in their credentials. There are approximately 2100 fellows, representing nursing's leaders in education, management, practice, and research. This is a very prestigious organization, and fellows have demonstrated their leadership. AAN also publishes the journal *Nursing Outlook*.

Examples of some of the AAN's current projects follow (AAN, 2013a):

- *Raise the Voice* is a campaign to ensure that more Americans hear about and understand the new possibilities for transforming the healthcare system. ANA fellows are working in partnership with other organizations in this initiative. Practical innovators are identified known as Edge Runners.
- The ANA provides expert panels to address current healthcare concerns.
- The Council for the Advancement of Nursing Science serves as a voice for nurse scientists and supports development of nursing science.
- The Geropsychiatric Nursing Collaborative's goal is to improve nursing education regarding the care of elders who have depression, dementia, and other mental health disorders.

American Nurses Credentialing Center. The American Nurses Credentialing Center (ANCC) was established by the ANA in 1973 to develop and implement a program that would provide tangible recognition of professional achievement. Through this program, many nurses meet certification requirements and pass certification exams in specific nursing practice areas—for example, pediatric nursing, adult psychiatric and mental health nursing, nurse executive, gerontological nursing, informatics nursing, and many more. After receiving certification, nurses must continue to adhere to specific requirements, such as completion of continuing education.

The ANCC engages in the following major activities (ANCC, 2013):

- *Accreditation Program*: The ANCC Accreditation program recognizes the importance of high-quality continuing nursing education (CNE) and skills-based competency programs. Around the world, ANCC-accredited organizations provide nurses with the knowledge and skills to help improve care and patient outcomes.

- *Certification Program*: ANCC's Certification Program enables nurses to demonstrate their specialty expertise and validate their knowledge to employers and patients. Through targeted exams that incorporate the latest nursing practice standards, ANCC certification empowers nurses with pride and professional satisfaction.
- *Pathway*: The Pathway to Excellence Program recognizes a healthcare organization's commitment to creating a positive nursing practice environment. The Pathway to Excellence in Long Term Care program is the first to recognize this type of supportive work setting, specifically in long-term care facilities. Pathway organizations focus on collaboration, career development, and accountable leadership to empower nurses.
- *Magnet Recognition Program*: ANCC's Magnet Recognition Program is the most prestigious distinction a healthcare organization can receive for nursing excellence and quality patient outcomes. Organizations that achieve Magnet recognition are part of an esteemed group that demonstrates superior nursing practices and outcomes.
- *Credentialing Knowledge Center*: ANCC's Credentialing Knowledge Center provides educational materials and guidance to support nurses and organizations in their quest to achieve success through its credentialing programs.

National League for Nursing. NLN is a nursing organization that focuses on excellence in nursing education. Its membership is primarily composed of schools of nursing and nurse educators. The NLN began in 1893 as the American Society of Superintendents of Training Schools. Its major publication is *Nursing Outlook*. It holds a number of educational meetings annually and provides continuing education and certification for nurse educators.

This organization has four major goals (NLN, 2013):

- *Goal I—Leader in Nursing Education*: Enhance the NLN's national and international impact as the recognized leader in nursing education.
- *Goal II—Commitment to Members*: Build a diverse, sustainable, member-led organization with the capacity to deliver the NLN's mission effectively, efficiently, and in accordance with the NLN's values.
- *Goal III—Champion for Nurse Educators*: Be the voice of nurse educators and champion their interests in political, academic, and professional arenas.
- *Goal IV—Advancement of the Science of Nursing Education*: Promote evidence-based nursing education and the scholarship of teaching.

American Association of Colleges of Nursing. AACN is the national organization for educational programs at the baccalaureate level and higher. The organization is particularly concerned with development of standards and resources and promotes innovation, research, and practice to advance nursing education (AACN, 2013). The organization represents more than 725 schools of nursing at the baccalaureate and higher levels. The dean or director of a school of nursing serves as a representative to the AACN. The organization holds annual meetings for nurse educators that focus on different levels of nursing education. The AACN has been involved in creating and promoting new roles and educational programs, which will be discussed in other chapters of this text. Examples of these roles are the clinical nurse leader (CNL) and the doctor of nursing practice (DNP). The major AACN publication is the *Journal of Professional Nursing*.

This organization's strategic goals and objectives for 2014–2016 are as follows (AACN, 2013):

- *Goal 1*: Provide strategic leadership that advances professional nursing education, research, and practice.
  - *Objective 1*: Lead innovation in baccalaureate and graduate nursing education that

promotes high-quality health care and new knowledge generation.

- *Objective 2*: Establish collaborative relationships and form strategic alliances to advance baccalaureate and graduate nursing education.
- *Objective 3*: Increase the visibility and participation of nursing's academic leaders as advocates for innovation in nursing.

■ *Goal 2*: Develop faculty and other academic leaders to meet the challenges of changing healthcare and higher education environments.

- *Objective 1*: Provide opportunities for academic leaders to strengthen leadership and administrative expertise.
- *Objective 2*: Expand initiatives that recruit and develop a diverse community of nurse educators throughout their academic careers.
- *Objective 3*: Increase opportunities for all members of the nursing academic unit to participate in AACN programs and initiatives.

■ *Goal 3*: Leverage AACN's policy and programmatic leadership on behalf of the profession and discipline.

- *Objective 1*: Serve as the primary voice for baccalaureate and graduate nursing education through media outreach, advocacy, policy development, and data collection.
- *Objective 2*: Respond to the needs of a diverse membership and external stakeholders.
- *Objective 3*: Implement initiatives to increase diversity among nursing students, faculty, and the workforce.

National Organization for Associate Degree Nursing. The National Organization for Associate Degree Nursing (N-OADN) represents associate degree (AD) nurses, AD nursing programs, and individual member nurse educators. The organization focuses on enhancing the quality of AD nursing education, strengthening the professional role of the AD nurse,

and protecting the future of AD nursing in the midst of healthcare changes. Its major goals follow (N-OADN, 2011):

- *Collaboration Goal:* Advance associate degree nursing education through collaboration with a diversity of audiences.
- *Education Goal:* Advance associate degree nursing education.
- *Advocacy Goal:* Advocate for issues and activities that support the organization's mission.

Sigma Theta Tau International. Sigma Theta Tau International (STTI) is a not-for-profit international organization based in the United States. This nursing honor society was created in 1922 by a small group of nursing students at what is now the Indiana University School of Nursing. Its mission is to provide leadership and scholarship in practice, education, and research to improve the health of all people (STTI, 2013). Membership in this organization is by invitation to baccalaureate and graduate nursing students who demonstrate excellence in scholarship and to nurse leaders who demonstrate exceptional achievements in nursing. STTI has 405,000 members, approximately 130,000 of whom are active members, and 86 countries are represented in its membership.

Schools of nursing form association chapters. The chapters are where most of the work of the organization takes place. There are 488 chapters, which include schools in Australia, Botswana, Brazil, Canada, Colombia, England, Ghana, Hong Kong, Japan, Kenya, Malawi, Mexico, the Netherlands, Pakistan, Portugal, Singapore, South Africa, South Korea, Swaziland, Sweden, Taiwan, Tanzania, Wales, and the United States. This is an important organization, and students should learn more about their school's chapter (if the school has one) and aspire to an invitation for induction into STTI. Inductees meet specific academic and leadership standards.

The major STTI publications are *Journal of Nursing Scholarship, Reflections on Nursing Leadership,* and the newest publication, *Worldviews on Evidence-Based Nursing*. The organization manages the major online library for nursing resources, the Virginia Henderson International Nursing Library, through its website.

International Council of Nurses. The International Council of Nurses (ICN), founded in 1899, is a federation of 130 national nurses associations representing approximately 16 million nurses worldwide (ICN, 2013). This organization is the international voice of nursing and focuses on activities to better ensure quality care for all and sound health policies globally. It has three major goals:

- To bring nursing together worldwide
- To advance nurses and nursing worldwide
- To influence health policy

The ICN focuses primarily on professional nursing practice (specific health issues, International Classification of Nursing Practice), nursing regulation (regulation and credentialing, ethics, standards, continuing education), and socioeconomic welfare for nurses (occupational health and safety, salaries, migration, and other issues). The ICN headquarters is in Geneva, Switzerland. This organization represents more than 130 national nurse associations, such as the ANA, and more than 16 million nurses.

National Student Nurses Association. The National Student Nurses Association (NSNA) has a membership of approximately 60,000 students enrolled in diploma, AD, baccalaureate, and general graduate nursing programs (NSNA, 2013). It is a national organization with chapters within schools of nursing. Its major publication is *Imprint.* Joining the NSNA is a great way to get involved and to begin to develop professional skills needed for the future (such as learning more about being a leader and a follower, critical roles for practicing nurses). The NSNA website provides an overview of the organization and its activities. (See "Linking to the Internet.") Attending a national convention is also a great way to find out about nursing in other areas

of the country and to network with other nursing students. Annual conventions attract more than 3000 nursing students and are held at different sites each year. This professional networking affords students opportunities to learn about graduate education, specialty groups, and nursing careers. Through NSNA, students can also get involved in the NSNA Leadership University (http://www.nsna.org/Membership/LeadershipUniversity.aspx). Through this program, students have the opportunity to be recognized for the leadership and management skills that they develop in NSNA and to earn academic credit for this experience.

Why Belong to a Nursing Professional Organization?

The previous section described many nursing professional organizations, as noted in in Exhibit 1-2, and there is further information in the *Nursing Education, Accreditation, and Regulation* chapter about some of these organizations. Why is it important to belong to a professional organization? Belonging to a nursing association requires money for membership and commitment to the association. Commitment involves being active, which means that it takes time. Membership, and it is hoped active involvement, can help nurses develop leadership skills, improve networking, and find mentors. Additionally, membership gives nurses a voice in professional issues and, in some cases, health policy issues, and it provides opportunities for professional development. Nurses who attend meetings, hold offices, and serve on committees or as delegates to large meetings benefit more from membership than those who do not participate. Submitting abstracts for a presentation or poster at a meeting is excellent experience for nurses and offers even more opportunities for networking with other nurses who might also provide resources and mentoring for professional development.

Joining a professional organization and becoming active in the work of such an organization is a professional obligation. Nurses represent the single largest voting bloc in any state. By using this political power through nursing and other professional organizations, nurses can speak in one powerful voice. Yet as nurses, we have often failed to pull together. Membership in a professional organization is one way to develop one strong voice.

Students can begin to meet this professional obligation by joining local student organizations and developing skills that can then be used after graduation, when they join professional organizations. Membership offers opportunities to serve as a committee member and even chair a committee. Organization communication methods can be observed, and the student can participate in the processes.

Nursing organizations give members the opportunity to participate in making decisions about nursing and health care in general. When new nurses enter the profession today, they find a healthcare system that is struggling to improve its quality and keep up with medical changes; one of the key issues impacting this struggle is the variation in the nursing shortage over time. To demonstrate the critical concern about this issue, the following is an example of how professional organizations can come together and advocate for patient care.

The Americans for Nursing Shortage Relief Alliance (ANSR) represents a diverse cross-section of healthcare and professional organizations. The ANSR includes 54 nursing organizations collectively representing approximately 2.7 million nurses, healthcare providers, and supporters of nursing issues who have united to address the national nursing shortage. As an example, the ANSR sent letters to both the U.S. Senate and the U.S. House of Representatives in June 2013, urging the following: "As you begin your consideration of the FY 2014 Labor, Health and Human Services, and Education (LHHS) Appropriations bill, the undersigned members of the ANSR (Americans for Nursing Shortage Relief) Alliance urge you to fund $251 million for the Title VIII—Nursing Workforce Development programs at the Health Resources

and Services Administration (HRSA) as well as $20 million for the Nurse Managed Health Clinics (NMHCs) as authorized under Title III of the Public Health Service Act" (ANSR, 2013).

The example set by this organization shows how nursing can band together to have a greater voice about critical healthcare policy issues such as the need to expand the nursing profession. Nursing is one of the largest healthcare professions, and nurses have many opportunities to serve as leaders in health care. Nurses work in a variety of settings, such as hospitals, clinics, home health care, nursing care facilities (long-term care, rehabilitation), physician offices, school health, hospice care, employment services, and numerous other service sites. The majority of nurses work in acute care hospital settings, but this is changing as more care moves into the community.

According to the Bureau of Labor Statistics' employment projections for 2010–2020 released in February 2012, the registered nursing workforce is expected to be the top occupation in terms of job growth through 2020. The number of employed nurses is predicted to grow from 2.74 million in 2010 to 3.45 million in 2020, an increase of 712,000 or 26%. Over this period, another 495,500 nursing workforce replacements are expected to be needed, bringing the total number of job openings for nurses due to growth and replacements to 1.2 million by 2020 (U.S. Bureau of Labor Statistics, 2012). In the past five years, there has been a nursing shortage, but this mismatch in supply and demand has decreased for now. The Tri-Council for Nursing, in a statement in 2010, cautioned that while increases in the nursing shortage slowed because of the economic downturn, during which fewer nurses left their jobs, and with some increase in enrollment numbers in nursing programs throughout the United States, we have not resolved the long-term problem of the nursing shortage. As the number of nurses in practice and nursing school enrollments fluctuate, the nursing shortage will impact access to care in the years to come (Tri-Council for Nursing,

2010). Because of demographic changes, the older adult population in the United States is increasing rapidly, and the Affordable Care Act promises to extend insurance coverage to more people; taken together, these developments signal that the demand for nurses will increase. The greater demand, in turn, is expected to lead to more nursing shortage problems as well as shortages of other healthcare professionals.

Nursing is a profession. It meets all the requirements for a profession. In the early part of its history, nursing was not viewed as such, as the review of nursing history described earlier in this chapter, but it is now recognized as a profession built on a "core body of knowledge that reflects its dual components of science and art" (ANA, 2010c, p. 22). O'Rourke (2003) explains that the profession of nursing "subscribes to the notion that the service orientation and ethics of its members is the basis for justifying the privilege of self-regulation," and "that the profession is responsible for developing a body of knowledge and techniques that can be applied in practice along with providing the necessary training to master such knowledge and skill" (pp. 97–98). The *Essence of Nursing: Knowledge and Caring* chapter explores the art and science of the profession of nursing.

THE IMAGE OF NURSING

Image may appear to be an unusual topic for a nursing text, but it is not. Image is part of any profession. It is the way a person appears to others, or in the case of a profession, the way that a profession appears to other disciplines and to the general public—in nursing's case, consumers of health care. Image and the perception of the profession affect recruitment of students, the view of the public, funding for nursing education and research, relationships with healthcare administrators and other

healthcare professionals, government agencies and legislators at all levels of government, and ultimately the profession's self-identity. Just as individuals may feel depressed or less effective if others view them negatively, so professionals can experience similar reactions if their image is not positive. Image influences everything the profession does or wishes to do. How nurses view themselves—their professional self-image—has an impact on professional self-esteem (Buresh & Gordon, 2006). How one is viewed has an impact on whether others seek that person out and how they view the effectiveness of what that person might do. Every time a nurse says to family, friends, or members of the public that he or she is a nurse, the nurse is representing the profession. Gordon stated, "We cannot expect outsiders to be the guardians of our visibility and access to public media and health policy arenas. We must develop the skills of presenting ourselves in the media and to the media—we have to take the responsibility for moving from silence to voice" (Buresh & Gordon, 2000, p. 15).

"Although nurses comprise the majority of healthcare professionals, they are largely invisible. Their competence, skill, knowledge, and judgment are—as the word 'image' suggests—only a reflection, not reality" (Sullivan, 2004, p. 45). The public views of nursing and nurses are typically based on personal experiences with nurses, which can lead to a narrow view of a nurse often based on only a brief personal experience. This experience may not provide an accurate picture of all that nurses can and do provide in the healthcare delivery process. In addition, this view is influenced by the emotional response of a person to the situation and the encounter with a nurse.

But the truth is that most often the nurse is invisible. Consumers may not recognize that they are interacting with a nurse, or they may think someone is a nurse who is not. When patients go to their doctor's office, they interact with staff, and often these patients think that they are interacting with a registered nurse. Most likely, they are not—the staff person is more likely to be a medical assistant of some type or a licensed practical/vocational nurse. When in the hospital, patients interact with many staff members, and there is little to distinguish one from another, so patients may refer to most staff as nurses. Uniforms do not even help identify roles, as many staff wear scrub clothes and lab clothes, and there has been less emphasis placed on professional attire.

This does not mean that the public does not value nurses—quite the contrary. When a person tells another that he or she is a nurse, the typical response is positive. However, many people do not know about the education required to become a nurse and to maintain current knowledge, or about the great variety of educational entry points into nursing that all lead to the RN qualification. Consumers generally view nurses as good people who care for others. For the 11th consecutive year, an annual Gallup Poll found that nursing ranked as number one in the annual list of occupations rated for honesty and ethical standards, with 81% of respondents agreeing with this assessment. This high vote of confidence has been a consistent annual result in the poll (Jones, 2010). What is not mentioned is that knowledge and competency are required to do the job properly.

You might wonder why it is so important for nurses to make themselves more visible. You chose nursing, so you know that it is an important profession. Nevertheless, many students have a narrow view of the profession, much closer to what is portrayed in the media—the nurse who cares for others, albeit with less understanding of the knowledge base required and competency needed to meet the complex needs of patients. There is limited recognition that nursing is a scientific field. The profession needs to be more concerned about visibility because nursing is struggling to attract qualified students and keep current nurses in practice.

The nurse's voice is typically silent, and this factor has demoralized nursing (Pike, 2001). This is a strong statement and may be a confusing one. What is the nurse's voice? It is the "unique perspectives and contributions that nurses bring to patient care" (Pike, 2001, p. 449). Nurses have all too often been silent about what they do and how they do it, but this has been a choice that nurses have made—to be silent or to be more visible. Both external and internal factors have impacted the nurse's voice and this silence. The external factors include the following (Pike, 2001):

- Historical role of nurse as handmaiden (not an independent role)
- Hierarchical structure of healthcare organizations (has often limited the role of nursing in decision making and leadership)
- Perceived authority and directives of physicians (has limited the independent role of nurses)
- Hospital policy (has often limited nursing actions and leadership)
- Threat of disciplinary or legal action or loss of job (might limit a nurse when he or she needs to speak out—advocate)

Nurses who can deal with the internal factors can be more visible and less silent about nursing. The internal factors to consider include these:

- Role confusion
- Lack of professional confidence
- Timidity
- Fear
- Insecurity
- Sense of inferiority

Nurses' loss of professional pride and self-esteem can also lead to a more serious professional problem: Nurses feel like victims and then act like victims. Victims do not take control, but rather see others as being in control; they abdicate responsibility. They play passive–aggressive games to exert power. This can be seen in the public image of nurses, which is predominantly driven by forces outside the profession. It also affects the nurse's ability to collaborate with others—both other nurses and other healthcare professionals. It is all too easy for nurses to feel like victims, and this perception has led in many ways to nurses viewing physicians in a negative light, emphasizing that "Physicians have done this to us." As a consequence, nurses have problems saying that they are colleagues with other healthcare professionals and acting like colleagues. "**Colleagueship** [boldface added] involves entering into a collaborative relationship that is characterized by mutual trust and response and an understanding of the perspective each partner contributes" (Pike, 2001, p. 449). Colleagues have the following characteristics:

- Do not let interprofessional or intraprofessional competition and antagonism from the past drive the present and the future
- Integrate their work to provide the best care
- Acknowledge that they share a common goal: quality patient care
- Recognize interdependence
- Share responsibility and accountability for patient care outcomes
- Recognize that collegial relationships are safe
- Handle conflict in a positive manner

What is unexpected is how nurses' silence may actually have a negative impact on patient care. This factor may influence how a nurse speaks out or advocates for care that a patient needs; how effective a nurse can be on the interprofessional treatment team; and how nurses participate in healthcare program planning on many levels. Each nurse has the responsibility and accountability to define himself or herself as a colleague, and empowerment is part of this process.

The role of nursing has experienced many changes, and many more will occur in the future. How has nursing responded to these changes and communicated them to the public and other healthcare professionals? Suzanne Gordon, a journalist who has written extensively about the nursing profession, noted that often the media are accused of representing nursing poorly when, in reality, the media are simply reflecting the public image of nursing (Buresh & Gordon, 2006). Nurses have not taken the lead in standing up and discussing their own image of nursing—what it is and what it is not. It is not uncommon for a nurse to refuse to talk to the press because the nurse feels no need to do so or sometimes because the nurse fears reprisals from his or her employer. When nurses do speak to the press, often when being praised for an action, they say, "Oh, I was just doing my job." This statement undervalues the reality that critical quick thinking on the part of nurses saves lives every day. What is wrong with taking that credit? Because of these types of responses in the media, nursing is not directing the image, but rather accepting how those outside profession describe nursing.

Gordon and Nelson (2005) comment that nursing needs to move "away from the 'virtue script' toward a knowledge-based identity" (p. 62). The "virtue script" continues to be present in current media campaigns that are supported by the profession. For example, a video produced by the National Student Nurses Association mentions knowledge but not many details; instead, it includes statements such as "[Nursing is a] job where people will love you" (Gordon & Nelson, 2005). How helpful is this approach? Is this view of being loved based on today's nursing reality? Nursing practice involves highly complex care; it can be stressful, demanding, and at times rewarding, but it is certainly not as simple as "everyone will love you." Why do nurses continue to describe themselves in this way? "One reason nurses may rely so heavily on the virtue script is that many believe this is their only legitimate source of status, respect, and self-esteem" (Gordon & Nelson, 2005, p. 67). This, however, is a view that perpetuates the victim mentality.

Landscape © f9photos/Shutterstock, Inc.

CONCLUSION

This chapter has highlighted the history of nursing, societal trends, image of nursing, and other influences that shape nursing as a profession. It presented an overview of the remainder of this text. Professional nursing includes many key aspects that will be discussed in more detail: art and science of nursing; education; critical issues related to health care, such as those involving consumers; the continuum of care; the healthcare delivery system; policy, and legal and ethical concerns; the five core competencies; and current issues regarding the practice of nursing.

Landscape © f9photos/Shutterstock, Inc.

CHAPTER HIGHLIGHTS

1. Nursing history provides a framework for understanding how nursing is practiced today.
2. The history of nursing is complex and has been influenced by social, economic, and political factors.
3. Florence Nightingale was instrumental in changing the view of nursing and education to improve care delivery.
4. Nursing meets the critical requirements for a profession.

5. The sources of professional direction include ANA documents that describe the scope of practice, accountability, and an ethical code.
6. Professional organizations play a key role in shaping nursing as a profession.
7. The image of nursing is formulated in many ways by the public, the media, interprofessional colleagues, and nurses. Nursing's image as a profession has both positive and negative aspects.

Landscape © f9photos/Shutterstock, Inc.

DISCUSSION QUESTIONS

1. How might knowing more about nursing history affect your personal view of nursing?
2. How did the image of nursing in Nightingale's time influence nursing from the 1860s through the 1940s?
3. How would you compare and contrast accountability, autonomy, and responsibility?
4. Based on content in this chapter, how would you define professionalism in your own words?

5. Why are standards important to the nursing profession and to healthcare delivery?
6. Review the ANA standards of practice and professional performance. Are you surprised by any of the standards? If so, why?
7. How would you explain to someone who is not in health care the reason that nursing emphasizes its social policy statement?

Landscape © f9photos/Shutterstock, Inc.

CRITICAL THINKING ACTIVITIES

1. Describe how the Nightingale Pledge has relevance today and how it might be altered to be more relevant. Work with a team of students to accomplish this activity and arrive at a consensus statement.

2. Interview two nurses and ask them if they think nursing is a profession, and determine the rationale for their viewpoint. How does what they say compare with what you have learned about professionalism in this chapter?

3. Attend a National Student Nurses Association meeting at your school. What did you learn about the organization? What did you observe in the meeting about leadership and nursing? Do you have any criticisms of the organization and how might it be improved?

4. Complete a mini-survey of six people (non-nurses), asking them to describe their image of nursing and nurses. Try to pick a variety of people. Summarize and analyze your data to identify any themes and unusual views. How does what you learned relate to the content in this chapter? List the similarities and differences, and then discuss your findings with a group of your classmates and compare with their findings.

5. Analyze a television program that focuses on a healthcare situation/story line. How are nurses depicted compared with other healthcare professionals? Compose a letter to the program describing your analysis, and document your arguments to support your viewpoint. This could be done with a team of students; watch the same program and then discuss opinions and observations.

ELECTRONIC Reflection Journal

Circuit Board: ©Photos.com

You are asked to develop an Electronic Reflection Journal that you will use after you complete each chapter. This is the place for you to comment on some aspect identified at the end of the chapter. You may also keep notes about issues that you want to expand on—reflect on—as you progress through your nursing education. If you are using technology that allows you to make visuals, use drawings and graphics to expand your journal thoughts.

In your first entry in your Electronic Reflection Journal, consider the following questions related to the image of nursing. Connect your responses so that you can better understand the importance of image to the profession and the meaning of profession.

1. Why is the image of nursing important to the profession? To health care in general?

2. What role do you think you might have as a nurse in influencing the image of nursing? Provide specific examples.

3. What is your opinion about nursing uniforms, and how do you think they influence the image of nursing?

4. What stimulated your interest in nursing as a profession? Was the image of nursing in any way related to your decision, and in what way did it impact your decision?

5. **Special assignment for this chapter:** Write your own definition of nursing and include it in your Electronic Reflection Journal. Work on this definition throughout this course as you learn more about nursing. Save the final draft, and at the end of each semester or quarter, go back to your definition and make any changes you feel are necessary. Keep a draft of each definition so that you can see your changes. When you graduate, review all your definitions; see how you have developed your view of professional nursing. Ideally, you would then review your definition again one year post graduation.

Landscape © f9photos/Shutterstock, Inc.

LINKING TO THE INTERNET

- American Association for the History of Nursing: http://www.aahn.org
- Directory of Links: http://dmoz.org/health/nursing/history
- Barbara Bates Center for the Study of the History of Nursing, University of Pennsylvania: http://www.nursing.upenn.edu/history/Pages/default.aspx
- Experiencing War: Women at War (Includes nurses): http://www.loc.gov/vets/stories/ex-war-womenatwar.html
- National Student Nurses Association: http://www.nsna.org
- American Assembly of Men in Nursing: http://aamn.org
- Nursing: The Ultimate Adventure pamphlet (NSNA): http://www.nsna.org/Publications/Ultimate_Adventure.aspx

CASE STUDIES

Landscape © f9photos/Shutterstock, Inc.

Case Study 1

You and your friends in the nursing program are having lunch after a class that covered content found in this chapter. One of your friends says, "I was bored when we got to all that information on professionalism and nursing organizations. What a waste of time. I just want to be a nurse." All of you are struggling to figure out what you have gotten yourself into. You turn to your friends and suggest it might be helpful to have an open discussion on the comment just made. So over lunch you all talk about the comment made by one of your friends. It was clear that the students who had read the chapter were better able to discuss the issue, but everyone had an opinion.

Case Questions

Here are some questions to consider:

1. What is the purpose of nursing organizations?
2. What role should professional organizations assume to increase nursing status in the healthcare system?
3. What are some of the advantages and disadvantages to joining a professional organization?
4. What do you know about your school's NSNA chapter? How would you join your school's student nursing association?
5. Which nursing organization mentioned in this chapter interests you and why? Compare your response with those of your other classmates.
6. Search on the Internet for a specialty nursing organization and pick one that interests you. What can you find out about the organization?

(continues)

CASE STUDIES (CONTINUED)

Case Study 2

The NSNA chapter in your school wants to help the school develop a campaign to increase enrollment. You have volunteered along with three other members to meet with the associate dean to discuss ideas for the campaign. The associate dean tells you that the school is going to use its standard marketing materials. She shows them to you. The materials focus on the importance of being a caring person to be a "good" nurse. When you ask to see print materials and materials to go on the Internet, you are told that the focus is on print and you see a photo of a nurse holding a patient's hand.

Case Questions

1. How do you respond to this marketing material?
2. Which recommendations would you make?
3. How might you get data from fellow students to support your recommendations?

Words of Wisdom

Jamie White, MSN, RN
Staff Nurse, Neonatal Intensive Care Unit, University of Oklahoma Medical Center, Oklahoma City, Oklahoma

What would have made the transition to your first nursing job easier?

The transition to my job was very easy. What made it this way was working in the unit for a year and a half as a nurse partner and clerk. If you already know the basics of the unit, then transition is much easier.

What things were included in your education that were most helpful? Least helpful?

The most helpful educational tool was the group/team work. Nursing is all about being a member of a team and relying on others to help you perform your job more efficiently. The other helpful experience was how nursing school changes your mind-set of school and work. Nursing is ever changing, and so is nursing school. I remember being stressed out my first semester due to the ever-changing environment and no clear line. Now, I understand why it's that way—because nursing is that way. I cannot tell you the least helpful, only because for everything I thought at the time had no purpose, I found the purpose when I entered the field.

What advice would you give entering students?

My advice would be to come into nursing if you truly want to touch people's lives. Nursing is full of frustrations and politics, but if you are in it for the love of people, then you will do fine. The best feeling I get is to hand a family their sick infant for the first time and to see the hope and love that is expressed.

Landscape © f9photos/Shutterstock, Inc.

REFERENCES

American Academy of Nursing (AAN). (2013a). AAN initiatives. Retrieved from http://www.aannet.org/initiatives-policy

American Academy of Nursing (AAN). (2013b). About AAN. Retrieved from http://www.aannet.org/about-the-academy

American Association of Colleges of Nursing (AACN). (2004, September 20). *AACN endorses the Sullivan Commission report on increasing diversity in the health professions* (press release). Washington, DC: Author.

American Association of Colleges of Nursing (AACN). (2013). Strategic plan. Retrieved from http://www.aacn.nche.edu/about-aacn/strategic-plan

American Nurses Association. (2010a). *Guide to the code of ethics for nurses. Interpretation and application.* Silver Spring, MD: Nursesbooks.org

American Nurses Association (ANA). (2010b). *Nursing: Scope and standards of practice.* Silver Spring, MD: Author.

American Nurses Association (ANA). (2010c). *Nursing's social policy statement.* Silver Spring, MD: Author.

American Nurses Association (ANA). (2012). *ANA 2012 annual report.* Silver Spring, MD: Author. Retrieved from http://www.nursingworld.org/FunctionalMenuCategories/AboutANA/2012-AnnualReport.pdf

American Nurses Association (ANA). (2013). About ANA. Retrieved from http://www.nursingworld.org/FunctionalMenuCategories/AboutANA

American Nurse Credentialing Center (ANCC). About ANCC. Retrieved from http://www.nursecredentialing.org/FunctionalCategory/AboutANCC

American Nurses Foundation (ANF). (2012). Retrieved from http://www.anfonline.org/Main/AboutANF/2012-Report.html

Americans for Nursing Shortage Relief (ANSR). (2013). ANSR health policy. Retrieved from http://www.ansralliance.org/index.html

Ashley, J. (1976). *Hospitals, paternalism, and the role of the nurse.* New York, NY: Teachers College Press.

Benner, P., Sutphen, M., Leonard, V., & Day, L. (2010). *Educating nurses: A call for radical transformation.* San Francisco, CA: Jossey-Bass.

Bixler, G., & Bixler, R. (1959). The professional status of nursing. *American Journal of Nursing, 59,* 1142–1147.

Boughn, S. (2001). Why women and men choose nursing. *Nursing and Healthcare Perspectives, 22,* 14–19.

Brooks, J. A., & Kleine-Kracht, A. E. (1983). Evolution of a definition of nursing. *Advances in Nursing Science, 5*(4), 51–63.

Bullough, V. (2006). Nursing at the crossroads: Men in nursing. In P. Cowen & S. Moorhead (Eds.), *Current issues in nursing* (7th ed., pp. 559–568). St. Louis, MO: Mosby.

Bullough, V., & Bullough, B. (1978). *The care of the sick: The emergence of modern nursing.* New York, NY: Prodist.

Buresh, B., & Gordon, S. (2006). *From silence to voice: What nurses know and must communicate to the public* (2nd ed.). Toronto, Ontario: Canadian Nurses Association.

Chinn, P. (2001). Feminism and nursing. In J. Dochterman & H. Grace (Eds.), *Current issues in nursing* (6th ed., pp. 441–447). St. Louis, MO: Mosby.

Cleary, B. (2007, July). Report given at the American Academy of Nursing Workforce Commission Committee on Preparation of the Nursing Workforce, Chicago, IL.

Cohen, S. (2007). The image of nursing. *American Nurse Today, 2*(5), 24–26.

Connolly, C. (2004). Beyond social history: New approaches to understanding the state of and the state in nursing history. *Nursing History Review, 12,* 5–24.

Dietz, D., & Lehozky, A. (1963). *History and modern nursing.* Philadelphia, PA: Davis.

Donahue, M. (1985). *Nursing: The finest art.* St. Louis, MO: Mosby.

Finkelman, A. (2012). *Leadership and management for nurses: Competencies for quality care.* (2nd ed.). Upper Saddle River, NJ: Pearson Education.

Freeman, L. (2007). Commentary. *Nursing History Review, 15,* 167–168.

Gordon, S. (2005). *Nursing against the odds.* Ithaca, NY: Cornell University Press.

Gordon, S., & Nelson, S. (2005). An end to angels. *American Journal of Nursing, 105*(5), 62–69.

Gorenberg, B. (1983). The research tradition of nursing: An emerging issue. *Nursing Research, 32,* 347–349.

Huber, D. (Ed.). (2014). *Leadership and nursing care management* (5th ed.). Philadelphia, PA: Saunders.

International Council of Nurses (ICN). (2013). Our mission. Retrieved from http://www.icn.ch/about-icn/ics-mission

Jacobs, M. K., & Huether, S. E. (1978). Nursing science: The theory practice linkage. *Advances in Nursing Science, 1,* 63–78.

Jones, J. (2010, December 3). Nurses top honesty and ethics for 11th year: Lobbyists, car salespeople, members of Congress get the lowest ratings. *Gallup.* Retrieved from http://www.gallup.com/poll/145043/Nurses-Top-Honesty-Ethics-List-11-Year.aspx

Kalisch, P., & Kalisch, B. (1986). *The advance of American nursing* (2nd ed.). Boston, MA: Little, Brown.

Kalisch, P., & Kalisch, B. (2005). Perspectives on improving nursing's public image. *Nursing Education Perspectives, 26*(1), 10–17.

Keller, M. C. (1979). The effect of sexual stereotyping on the development of nursing theory. *American Journal of Nursing, 79,* 1584–1586.

Kidd, P., & Morrison, E. (1988). The progression of knowledge in nursing: A search for meaning. *Image, 20,* 222–224.

Kupperschmidt, B. (2004). Making a case for shared accountability. *Journal of Nursing Administration, 34*, 114–116.

Lindberg, B., Hunter, M., & Kruszewski, K. (1998). *Introduction to nursing* (3rd ed.). Philadelphia, PA: Lippincott.

Lynaugh, J. E., & Fagin, C. M. (1988). Nursing comes of age. *Image, 20*, 184–190.

Masters, K. (2005). *Role development in professional nursing practice*. Sudbury, MA: Jones and Bartlett.

National League for Nursing (NLN). (2013). Mission/goals/core values. Retrieved from http://www.nln.org/aboutnln/ourmission.htm

National Organization for Associate Degree Nursing (N-OADN). (2011). Vision, mission and goals. Retrieved from http://www.noadn.org/about/mission-and-goals.html

National Student Nurses Association (NSNA). (2013). Welcome to NSNA! Retrieved from http://www.nsna.org

Nightingale, F. (1858a). *Notes on matters affecting the health, efficiency, and hospital administration of the British army*. London, UK: Harrison and Sons.

Nightingale, F. (1858b). *Subsidiary notes as to the introduction of female nursing into military hospitals*. London, UK: Longman, Green, Longman, Roberts, and Green.

Nightingale, F. (1859). *Notes on hospitals*. London, UK: Harrison and Sons.

Nightingale, F. (1992). *Notes on nursing: What it is, and what it is not* (Commemorative ed.). Philadelphia, PA: Lippincott Williams & Wilkins. (Original work published 1860).

O'Rourke, M. (2003). Rebuilding a professional practice model: The return of role-based practice accountability. *Nursing Administrative Quarterly, 27*, 95–105.

Perry, J. (1985). Has the discipline of nursing developed to the stage where nurses do "think nursing"? *Journal of Advanced Nursing, 10*, 31–37.

Pike, A. (2001). Entering collegial relationships. In J. Dochterman & H. Grace (Eds.), *Current issues in nursing* (6th ed., pp. 448–452). St. Louis, MO: Mosby.

Quinn, C., & Smith, M. (1987). *The professional commitment: Issues and ethics in nursing*. Philadelphia, PA: Saunders.

Ritter-Teitel, J. (2002). The impact of restructuring on professional nursing practice. *Journal of Nursing Administration, 32*, 31–41.

Rosen, G. (1958). *A history of public health*. New York, NY: M.D. Publications.

Schein, E., & Kommers, D. (1972). *Professional education*. New York, NY: McGraw-Hill.

Seymer, L. (Ed.). (1954). *Selected writings on Florence Nightingale*. New York, NY: Macmillan.

Shames, K. H. (1993). *The Nightingale conspiracy: Nursing comes to power in the 21st century.* Montclair, NJ: Enlightenment Press.

Shaw, M. (1993). The discipline of nursing: Historical roots, current perspectives, future directions. *Journal of Advanced Nursing, 18,* 1651–1656.

Sigma Theta Tau International (STTI). (2013). STTI organizational fact sheet. Retrieved from http://www.nursingsociety.org/aboutus/mission/Pages/factsheet.aspx

Slater, V. (1994). The educational and philosophical influences on Florence Nightingale, an enlightened conductor. *Nursing History Review, 2,* 137–151.

Sochalski, J. (2002). Nursing shortage redux: Turning the corner on an enduring problem. *Health Affairs, 21,* 157–164.

Sullivan, E. (2002). In a woman's world. *Reflections on Nursing Leadership, 28*(3), 10–17.

Sullivan, E. J. (2004). *Becoming influential: A guide for nurses.* Upper Saddle River, NJ: Pearson Education.

Sullivan, L., & Sullivan Commission. (2004). *Missing persons: Minorities in the health professions.* Battle Creek, MI: W. K. Kellogg Foundation.

Tri-Council for Nursing. (2010). *Joint statement from the Tri-Council for Nursing on recent registered nurse supply and demand projections.* Washington, DC: American Association of Colleges of Nursing.

U.S. Bureau of Labor Statistics. (2012). Employment projection. Retrieved from http://www.bls.gov/news.release/ecopro.t06.htm

U.S. Department of Health and Human Services, Health Resources and Services Administration, Bureau of Health Professions. (2010). The registered nurse population: Findings from the March 2008 national sample survey of registered nurses. Retrieved from http://datawarehouse.hrsa.gov/nursingsurvey.aspx

Wall, B. (2003). Science and ritual: The hospital as medical and sacred space, 1865–1920. *Nursing History Review, 11,* 51–68.

Widerquist, J. (1997). Sanitary reform and nursing. *Nursing History Review, 5,* 149–159.

Woodham-Smith, C. (1951). *Florence Nightingale: 1820–1910.* New York, NY: McGraw-Hill.

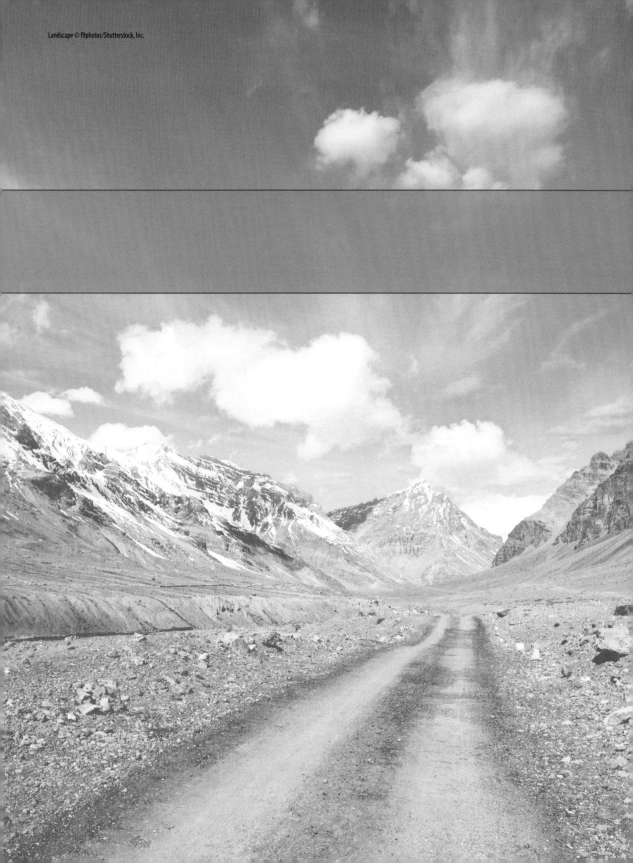

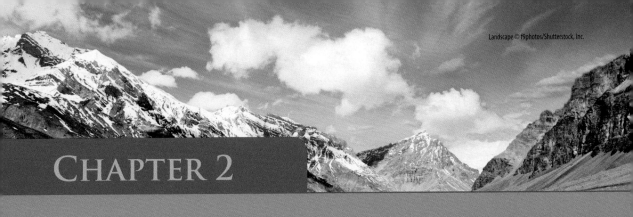

CHAPTER 2

The Essence of Nursing: Knowledge and Caring

CHAPTER OBJECTIVES

At the conclusion of this chapter, the learner will be able to:

- Discuss issues related to defining nursing
- Examine the knowledge–caring dyad
- Describe knowledge, knowledge workers, and knowledge management
- Explain the meaning of caring to nursing
- Discuss the relevance of scholarship to nursing
- Describe the relationship of theory to nursing and to critical nursing theories
- Discuss the importance of research to nursing
- Illustrate how professional literature and new modalities of scholarship are part of nursing scholarship
- Compare and contrast the major nursing roles

CHAPTER OUTLINE

KEY TERMS

Advocate	Identity	Research
Caring	Intuition	Researcher
Change agent	Knowledge	Role
Clinical reasoning and judgment	Knowledge management	Role transition
Collaboration	Knowledge worker	Scholarship
Counselor	Leader	Status
Critical thinking	Provider of care	Theory
Educator	Reality shock	
Entrepreneur	Reflective thinking	

INTRODUCTION

In 2007, Dr. Pamela Cipriano, editor in chief of *American Nurse Today*, wrote an editorial in honor of Nurses Week entitled, "Celebrating the Art and Science of Nursing." This is the topic of this chapter, although its title is "The Essence of Nursing: Knowledge and Caring." Knowledge represents the science of nursing, and caring represents the art of nursing. A 2006 publication by Nelson and Gordon, *The Complexities of Care: Nursing Reconsidered*, expanded on this topic. The authors stated, "Because we take caring seriously, we (the authors) are concerned that discussions of nursing care tend to sentimentalize and decomplexify the skill and knowledge involved in nurses' interpersonal or relational work with patients" (p. 3). Nelson and Gordon make a strong case that there is an ongoing problem of nurses devaluing the care they provide, particularly regarding the required knowledge component of nursing care and technical competencies needed to meet patient care needs and focus on the caring. This chapter explores the knowledge and caring of nursing practice. Both must be present, and both are important for quality nursing care. Content includes the effort to define nursing, knowledge and caring, competency, scholarship in nursing, the major nursing roles, and leadership.

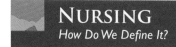

NURSING
How Do We Define It?

Defining nursing is relevant to this chapter and requires further exploration. Can nursing be defined, and if so, why is it important to define it? Before this discussion begins, you should review your personal definition of nursing. You may find it strange to spend time on the question of a definition of nursing, but the truth is, there is no universally accepted definition by healthcare professionals and patients. The easy first approach to developing a definition is to describe what nurses do; however, this approach leaves out important aspects and essentially reduces nursing to tasks. More consideration needs to be given to (1) what drives nurses to do what they do, (2) why they do what they do (rationales, evidence-based practice [EBP]), and (3) what is achieved by what they do (outcomes) (Diers, 2001). Diers noted that even Florence Nightingale's and Virginia Henderson's definitions are not definitions of what nursing *is*, but more of what nurses *do*. Henderson's definition is more of a personal concept than a true definition. Henderson herself even said that what she wrote was not the complete definition of nursing (Henderson, 1991). Diers also commented that there really are no full definitions for most disciplines.

Yet nursing is still concerned with a definition. Having a definition serves several purposes that really drive what that definition will look like (Diers, 2001):

- Providing an operational definition to guide research
- Acknowledging that changing laws requires a definition that will be politically accepted—for example, in relationship to a nurse practice act
- Convincing legislators about the value of nursing—for example, to gain funds for nursing education
- Explaining what nursing is to consumers/patients (although no definition is totally helpful because patients/consumers will respond to a description of the work, not a definition)
- Explaining to others in general what one does as a nurse (then the best choice is a personal description of what nursing is)

One could also say that a definition is helpful in determining what to include in a nursing curriculum, but nursing has been taught for years without a universally accepted definition. The American Nurses Association (ANA, 2010a) defines nursing as "the protection, promotion, and optimization of health and abilities, prevention of illness and injury, alleviation of suffering through the diagnosis and treatment of human response, and advocacy in the care of individuals, families, communities, and populations" (p. 66). Some of the critical terms in this definition include the following:

- *Promotion of health:* "Mobilize healthy patterns of living, foster personal and family development, and support self-defined goals of individuals, families, communities, and populations" (ANA, 2010a, p. 23).
- *Health:* "An experience that is often expressed in terms of wellness and illness, and may occur in the presence or absence of injury" (ANA, 2010a, p. 65).
- *Prevention of illness and injury:* Interventions taken to keep illness or injury from occurring—for example, immunization for tetanus or teaching parents how to use a car seat.
- *Illness:* "The subjective experience of discomfort" (ANA, 2010a, p. 65).
- *Injury:* Harm to the body—for example, a broken arm caused by a fall from a bicycle.
- *Diagnosis:* "A clinical judgment about the patient's response to actual or potential health conditions or needs. The diagnosis provides the basis for determination of a plan to achieve expected outcomes. Registered nurses utilize nursing and medical diagnosis depending upon educational and clinical preparation and legal authority" (ANA, 2010a, p. 64).
- *Human response:* The phenomena of concern to nurses that include any observable need, concern, condition, event, or fact of interest actual or potential health problems (ANA, 2010b, p. 40).
- *Treatment:* To give care through interventions—for example, administering medication, teaching a patient how to give himself or herself insulin, wound care, preparing a patient for surgery, and ensuring that the patient is not at risk for an infection.
- *Advocacy:* The act of pleading for or supporting a course of action on behalf of individuals, families, communities, and populations—for example, a nurse who works with the city council to improve health access for a community.

Seven essential features of professional nursing have been identified from definitions of nursing (ANA, 2010b, p. 9):

1. Provision of a **caring relationship** that facilitates health and healing
2. **Attention** to the range of human experiences and responses to health and illness within the physical and social environments
3. **Integration of assessment data with knowledge** gained from an appreciation of the patient or the group

4. **Application of scientific knowledge** to the processes of diagnosis and treatment through the use of judgment and critical thinking
5. Advancement of professional nursing knowledge through **scholarly inquiry**
6. Influence on social and public policy to **promote social justice**
7. **Assurance of safe, quality, and evidence-based practice**

In this list, terms that indicate the importance of knowledge and caring to nursing are in bold. Knowledge and caring are the critical dyad in any description or definition of nursing, and both relate to nursing scholarship and leadership.

The North American Nursing Diagnosis Association (NANDA, 2011) has described nursing interventions and developed the Nursing Interventions Classification (NIC; University of Iowa, 2011) and the Nursing Outcomes Classification (NOC) as part of its attempts to define the work of nursing (University of Iowa, 2011). Maas (2006) discussed the importance of these initiatives, which she described as the building blocks of nursing practice theory, and noted that "rather than debating the issues of definition, nursing will be better served by focusing those energies on its science and the translation of the science of nursing practice" (p. 8). Three conclusions are that (1) no universally accepted definition of nursing exists, although several definitions have been developed by nursing leaders and nursing organizations; (2) individual nurses may develop their own personal description of nursing to use in practice; and (3) a more effective focus is the pursuit of nursing knowledge to build nursing scholarship. The first step is to gain a better understanding of knowledge and caring in relationship to nursing practice.

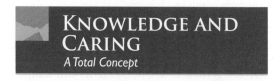

KNOWLEDGE AND CARING
A Total Concept

Understanding how knowledge and caring form the critical dyad for nursing is essential to providing effective quality care. **Knowledge** is specific information about something, and **caring** is behavior that demonstrates compassion and respect for another. But these are very simple definitions. The depth of nursing practice goes beyond basic knowledge and the ability to care. Nursing encompasses a distinct body of knowledge coupled with the art of caring. As stated in Butcher, "A unique body of knowledge is a foundation for attaining the respect, recognition, and power granted by society to a fully developed profession and scientific discipline" (2006, p. 116). Nurses use critical thinking as they apply knowledge, evidence, and caring to the nursing process and become competent. Experts such as Dr. Patricia Benner, who led the Carnegie Foundation Study on nursing education (Benner, Sutphen, Leonard, & Day, 2010), suggest that we often use the term *critical thinking*, but there is high variability and little consensus on what constitutes critical thinking. **Clinical reasoning and judgment** are also very important and include critical thinking.

Knowledge

Knowledge can be defined and described in a number of ways. There are five ways of knowing (Cipriano, 2007) that are useful in understanding how one knows something. A nurse might use all or some of these ways of knowing when providing care.

1. Empirical knowing focuses on facts and is related to quantitative explanations—predicting and explaining.
2. Ethical knowing focuses on a person's moral values—what should be done.
3. Personal knowing focuses on understanding and actualizing a relationship between a nurse and a patient, including knowledge of self (nurse).
4. Aesthetic knowing focuses on the nurse's perception of the patient and the patient's needs, emphasizing the uniqueness of each relationship and interaction.

5. Synthesizing, or pulling together the knowledge gained from the four types of knowing, allows the nurse to understand the patient better and to provide higher-quality care.

The ANA (2010b) identified the key issues related to the knowledge base for nursing practice, including both theoretical and evidence-based knowledge:

- Promotion of health and wellness
- Promotion of safety and quality of care
- Care, self-care processes, and care coordination
- Physical, emotional, and spiritual comfort, discomfort, and pain
- Adaptation to physiologic and pathophysiologic processes
- Emotions related to experiences of birth, growth and development, health, illness, disease, and death
- Meanings ascribed to health and illness, and other concepts
- Linguistic and cultural sensitivity
- Health literacy
- Decision making and the ability to make choices
- Relationships, role performance, and change processes within relationships
- Social policies and their effects on health
- Healthcare systems and their relationships to access, cost, and quality of health care
- The environment and the prevention of disease and injury

This is the basic knowledge that every nurse should have to practice. Nurses use this knowledge base in collaboration with patients to assess, plan, implement, and evaluate care (ANA, 2010b, pp. 13–14).

Knowledge Management

Knowledge work is a critical component of healthcare delivery today, and nurses are knowledge workers. Forty percent or more of workers in knowledge-intensive businesses, such as a healthcare organization, are **knowledge workers** (Sorrells-Jones &

Weaver, 1999). **Knowledge management** includes both routine work (such as taking vital signs, administering medications, and walking a patient) and nonroutine work, which (1) involves exceptions, (2) requires judgment and use of knowledge, and (3) may be confusing or not fully understood. In a knowledge-based environment, a person's title is not as important as the person's expertise, and use of knowledge and learning are important. Knowledge workers actively use the following skills:

- Collaboration
- Teamwork
- Coordination
- Analysis
- Critical thinking
- Evaluation
- Willingness to be flexible

Knowledge workers recognize that change is inevitable and that the best approach is to be ready for change and to view it as an opportunity for learning and improvement. Nurses use knowledge daily in their work—both routine and nonroutine—and must have the characteristics of the knowledge worker. They work in an environment that expects healthcare providers to use the best evidence in providing care. "Transitioning to an evidence-based practice requires a different perspective from the traditional role of nurse as 'doer' of treatments and procedures based on institutional policy or personal preference. Rather, the nurse practices as a 'knowledge worker' from an updated and ever-changing knowledge base" (Mooney, 2001, p. 17). The knowledge worker focuses on acquiring, analyzing, synthesizing, and applying evidence to guide practice decisions (Dickenson-Hazard, 2002). The knowledge worker uses synthesis, competencies, multiple intelligences, a mobile skill set, outcome practice, and teamwork, as opposed to the old skills of functional analysis, manual dexterity, fixed skill set, process value, process practice, and unilateral performance (Porter-O'Grady & Malloch, 2007). This nurse is a clinical scholar. The employer and patients value a nurse for what the nurse knows and how this knowledge is used to meet patient care outcomes—not just for technical expertise or caring, although these aspects of performance are also important (Kerfoot, 2002).

This change in a nurse's work is also reflected in the Carnegie Foundation Report on nursing education, as reported by Patricia Benner and colleagues (2010). Benner suggested that instead of focusing on content, nurse educators need to focus on teaching nurses how to access information, use and manipulate data (such as those data available from patient information systems), and document in the electronic interprofessional format.

Reflective Thinking, Intuition, and Clinical Thinking and Judgment: Impact on Knowledge Development and Application

Critical thinking, reflective thinking, and intuition are different approaches to thinking and can be used in combination. Nurses use all of them to explore, understand, develop new knowledge, and apply knowledge. What they mean and how are they used in nursing follows.

Critical Thinking. **Critical thinking** is clearly a focus of nursing. The ANA standards state that the nursing process is a critical thinking tool, albeit not the only one used in nursing (ANA, 2010a). This skill emphasizes purposeful thinking, rather than sudden decision making that is not based on thought and knowledge. Alfaro-LeFevre (2011) identified four key critical thinking components of critical thinking:

- Critical thinking characteristics (attitudes/behaviors)
- Theoretical and experiential knowledge (intellectual skills/competencies)
- Interpersonal skills/competencies
- Technical skills/competencies

In reviewing each of these components, one can easily identify the presence of knowledge, caring (interpersonal relationships, attitudes), and technical expertise.

A person uses four key intellectual traits in critical thinking (Paul, 1995). Each of the traits can be learned and developed.

- *Intellectual humility:* Willingness to admit what one does not know. (This is difficult to do, but it can save lives. A nurse who cannot admit that he or she does not know something and yet proceeds is taking a great risk. It is important for students to be able to use intellectual humility as they learn about nursing.)
- *Intellectual integrity:* Continual evaluation of one's own thinking and willingness to admit when your thinking is not adequate. (This type of honesty with self and others can make a critical difference in care.)
- *Intellectual courage:* Ability to face and fairly address ideas, beliefs, and viewpoints for which one may have negative feelings. (Students enter into a new world of health care and do experience confusing thoughts about ideas, beliefs, and viewpoints, and sometimes their personal views may need to be put aside in the interest of the patient and safe, quality care.)
- *Intellectual empathy:* Conscious effort to understand others by putting one's own feelings aside and imagining oneself in another person's place.

Caring and critical thinking are also connected in that caring stimulates critical thinking (Zimmerman & Phillips, 2000). Nurses, first as students and then as professional nurses, think more about the work they are doing when they appreciate the experience of caring.

Critical thinking skills that are important to develop include affective learning; applied moral reasoning and values (relates to ethics); comprehension; application, analysis, and synthesis; interpretation; knowledge, experience, judgment, and evaluation; learning from mistakes when they happen; and self-awareness (Finkelman, 2001). This type of thinking helps to reduce the tendency toward dichotomous thinking and groupthink. Dichotomous thinking leads one to look at an issue, situation, or problem as one way or the other, such as good or bad, black or white. This narrowing of scope limits choices. Groupthink occurs when all group or team members think alike. While all of the team members might be working together smoothly, groupthink limits choices, discourages open discussion of possibilities, and diminishes the ability to consider alternatives. Problem solving is not a critical thinking skill, but effective problem solvers use critical thinking.

The following methods will help develop your critical thinking skills (Finkelman, 2001, p. 196):

1. Seek the best information and data possible to allow you to fully understand the issue, situation, or problem. Questioning is critical. Examples of some questions that might be asked are: What is the significance of _____? What is your first impression? What is the relationship between and _____? What impact might _____ have on _____? What can you infer from the information/data?

2. Identify and describe any problems that require analysis and synthesis of information—thoroughly understand the information/data.

3. Develop alternative solutions—more than two is better because this forces you to analyze multiple solutions even when you discard one of them. Be innovative and move away from proposing only typical or routine solutions.

4. Evaluate the alternative solutions and consider the consequences for each one. Can the solutions really be used? Do you have the resources you need? How much time will it take? How well will the solution be accepted? Identify pros and cons.

5. Make a decision, choosing the best solution, even though there is risk in any decision making.

6. Implement the solution but continue to question.

7. Follow up and evaluate; plan for evaluation from the very beginning. Self-assessment of critical thinking skills is an important part of using critical thinking. How does one use critical thinking, and is it done effectively?

Reflective Thinking. Throughout one's nursing education experience and practice, **reflective thinking** needs to become a part of daily learning and practice. Conway (1998) noted that nurses who use reflective thinking implement care based on the individualized care needs of the patient, whereas nurses who use reflective thinking less tend to provide illness-oriented care. Reflection is seen as a part of the art of nursing, which requires "creativity and conscious self-evaluation over a period of time" (Decker, 2007, p. 76). Reflection helps nurses cope with unique situations. The following questions might be asked (Johns, 2004, p. 18):

- Empirical: "What knowledge informed or might have informed you?"
- Aesthetic: "Which particular issues seem significant to pay attention to?"
- Personal: "Which factors influenced the way you felt, thought, or responded?"
- Ethical: "To what extent did you act for the best and in tune with your values?"

Responding to these questions leads to reflection: "How might you respond more effectively if you encounter this situation again?"

Critical reflection requires that the student or nurse examine the underlying assumptions and really question or even doubt the arguments, assertions, or facts of a situation or case (Benner, Hughes, & Sutphen, 2008). This allows the nurse to better grasp the patient's situation.

The skills needed for reflective thinking are the same skills required for critical thinking—the ability to monitor, analyze, predict, and evaluate (Pesut & Herman, 1999), and to take risks, be open, and have imagination (Westberg & Jason, 2001). Guided reflection with faculty who assist students in using reflective thinking during simulated learning experiences can enhance student learning and help students learn reflective learning skills. It is recommended (Johns, 2004) that this process be done with faculty to avoid negative thoughts that a student may experience (Decker, 2007). The student should view the learning experience as an opportunity to improve and see the experience from different perspectives. Some strategies that might be used to develop reflective thinking are keeping a journal (such as the Electronic Reflective Journal it is suggested that you keep in conjunction with this text), engaging in one-to-one dialogue with a faculty facilitator, engaging in e-mail dialogues, and participating in structured team/group forums. Team/group forums help you learn more about constructive feedback and can also be conducted online in the form of discussion forums. Reflective thinking strategies are not used for grading or evaluation, but rather are intended to help you think about your learning experience in an open manner.

Intuition. **Intuition** is part of thinking. Including intuition in critical thinking helps to expand the person's ability to know (Hansten & Washburn, 2000). The most common definition of intuition is having a gut feeling about something. Nurses often have this feeling as they provide care—"I just have this feeling that Mr. Wallace is heading for problems." It is hard to explain what this is, but it happens. The following are examples of thoughts that a person might relate to intuition (Rubenfeld & Scheffer, 2009):

- I felt it in my bones.
- I couldn't put my finger on why, but I thought instinctively I knew.
- My hunch was that … .
- I had a premonition/inspiration/impression.
- My natural tendency was to … .
- Subconsciously I knew that.
- Without thought I figured it out.
- Automatically I thought that.
- While I couldn't say why, I thought immediately that … .
- My sixth sense said I should consider … .

Intuition is not science, but sometimes intuition can stimulate research and lead to greater knowledge and questions to explore. Intuition is related to experience. A student would not likely experience intuition about a patient care situation, but over time, as nursing expertise is gained, the student may be better able to use intuition. Benner's

(2001) work, *From Novice to Expert*, suggests that intuition for nurses is really the putting together of the whole picture based on scientific knowledge and clinical expertise, not just a hunch, and that intuition continues to be an important part of the nursing process (Benner et al., 2008).

Caring

There is no universally accepted definition for caring in nursing, but it can be described from four perspectives (Mustard, 2002). The first is the sense of caring, which is probably the most common perspective for students to appreciate. This perspective emphasizes compassion, or being concerned about another person. This type of caring may or may not require knowledge and expertise, but in nursing, effective caring requires both knowledge and expertise. The second perspective is doing for other people what they cannot do for themselves. Nurses do this all the time, and it requires knowledge and expertise to be effective. The third perspective is to care for the medical problem; this, too, requires knowledge of the problem, interventions, and so on, as well as expertise to provide the care. Providing wound care or administering medications is an example of this type of caring. The fourth perspective is "competence in carrying out all the required procedures, personal and technical, with true concern for providing the proper care at the proper time in the proper way" (Mustard, 2002, p. 37). Not all four types of caring must be used at one time to be described as caring. Caring practices have been identified by the American Association of Critical-Care Nurses in the organization's synergy model for patient care (2011) as "nursing activities that create a compassionate, supportive, and therapeutic environment for patients and staff, with the aim of promoting comfort and healing and preventing unnecessary suffering."

Nursing theories often focus on caring. Theories are discussed later in this chapter. One theory in particular is known for its focus on caring—Watson's theory on caring. Watson (1979) defined nursing "as the science of caring, in which caring is described as transpersonal attempts to protect, enhance, and preserve life by helping find meaning in illness and suffering, and subsequently gaining control, self-knowledge, and healing" (Scotto, 2003, p. 289).

Patients today need caring. They feel isolated and are often confused by the complex medical system. Many patients have chronic illnesses such as diabetes, arthritis, and cardiac problems that require long-term treatment, and these patients need to learn how to manage their illnesses and be supported in the self-management process. Even many patients with cancer who have longer survival rates today are now described as having a chronic illness.

How do patients view caring? Patients may not see the knowledge and skills that nurses need, but they can appreciate when a nurse is there with them. The nurse–patient relationship can make a difference when the nurse uses caring consciously (Schwein, 2004). Characteristics of the patient-centered relationship are as follows:

- Being physically present with the patient
- Having a dialogue with the patient
- Showing a willingness to share and hear— to use active listening
- Avoiding assumptions
- Maintaining confidentiality
- Showing intuition and flexibility
- Believing in hope

Caring is offering of self. This means "offering the intellectual, psychological, spiritual, and physical aspects one possesses as a human being to attain a goal. In nursing, this goal is to facilitate and enhance patients' ability to do and decide for themselves (i.e., to promote their self-agency)" (Scotto, 2003, p. 290). According to Scotto, "Nurses must prepare themselves in each of the four aspects to be competent to care" described as (pp. 290–291):

- The intellectual aspect of nurses consists of an acquired, specialized body of knowledge, analytical thought, and clinical judgment, which are used to meet human health needs.
- The psychological aspect of nurses includes the feelings, emotions, and memories that are part of the human experience.

- The spiritual aspect of nurses, as for all human beings, seeks to answer the questions, "Why? What is the meaning of this?"
- The physical aspect of nurses is the most obvious. Nurses go to patients' homes, the bedside, and a variety of clinical settings where they apply their strength, abilities, and skills to attain a goal. For this task, nurses first must care for themselves, and then they must be accomplished and skillful in nursing interventions.

For students to be able to care for others, they need to care for themselves. This is also important for practicing nurses. It takes energy to care for another person, and this effort is draining. Developing positive, healthy behaviors and attitudes can protect a nurse later when more energy is required in the practice of nursing.

As students begin their nursing education program (and indeed throughout the program), the issue of the difference between medicine and nursing often arises. Caring is something that only nurses do, or so nurses say. Many physicians would say that they also care for patients and have a caring attitude. Nurses are not the only healthcare professionals who can say that caring is part of their profession. However, what has happened with nursing (which may not have been so helpful) is that when caring is discussed in relation to this profession, it is described only in emotional terms (Moland, 2006). This ignores the fact that caring often involves competent assessment of the patient to determine what needs to be done, and the ability to subsequently provide that care; for both of these endeavors to be effective, the healthcare provider must have knowledge. The typical description of medicine is curing; for nursing, it is caring. This type of extreme dichotomy is not helpful for either profession individually and also has implications for the interrelationship between the two professions, adding conflict and creating difficulty in communication in the interprofessional team.

The use of technology in health care has increased steadily since 1960, particularly since the end of the 20th century. Nurses work with technology daily, and more and more care involves some type of technology. This has had a positive impact on care; however, some wonder about the negative impact of technology on caring. Does technology create a barrier between the patient and the nurse that interferes with the nurse–patient relationship? Because of this concern, "nurses are placing more emphasis on the 'high touch' aspect of a 'high tech' environment, recognizing that clients (patients) require human interactions, such as warmth, care, acknowledgement of self-worth, and collaborative decision-making" (Kozier, Erb, & Blais, 1997, p. 10). There must be an effort to combine technology and caring because both are critical to positive patient outcomes. This synergistic relationship is referred to as "technological competency as caring" in nursing (Locsin, 2005). Nurses who use technology but ignore the patient as a person are just technologists; they are not nurses who use knowledge, caring, critical thinking, technological skills, and recognition of the patient as a person as integral parts of the caring process. For example, the nurse who focuses on the computer monitor in the room and does not engage the patient is not caring in an effective manner.

Competency

Competency is the behavior that a student is expected to demonstrate. The ANA standards define competency as "an expected and measurable level of nursing performance that integrates knowledge, skills, abilities, and judgment based on established scientific knowledge and expectations for nursing practice" (2010a, p. 64). The ultimate goal of competence is to promote patient safety and quality care. The major Institute of Medicine (IOM) report on nursing, *The Future of Nursing* (2010), identifies in its eight recommendations the need for all nurses to engage in lifelong learning. Competency levels change over time as students gain more experience. Development of competencies continues throughout a nurse's career. Nurses in practice have to demonstrate certain competencies to continue practice. This is typically done by meeting staff development/education requirements. Students, however, must satisfy competency requirements to progress through the nursing program and graduate. Competencies include elements of knowledge, caring, and technical skills.

After a number of IOM reports described serious problems with health care, including errors and poor-quality care, an initiative was developed to identify core competencies for all healthcare professions, including nursing, to build a bridge across the quality chasm to improve care (IOM, 2003). It is hoped that these competencies will have an impact on education for, and practice in, health professions (Finkelman & Kenner, 2012). The core competencies are summarized here:

1. *Provide patient-centered care:* Identify, respect, and care about patients' differences, values, preferences, and expressed needs; relieve pain and suffering; coordinate continuous care; listen to, clearly inform, communicate with, and educate patients; share decision making and management; and continuously advocate disease prevention, wellness, and promotion of healthy lifestyles, including a focus on population health. The description of this core competency relates to content found in definitions of nursing, nursing standards, nursing social policy statement, and nursing theories.

2. *Work in interdisciplinary/interprofessional teams:* Cooperate, collaborate, communicate, and integrate care in teams to ensure that care is continuous and reliable. There is much knowledge available about teams and how they impact care. Leadership is a critical component of working on teams—both as team leader and as followers or members. Many of the major nursing roles that are discussed in this chapter require working with teams.

3. *Employ evidence-based practice:* Integrate best research with clinical expertise and patient values for optimal care, and participate in learning and research activities to the extent feasible. EBP has been mentioned in this chapter about knowledge and caring as it relates to research.

4. *Apply quality improvement:* Identify errors and hazards in care; understand and implement basic safety design principles, such as standardization and simplification; continually understand and measure quality of care in terms of structure, process, and outcomes in relation to patient and community needs; and design and test interventions to change processes and systems of care, with the objective of improving quality. Understanding how care is provided and which problems in providing care arise often leads to the need for additional knowledge development through research.

5. *Utilize informatics:* Communicate, manage knowledge, mitigate error, and support decision making using information technology. This chapter focuses on knowledge and caring, both of which require use of informatics to meet patient needs.

SCHOLARSHIP IN NURSING

There is a great need to search for better solutions and knowledge and to disseminate knowledge. This discussion about scholarship in nursing explores the meaning of scholarship, the meaning and impact of theory and research, use of professional literature, and new scholarship modalities.

What Does Scholarship Mean?

The American Association of Colleges of Nursing (AACN) defines **scholarship** in nursing "as those activities that systematically advance the teaching, research, and practice of nursing through rigorous inquiry that: (1) is significant to the profession, (2) is creative, (3) can be documented, (4) can be replicated or elaborated, and (5) can be peer-reviewed through various methods" (2005, p. 1). The common response when asking which activities might be considered scholarship is "research." Boyer (1990), however, questioned this view of scholarship, suggesting that other activities may also be scholarly:

- Discovery, in which new and unique knowledge is generated (research, theory development, philosophical inquiry)
- Teaching, in which the teacher creatively builds bridges between his or her own understanding and the students' learning
- Application, in which the emphasis is on the use of new knowledge in solving society's problems (practice)
- Integration, in which new relationships among disciplines are discovered (publishing, presentations, grant awards, licenses, patents, or products for sale; must involve two or more disciplines, thus advancing knowledge over a broader range)

These four aspects of scholarship are critical components of academic nursing and support the values of a profession committed to both social relevance and scientific advancement.

Some nurses think that the AACN definition of scholarship limits scholarship to educational institutions only. Mason (2006) commented that this is a problem for nursing; science needs to be accessible to practitioners. She defined scholarship as "an in-depth, careful process of exploring current theory and research with the purpose of either furthering the science or translating its findings into practice or policy" (Mason, 2006, p. 11). The better approach, then, is to consider scholarship in both the education and practice arenas and still emphasize that nursing is a patient-centered practice profession. Nursing theory and research have been mentioned in this chapter and by Mason as part of knowledge and caring and scholarship of nursing. Understanding what they are and how they have an impact on practice is important if all nurses are to be scholars and leaders.

Nursing has a long history of scholarship, although some periods seem to have been more active than others in terms of major contributions to nursing scholarship. **Exhibit 2-1** describes some of the milestones that are important in understanding nursing scholarship.

Exhibit 2-1	A Brief History of Selected Nursing Scholarship Milestones

1850	Nightingale conducted first nursing research by collecting healthcare data during the Crimean War.
1851	Florence Nightingale, age 32, went to the Institution of Deaconesses at Kaiserswerth to train in nursing. She was interested in care focused on spirituality and healing.
1854–1855	Nightingale created the first standards for care.
1854–1856	Nightingale applied knowledge of statistics and care training. She took charge of lay nurses and the anglican sisters; nurses had to wear uniforms: loose gray dresses, a jacket, cap, and sash. This dress was practical because halls and rooms were drafty and cool.
1860	The first training school was founded in London.
1860	*Notes on Nursing* by Nightingale was published.
	Prior to the 1860s and the Civil War, religious orders (primarily of the Catholic Church) cared for the sick. These early times were characterized by several significant historical events:
	▪ A lack of organized nursing and care led to the development of Bellevue Hospital, which was founded in 1658 in New York.
	▪ In 1731, the Philadelphia Almshouse was started by the Sisters of Charity, spearheaded by Elizabeth Ann Bayley Seton, a physician's daughter who married, was widowed, and then entered religious life and provided nursing care.
	▪ Charity Hospital in New Orleans, Louisiana, was founded in 1736 and funded by private endowment.
1860–1865	The Civil War broke out. Dorothea Dix, Superintendent of Female Nurses for the Union Army, needed help with the wounded. She set the first qualifications for nurses.
1860s	Dr. Elizabeth Blackwell, first female U.S. physician, started the Women's Central Association for Relief in New York City, which later became the Sanitary Commission.
	The New England Hospital for Women and Children in Boston, Massachusetts, opened in 1860. During its early years there was no structured care.
	Woman's Hospital of Philadelphia opened in 1861, also with no structured care.
	In 1863, the state of Massachusetts began the first board of nursing, the first attempt at regulation of the practice of nursing.
1870s	The first U.S. nursing school graduate was Linda Richards in 1873 from the New England Hospital for Women and Children in Boston, Massachusetts.
	Although a plea for attention to the hospital environment had been made by Nightingale, it was not until the 1870s that lights were introduced.
	Written patient reports were instituted during this time, replacing the verbal reports previously used.
	Hospitals began to examine the causes of mortality among their patient population.
	Mary Mahoney, the first black nurse, graduated in 1879.

Exhibit 2-1 (*continued*)

1873	Three nursing schools were founded:
	▪ The Bellevue Training School in New York City, New York
	▪ The Connecticut Training School in New Haven, Connecticut
	▪ The Boston Training School in Boston, Massachusetts
1882	Clara Barton, a schoolteacher, founded the American Red Cross.
1884	Isabel Hampton Robb wrote *Nursing: Its Principles and Practice for Hospital and Private Use.*
1885	The first nursing text was published: *A Textbook of Nursing for the Use of Training Schools, Families and Private Students.*
1890s	The Visiting Nurses Group started in England.
1893	The American Society of Superintendents of Training Schools was formed.
	Lillian Wald founded the Henry Street Settlement, a community center in New York City. This was the beginning of community-based care.
	The Nightingale Pledge was written by Mrs. Lystra E. Gretter, which was a modification of the doctor's Hippocratic Oath. The pledge was written for the Farrand Training School for Nurses, Detroit, Michigan.
1897	The University of Texas at Galveston moved undergraduate nursing education into the university setting.
1900–1930s	A shortage of funds put nursing education under the control of doctors and hospitals. This situation resulted from:
	▪ Leaders believing that the only way to change was to organize
	▪ The need to provide protection for the public from poorly educated nurses
	▪ A lack of sanitation
	▪ Schools providing cheap services for hospitals
1900s–1940s	As nursing became more ensconced in university settings, nursing research became more important for well-educated nurses to study. The first research studies focused on nursing education.
1900	Columbia Teachers College offered the first graduate nursing degree.
	As nursing moved from a practice-based discipline to a university program, subjects such as ethics were introduced for the first time. Isabel Hampton Robb, considered the architect of American nursing, wrote *Nursing Ethics*, the first ethics text for nurses.
	Both textbooks and journals for nurses became available. Among the first of the journals was the *American Journal of Nursing*.
1901	Mary Adelaide Nutting started a 3- to 6-month preparatory course for nurses; by 1911, 86 schools had some form of formalized, structured nurse training.
1907	Mary Adelaide Nutting became the first nursing professor and began the first state nursing association in Maryland. At this time nursing was moving toward a more formal educational system, similar to that of the discipline of medicine. A professional organization at a state level gave recognition to nursing as a distinct discipline.

(*continues*)

Exhibit 2-1 (continued)

	Now a distinct discipline, nursing needed standards to guide practice and education. Isabel Hampton Robb wrote *Educational Standards for Nurses.*
1908	Other professional organizations grew, including the National Association of Colored Graduate Nurses.
1909	The first bachelor's degree program in nursing was started at the University of Minnesota.
1911	The concept of specialties within nursing began with Bellevue Hospital's midwifery program.
1912	The American Society of Superintendents of Training Schools became the National League for Nursing Education (NLNE).
	The National Organization for Public Health Nursing was founded.
	The *Public Health Nursing* journal was started.
1917	The National League for Nursing Education identified its first *Standard Curriculum for Schools of Nursing*, a remedy for the lack of standards in nursing education.
1920	The first master's program in nursing began at Yale School of Nursing.
1922	Sigma Theta Tau International (STTI), the nursing honor society, was formed.
1923	The Goldmark Report called for nursing education to be separate from (and precede) employment; it also advocated nursing licensure and proper training for faculty at nursing institutions.
1925	Mary Breckenridge founded the Frontier Nursing Service in Kentucky. Her intent was to provide rural health care; this organization was the first to employ nurses who could also provide midwifery services.
	As the status of women increased, nurses were among the first women to lead the women's rights movements in the United States.
1930	A total of 41 (out of 48) states established regulatory state boards of nursing.
1931	The Association of Collegiate Schools of Nursing formed, eventually becoming the Department of Baccalaureate and Higher Degrees of the NLN.
1934	New York University and the Teachers College started PhD and EdD in programs in nursing.
1940	The Nursing Council on National Defense, formed after World War I (1917–1918), underwent changes during 1940.
1942	The American Association of Industrial Nurses (AAIN) was founded.
1948	The Brown Report recommended that nursing education programs be located in universities; this report also formed the basis for evaluating nursing programs.
1950s–1960s	Early nursing theory was developed.
1950	The American Nurses Association (ANA) published the first edition of the *Code for Nurses.*
	Graduate nursing education began programs to prepare clinical nurse specialists.

Exhibit 2-1 *(continued)*

1952	The NLNE changed its name to the National League for Nursing (NLN).
	Publication of *Nursing Research* began under the direction of the ANA.
	Mildred Montag started the first associate degree nursing programs. These were designed as pilots to create a technical nurse below the level of the professional nurse, but with training beyond that of a practical nurse.
1954	The University of Pittsburgh started a PhD program in nursing (academic doctorate).
1955	The American Nurses Foundation was formed to obtain funds for nursing research.
1956	Columbia University granted its first master's degree in nursing.
1960	The doctorate in nursing science (DNS) degree was started at Boston University (professional doctorate).
1960s	Federal monies were made available for doctoral study for nurse educators.
1963	The initial publication of *International Journal of Nursing Studies* became available.
1964	Loretta Ford established the first nurse practitioner program at the University of Colorado.
1965	The first nursing research conference was held.
	The ANA made the statement that a baccalaureate degree should represent the entry level for nursing practice. As of 2014, this recommendation was still not fully implemented, although there has been significant improvement in the last five years.
1967	The STTI launched its publication *Image*.
1969	The American Association of Colleges of Nursing (AACN) formed, with its 123 members serving as representation for bachelor's degree and higher education nursing programs.
1970s–1990s	This period of development saw the birth of most nursing theories; some of these theories have been tested and expanded upon.
1973	The first nursing diagnosis conference was held.
	The American Academy of Nursing (AAN) was formed under the aegis of the ANA to recognize nursing leaders.
	The ANA published the first edition of *Standards of Nursing Practice*.
1978–1979	Several new nursing research journals had their initial publication.
1985	The National Center for Nursing Research was established at the National Institutes of Health, later to become the National Institute of Nursing Research (NINR).
1990s	Evidence-based practice became a major focus.

(continues)

Exhibit 2-1 *(continued)*	
1993	The ANA published its position statement on nursing education.
	The Commission on Collegiate Nursing Education (CCNE) was formed to accredit nursing programs, with an emphasis on bachelor's and master's degree programs.
	The Cochrane Collaborative was formed to develop and publish systematic reviews; it was named after British epidemiologist Archie Cochrane.
1995	The ANA published the first edition of *Nursing's Social Policy Statement*.
1996	The Joanna Briggs Institute for Evidence-Based Practice was founded in Adelaide, Australia.
1997	The National League for Nursing Accrediting Commission (NLNAC) became a separate corporation from the NLN. (It changed its name to the Accreditation Commission for Education in Nursing [ACEN] in 2013.)
1999	The AACN published its position statement on nursing research.
2004	The NLN established Centers for Excellence in Nursing Education to recognize exemplar schools of nursing.
	The AACN endorsed the development of and called for pilot schools to create the Clinical Nurse Leader (CNL).
	The Columbia University School of Nursing offered the first doctor of nursing practice (DNP) degree.
2007	The NLN established the Academy of Nursing Education to recognize nursing education leaders.
2010	The landmark nursing education report, *Educating Nurses: A Call for Radical Transformation* (Benner, Sutphen, Leonard, and Day), was published.
	A significant Institute of Medicine report, *The Future of Nursing: Leading Change, Advancing Health*, was published.

Nursing Theory

A simple description of a **theory** is "words or phrases (concepts) joined together in sentences, with an overall theme, to explain, describe, or predict something" (Sullivan, 2006, p. 160). Theories help nurses understand and find meaning in nursing. A number of nursing theories have been developed since Nightingale's contributions to nursing, particularly during the 1960s through 1980s. These theories vary widely in their scope and approach. This surge in development of nursing theories was related to the need to "justify nursing as an academic discipline"—the need to develop and describe nursing knowledge (Maas, 2006, p. 7). Some of the major theories are described in **Exhibit 2-2** from the perspective of how each description, beginning with Nightingale, responds to the following concepts:

- The person
- The environment
- Health
- Nursing

Since the late 1990s, nursing education has placed less emphasis on nursing theory. This change has been controversial. Theories may be used to

Exhibit 2-2   Overview of Major Nursing Theories and Models

Theories and Models	Person	Environment	Health	Nursing
Systematic approach to health care Florence Nightingale	Recipient of nursing care.	External (temperature, bedding, ventilation) and internal (food, water, and medications).	Health is "not only to be well, but to be able to use well every power we have to use" (Nightingale, 1969 [reissue], p. 24).	Alter or manage the environment to implement the natural laws of health.
Theory of caring in nursing Jean Watson	A "unity of mind body spirit/ nature" (Watson, 1996, p. 147).	A "field of connectedness" at all levels (p. 147).	Harmony, wholeness, and comfort.	Reciprocal transpersonal relationship in caring moments guided by curative factors.
Science of unitary human beings Martha E. Rogers	An irreducible, irreversible, pandimensional, negentropic energy field identified by pattern; a unitary human being develops through three principles: helicy, resonancy, and integrality (Rogers, 1992).	An irreducible, pandimensional, negentropic energy field, identified by pattern and manifesting characteristics different from those of the parts and encompassing all that is other than any given human field (Rogers, 1992).	Health and illness area a part of a continuum (Rogers, 1970).	Seeks to promote symphonic interaction between human and environmental fields, to strengthen the integrity of the human field, and to direct and redirect patterning of the human and environmental fields for realization of maximum health potential (Rogers, 1970).
Self-care deficit nursing theory Dorothea E. Orem	A person under the care of a nurse; a total being with universal, developmental needs, and capable of self-care (patient).	Physical, chemical, biologic, and social contexts with which human beings exist; environmental components include environmental factors, environmental conditions, and developmental environment (Orem, 1985).	"A state characterized by soundness or wholeness of developed human structures and of bodily and mental functioning" (Orem, 1995, p. 101).	Therapeutic self-care designed to supplement self-care requisites. Nursing actions fall into one of three categories: wholly compensatory, partly compensatory, or supportive educative system (Orem, 1985).
Roy adaptation model Callista Roy	"A whole with parts that function as a unity" (Roy & Andrews, 1999, p. 31).	Internal and external stimuli; "the world within and around humans as adaptive systems" (p. 51).	"A state and process of being and becoming an integrated and whole human being" (p. 54).	Manipulation of stimuli to foster successful adaptation.

(continues)

Exhibit 2-2 (continued)   Overview of Major Nursing Theories and Models

Theories and Models	Person	Environment	Health	Nursing
Neuman systems model Betty Neuman	A composite of physiological, psychological, sociocultural, developmental, and spiritual variables in interaction with the internal and external environment; represented by central structure, lines of defense, and lines of resistance.	All internal and external factors of influences surrounding the client system.	A continuum of wellness to illness.	Prevention as intervention; concerned with all potential stressors.
Systems framework and theory of goal attainment Imogene M. King	A personal system that interacts with interpersonal and social systems (human being).	A context "within which human beings grow, develop, and perform daily activities" (King, 1981, p. 18). "The internal environment of human beings transforms energy to enable them to adjust to continuous external environmental changes" (p. 5).	"Dynamic life experiences of a human being, which implies continuous adjustment to stressors in the internal and external environment through optimum use of one's resources to achieve maximum potential for daily living" (p. 5).	A process of human interaction; the goal of nursing is to help patients achieve their goals.
Behavioral systems model Dorothy Johnson	A biophysical being who is a behavioral system with seven subsystems of behavior (human being).	Includes internal and external environment.	Efficient and effective functioning of system; behavioral system balance and stability.	An external regulatory force that acts to preserve the organization and integrity of the patient's behavior at an optimal level under those conditions in which the behavior constitutes a threat to physical or social health or in which illness is found (Johnson, 1980, p. 214).

Theory of human becoming Rosemarie Parse	An open being, more than and different from the sum of parts in mutual simultaneous interchange with the environment, who chooses from options and bears responsibility for choices (Parse, 1987, p. 160).	In mutual process with the person.	Continuously changing process of becoming.	Use of true presence to facilitate the becoming of the participant.
Transcultural nursing model Madeleine Leininger	Human beings, family, group, community, or institution.	"Totality of an event, situation, or experience that gives meaning to human expressions, interpretations, and social interactions in physical, ecological, sociopolitical, and/or cultural settings" (Leininger, 1991, p. 46).	"A state of well-being that is culturally defined, valued, and practiced" (Leininger, 1991, p. 46).	Activities directed toward assisting, supporting, or enabling with needs in ways that are congruent with the cultural values, beliefs, and lifeways of the recipient of care (Leininger, 1995).
Interpersonal relations model Hildegard Peplau	"Encompasses the patient (one who has problems for which expert nursing services are needed or sought) and the nurse (a professional with particular expertise)" (Peplau, 1952, p. 14).	Includes culture as important to the development of personality.	"Implies forward movement of personality and other ongoing human processes in the direction of creative, productive, personal, and community living" (Peplau, 1952, p. 12).	The therapeutic, interpersonal process between the nurse and the patient.

Sources: Johnson, D. (1980). The behavioral systems model for nursing. In J. Riehl & C. Roy (Eds.), *Conceptual models for nursing practice* (2nd ed., pp. 207–216). New York, NY: Appleton-Century-Crofts; King, I. M. (1981). *A theory of nursing: Systems, concepts, process.* New York, NY: Wiley; Leininger, M. M. (1991). *Culture care diversity and universality: A theory of nursing.* New York, NY: National League for Nursing; Leininger, M. M. (1995). Transcultural nursing perspectives: Basic concepts, principles, and culture care incidents. In M. M. Leininger (Ed.), *Transcultural nursing: Concepts, theories, research, and practices* (2nd ed., pp. 57–92). New York, NY: McGraw-Hill; Nightingale, F. (1969 [reissue]) *Notes on nursing: What it is and what it is not.* New York, NY: Dover; Orem, D. (1985). *Nursing: Concepts of practice* (3rd ed.). St. Louis, MO: Mosby; Orem, D. (1995). *Nursing: Concepts of practice* (5th ed.). St. Louis, MO: Mosby; Parse, R. R. (1987). *Nursing science: Major paradigms, theories, and critiques.* Philadelphia, PA: Saunders; Peplau, H. (1952). *Interpersonal relations in nursing.* New York, NY: G. P. Putnam's Sons; Rogers, M. E. (1970). *An introduction to the theoretical basis of nursing.* Philadelphia, PA: Davis; Rogers, M. E. (1992). Nursing science and the space age. *Nursing Science Quarterly, 5,* 27–34; Roy, C., & Andrews, H. A. (1999). *The Roy adaptation model.* New York, NY: Appleton-Lange; Watson, J. (1996). Watson's philosophy and theory of human caring in nursing. In J. P. Riehl-Sisca (Ed.), *Conceptual models for nursing practice* (pp. 219–235). Norwalk, CT: Appleton & Lange, as cited in K. Masters (2005). *Role development in professional nursing practice.* Sudbury, MA: Jones and Bartlett.

provide frameworks for research studies and to test their applicability. In addition, practice may be guided by one of the nursing theories. In hospitals and other healthcare organizations, the nursing department may identify a specific theory or a model on which the staff bases its mission. In these organizations, it is usually easy to see how the designated theory is present in the official documents about the department, but it is not always so easy to see how the theory impacts the day-to-day practice of nurses in the organization. It is important to remember that theories do not tell nurses what they must do or how they must do something; rather, they are guides—abstract guides. **Figure 2-1** describes the relationship between theory, research, and practice.

Most of the existing nursing theories were developed in the 1970s through 1990s, so which issues might future theories address? In 1992, the following were predicted as possible areas to be included in nursing theories (Meleis, 1992):

- The human science underlying the discipline that "is predicated on understanding the meanings of daily lived experiences as they are perceived by the members or the participants of the science" (p. 112)
- The increased emphasis on practice orientation, or actual, rather than "ought-to-be," practice

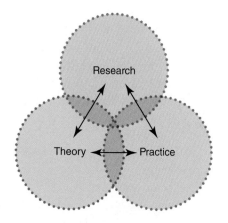

Figure 2-1   Relationship Theory, Research, Practice

Source: Masters, K. (2005). *Role development in professional nursing practice.* Sudbury, MA: Jones and Bartlett.

- The mission of nursing to develop theories to empower nurses, the discipline, and clients (patients)
- "Acceptance of the fact that women may have different strategies and approaches to knowledge development than men" (p. 113)
- Nursing's attempt to "understand consumers' experiences for the purpose of empowering them to receive optimum care and to maintain optimum health" (p. 114)
- "The effort to broaden nursing's perspective, which includes efforts to understand the practice of nursing in third world countries" (p. 114)

These potential characteristics of nursing are somewhat different from those evidenced in past theories. Consumerism is highlighted through better understanding consumers/patients and empowering them. Empowering nurses is also emphasized. The suggestion that female nurses and male nurses might approach care issues differently has not really been addressed in the past. The effort to broaden nursing's perspective is highly relevant today, given the increase in globalization and the emphasis on culturally appropriate care. Developed and developing countries can share information via the Internet in a matter of seconds. There are fewer boundaries than ever before, such that better communication and information exchange have become possible. A need for nursing to expand its geographic scope certainly exists because the nursing issues and care problems are often the same or very similar worldwide. Indeed, a global effort to solve these problems on a worldwide scale is absolutely necessary. Take, for example, issues such as infectious diseases: Because of the ease of travel, they can quickly spread from one part of the world to another in which the disease is relatively unknown.

In conclusion, it is not really clear what role nursing theories might play and how theories might change in the future, although theory development is not as active today as it was in the past.

Nursing Research

Nursing **research** is "systematic inquiry that uses disciplined methods to answer questions and solve problems" (Polit & Beck, 2013, p. 4). The major purpose of doing research is to expand nursing knowledge to improve patient care and outcomes. That is, research helps to explain and predict care that nurses provide. Two major types of research exist: basic and applied. Basic research is conducted to gain knowledge for knowledge sake; however, basic research results may then be used in applied or clinical research.

Nursing has not connected research with practice as much as it should, although this situation has changed somewhat in recent years. This type of approach separates the practitioner from the research process too much. Nursing needs to know more about "whether and how nurses produce knowledge in their practice" (Reed, 2006, p. 36). Nursing—indeed, all health care—needs to be patient-centered (IOM, 2003), and research should not be an exception. This does not mean that there is no need for research in administration/management and in education, because there are critical needs in these areas; rather, it means that nursing needs to gain more knowledge about the nursing process with patients as the center. Because of these issues, evidence-based practice has become more central in nursing practice. The research process is similar to the nursing process in that there is a need to identify a problem using data, determine goals, describe what will be done, and then assess results.

Professional Literature

Professional literature is an important part of nursing scholarship, but it is important to remember that "because of the changing health care environment and the proliferation of knowledge in health care and nursing, much of the knowledge acquired in your nursing education program may be out of date 5 years after you graduate" (Zerwekh & Claborn, 2006, p. 197). This literature is found in textbooks and in professional journals. It represents a repository of nursing knowledge that is accessible to nursing students and nurses. It is important that nurses keep up with the literature in their specialty areas, given the increased emphasis on EBP. Increased access to journals is now available through the Internet; this is a positive change because it makes knowledge more accessible when it is needed, including e-books.

Textbooks typically are a few years behind current information because of the length of the publication schedule. Although this gap is improving, it still takes significantly longer to publish a textbook than a journal. It is also more expensive to publish a book, so new editions do not come out annually. The content found in textbooks provides the background information and detail on particular topics. A textbook is peer reviewed when content is shared with experts on the topic for feedback to the author(s). Today, many textbook publishers offer companion websites to provide additional material and, in some cases, more updated content or references. More publishers are publishing textbooks in e-book format; some offer both hard-copy and e-books, and others offer only e-books. This change might reduce the delay in getting textbooks published and provide a method for updating content quickly.

Content in journals is typically more current than that in textbooks and usually focuses on a very specific topic in less depth than a textbook. Higher-quality journals are peer reviewed. This means that several nurses who have expertise in the manuscript's topic review submitted manuscripts. A consensus is then reached with the editor regarding whether to publish the manuscript. Online access to journal articles has made this literature increasingly available to nurses.

Nursing professional organizations often publish journals. Studies published in the last 25 years in scientific nursing journals have primarily focused on adults and psychological factors, with a decrease in theory-based studies and an increase in qualitative studies being noted (Oermann & Jenerette, 2013). Any nurse with expertise in an area can submit an article for publication; however, this does not mean all manuscripts are published. The profession needs more nurses publishing, particularly in journals. **Exhibit 2-3** identifies examples of nursing journals.

Exhibit 2-3	Examples of Nursing Journals

American Journal of Nursing (AJN)

American Nursing Today

Archives of Psychiatric Nursing

Emergency Room Nursing

Home Healthcare Nurse

Image: The Journal of Nursing Scholarship

Journal of Cardiovascular Nursing

Journal of Nursing Administration

Journal of Nursing Care Quality

Journal of Nursing Informatics

Journal of Nursing Management

Journal of Nursing Scholarship

Journal of Pediatric Nursing

Journal of Perinatal and Neonatal Nursing

Journal of Professional Nursing

Journal of Psychiatric Nursing and Mental Health Nursing

Nurse Leader

Nursing Management

Nursing Outlook

Nursing Research

Nursing 2014

Oncology Nursing

Online Journal of Nursing

World Views of Evidence-Based Nursing

New Modalities of Scholarship

Scholarship, as noted previously, includes publications, copyrights, licenses, patents, or products for sale. Nursing is expanding into a number of new modalities that can be considered scholarship. Many of these modalities relate to web-based learning—including course development and learning activities, and products such as case software for simulation experiences—and involve other technology, such as tablets and podcasting. Most of these new modalities relate to teaching and learning in academic programs, although many have expanded into staff development/education and continuing education. In developing these modalities, nurses are creating innovative teaching methods, developing programs and learning outcomes, improving professional development, applying technical skills, and sharing scholarship in a more timely manner. When interprofessional approaches are used, integrative scholarship occurs. The Sigma Theta Tau International provides a number of continuing education programs offered through the Internet supporting use of best evidence to improve care and management; some are identified in **Box 2-1**.

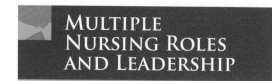

MULTIPLE NURSING ROLES AND LEADERSHIP

Nurses use knowledge and caring as they provide care to patients; however, there are other aspects of nursing that are important. Nurses function in multiple roles, sometimes at the same time. As nurses function in these roles, they need to demonstrate leadership.

Key Nursing Roles

Before discussing nursing roles, it is important to discuss some terminology related to roles. A role can vary depending on the context. **Role** means the

Box 2-1	Examples of a Continuing Education Program Promoting Evidence-Based Practice at the Bedside

Sigma Theta Tau International offers continuing education courses for nurses; examples of content include:

- Evidence-Based Nursing: The Joanna Briggs Approach Parts 1, 2, and 3
- Nurse Manager Certificate Program: The Use of Evidence to Guide Decision Making and Management Practices
- Nurse Manager Certificate Program: Facilitating Staff Development
- Inflammation and Disease
- Living with Illness

Source: Sigma Theta Tau International. Continuing education program promoting clinical scholars at the bedside. Retrieved from http://www.nursingknowledge.org/knowledge.html?product_type=107

expected and actual behaviors that one would associate with a position such as a nurse, physician, teacher, pharmacist, and so on. Connected to role is **status**, which is a position in a social structure, with rights and obligations—for example, a nurse manager. As a person takes on a new role, the person experiences **role transition**. Nursing students are in role transition as they gradually learn the nursing roles. All nursing roles are important in patient care, and typically these roles are interconnected in practice. Students learn about the roles and what is necessary to be competent to meet role expectations. **Identity** also is involved: "Identity is foundational to professional nursing practice. Identity in nursing can be defined as the development within nurses of an internal representation of people–environment interactions in the exploration of human responses to actual or potential health problems. Professional identity is foundational to the assumption of various nursing roles" (Cook, Gilmer, & Bess, 2003, p. 311).

Nursing is a complex profession and involves multiple types of consumers of nursing care (e.g., individuals, families, communities, and populations), multiple types of problems (e.g., physical, emotional, sociological, economic, and educational), and multiple settings (e.g., hospitals, clinics, communities, and schools), and specialties within each of these dimensions. Some roles such as teaching,

administration, and research do not focus as much on direct patient care. Different levels of knowledge, caring, and education may be required for different roles. There are many nursing roles, and all of them require leadership. The key roles found in nursing are discussed in the following sections.

Provider of Care

The **provider of care** role is probably what students think nursing is all about—this is the role typically seen in the hospital setting and the role that most people think of when they think of a nurse. Caring is attached most to this role, but knowledge is critical to providing safe, quality care. When the nurse is described, it is often the caring that is emphasized, with less emphasis on the knowledge and expertise required to provide quality care. This perspective is not indicative of what really happens because nurses need to use knowledge and be competent, as discussed earlier in this chapter. Providing care has moved far beyond the hospital, with nurses providing care in clinics, schools, the community, homes, industry, and at many more sites.

Educator

Nurses spend a lot of time teaching—teaching patients, families, communities, and populations. In the **educator** role, nurses focus on health promotion and prevention and helping the patient (individuals, families, communities, and populations) cope with illness and injury. Teaching needs to be planned and based on needs, and nurses must know about teaching principles and methods. Some nurses teach other nurses and healthcare providers in healthcare settings—an activity called staff development or staff education. Other nurses teach in nursing schools. Nursing education is now considered to be a type of nursing specialty/advanced practice.

Counselor

A nurse may act as a **counselor**, providing advice and counseling to patients, families, communities, and populations. This is often done in conjunction with other roles.

Manager

Nurses act as managers daily in their positions, even if they do not have a formal management position. Management is the process of getting something done efficiently and effectively through and with other people. Nurses might do this by ensuring that a patient's needs are addressed. For example, the nurse might ensure that the patient receives needed laboratory work or a rehabilitation session. The nurse plans who will give care (and when and how), evaluates outcomes, and so forth. Managing care involves critical thinking, clinical reasoning and judgment, planning, decision making, delegating, collaborating, coordinating, communicating, working with interprofessional teams, and leadership.

Researcher

Only a small percentage of nurses are actual nurse **researchers**; however, nurses may participate in research in other ways. The most critical means is by using EBP or evidence-based management (EBM), which is one of the five core healthcare professional competencies. Some nurses now hold positions in research studies that may or may not be nursing research studies. These nurses assist in data collection and even manage data collection projects.

Collaborator

Every nurse is a collaborator. "**Collaboration** [boldface added] is a cooperative effort that focuses on a win-win strategy. Collaboration depends on each individual recognizing the perspective of others who are involved and eventually reach a consensus of common goal(s)" (Finkelman, 2012, p. 353). A nurse collaborates with other healthcare providers, members of the community, government agencies, and many other individuals and organizations. Teamwork is a critical component of daily nursing practice.

Change Agent (Intrapreneur)

It is difficult to perform any of the nursing roles without engaging in change. This change may be found in how care is provided; where care is provided and when; to whom care is provided; and why care is provided. Change is normal today. The healthcare delivery system experiences constant change. Nurses deal with change wherever they work, but they may also initiate change for care improvement. When a nurse acts as a **change agent** within the organization where the nurse works, the nurse is an intrapreneur. This requires risk and the ability to see change in a positive light. An example of a nurse acting as a change agent would be a nurse who sees the value in extending visiting hours in the intensive care unit. The nurse reviews the literature on this topic to support EBP interventions and then approaches management with the suggestion about making a change. The nurse then works with the interprofessional team to plan, implement, and evaluate this change to assess the outcomes.

Entrepreneur

The **entrepreneur** role is not as common as other roles, but it is becoming increasingly prominent. The entrepreneur works to make changes in a broader sense. Examples include nurses who are healthcare consultants and legal nurse consultants, and nurses who establish businesses related to health care, such as a staffing agency, a business to develop a healthcare product, a healthcare media business, or a collaboration with a technology venture such as engineering.

Patient Advocate

Nurses serve as the patient and family **advocate**. The nurse may advocate on behalf of an individual, a family, a community, or a population. In this role, the nurse acts as a change agent and a risk taker. The nurse speaks for the patient but does not take away the patient's independence. A nurse caring for a patient in the hospital, for example, might advocate with the physician to alter care so as to allow a dying patient to spend more time with family. A nurse might also advocate for better health coverage by writing to the local congressional representative or by attending a meeting about care in the community.

Leader

In all of these roles, nurses need to act as **leaders**; however, it is important to recognize that being a leader is a role that nurses assume, either formally by taking an administrative position or informally as others recognize that they have leadership characteristics.

Summary Points: Roles and What Is Required

To meet the demands of these multiple roles, nurses need to be prepared and competent. Prerequisites and the nursing curriculum, through its content, simulation laboratory experiences, and clinical experiences, help students to transition to these roles. The prerequisites provide content and experiences related to biological sciences, English and writing, sociology, government, languages, psychology, and mathematics and statistics. In nursing, course content relates to the care of diverse patients in the hospital, in homes, and in communities; planning and implementing care; communication and interpersonal relationships; culture; teaching; community

health; epidemiology; issues related to safe, quality care; research and EBP; health policy; and leadership and management. As discussed earlier in this chapter, this content relates to the required knowledge base.

When students transition to the work setting as registered nurses, they should be competent as beginning nurses; even so, the transition is often difficult. **Reality shock** may occur. This reaction may occur when a new nurse is confronted with the realities of the healthcare setting and nursing, which are typically very different from what the nurse has experienced in school (Kramer, 1985). Knowledge and competency are important, but new nurses also need to build self-confidence, and they need time to adjust to the differences between the academic world and real-life practice. Some schools of nursing, in collaboration with hospitals, now offer internship/externship and residency programs for new graduates to decrease reality shock. The major nursing roles that you will learn about in your nursing programs are important in practice, but it is also important for you to learn about being an employee, working with and in teams, communicating in real situations, and functioning in complex organizations.

More nurses—particularly new graduates—work in hospitals than in other healthcare settings, although the number of nurses working in hospitals is decreasing. Hospital care has changed since 1996, with sicker patients staying in the hospital for shorter periods and with greater use of complex technology. These changes have an impact on what is expected of nurses—namely, in terms of competencies.

Nursing standards, nurse practice acts, professional ethics, and the nursing process influence nursing roles. Health policy also has an impact on roles; for example, legislation and changes in state practice guidelines were required before the advanced practice nurse could have prescriptive authority (ability to prescribe medications). This type of role change requires major advocacy efforts from nurses and nursing organizations.

Landscape © f9photos/Shutterstock, Inc.

CONCLUSION

This chapter has highlighted the definitions of nursing, description of nursing roles, the changing skills sets needed by nurses, ways of knowing, and the need for a movement toward recognition of nurses as knowledge workers. Some key nursing theories were also described. Scholarship in nursing includes knowledge, research, and publications, all of which provide the profession with a framework for effective evidence-based practice.

Landscape © f9photos/Shutterstock, Inc.

CHAPTER HIGHLIGHTS

1. The definition of nursing varies depending on the source.
2. The need to define nursing relates to the ability to describe what nursing is and what it does.
3. Caring and knowledge are critical components of the nursing profession.
4. Today, the trend is toward preparing nurses to serve as knowledge workers.
5. Competency is defined by and related to the new skills that a nurse needs to function in today's healthcare environment.
6. Nursing scholarship is demonstrated in nursing theory, research, and professional literature.
7. The key roles of the nurse are care provider, educator, manager, advocate, counselor, researcher, collaborator, change agent (intrapreneur), entrepreneur, and leader.

Landscape © f9photos/Shutterstock, Inc.

DISCUSSION QUESTIONS

1. Discuss the relationship between knowledge and caring in nursing.
2. How might knowing the definition of nursing impact how you practice?
3. What does *knowledge worker* mean?
4. What are the characteristics of a nurse manager?
5. Why is leadership important in nursing?
6. Describe the nurse's role in today's healthcare system.
7. Why are competencies important?
8. Discuss the role of critical thinking in nursing education and explain why there is little agreement about what constitutes critical thinking. What is the importance of clinical reasoning and judgment? Identify examples from your own practice that apply to critical thinking and clinical reasoning and judgment.

Landscape © f9photos/Shutterstock, Inc.

CRITICAL THINKING ACTIVITIES

1. Based on what you have learned about critical thinking, assess your own ability to use critical thinking. Make a list of your strengths and limitations regarding using critical thinking. Determine several strategies that you might use to improve your critical thinking. Write down these strategies and track your improvement over the semester. Apply the critical thinking skills mentioned in this chapter to guide you in this activity.

2. Review the descriptions of the nursing theories found in Exhibit 2-2. Compare and contrast the theories in relationship to their views of person, environment, health, and nursing. Identify two similarities and dissimilarities in the theories. Select a theory that you feel represents your view of nursing at this time. Why did you select this theory?

3. Caring is a concept central to nursing. Review the description of the nursing theories found in Exhibit 2-2. Identify which theories emphasize caring, and describe how this is demonstrated in the theory.

4. Go to the National Institute of Nursing Research website (http://www.ninr.nih.gov/AboutNINR/) and click Mission & Strategic Plan. Explore the Ongoing Research Interests section. What are some of the interests? Do any of them intrigue you? If so, why? What is the NINR's current strategic plan? What can you learn about past and current nursing research? Did you think of these areas of study as part of nursing before this course? Why or why not? What impressed you about the research? Do you think these results are practice oriented?

5. Do you think nursing scholarship is important? Provide your rationale for your response.

6. Select one of the major nursing roles and describe it. Explain why you would want to function in this role.

7. Interview a staff nurse, a nurse manager, and an educator and ask for their definition of nursing. Compare their answers. Why do you believe there are differences? How do these definitions relate to what you have learned in this chapter?

8. How do you respond to the following: You are told that the profession of nursing needs to abandon its image of nurses as angels and promote an image of nurses as competent professionals who are both knowledgeable and caring (Rhodes, Morris, & Lazenby, 2011). Debate this issue in class.

9. Ask a patient to describe the role of a nurse; then compare it with your view of nursing. Is it similar or different, and why?

ELECTRONIC *Reflective Journal*

Circuit Board: ©Photos.com

What does *caring* mean to you? How does your view of caring compare with what you have learned in this chapter?

Landscape © f9photos/Shutterstock, Inc.

LINKING TO THE INTERNET

- National Institutes of Health: http://www.nih.gov
- National Institute of Nursing Research: http://www.ninr.nih.gov/
- American Nurses Association: http://www.nursingworld.org
- North American Nursing Diagnosis International (NANDA): http://www.nanda.org
- Nursing Interventions Classification: (NIC) http://www.nursing.uiowa.edu/excellence/nursing_knowledge/clinical_effectiveness/nic.htm
- Nursing-Sensitive Outcomes Classification (NOC): http://www.nursing.uiowa.edu/excellence/nursing_knowledge/clinical_effectiveness/nocpubs.htm
- Our Concept of Critical Thinking: http://www.criticalthinking.org/aboutCT/ourConceptCT.cfm
- Defining Critical Thinking: http://www.criticalthinking.org/aboutCT/definingCT.cfm
- Sigma Theta Tau International: Nursing Knowledge International: http://www.nursingknowledge.org/Portal/main.aspx?PageID=32
- Nursing Theory Information: http://www.sandiego.edu/nursing/research/nursing_theory_research.php

CASE STUDIES

Landscape © f9photos/Shutterstock, Inc.

Case Study 1

A nurse who works in a community clinic has a busy day ahead of her. The first half of the day is focused on seeing four patients as follow-up to their appointments last week for high blood pressure (hypertension). The nurse checks each patient's blood pressure, asks about symptoms, weighs each patient, and asks if the patient has any questions. If there are negative changes, the patient sees the physician. The nurse also assists the physician with physical exams as needed. Two new patients require patient education about their diets. A dietician appointment is scheduled for one patient who needs more intensive assistance. In the afternoon, the nurse leads a group for diabetic patients. At the end of the day, the nurse meets with her nurse manager for her annual performance evaluation, and the nurse manager tells the nurse that she should write a journal article about the group for patients with diabetes. The nurse is getting into her car to go home and thinks to herself, "Now when would I have time to write a journal article!"

Case Questions

1. Which ways of knowing did the nurse use in providing care?
2. What makes this nurse a knowledge worker?
3. Identify what the nurse did that was routine and nonroutine (knowledge management).
4. How did change impact this nurse?

CASE STUDIES (CONTINUED)

Case Study 2

A Historical Event to Demonstrate the Importance of the Art and Science of Nursing, Nursing Roles, and Leadership

The following case is a summary of a change in healthcare delivery that impacted nurses. After reading the case, respond to the questions.

In the 1960s, something significant began to happen in hospital care, and ultimately in the nursing profession. But first, let's go back to the 1950s for some background information. There was increasing interest in coronary care during this time, particularly for acute myocardial infarctions. It is important to remember that changes in health care are certainly influenced by changes in science and technology, but incidents and situations within the country as a whole also drive change and policy decisions. This situation was no exception. Presidents Dwight D. Eisenhower and Lyndon B. Johnson both had acute myocardial infarctions, which received a lot of press coverage. The mortality rate from acute myocardial infarctions was high. There were also significant new advances in care monitoring and interventions: cardiac catheterization, cardiac pacemakers, continuous monitoring of cardiac electrical activity, portable cardiac defibrillators, and external pacemakers. This really was an incredible list to come onto the scene at the same time.

Now, what was happening with nursing in the 1950s regarding the care of cardiac patients? Even with advances, nurses were providing traditional care, and the boundaries between physicians and nurses were very clear.

Physicians

- Examined the patient
- Took the electrocardiogram
- Drew blood for lab work
- Diagnosed cardiac arrhythmias
- Determined interventions

Nurses

- Made the patient comfortable
- Took care of the patient's belongings
- Answered the family's questions
- Took vital signs (blood pressure, pulse, and respirations)
- Made observations and documented them
- Administered medications
- Provided the diet ordered and rest

In the 1960s, change began to happen. Dr. Hughes Day, a physician at Bethany Hospital in Kansas City, had an interest in cardiac care. The hospital redesigned its units, moving away from open wards to private and semiprivate rooms. This was nice for the patients, but it made it difficult for nurses to observe patients. (This is a good example of how environment and space influence care.) Dr. Day established a Code Blue to communicate the need for urgent response to patients having critical cardiac episodes (Day, 1972). This was a great idea, but the response often came too late for many patients who were not observed early enough. Dr. Day then instituted monitoring of patients

(continues)

CASE STUDIES (CONTINUED)

with cardiac problems who were unstable. Another good idea, but if there was a problem, what would happen? Who would intervene, and how? Dr. Day would often be called, even at home at night, but in such a critical situation how could he get to the hospital in time? Nurses had no training or experience with the monitoring equipment or in recognizing arrhythmias, or knowledge about what to do if there were problems. Dr. Day was beginning to see that his ideas needed revision.

At the same time that Dr. Day was exploring cardiac care, Dr. L. Meltzer was involved in similar activity at Presbyterian Hospital in Philadelphia. Each of these physicians did not know of the work that the other was doing. Dr. Meltzer went about the problem a little differently. He knew that a separate unit was needed for cardiac patients, but he was less sure about how to design it and how it would function. Dr. Meltzer approached the Division of Nursing, U.S. Public Health Services, for a grant to study the problem. He wanted to establish a two-bed cardiac care unit (CCU). His research question was *Will nurse monitoring and intervention reduce the high incidence of arrhythmic deaths from acute myocardial infarctions?* At this time (and in a development that was good for nursing), Faye Abdella, PhD, RN, was leading the Division of Nursing. She really liked the study proposal but felt that something important was missing. To receive the grant, Dr. Meltzer needed to have a nurse lead the project. Dr. Meltzer proceeded to look for that nurse. He turned to the University of Pennsylvania and asked the dean of nursing for a recommendation. Rose Pinneo, MSN, RN, a nurse who had just completed her master's degree and had experience in cardiac care, was selected. Dr. Meltzer and Pinneo became a team. Pinneo liked research and wanted to do this kind of work. By chance, she had her opportunity. What she did not know was that this study and its results would have a major long-term impact on cardiac care and the nursing profession.

Dr. Zoll, who worked with Dr. Meltzer, recognized the major barrier to success in changing patient outcomes: Nurses had no training in what would be required of them in the CCU. This represented a major shift in what nurses usually did. If this was not changed, no study could be conducted based on the research question that they had proposed. Notably, Dr. Meltzer proposed a new role for nurses in the CCU:

- The nurse has specific skills in monitoring patients using the new equipment.
- Registered nurses (RNs) would provide all the direct care. Up until this time, the typical care organization consisted of a team of licensed practical nurses and aides, who provided most of the direct care, led by an RN (team nursing). This had to change with the proposed CCU staffing, increasing the need for more qualified RNs in CCU.
- RNs would interpret heart rhythms using continuous-monitoring electrocardiogram data.
- RNs would initiate emergency interventions when needed.
- RNs, not physicians, would be central in providing care in CCU 24 hours a day, 7 days a week, but they must practice with the physicians.

There were questions as to whether RNs could be trained for this new role, but Dr. Meltzer had no doubt that they could be.

CASE STUDIES (CONTINUED)

Based on Dr. Meltzer's plan and the new role, Pinneo needed to find the nurses for the units. She wanted nurses who were ready for a challenge and who were willing to learn the new knowledge and skills needed to collect data. Collecting data would be time consuming, plus the nurses had to provide care in a very new role. The first step after finding the nurses was training. This, too, was unique. An interprofessional approach was taken, and it took place in the clinical setting, the CCU. Clinical conferences were held to discuss patients and their care once the unit opened.

The nurses found that they were providing care for highly complex problems. They were assessing and diagnosing, intervening, and having to help patients with their psychological responses to having had an acute myocardial infarction. Clearly, knowledge and caring were important, but added to this was curing. With the interventions that nurses initiated, they were saving lives. Standing orders telling nurses what to do in certain situations based on data they collected were developed by Dr. Meltzer and used by the CCU staff. House staff—physicians in training—began to turn to the nurses to learn because the CCU nurses had experience with these patients. Dr. Meltzer called his approach the scientific team approach. In 1972, he wrote, "Until World War II even the recording of blood pressure was considered outside the nursing sphere and was the responsibility of a physician. As late as 1962, when coronary care was introduced, most hospitals did not permit their nursing staff to perform venipunctures or to start intravenous infusions. That nurses could interpret the electrocardiograms and defibrillate patients indeed represented a radical change for all concerned" (Meltzer, Pinneo, & Kitchell, 1972, p. 8).

What were the results of this study? Nurses could learn what was necessary to function in the new role. Nurses who worked in CCU gained autonomy, but now the boundaries between physicians and nurses were less clear, and this began to spill over into other areas of nursing. There is no doubt that nursing began to change. CCUs opened across the country. They also had an impact on other types of intensive care.

Case Questions

If you do not know any terms in this case, look them up in a medical dictionary. Based on this case, discuss the implications of the art and science of nursing.

1. What were the differences in how Dr. Day and Dr. Meltzer handled their interests in changing cardiac care?
2. Who led this initiative? Why is this significant?
3. Compare and contrast the changes in nursing roles before the Meltzer and Day studies. What was the role supported by their work?
4. What about this case is unique and unexpected?
5. What does this case tell you about the value of research?

Sources: Day, H. (1972). History of coronary care units. American Journal of Cardiology, 30, 405; Meltzer, L., Pinneo, R., & Kitchell, J. (1972). Intensive coronary care: A manual for nurses. Philadelphia, PA: Charles Press.

Words of Wisdom

© Roobcio/Shutterstock, Inc.

Nancy Batchelor, DNP, MSN, RNC, CNS

Assistant Professor, Clinical Nursing, University of Cincinnati College of Nursing Staff Nurse, Hospice of Cincinnati, East Inpatient Unit, Cincinnati, Ohio

Hospice nursing is different from any other type of nursing. Some feel that it is a ministry. The focus is on providing holistic care for the patient diagnosed with terminal disease and the family. Hospice and palliative care nurses care for patients who have incurable disease. The hospice nurse manages symptoms to allow the patient the highest quality of life possible while moving along life's continuum toward death. Hospice and palliative care nursing is a growing specialty, and it will continue to grow as the population ages and as individuals cope with chronic disease. Hospice and palliative care nurses deliver care based on principles identified by Florence Nightingale: caring, comfort, compassion, dignity, and quality.

As a hospice inpatient care center nurse, I care for my patients using the principles described. Besides using my technical nursing skills, I am able to spend time with the patients doing the little things that make them more comfortable—whether it is holding their hand, giving a massage, sharing a snack, reminiscing about their lives, alleviating the burden of care from the family, praying, or just providing a caring presence. Depending on the situation, I may prepare my patients to return home with family, to a level of long-term care, or to the hereafter. I feel totally blessed and privileged to minister, to alleviate suffering, to facilitate bereavement, and to prepare for transition from life to death.

Landscape © f9photos/Shutterstock, Inc.

REFERENCES

Alfaro-LeFevre, R. (2011). *Applying nursing process: A tool for critical thinking*. Philadelphia, PA: Lippincott Williams & Wilkins.

American Association of Colleges of Nursing (AACN). (2005). *Position statement on defining scholarship for the discipline of nursing*. Washington, DC: Author.

American Association of Critical-Care Nurses. (2011). The AACN synergy model for patient care. Retrieved from http://www.aacn.org:88/wd/certifications/content/synmodel.pcms?pid=1&&menu=

American Nurses Association (ANA). (2010a). *Nursing scope and standards of practice* (2nd ed.). Silver Spring, MD: Author.

American Nurses Association (ANA). (2010b). *Nursing's social policy statement*. Silver Spring, MD: Author.

Benner, P. (2001). *From novice to expert: Excellence and power in clinical nursing practice* (commemorative ed.). Upper Saddle River, NJ: Prentice Hall.

Benner, P., Hughes, R., & Sutphen, M. (2008). Clinical reasoning, decision making, and action: Thinking critically and clinically. In R. Hughes (Ed.), *Patient safety and quality:*

An evidence-based handbook for nurses (pp. 103–125). Rockville, MD: Agency for Health Research and Quality. AHRQ Publication #08-0043

Benner, P., Sutphen, M., Leonard, V., & Day, L. (2010). *Educating nurses: A call for radical transformation*. San Francisco, CA: Jossey-Bass.

Boyer, E. (1990). *Scholarship reconsidered: Priorities for the professionate*. Princeton, NJ: Carnegie Foundation for the Advancement of Teaching.

Butcher, H. (2006). Integrating nursing theory, nursing research, and nursing practice. In J. P. Cowen & S. Moorehead (Eds.), *Current issues in nursing* (7th ed., pp. 112–122). St. Louis, MO: Mosby.

Cipriano, P. (2007). Celebrating the art and science of nursing. *American Nurse Today, 2*(5), 8.

Conway, J. (1998). Evolution of the species "expert nurse": An examination of practical knowledge held by expert nurses. *Journal of Clinical Nursing, 7*(1), 75–82.

Cook, T., Gilmer, M., & Bess, C. (2003). Beginning students' definitions of nursing: An inductive framework of professional identity. *Journal of Nursing Education, 42*(7), 311–317.

Decker, S. (2007). Integrating guided reflection into simulated learning. In P. Jeffries (Ed.), *Simulation in nursing education* (pp. 73–85). New York, NY: National League for Nursing.

Dickenson-Hazard, N. (2002). Evidence-based practice: "The right approach." *Reflections in Nursing Leadership, 28*(2), 6.

Diers, D. (2001). What is nursing? In J. Dochterman & H. Grace (Eds.), *Current issues in nursing* (pp. 5–13). St. Louis, MO: Mosby.

Finkelman, A. (2001, December). Problem-solving, decision-making, and critical thinking: How do they mix and why bother? *Home Care Provider*, 194–199.

Finkelman, A. (2012). *Leadership and management for nurses: Core competencies for quality care* (2nd ed.). Upper Saddle River, NJ: Pearson Education.

Finkelman, A., & Kenner, C. (2012). *Teaching IOM: Implications of the Institute of Medicine reports for nursing education* (3rd ed.). Silver Spring, MD: American Nurses Association.

Hansten, R., & Washburn, M. (2000). Intuition in professional practice: Executive and staff perceptions. *Journal of Nursing Administration, 30*, 185–189.

Henderson, V. (1991). *The nature of nursing: Reflections after 25 years.* Geneva, Switzerland: International Council of Nurses.

Institute of Medicine (IOM). (2003). *Health professions education: A bridge to quality.* Washington, DC: National Academies Press.

Institute of Medicine (IOM). (2010). *The future of nursing: Leading change, advancing health.* Washington, DC: National Academies Press.

Johns, C. (2004). *Becoming a reflective practitioner* (2nd ed.). Malden, MA: Blackwell.

Kerfoot, K. (2002). The leader as chief knowledge officer. *Nursing Economics, 20*(1), 40–41, 43.

Kozier, B., Erb, G., & Blais, K. (1997). *Professional nursing practice: Concepts and perspectives.* Menlo Park, CA: Addison Wesley Longman.

Kramer, M. (1985). Why does reality shock continue? In J. McCloskey & H. Grace (Eds.), *Current issues in nursing* (pp. 891–903). Boston, MA: Blackwell Scientific.

Locsin, R. (2005). *Technological competency as caring in nursing: A model for practice.* Indianapolis, IN: Sigma Theta Tau International.

Maas, M. (2006). What is nursing, and why do we ask? In P. Cowen & S. Moorhead (Eds.), *Current issues in nursing* (7th ed., pp. 5–10). St. Louis, MO: Mosby.

Mason, D. (2006). Scholarly? AJN is redefining a crusty old term. *American Journal of Nursing, 106*(1), 11.

Meleis, A. (1992). Directions for nursing theory development in the 21st century. *Nursing Science Quarterly, 5*, 112–117.

Moland, L. (2006). Moral integrity and regret in nursing. In S. Nelson & S. Gordon (Eds.), *The complexities of care: Nursing reconsidered* (pp. 50–68). Ithaca, NY: Cornell University Press.

Mooney, K. (2001). Advocating for quality cancer care: Making evidence-based practice a reality. *Oncology Nursing Forum, 28*(suppl 2), 17–21.

Mustard, L. (2002). Caring and competency. *JONA's Healthcare Law, Ethics, and Regulation, 4*(2), 36–43.

Nelson, S., & Gordon, S. (Eds.). (2006). *The complexities of care: Nursing reconsidered.* Ithaca, NY: Cornell University Press.

North American Nursing Diagnosis Association (NANDA). (2011). Nursing diagnoses: Definitions and classification. Retrieved from http://www.nanda.org/DiagnosisDevelopment/DiagnosisSubmission/PreparingYourSubmission/GlossaryofTerms.aspx

Oermann, M., & Jenerette, C. (2013). Scientific nursing journals over 25 years: Most studies continue to focus on adults and psychological variables, with a decline in theory-testing–based studies and an increase in qualitative studies. *Evidence-Based Nursing, 16*(4), 117–118.

Paul, R. (1995). *Critical thinking: How to prepare students for a rapidly changing world.* Santa Rosa, CA: Midwest.

Pesut, D., & Herman, J. (1999). *Clinical reasoning: The art and science of critical and creative thinking.* Albany, NY: Delmar.

Polit, D., & Beck, C. (2013). *Essentials of nursing research.* Philadelphia, PA: Lippincott Williams & Wilkins.

Porter-O'Grady, T., & Malloch, K. (2007). *Quantum leadership: A resource for health care innovation* (2nd ed.). Sudbury, MA: Jones and Bartlett.

Reed, P. (2006). The practitioner in nursing epistemology. *Nursing Science Quality, 19*(1), 36–38.

Rhodes, M., Morris, A., & Lazenby, R. (2011, May). Nursing at its best: Competent and caring. *OJIN, 16.* Retrieved from http://www.nursingworld.org/MainMenuCategories/ANAMarketplace/ANAPeriodicals/OJIN/TableofContents/Vol-16-2011/No2-May-2011/Articles-Previous-Topics/Nursing-at-its-Best.html

Rubenfeld, M., & Scheffer, B. (2009). *Critical thinking tactics for nurses* (2nd ed.). Sudbury, MA: Jones and Bartlett.

Schwein, J. (2004). The timeless caring connection. *Nursing Administration Quarterly, 28*(4), 265–270.

Scotto, C. (2003). A new view of caring. *Journal of Nursing Education, 42*, 289–291.

Sullivan, A. (2006). Nursing theory. In J. Zerwekh & J. Claborn (Eds.), *Nursing Today* (pp. 159–178). St. Louis, MO: Elsevier.

Sorrells-Jones, J. & Weaver, D. (1999). Knowledge workers and knowledge-intense organizations, Part 1: A promising framework for nursing and health care. *JONA, 29*(7/8), 12–18.

University of Iowa, College of Nursing. (2011). Center for Nursing Classification and Clinical Effectiveness. Retrieved from http://www.nursing.uiowa.edu/excellence/nursing_knowledge/clinical_effectiveness/index.htm

Watson, J. (1979). *Nursing: The philosophy and science of caring.* Boston, MA: Little, Brown.

Westberg, J., & Jason, H. (2001). *Fostering reflection and providing feedback.* New York, NY: Springer.

Zerwekh, J., & Claborn, J. (2006). *Nursing today: Transition and trends.* St. Louis, MO: Saunders.

Zimmerman, B., & Phillips, C. (2000). Affective learning: Stimulus to critical thinking and caring practice. *Journal of Nursing Education, 39*(9), 422–423.

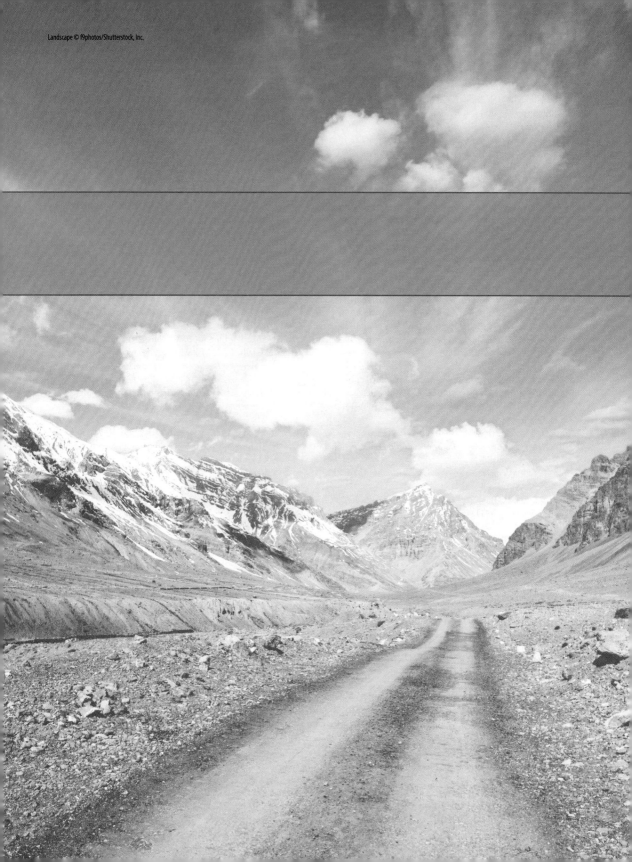

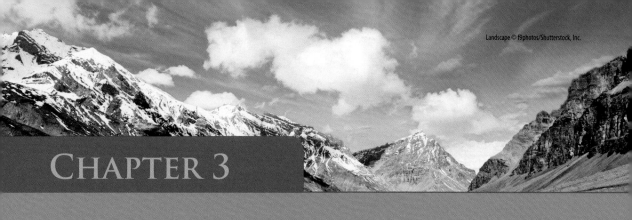

CHAPTER 3

Nursing Education, Accreditation, and Regulation

CHAPTER OBJECTIVES

At the conclusion of this chapter, the learner will be able to:

- Discuss the differences between nursing education and other types of education
- Compare the types of nursing programs and degrees
- Examine the roles of major nursing organizations that affect nursing education
- Describe the nursing education accreditation process and explain its importance marked in previous pass

- Explain requirements and issues related to quality nursing education
- Discuss the faculty shortage problem and the need for more sites for student clinical experiences
- Discuss the importance of regulation and the regulatory process, and identify critical issues related to them

KEY TERMS

Accreditation
Advanced practice nurse
Apprenticeship
Articulation
Associate degree in nursing
Baccalaureate degree in nursing

Continuing education
Curriculum
Diploma schools of nursing
Distance education
Master's degree in nursing
Nurse practice act

Practicum
Preceptor
Prescriptive authority
Regulation
Self-directed learning
Standard
Training

INTRODUCTION

This chapter focuses on three critical concerns in the nursing profession: (1) nursing education, (2) accreditation of nursing programs, and (3) regulatory issues such as licensure. These concerns are interrelated because they change and require input from the nursing profession. Even after graduation, nurses should be aware of educational issues, such as appropriate and reasonable accreditation of nursing programs and ensuring that regulatory issues support the critical needs of the public for quality health care and the needs of the profession. The Tri-Council for Nursing—an alliance of four nursing organizations (American Association of Colleges of Nursing [AACN], American Nurses Association [ANA], American Organization

of Nurse Executives [AONE], and National League for Nursing [NLN])—issued a consensus policy statement in 2010 following Congress's passage of healthcare reform legislation. In part, this policy statement reads as follows:

> Current healthcare reform initiatives call for a nursing workforce that integrates evidence-based clinical knowledge and research with effective communication and leadership skills. These competencies require increased education at all levels. At this tipping point for the nursing profession, action is needed now to put in place strategies to build a stronger nursing workforce. Without a more educated nursing workforce, the nation's health will be further at risk. (Tri-Council for Nursing, 2010, p. 1)

This statement is in line with the Institute of Medicine (IOM) recommendations for healthcare professions education. **Figure 3-1** highlights the components of the education-to-practice process.

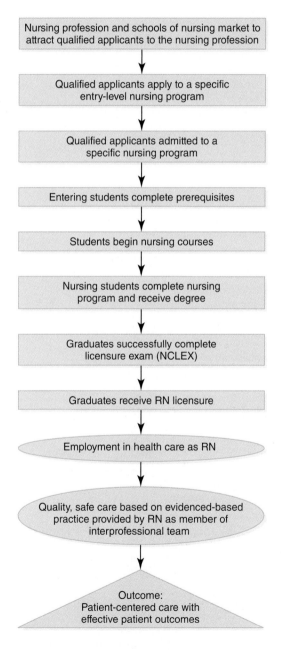

Nursing profession and schools of nursing market to attract qualified applicants to the nursing profession

Qualified applicants apply to a specific entry-level nursing program

Qualified applicants admitted to a specific nursing program

Entering students complete prerequisites

Students begin nursing courses

Nursing students complete nursing program and receive degree

Graduates successfully complete licensure exam (NCLEX)

Graduates receive RN licensure

Employment in health care as RN

Quality, safe care based on evidenced-based practice provided by RN as member of interprofessional team

Outcome: Patient-centered care with effective patient outcomes

Figure 3-1 From Education to Practice

NURSING EDUCATION

A nursing student might wonder why a nursing text has a chapter that includes content about nursing education. By the time students are reading this text, they will have selected a nursing program and enrolled. This content is not included here to help someone decide whether to enter the profession, or which nursing program to attend. Rather, it is essential because education is a critical component of the nursing profession. Nurses need to understand the structure and process of the profession's education, quality issues, and current issues and trends. **Exhibit 3-1** provides an extensive glossary of nursing education terms.

Data from 2013 indicate that nursing students represent more than half of all healthcare professionals (AACN, 2014). The number of students enrolling in entry-level baccalaureate programs increased by 2.6% from 2012 to 2013. Although there was growth over this one-year period, it represented the lowest increase in enrollment in the past five years. Enrollment in baccalaureate nursing programs reached 259,100 in 2013, an increase from 238,799 in 2010. Over the same period, AACN reports, there were enrollment increases of 4.4% in master's programs and 8.3% in other graduate nursing programs. Doctor of nursing practice (DNP) programs experienced a 21.6% enrollment increase, and the number of students in research-focused doctorate programs grew by 1.7%.

A key concern for nurse educators is not only the need to increase enrollment and completion rates, but also the need to reduce the number of qualified applicants who are not able to enroll because nursing programs do not have places for them, typically due to faculty shortages, lack of clinical placement sites, and/or limited funding. For 2013, preliminary data indicate that 53,667 qualified applicants could not enroll in 610 entry-level baccalaureate programs (AACN, 2014). The percentage of minorities enrolling

Exhibit 3-1   Definition of Nursing Education Terms

Nonbaccalaureate Programs

Licensed practical nursing (LPN or LVN) program: A program that requires at least 1 year of full-time equivalent coursework and awards the graduate a diploma or certificate of completion as an LPN/LVN.

LPN (LVN) to associate degree in nursing program: A program that admits licensed practical nurses and awards an associate degree in nursing at completion.

Diploma nursing program: Offers the required curriculum for a registered nurse but does not offer an associate or baccalaureate degree; take same registered nurse licensure exam as associate degree or baccalaureate degree graduate. Many of these programs have closed, and those that remain open now often partner with community colleges and in some cases universities to offer academic degrees.

Associate degree in nursing: A program that requires at least 2 academic years of college academic credit and awards an associate degree (ADN) in nursing. Graduates take the same registered nurse licensure exam as baccalaureate graduates.

Baccalaureate Programs

Generic (basic or entry-level) baccalaureate program: Admits students with no previous nursing education and awards a baccalaureate nursing (BS or BSN) degree. Program requires at least 4 but not more than 5 academic years of college academic credit.

Accelerated baccalaureate/direct entry for non-nursing college graduates program: Admits students with baccalaureate degrees or higher in other disciplines and no previous nursing education and awards a baccalaureate nursing degree. The curriculum is designed for completion in less time than the generic baccalaureate program, usually through a combination of bridge or transition courses.

LPN/LVN to baccalaureate in nursing program: Admits licensed practical nurses and awards a baccalaureate nursing degree.

RN to baccalaureate in nursing (RN baccalaureate; RN completion) program: Admits RNs with associate degrees or diplomas in nursing and awards a baccalaureate nursing degree.

Master's Programs

Master of science (MS/MSN) in nursing program: Admits students with baccalaureate nursing degrees and awards a master of science in nursing degree. This degree typically focuses on advanced practice in a specialty area—for example, acute care adult nurse practitioner, primary care pediatrics nurse practitioner—but it can also include specializations such as nursing anesthesia (CRNA), nurse–midwifery (CNM), nursing administration, and nursing education.

Accelerated baccalaureate to master's program: Admits students with baccalaureate nursing degrees and awards a master's in nursing degree. The curriculum is designed for completion in less time than a traditional master's program, usually through a combination of bridge or transition courses and core courses.

Master of arts in nursing program: Admits students with baccalaureate nursing degrees and awards a master of arts degree in nursing.

Master of science with a major in nursing program: Admits students with baccalaureate nursing degrees and awards a master of science degree with a major in nursing.

LPN/LVN to master's degree program: Admits RNs without baccalaureate degrees in nursing and awards a master's degree in nursing. Graduates meet requirements for a baccalaureate nursing degree as well.

Exhibit 3-1 (continued)

RN to master's degree program: Admits RNs without baccalaureate degrees in nursing and awards a master's degree in nursing. Students may or may not receive a BSN degree, although they complete the coursework related to BSN.

Master's degree for non-nursing college graduates (accelerated or direct entry/entry-level/second-degree master's) program: Admits students with baccalaureate degrees in other disciplines and no previous nursing education. The program prepares graduates for entry into the profession and awards a master's degree in nursing. Although these programs generally require a baccalaureate degree, a few programs admit students without baccalaureate degrees. Students must complete baccalaureate nursing degree requirements in addition to master's requirements.

Dual-degree master's programs: Admits RNs with baccalaureate degrees in nursing and awards a master's degree in another field (e.g., master of business administration, master of public health degree, master of public administration degree, master of hospital administration degree, master of divinity degree, or Juris Doctor); graduates may also receive a master's degree in nursing.

Doctoral Programs

Doctor of nursing practice (DNP): Admits nurses who want to pursue a doctoral degree that focuses on practice rather than research. This practice-focused doctoral program prepares graduates for the highest level of nursing practice beyond the initial preparation in the discipline and is a terminal degree. This degree program may admit students with a master's degree or, in some cases, with a BSN. For example, CRNA programs are transitioning from master's programs to BSN-DNP programs.

Doctoral (research-focused) program: Admits RNs with a master's degree in nursing and awards a doctoral degree. This program prepares students to pursue intellectual inquiry and conduct independent research for the purpose of extending knowledge. In the academic community, the PhD (doctor of philosophy degree) is the most commonly offered research-focused doctoral degree. However, some schools, for a variety of reasons, may award a doctor of nursing science (DNS or DNSc) degree as the research-focused doctoral degree, although most of these programs have closed. Some doctoral programs are now admitting students with BSN degrees; these students complete all graduate-level requirements and receive a PhD.

Other Programs

Clinical nurse specialist program: A graduate, master's-level program in which a defined curriculum includes theory, research, and clinical preparation for competency-based specialty practice.

Nurse practitioner program: A graduate, master's-level preparation in which a defined curriculum includes theory, research, and clinical preparation for competency-based primary care or acute care. Graduates are awarded a master's degree in nursing and are eligible to sit for a national nurse practitioner certification examinations offered for a wide variety of specializations.

Clinical nurse leader program: A graduate, master's-level program in which a defined curriculum includes leadership content focused on direct patient care.

Post-master's nurse practitioner certificate program: A formal postgraduate program for the preparation of nurse practitioners that admits registered nurses with master's degrees in nursing. At completion, students are awarded a certificate or other evidence of completion, such as a letter from the program director. These students are eligible to sit for the national NP examinations.

(continues)

Exhibit 3-1 (*continued*)

Nurse practitioner: A registered nurse who, through a graduate degree program in nursing, functions in an independent care provider role and addresses the full range of patient/client health problems and needs within an area of specialization.

Nursing students: Students who have been formally accepted into a nursing program regardless of whether they have taken any nursing courses.

Pre-nursing students: Students who have not yet been formally accepted into an entry-level nursing program.

Source: American Association of Colleges of Nursing. (2007). *2006–2007 enrollment and graduations in baccalaureate and graduate programs in nursing.* Washington, DC: Author.

---

in such programs has increased (2013). Nursing students from minority backgrounds represented 28.3% of students in entry-level baccalaureate programs, 29.3% of master's students, and 27.7% of students in research-focused doctoral programs.

The lack of clinical placement settings continues to be a major problem (NLN, 2013a).

This snapshot of data indicates that there has been improvement in the number of applicants to the various nursing degree programs and in enrollment rates, but much work remains to reach the desired levels so as to meet the needs of the healthcare delivery system for qualified nurses. **Figure 3-2** illustrates the current distribution of RNs in the United States according to initial nursing degree.

Given the critical issues of a changing nursing shortage and the consequent need to attract more students to nursing programs, this section focuses on nursing education to facilitate a better understanding of current and future concerns. The nursing shortage has been a recurring issue throughout the modern history of nursing.

A Brief History of Nursing Education

It is impossible to discuss the history of nursing education without reflecting on the history of the

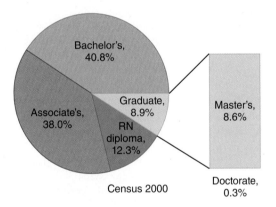

Census 2000

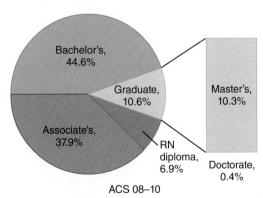

ACS 08–10

Figure 3-2 Highest Degree Held by RNs, Census 2000 and ACS 2008 to 2010

Source: Reproduced from Health Resources Services Administration, Bureau of Health Professions, National Center for Health Workforce Analysis. (April, 2013). *The U.S. Nursing Workforce: Trends in Supply and Education.* Retrieved from http://bhpr.hrsa.gov/healthworkforce/reports/nursingworkforce/nursingworkforcefullreport.pdf

profession and the history of health care. All three are interconnected.

A key historical nursing leader was Florence Nightingale. She changed not only the practice of nursing but also nursing **training**, which eventually came to be called education rather than training. Training focuses on fixed habits and skills; uses repetition, authority, and coercion; and emphasizes dependency (Donahue, 1983). Education focuses more on self-discipline, responsibility, accountability, and self-mastery (Donahue, 1983). Up until the time that Nightingale became involved in nursing, there was little, if any, training for the role. **Apprenticeship** was used to introduce new recruits to nursing, and often it was not done effectively. As nursing changed, so did the need for more information and skills, leading to increasingly structured educational experiences. This did not occur without debate and disagreement regarding the best approach. What did happen, and how does it impact nursing education today?

In 1860, Nightingale established the first school of nursing, St. Thomas, in London, England. She was able to do this because she had received a very good education in the areas of math and science, which was highly unusual for women of her era. With her experience in the Crimean War, Nightingale recognized that many soldiers were dying not just because of their wounds but also because of infection and failure to place them in the best light for healing. In turn, she devoted her energies to upgrading nursing education; she placed less focus on on-the-job training and more focus on a structured educational program of study, creating the training school. This training school and those that quickly followed also became a source of cheap labor for hospitals. Students were provided with some formal nursing education, but they also worked long hours in the hospitals and were the largest staff source. The apprenticeship model, as it was called, continued, but it became more structured and included a more formal educational component. This educational component was far from ideal, but over time, it

expanded and improved. During the same era, similar programs opened in the United States. These programs were called diploma schools, and some of the first schools in the United States were Johns Hopkins (Baltimore, Maryland), the New England Hospital for Women and Children (Boston, Massachusetts), Women's Hospital (Philadelphia, Pennsylvania), and Bellevue Hospital (New York City). During this period, Canada also developed similar programs.

Hospitals across the United States began to open schools as they realized that students could be used as staff in the hospitals. The quality of these schools varied widely because there were no standards aside from what the individual hospital wanted to do. A few schools recognized early on the need for more content and improved teaching; some of these schools were creative and formed partnerships with universities so that students could receive some content through an academic institution. Despite these small efforts to improve, the schools continued to be very different, and there were concerns about the quality of nursing education.

Major Nursing Reports: Improving Nursing Education

In 1918, an important step was taken through an initiative supported by the Rockefeller Foundation to address the issue of the diploma schools. This initiative culminated in the *Goldmark Report*, the first of several major reports about U.S. nursing education. This report included the following key points (Goldmark, 1923):

- Hospitals controlled the total education hours, offering minimal content and, in some cases, no content even when that content was needed.
- Science, theory, and practice of nursing were often taught by inexperienced instructors with few teaching resources.
- Students were supervised by graduate nurses who had limited experience and time to assist the students in their learning.

- Classroom experiences frequently occurred after the students had worked long hours, even during the night.
- Students typically were able to only get the experiences that their hospital provided, with all clinical practice being located in one hospital. As a consequence, students might not get experiences in specialties such as obstetrics, pediatrics, and psychiatric–mental health.

The *Goldmark Report* had an impact, particularly through its key recommendations: (1) separating university schools of nursing from hospitals (this represented only a minority of the schools of nursing); (2) changing the control of hospital-based programs to schools of nursing; and (3) requiring a high school diploma for entry into any school of nursing. These recommendations represented major improvements in nursing education.

Changes were made, but slowly. The National League for Nursing started developing and implementing standards for schools, but it took more than 20 years to accomplish this mission. New schools opened based on the Goldmark recommendations, such as Yale University (New Haven, Connecticut) and Case Western Reserve University (Cleveland, Ohio).

A second report that had a major impact on improving nursing education was the *Brown Report* (Brown, 1948), which also focused on the quality and structure of nursing education. This report led to the establishment of a formalized process, to be conducted by the NLN, to accredit nursing schools. Accreditation is discussed in more detail later in this chapter. It represented a critical step toward improving schools of nursing and the practice of nursing because it established standards across schools.

The third report on the assessment of nursing education was published in 2010, *Educating Nurses: A Call for Radical Transformation* (Benner, Sutphen, Leonard, & Day, 2010). This report addressed the need to better prepare nurses to practice in a rapidly changing healthcare system in order to

ensure quality care. The conclusion of this qualitative study of nursing education was that there is need for great improvement. Students should be engaged in the learning process. There needs to be more connection between classroom experience and clinical experience, with a greater emphasis on practice throughout the nursing curriculum. Students need to be better prepared to use clinical reasoning and judgment and to understand the trajectory of illness. To meet the recommendations of this landmark report, nursing education must make major changes and improvements. **Exhibit 3-2** describes the report's recommendations.

The most recent report released by the Institute of Medicine (IOM), *The Future of Nursing: Leading Change, Advancing Health* (2010), delineated several key messages for nurses and nursing education. Nurses should practice to the fullest extent possible based on their level of education. There should be mechanisms for nurses to advance their education easily, to act as full partners in healthcare delivery, and to be involved in policy making especially as it relates to the healthcare workforce. This report, along with the Carnegie report by Benner and colleagues (2010), is transforming nursing's role in health care and calling for radical changes in nursing education.

Entry into Practice: A Debate

The challenges in making changes in the entry into practice debate were great when one considers that a very large number of hospitals in communities across the country had diploma schools based on the old model, and these schools were part of, and funded by, their communities. It was not easy to change these schools or to close them without major nursing and community debate and conflict. These schools constituted the major type of nursing education in the United States through the 1960s, and some schools still exist today. The number of diploma schools has decreased primarily because of the critical debate over what type of education

Exhibit 3-2   Recommendations from *Educating Nurses: A Call for Radical Transformation*

Entry and Pathways

- Come to agreement about a set of clinically relevant prerequisites.
- Require the BSN for entry to practice.
- Develop local **articulation** programs to ensure a smooth, timely transition from ADN to BSN programs.
- Develop more ADN-to-MSN programs.

Student Population

- Recruit a more diverse faculty and student body.
- Provide more financial aid, whether from public or private sources, for all students, at all levels.

The Student Experience

- Introduce pre-nursing students to nursing early in their education.
- Broaden the clinical experience.
- Preserve post-clinical conferences and small patient-care assignments.
- Develop pedagogies that keep students focused on the patient's experience.
- Vary the means of assessing student performance.
- Promote and support learning the skills of inquiry and research.
- Redesign the ethics curricula.
- Support students in becoming agents of change.

Teaching

- Fully support ongoing faculty development for all who educate student nurses.
- Include teacher education courses in master's and doctoral programs.
- Foster opportunities for educators to learn how to teach students to reflect on their practice.
- Support faculty in learning how to coach students.
- Support educators in learning how to use narrative pedagogies.
- Provide faculty with resources to stay clinically current.
- Improve the work environment for staff nurses, and support them in learning to teach.
- Address the faculty shortage.

Entry to Practice

- Develop clinical residencies for all graduates.
- Change the requirements for licensure.

National Oversight

- Require performance assessments for licensure.
- Cooperate on accreditation.

Source: Summary of Recommendations from Benner, P., Sutphen, M., Leonard, V., & Day, L. (2010). *Educating nurses: A call for radical transformation.* San Francisco, CA: Jossey-Bass. Reprinted with permission of John Wiley & Sons, Inc.

nurses need for entry into practice. The drive to move nursing education into college and university settings was great, but there was also great support to continue with the diploma schools of nursing.

In 1965, the National League for Nursing and the American Nurses Association came out with strong statements endorsing college-based nursing education as the entry point into the profession. The ANA (1965) stated that "minimum preparation for beginning technical (bedside) nursing practice at the present time should be associate degree education in nursing" (p. 107). The situation was very tense. The two largest nursing organizations at the time—one primarily focused on education (NLN) and the other more on practice (ANA)—clearly took a stand. From the 1960s through the 1980s, these organizations tried to alter accreditation, advocated for the closing of diploma programs, and lobbied all levels of government (Leighow, 1996). This was a very emotional issue, and even today it continues to be a tense topic because it has not been fully resolved, although stronger statements were made in 2010–2011 to change to a baccalaureate entry level (Benner et al., 2010; IOM, 2010).

Since 1965, many changes have been made in the educational preparation of nurses:

- The number of diploma schools gradually decreased, but they still exist.
- The number of associate degree in nursing (ADN) programs grew. However, there was, and continues to be, concern over the potential development of a two-level nursing system—ADN and bachelor of science in nursing (BSN)—with one viewed as technical and the other as professional. However, this really has not happened. In fact, ADN programs continue to increase, and there has been no change in licensure for any of the nursing programs. All graduates of diploma programs, associate degree programs, and baccalaureate programs continue to take the same exam that made nursing the first health-care profession to have a single national exam.

- BSN programs continued to grow but still have not outpaced ADN programs.

The two major current reports on nursing, *Nursing Education* (Benner et al., 2010) and *The Future of Nursing* (IOM, 2010) both recommend that entry to practice require the BSN. The IOM report recommended that the proportion of practicing nurses with BSN increase by 80% by 2020—a call that has led to an increase in the number of RN-BSN programs and increased enrollment in these programs, many of which are offered online.

In addition, because of the movement of many nursing schools into the university setting, nursing programs lost their strong connection with hospitals. Rather than establish different educational models with hospitals, the nursing education community sought to get away from the control of hospitals and move to an academic setting; however, now nursing educators and students are visitors in hospitals with little feeling of partnership and connection. This has had an impact on clinical experiences, in some cases limiting effective clinical learning.

Differentiated Nursing Practice

Another issue related to entry into practice is differentiated nursing practice. According to Rick (2003), "[L]eaders have yet to fully step up to the plate to determine and articulate what is really needed for nursing in the full spectrum of practice environments. Practice settings should offer differentiated nursing roles with distinct and complementary responsibilities" (p. 11). Differentiated practice is not a new idea; it has been discussed in the literature since the 1990s. Differentiated practice is described as a "philosophy that structures the roles and functions of nurses according to their education, experience, and competence," or "matching the varying needs of clients with the varying abilities of nursing practitioners" (American Organization of Nurse Executives, 1990, as cited in Hutchins, 1994, p. 52). This is clearly not a new issue, but it is an issue that is still not resolved.

How does this actually work in practice? Does a clinical setting distinguish between RNs who have a diploma and those who have a BSN degree? Does this impact role function and responsibilities? Does the organization even acknowledge degrees on name badges? Most healthcare organizations do note differences when it comes to RNs with graduate degrees, but many do not necessarily note degrees for other nurses. This approach does not recognize that there are differences in the educational programs that award each degree or diploma. The ongoing debate remains difficult to resolve because all RNs, regardless of the type and length of their basic nursing education program, take the same licensing exam. Patients and other healthcare providers rarely understand the differences or even know that differences exist.

In 1995, a joint report was published by the AACN in collaboration with the American Organization of Nurse Executives and the National Organization (AONE) and the National Organization for Associate Degree Nursing (N-OADN). This document described the two roles of the BSN and the ADN graduate (p. 28):

- The BSN graduate is a licensed RN who provides direct care that is based on the nursing process and focused on patients/clients with complex interactions of nursing diagnoses. Patients/clients include individuals, families, groups, aggregates, and communities in structured and unstructured healthcare settings. The unstructured setting is a geographical or a situational environment that may not have established policies, procedures, and protocols and has the potential for variations requiring independent nursing decisions.
- The ADN graduate is a licensed RN who provides direct care that is based on the nursing process and focused on individual patients/clients who have common, well-defined nursing diagnoses. Consideration is given to the patient's/client's relationship within the family. The ADN functions in a structured healthcare setting, which is a geographical

or situational environment where the policies, procedures, and protocols for provision of health care are established. In the structured setting, there is recourse to assistance and support from the full scope of nursing expertise.

Despite increased support, such as from AONE, for making the BSN the entry-level educational requirement, this question continues to be one of the most frustrating issues in the profession and has not been clearly resolved (AACN, 2005a). The AACN believes that:

> education has a direct impact on the skills and competencies of a nurse clinician. Nurses with a baccalaureate degree are well-prepared to meet the demand placed on today's nurse across a variety of settings and are prized for their critical thinking, leadership, case management, and health promotion skills. (AACN, 2005a, p. 1)

Since 2001, there has been an increase in the number of students enrolling in entry-level BSN programs, and the number of RNs returning to school for their BSN also continues to increase. The result has been nine years of steady growth in the number of RNs with baccalaureate degrees (ANA, 2011). A study by Aiken, Clarke, Cheung, Sloane, and Silber (2003) indicates that there is a "substantial survival advantage" for patients in hospitals with a higher percentage of BSN RNs. Other studies (Estabrooks, Midodzi, Cummings, Ricker, & Giovannetti, 2005) support these outcomes. McHugh and Lake (2010) examined how nurses rate their level of expertise as a beginner, competent, proficient, advanced, and expert and how often they were selected as a preceptor or consulted by other nurses for their clinical judgment. The survey, which was actually done in 1999, included 8611 nurses. More highly educated nurses rated themselves as having more expertise than less educated nurses, and this correlated with how frequently they were asked to be preceptors or consulted by other nurses. The long-term impact of these types of studies on the entry into practice is unknown, but there is more evidence now to support the decision made in 1965 along with recommendations from major reports (Benner et al., 2010; IOM, 2010).

Aiken and colleagues published a study in 2014 addressing nurse staffing and hospital mortality in nine European countries. This study received major recognition by healthcare organizations and through the media. The sample included discharge data for 422,730 patients aged 50 years or older who had common surgeries in the nine countries. The survey included 26,516 nurses in the study hospitals. The findings indicate that increasing a nurse's workload by one patient increased the likelihood of an inpatient dying within 30 days of admission by 7%; in contrast, every 10% increase in the number of nurses with bachelor's degrees was associated with a 7% decrease in the likelihood of an inpatient dying within 30 days of admission. These associations imply that patients receiving care in hospitals in which 60% of nurses had bachelor's degrees and nurses cared for an average of six patients would have almost 30% lower mortality than patients in hospitals in which only 30% of nurses had bachelor's degrees and nurses cared for an average of eight patients. Thus there is value in using BSN-prepared nurses in these hospitals, whereas reducing nursing staff may have a negative impact on patient outcomes.

In the last few years, some hospitals have implemented initiatives to hire only RNs with BSN degrees and to encourage staff members without a BSN degree to return to school. This decision by hospitals is highly dependent on the availability of RNs with the BSN degree.

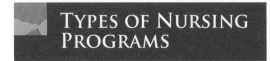

TYPES OF NURSING PROGRAMS

Nursing is a profession with a complex education pattern: It has many different entry-level pathways to licensure and many different graduate programs.

The following content provides descriptions of the major nursing education programs. Because several types of entry-level nursing programs exist, this complicates the issue and raises concerns about the best way to provide education for nursing students.

Diploma Schools of Nursing

Diploma schools of nursing still exist, though many now have partnerships with colleges or universities where students might take some of their courses. Many of these schools have closed, some have been converted into associate degree programs and even to baccalaureate programs, and some have partnered with BSN programs. However, there has been a slight increase in these programs because employers feel that their need for staff nurses is so great and degree programs are not meeting these needs. The Association of Diploma Schools of Professional Nursing represents these schools. Diploma schools are accredited by the NLN. Graduates take the same licensing exam as graduates from all the other types of nursing programs. The nursing curriculum is similar; the graduates need the same nursing content for the licensing exam. However, the students typically have fewer prerequisites, particularly in the liberal arts and sciences, though they do have some science content. There is variation in these schools because students may take some of their required courses in local colleges.

Associate Degree in Nursing

Programs awarding an **associate degree in nursing** (AD/ADN) began when Mildred Montag published a book on the need for a different type of nursing program—a 2-year program that would be established in community colleges (Montag, 1959). At the time that Montag created her proposal, the United States was experiencing a shortage of nurses after World War II. For students, ADN programs are less expensive and shorter. The programs are accredited by the NLN. The curriculum includes some liberal arts and sciences at the community college level and focuses more on technical nursing. Graduates take the same licensing exam as graduates from all other prelicensure nursing programs.

Recently, a variety of models and opportunities for ADN students and graduates have been introduced. Montag envisioned the ADN as a terminal degree; this perception has since changed, with the degree now being viewed more as part of a career mobility path. The RN-BSN or BSN completion programs that are found throughout the United States are a way for ADN graduates to complete the requirements for a BSN. Typically, these graduates work and then go back to school, often on a part-time basis, to complete a BSN in a university-level program. Typically, some prerequisite courses must be taken before these students enter most BSN programs. Additional nursing courses that these students may take are health assessment, public/community health with clinical practice, leadership and management, research/evidence-based practice, and health policy. Until recently, these students rarely took additional clinical courses, as this is not the major focus of the RN-BSN programs; now, however, all programs accredited by AACN must include clinical experiences or a **practicum**. The content typically included for the clinical experience is public/community health, focusing on what these students did not cover in their ADN program. Today, many of the RN-BSN programs are offered online, and greater efforts are made to facilitate the transition from the ADN program to the BSN program. The overall goal is to guide all ADN graduates back to school for a BSN, though this has not yet been accomplished. These graduates do not have to take the licensure exam because they are already RNs, but they are expected to be licensed to participate in a RN-BSN program.

Another change that has been taking place is the development of partnerships with ADN and BSN programs. In these partnerships, the ADN program has a clear relationship with a BSN program. This allows for a seamless transition from one program to the other. Students spend their first 2 years in the ADN program and then complete the last 2 years of the BSN degree in the partner program. In these types of programs, both the participating ADN and BSN programs collaborate on the curriculum and determine how to best transition the students. One benefit of this model is that students pay the community college fees, which are less costly than the university fees, for the first 2 years. If there is no BSN program in a community, students can stay within their own community for the first 2 years before transitioning to a more distant BSN program.

Baccalaureate Degree in Nursing

The idea for the **baccalaureate degree in nursing** was introduced in the *Goldmark Report* (Goldmark, 1923), although it took many years for this recommendation to have an impact on nursing education. The original programs took 5 years to complete, with the first 2 years being spent in liberal arts and sciences courses, followed by 3 years in nursing courses. The programs then began to change to a 4-year model, with variations of 2 years in liberal arts and sciences and then 2 years in nursing courses, though some 5-year programs still exist. Some schools introduce students to nursing content during the first 2 years, but typically the amount of nursing content is limited during this period. In many colleges of nursing, students are not admitted to the college/school of nursing until they complete the first 2 years, although the students are in the same university. These programs may be accredited by the NLN or through the AACN, both of which have accrediting services. (More information about accreditation appears later in the chapter.) BSN graduates take the same licensure exam as all other prelicensure nursing program graduates.

In the 1960s, BSN programs and enrollment grew rapidly. As discussed, the question of the educational level for entry into the profession continues to be unresolved, although since 1965, major nursing organizations have clearly stated that it is the BSN. The RN-BSN programs have grown in the last few years. A BSN is required for admission to a nursing graduate program. "Articulation agreements are important mechanisms that enhance access to baccalaureate level nursing education. These agreements support education mobility and facilitate the seamless transfer of academic credit between associate degree (ADN) and baccalaureate (BSN) nursing programs" (AACN, 2005c, p. 1). State law may mandate these agreements, which may be between individual schools, or they may be part of statewide articulation plans to facilitate more efficient transfer of credits. This helps students who want to take some courses in an ADN program or who have an ADN degree to enter BSN programs. However, as described earlier, there are several routes for students with degrees (undergraduate and graduate) in other areas to enter nursing programs.

Master's Degree in Nursing

Graduate education and the evolution of the **master's degree in nursing** have a long history. Early on, it was called postgraduate education, and the typical focus areas were public health, teaching, supervision, and some clinical specialties. The first formal graduate program was established in 1899 at Columbia University Teachers College (Donahue, 1983). The NLN supported the establishment of graduate nursing programs, and these programs were developed in great numbers. For example, some of the early programs, such as Yale School of Nursing, admitted students without a BSN who had a baccalaureate degree in another major. Today, this is very similar to the accelerated programs or direct entry programs in which students with other degrees are admitted to a BSN program that is shorter, covering the same content but with an accelerated approach. These students are typically categorized as graduate students because of their previous degree. Even so, they must complete prelicensure BSN requirements before they can take nursing graduate courses, and

in some cases, they are not admitted to the nursing graduate program automatically.

The master's programs in nursing have evolved since the 1950s. The typical length for a master's program is 2 years, and students may attend full time or part time. These programs are accredited by the NLN or AACN and, in some cases, by nursing specialty organizations, as discussed in this chapter. The following are examples of master's degree programs:

- Advanced practice nursing (APRN): This master's degree can be offered in any clinical area, but typical areas are adult health, pediatrics, family health, women's health, neonatal health, and psychiatric–mental health. Graduates take APRN certification exams in their specialty area and must then meet specific state requirements, such as for **prescriptive authority**, which gives them limited ability to prescribe medications. These nurses usually work in independent roles. The American Nurses Credentialing Center (ANCC) provides national certification exams for **advanced practice nurses** in a variety of areas.
- Clinical nurse specialist (CNS): This master's degree can be offered in any clinical area. Specialty exams may also be taken. These nurses usually work in hospital settings. The ANCC provides national certification for CNSs in a variety of areas, as discussed later in this chapter.
- Certified registered nurse anesthetists (CRNA): This master's degree is not offered at all colleges of nursing. It takes 2 years to complete and focuses on preparing nurses to deliver anesthesia. This is a highly competitive graduate program. The Council on Accreditation of Nurse Anesthesia Educational Program, as part of the American Association of Nurse Anesthetists, focuses on accreditation of these programs and certification. This educational program is now moving to the level of doctor of nursing practice (DNP); all

master's-level programs will be converted to DNP programs or closed by 2025.

- Certified nurse–midwife: This master's degree focuses on midwifery—pregnancy and delivery, as well as gynecologic care of women and family planning. These programs are accredited by the American College of Nurse–Midwives.
- Clinical nurse leader (CNL): This is one of the newer master's degrees, which prepares nurses for leadership positions that have a direct impact on patient care.

The CNL is a provider and a manager of care at the point of care to individuals and cohorts. The CNL designs, implements, and evaluates patient care by coordinating, delegating and supervising the care provided by the healthcare team, including licensed nurses, technicians, and other health professionals. (AACN, 2007, p. 6)

- Master's degree in a functional area: This type of master's degree focuses on the functional areas of administration or education. It was more popular in the past, but with the growing need for nursing faculty, there has been a resurgence of master's programs in nursing education. In some cases, colleges of nursing are offering certificate programs in nursing education. In these programs, a nurse with a nursing master's degree may take a certain number of credits that focus on nursing education and then, if the nurse successfully completes the NLN certification exam, the nurse will be a certified nurse educator. This provides the nurse with additional background and experience in nursing education.

Doctoral Degree in Nursing

The doctoral degree (doctor of philosophy—PhD) in nursing has had a complicated development history. The doctorate of nursing science (DNSc)

was first offered in 1960, but most of these degree programs have since transitioned to PhD programs. There were PhD programs in education in nursing as early as 1924, and New York University started the first PhD program in nursing in 1953. Not enough students are entering these programs, and this has had an impact on nursing faculty. Someone with a PhD is not always required to teach, but is encouraged to do so. Nurses with PhDs usually are involved in research because it is considered a research degree, although a nurse at any level can be involved in research and may or may not teach. Study for a PhD typically takes place after receiving a master's degree in nursing and includes coursework and a research-focused dissertation. This process can take 4 to 5 years to complete, and much depends on completion of the dissertation. Nurses with PhDs may be called "doctor"; this is not the same as the "medical doctor" title, but rather a designation or title indicating completion of doctoral work in the same way that an English professor with a doctorate is called "doctor."

Both types of doctoral programs are now offered as BSN-PhD or BSN-DNP options in some schools of nursing. This means the student does not have to obtain a master's degree prior to entering the program. The goal is to increase the number of nurses with doctoral degrees. In addition, the specialty of nurse anesthesia requires that all nurses pursuing this specialty do so via a BSN-DNP degree by 2015, so many nurse anesthesia master's programs have changed or are in the process of changing to conferring a BSN-DNP degree. The same is true for other specialties that have established the goal of a career pathway through the BSN-DNP by 2025, though nurse anesthesia has moved noticeably more quickly toward this change.

Doctor of Nursing Practice

The DNP is the newest nursing degree. The DNP is not a PhD program, although nurses with a DNP degree are also called "doctor." However, this does not represent the same title as someone with a PhD or a doctor or medicine. The DNP is a practice-focused doctoral degree program. This position has been controversial within nursing and within health care, particularly among physicians. Because this position is new, it is difficult to know what its long-term impact will be on the profession and on health care. The AACN has described the purpose of the DNP as follows:

> Transforming healthcare delivery recognizes the critical need for clinicians to design, evaluate, and continuously improve the context within which care is delivered. The core function of healthcare is to provide the best possible clinical care to individuals, families and communities. The context within which care is delivered exerts a major impact on the kinds of care that are provided and on the satisfaction and productivity of individual clinicians. Nurses prepared at the doctoral level with a blend of clinical, organizational, economic and leadership skills are most likely to be able to critique nursing and other clinical scientific findings and design programs of care delivery that are locally acceptable, economically feasible, and which significantly impact healthcare outcomes. (AACN, 2004, p. 7)

Practice-focused doctoral nursing programs prepare leaders for nursing practice. The long-term goal is to make the DNP the terminal practice degree for APRN preparation, including for CNSs, certified registered nurse anesthetists, certified nurse–midwifes, and nurse practitioners (AACN, 2004). This means that by 2015—a date identified by the AACN—and by 2025—a date identified by the American Association of Nurse Anesthetists—advanced practice registered nurses (APRNs) would not get master's degrees but rather DNP degrees. At this time it does not appear that the 2015 goal will be met, but many programs are in the midst

of a transition toward that goal. Some of the reasons that the DNP degree was developed relate to the process for obtaining an APRN master's degree, which requires a large number of credits and clinical hours. It was recognized that students should be getting more credit for their coursework and effort. Going on to a DNP program allows them to apply some of this credit toward a doctoral-level program. Practice-focused doctoral programs offer a number of benefits (AACN, 2004, pp. 7–8):

- Development of needed advanced competencies for increasingly complex clinical, faculty, and leadership roles
- Enhanced knowledge to improve nursing practice and patient outcomes
- Enhanced leadership skills to strengthen practice and healthcare delivery
- Better match of program requirements and credits and time with the credential earned
- Provision of an advanced educational credential for those who require advanced practice knowledge but do not need or want a strong research focus (e.g., clinical faculty)
- Parity with other health professions, most of which have a doctorate as the credential required for practice
- Enhanced ability to attract individuals to nursing from non-nursing backgrounds
- Increased supply of faculty for clinical instruction
- Improved image of nursing

Because the DNP is a new degree and represents a new nursing role, it is not clear at this time what its long-term impact will be on nursing and on healthcare delivery. Some have questioned the decision to confer such a degree in light of the need for a greater number of APRNs for primary care (Cronenwett, Dracup, Grey, McDauley, Meleis, & Salmon, 2011); others have questioned it because there is need for nurses with PhDs. There is concern that nurses who might have once considered a PhD will instead seek a DNP; indeed, data indicate that there is now greater enrollment in DNP programs, so this prediction has proved correct. As of 2011, there were no professional regulations that required a DNP in place of a master's degree, but this is now changing. For example, the master's in nurse anesthesia is moving to a DNP only. Advanced practice master's will, over time, migrate to DNP degrees. Regulation also will have an impact on final decisions about degree entry.

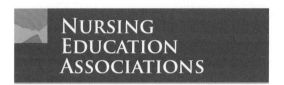

NURSING EDUCATION ASSOCIATIONS

There are three major nursing education organizations, each with a different program focus. These organizations are the NLN, the AACN, and the N-OADN.

National League for Nursing

The NLN is an older organization than the AACN. It "promotes excellence in nursing education to build a strong and diverse nursing workforce" (NLN, 2007a, p. 2). The NLN's goals for 2013 can be summarized as follows (NLN, 2013b):

1. *Leader in nursing education*: Enhance the NLN's national and international impact as the recognized leader in nursing education.
2. *Commitment to members*: Build a diverse, sustainable, member-led organization with the capacity to deliver the NLN's mission effectively, efficiently, and in accordance with its values.
3. *Champion for nurse educators*: Be the voice of nurse educators and champion their interests in political, academic, and professional arenas.
4. *Advancement of the science of nursing education*: Promote evidence-based nursing education and the scholarship of teaching.

The major difference between the AACN and the NLN is that the AACN represents only university-level nursing education programs (baccalaureate

to doctoral degrees). The NLN represents all nursing programs (ADN, BSN, master's) other than doctoral programs. The NLN accredits nursing programs through the Accreditation Commission for Nursing (ACEN); accreditation is discussed in a later section of this chapter. The NLN offers educational opportunities for its members (individual membership and school of nursing membership) and addresses policy and standards issues related to nursing education.

American Association of Colleges of Nursing

The AACN is the national organization that represents university and baccalaureate programs in nursing. It has approximately 725 members (schools/colleges of nursing). Its activities include educational research, government advocacy, data collection, publishing, and initiatives to establish standards for baccalaureate and graduate degree nursing programs, including implementation of the standards. Its goals for 2012–2014 are threefold: (1) provide strategic leadership that advances professional nursing education, research, and practice; (2) develop faculty and other academic leaders to meet the challenges of changing healthcare and higher education environments; and (3) leverage AACN's policy and programmatic leadership on behalf of the profession and discipline (AACN, 2013). The AACN is also involved in accreditation of university nursing programs through its Commission on Collegiate Nursing Education (CCNE; BSN including RN-BSN, master's, DNP).

National Organization for Associate Degree Nursing

The N-OADN is the organization that advocates for associate degree nursing education and practice (N-OADN, 2013). Its major goals are as follows:

1. *Collaboration*: Advance associate degree nursing education through collaboration with a diversity of audiences.

2. *Education*: Advance associate degree nursing education.

3. *Advocacy*: Advocate for issues and activities that support N-OADN's mission.

N-OADN began in 1952 when Mildred Montag proposed the ADN—a degree in nursing that took less time to acquire than the BSN, which is a 2-year program often based in a community college. The first programs opened in 1958. As of 2008, 63.2% of RN graduates were from ADN programs and 50% from BSN programs (ANA, 2011). In 2012, there were 59 diploma programs, 696 ADN programs, and 1084 BSN programs. This breakdown represented a change from the previous year marked by an increase of 19 BSN and 24 ADN programs (NLN, 2013b).

The N-OADN organization does not offer accreditation services. Accreditation of ADN programs is done through the NLN accrediting organization (ACEN).

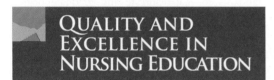

QUALITY AND EXCELLENCE IN NURSING EDUCATION

Nursing Education Standards

Nursing education **standards** are developed by the major nursing professional organizations that focus on education: NLN, AACN, and N-OADN. The accrediting bodies of the NLN and the AACN also set standards. State boards of nursing are involved as well. In addition, colleges and universities must meet certain standards for non-nursing accreditation at the overall college or university level. Standards guide decisions, organizational structure, process, policies and procedures, budgetary decisions, admissions and progress of students, evaluation/assessment (program, faculty, and student), curriculum, and other academic issues. Critical standard documents published by the AACN are *The Essentials* covering baccalaureate, master's, and DNP degrees (AACN, 2006, 2008, 2011).

NLN Excellence in Nursing Education Model

Recognition by the NLN as a Center of Excellence in Nursing Education identifies schools of nursing that demonstrate "sustained, evidence-based, and substantive innovation in the selected area; conduct ongoing research to document the effectiveness of such innovation; set high standards for themselves; and are committed to continuous quality improvement" (NLN, 2007b). These schools make a commitment to pursue excellence in (1) student learning and professional development, (2) development of faculty expertise in pedagogy, or (3) advancing the science of nursing education. This award is given to a school—not a program in a school—and remains in effect for 3 years. After this period, the school must be reviewed again for the Center of Excellence recognition. This NLN initiative is an excellent example of efforts to improve nursing education.

Another initiative to recognize excellence, also undertaken by the NLN, is the Academy of Nursing Education, which inducted its first nurse education fellows in 2007. The purpose of the Academy of Nursing Education is to foster excellence in nursing education by recognizing and capitalizing on the wisdom of outstanding individuals who have made enduring and substantial contributions to nursing education in one or more areas (teaching/learning innovations, faculty development, research in nursing education, leadership in nursing education, public policy related to nursing education, or collaborative education/practice/community partnerships) and who will continue to provide visionary leadership in nursing education and in the academy (NLN, 2007a). Nurses who are selected as fellows must document distinguished contributions in one or more areas: (1) teaching/learning innovations, (2) faculty development, (3) research in nursing education, (4) leadership in nursing education, (5) public policy related to nursing education, and (6) collaborative education/practice/community partnerships.

Focus on Competencies

The nursing curriculum should identify the competencies expected of students throughout the nursing program. There is greater emphasis today on implementing healthcare professions competencies, as noted by the IOM recognition that all healthcare professions should meet five core competencies: (1) provide patient-centered care; (2) work in interdisciplinary/professional teams; (3) employ evidence-based practice; (4) apply quality improvement; and (5) utilize informatics (IOM, 2003). This does not mean that profession-specific competencies are not relevant, but rather recognizes the existence of basic competencies that all healthcare professions should demonstrate.

You need to know what the expected competencies are so that you can be an active participant in your own learning to reach these competencies. The competencies are used in evaluation and to identify the level of learning or performance expected of the student. Nursing is a profession—a practice profession—so performance is a critical factor. Competency is "the application of knowledge and the interpersonal, decision-making, and psychomotor skills expected for the nurse's practice role, within the context of public health, welfare, and safety" (National Council of State Boards of Nursing [NCSBN], 2005, p. 1). The ANA defines competence as "an expected and measurable level of nursing performance that integrates knowledge, skills, abilities, and judgment, based on established scientific knowledge and expectations for nursing practice" (ANA, 2010, p. 64). Competencies should clearly state the expected parameters related to the behavior or performance. The curriculum should support the development of competencies by providing necessary prerequisite knowledge and learning opportunities to meet the competency. The ultimate goal is a competent RN.

Curriculum

A nursing program's **curriculum** is the plan that describes the program's philosophy, levels, terminal competencies for students (or what they are expected to accomplish by the end of the program), and course content (described in course syllabi). Also specified are the sequence of courses and a designation of course credits and learning experiences, such as didactic courses (typically offered in a lecture/classroom, seminar setting. or both venues) and clinical or practicum experiences. In addition, simulation laboratory experiences are included either at the beginning of the curriculum or throughout the curriculum. The nursing curriculum is very important. It informs potential students what they should expect in a program and may influence a student's choice of programs, particularly at the graduate level. It helps orient new students and is important in the accreditation of nursing programs. State boards of nursing also review the program curricula of schools of nursing in their state. To keep current, it is important that curricula are reviewed regularly by the faculty and in a manner that allows changes to be made as easily and quickly as possible.

The *Essentials of Baccalaureate Education for Professional Nursing* Practice provides guidelines for baccalaureate education, and CCNE accreditation requires that these guidelines be used to develop BSN curricula (AACN, 2008). This document was revised in 2008. The following paragraphs provide some history on this change.

The IOM published an important report, *Health Professions Education* (2003) that addressed the need for education in all major health professions to meet several common competencies to improve care. The development of this report was motivated by grave concerns about the quality of care in the United States and the need for healthcare education programs to prepare professionals who provide quality, safe care. "Education for health professions is in need of a major overhaul. Clinical education [for all healthcare professions] simply has not kept pace with or been responsive enough to shifting patient demographics and desires, changing health system expectations, evolving practice requirements and staffing arrangements, new information, a focus on improving quality, or new technologies" (IOM, 2001, as cited in IOM, 2003, p. 1). The IOM core competencies were also emphasized in the *Essentials of Baccalaureate Education* (AACN, 2008); however, schools of nursing need to make changes to include the competencies, and in some cases add new content to meet these needs.

Along with the call from the IOM to make major changes in health professions education, there is recognition that nursing education needs improvement and changes to make it more current with practice today. The NLN (2007a) has stated:

> Student-centered, interactive, and innovative programs and curricula should be designed to promote leadership in students, develop students' thinking skills, reflect new models of learning and practice, effectively integrate technology, promote a lifelong career commitment in students, include intra- and inter-professional learning experiences, and prepare students for the roles they will assume.

Didactic or Theory Content

Nursing curricula may vary as to titles of courses, course descriptions and objectives/learning outcomes, sequence, and number of hours of didactic content and clinical experiences, but there are some constants even within these differences. Nursing content needs to include the following broad topical areas:

- Adult health or medical–surgical nursing
- Psychiatric–mental health nursing
- Pediatrics
- Maternal–child nursing (obstetrics, women's health, neonatal care)
- Public/community health
- Gerontology
- Leadership and management
- Pharmacology
- Health assessment
- Evidence-based practice

- Research
- Health policy
- Legal and ethical issues
- Professional issues and trends

Many schools also offer courses in informatics and in genetics. Quality improvement content is often weak, even though it is now considered critical knowledge that every practicing nurse needs to have if care is to be improved.

Nursing content may be provided in clearly defined courses that focus on only one topical area, or it may be integrated with multiple topics. Clinical experiences/practicums may be blended with related didactic content—for example, pediatric content and pediatric clinical experience—such that they are considered one course; alternatively, the clinical/practicum and didactic content may be offered as two separate courses, typically in the same semester. Faculty who teach didactic content may or may not teach in the clinical setting.

Practicum or Clinical Experience

The hours for the practicum can be highly variable within one school and from school to school (i.e., the number of hours per week and sequence of days, such as practicum on Tuesdays and Thursdays from 8 a.m. to 3 p.m.). Many schools are now offering 12-hour clinical sessions. Twelve-hour work shifts may lead to fatigue and an increased number of errors. Some schools offer clinical experiences in the evenings, at night, and on weekends. It is important for students to understand the time commitment and scheduling, which have a great impact on students' personal lives and employment. In addition, these clinical experiences require preparation time. The types of clinical settings are highly variable and depend on the objectives and the available sites. Typical types of settings are acute care hospitals (all clinical areas); psychiatric hospitals; pediatric hospitals; women's health (may include obstetrics) clinics; community health clinics and other health agencies; home health agencies and patients' homes; hospice centers, including freestanding sites, hospital-based centers, and patients' homes; schools; camps; health-oriented consumer organizations such as the American Diabetes Association; health mobile clinics; homeless shelters; doctors' offices; clinics of all types; ambulatory surgical centers; emergency centers; Red Cross centers; businesses with occupational health services; and many more. In some of these settings—for example, in acute care—faculty remain with the students for the entire rotation time. In other settings, particularly public/community healthcare settings, faculty visit students at the site because typically only 1 to 4 students are in each site, compared with the larger group (8 to 10 students) usually assigned to a faculty member for hospital experiences. The number of hours per week in clinical experiences increases in a nursing program, with the most hours assigned at the end of the program.

Most schools of nursing use preceptors as part of the nursing curriculum at some time, in both undergraduate and graduate programs. In entry-level programs, preceptor experiences are typically used toward the end of the program, but some schools use preceptors throughout the program for certain courses such as master's programs. A **preceptor** is an experienced and competent staff member (an RN or a nurse practitioner or medical doctor for APRN, nurse anesthesia, and nurse–midwife graduate nursing students) who has received formal training to function in this role. The preceptor serves as a role model and a resource for the nursing student and guides learning. The student is assigned to work alongside the preceptor. Faculty provide overall guidance to the preceptor regarding the nature of, and objectives for, the student's learning experiences; monitor the student's progress by meeting with the student and the preceptor; and are on call for communication with the student and preceptor as needed. The preceptor participates in evaluations of the student's progress, along with the student, but the faculty member has the ultimate student evaluation responsibility. The state board of nursing may dictate how many total hours in the undergraduate nursing program may be devoted to preceptorship

experiences. At the graduate level, the number of preceptorship hours is much higher.

Distance Education

Distance education or online education has become quite common in nursing education, although not all schools offer courses in this manner. The AACN recognizes distance education as "a set of teaching and/or learning strategies to meet the learning needs of students separate from the traditional classroom and sometimes from traditional roles of faculty" (Reinert & Fryback, 1997). This definition is still applicable today, and distance education technologies have expanded over the last few years as technology developed. Some of the common distance education technologies that are used are email, fax, audiotaped instruction, audiocassette, conference by telephone or via Internet, CD-ROM, email lists (such as LISTSERV), interactive television, desktop video conference, and Internet-based programming. There is no doubt that these methods will continue to expand. The most common and increasingly more widely adopted education approach is online courses.

Distance education can be configured in several ways, including the following:

- Self-study or independent study
- Hybrid model—distance education combined with traditional classroom delivery (the most common configuration)
- Faculty-facilitated online learning with no classroom activities (the approach that is growing the most rapidly)

As stated by the AACN, "When utilizing distance learning methods, a program provides or makes available resources for the students' successful attainment of all program objectives" (2005b, p. 1). For schools to effectively offer courses or entire programs using technologies for distance education, they must ensure that the following supports are provided: registration, student affairs support, technology support, library access, and other support services such as tutoring.

Students who participate in distance education must have certain characteristics to be successful in this type of educational program. Most notably, they need to be responsible for their own learning, with faculty facilitating their learning. Computer competencies are critical for completing coursework and reducing student stress. Students must have required hardware and software. Students who are organized and able to develop and meet a schedule will be able to handle the course requirements. If students are assertive, ask questions, and ask for help, they will be more successful. Effective online learning also requires active, engaged competent faculty.

Self-directed learning is important for all nursing students because it leads to greater ability to achieve lifelong learning as a professional. There are a variety of definitions of self-directed learning, most of which are based on Knowles's (1975, p. 18, as cited in O'Shea, 2003, p. 62) definition: "a process in which individuals take the initiative, with or without the help of others, in diagnosing their learning needs, formulating learning goals, identifying human and material resources for learning, choosing and implementing appropriate learning strategies and evaluating learning outcomes." Student-centered learning approaches can assist students—for example, problem-based learning or team-based learning. This type of approach means that the faculty must also change how they teach. Faculty members assume the role of a facilitator of learning, which requires establishing a more collaborative relationship between faculty and students. Faculty work with students to develop active participation and goal setting: helping students to work on setting goals, making plans with clear strategies to meet the goals, and encouraging self-assessment. Flipped classroom approach is also new to nursing, for example with content provided online, in textbooks, etc. and the expectation that students come to class prepared so that they can actively participate in learning activities in the classroom rather than listening to lectures. Distance education typically emphasizes adult teaching and learning principles

more than the traditional classroom approach does, and approaches such as the flipped classroom focus more on these principles. Knowles (1984) originally described principles that emphasized how learners engage with this type of educational program:

- Accept responsibility for collaborating in the planning of their learning experiences
- Set goals
- Actively participate
- Pace their own learning
- Participate in monitoring their own progress; perform self-assessment

As noted in the 2010 report on nursing education (Benner et al., 2010), there is need for greater student engagement in the classroom.

The quality of distance education is as important as the quality of traditional classroom courses. Syllabi that provide the course description, credits, objectives or learning outcomes, and other information about the course should ensure that the same general structure is followed whether a course is taught using a traditional approach or through distance education. Student evaluation must be built into a distance education course just as it is in non-distant courses; however, more details are typically provided in distance education course materials and teaching–learning practices may be different. Schools should ensure that students provide anonymous evaluations of the course and faculty.

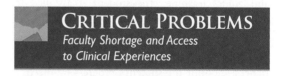

CRITICAL PROBLEMS
Faculty Shortage and Access to Clinical Experiences

Today, two critical problems that concern participants in nursing education programs are the growing faculty shortage and the need to find clinical experiences for students, particularly as efforts are made to increase enrollment. These complex problems require more than one solution, and they have a great impact on the quality of nursing education and student outcomes.

Faculty Shortage

The faculty shortage is part of the nursing shortage problem, because it means that fewer new nurses can enter the profession. "A particular focus on securing and retaining adequate numbers of faculty is essential to ensure that all individuals interested in—and qualified for—nursing school can matriculate in the year they are accepted" (Americans for Nursing Shortage Relief, 2007, p. 2). Aside from having a limited number of faculty, nursing programs struggle to provide space for clinical laboratories and to secure a sufficient number of clinical training sites at healthcare facilities.

A school's faculty should reflect a balance of expert clinicians who can teach, expert researchers and grant writers who can teach and meet research obligations, and expert teachers who are pedagogical scholars (NLN, 2007b). Today, schools of nursing, regardless of the type of program, are struggling to meet the demand for greater enrollment of students because of the limited number of faculty. Schools of nursing are having problems recruiting experienced faculty, and thus many faculty are new to teaching. This shortage comes at a time when there already is a fluctuating nursing shortage. Some of the same factors that affect the nursing shortage have an impact on the faculty shortage, such as retirement. This challenge will only increase in the future because a large number of nursing faculty members are approaching retirement age. It is also difficult to attract nurses to teaching because the pay is lower than for nursing practice; for this reason, nurses with graduate degrees often opt to stay in active practice. Attracting nurses to graduate school is an issue, particularly at the doctoral level. It is hoped that the DNP degree will attract more nurses to such advanced degree programs, but these nurses may not be interested in teaching—and the DNP program is not designed to prepare faculty but rather to prepare practitioners. However, even if more students do apply to DNP programs, many are likely to be denied admission due to the lack of sufficient faculty to teach in the programs. The Health Care Reform legislation of 2010 (Patient Protection and Affordable Care Act) offers some opportunities to expand nursing faculty by providing funding for education so that nurses can prepare for the faculty role.

Access to Clinical Experiences

With the drive to increase student enrollments, securing enough clinical sites to meet course objectives has proved a challenge for schools of nursing. If a number of nursing schools are located in the same area, there will also be competition for clinical slots. This is particularly pronounced in specialties that have fewer patients, which translates into tight demand for clinical slots—such is the case in pediatrics, obstetrics, and mental health, for example.

Schools of nursing have to be more innovative and recognize that every student may not get the same clinical experiences. For example, there has been increasing use of non–acute care pediatric settings. Some communities do not have pediatric hospitals and may have limited beds assigned to pediatric care. Other sites that might be used are pediatrician offices, pediatric clinics, schools, daycare centers, and camps. For obstetrics, possible clinical sites are birthing centers, obstetrician offices, and midwifery practices. Mental health clinical experiences may take place in clinics, at homeless shelters, in mental health emergency and crisis centers, and at a mental health association site.

This difficulty in getting sites has meant that some schools have been forced to move away from the traditional clinical hours offered—Monday through Friday during the day. Some schools are recognizing that operating on a 9-month basis with a long summer break affects the availability of clinical experiences. To accommodate the needs of all schools of nursing and the need to increase student enrollment, community-area healthcare providers are working with schools to determine how all these needs can be met effectively.

A Response and Innovation: Laboratory Experiences and Clinical Simulation

Laboratory and simulation experiences have become important teaching–learning settings for developing competencies, partly because of problems in accessing clinical experiences, but also as a result of the recognition that they provide effective learning experiences for students with no risk of harm to patients. The NCSBN (2005) defines simulation as "activities that mimic reality of a clinical environment and are designed to demonstrate procedures, decision making and critical thinking through techniques such as role playing and the use of devices such as interactive videos or mannequins" (p. 11). Simulation helps students develop confidence in their skills in a safe setting before they begin caring for real patients and can help students to develop teamwork abilities. The simulated environment provides opportunities for teams of nurses or, ideally, interprofessional students to work together to solve simulated clinical situations. Students can be evaluated and provided with feedback in more structured learning situations. Simulated experiences should be as close to real life as possible—although they are not, of course, totally real. However, this does not mean that these learning situations are not very helpful for student learning. Laboratories that are not as high-tech as simulation centers may be used to learn basic skills. Most schools do not have their own full simulation laboratories due to the expense of setting up and running such labs. Often the simulation laboratory is established through a partnership of multiple health practice education programs and/or hospitals to reduce the financial burden on each institution and to offer simulation to a variety of students, often in an interprofessional experience, and staff.

A simulation lab is expensive to develop and maintain. Students need to respect the equipment and supplies and follow procedures so that costs can be managed. Faculty supervision in the simulation lab may be based on a higher ratio of students to faculty than the required ratio for clinical experiences,

providing more cost-effective teaching and learning. With the development of more sophisticated technology, computer simulation can even be incorporated into distance education.

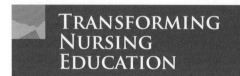

TRANSFORMING NURSING EDUCATION

The IOM reports on quality in healthcare delivery have resulted in greater urgency to institute changes in nursing education. In fact, the 2010 nursing education report identified preparation of nurses to meet these quality demands as a critical topic (Benner et al., 2010). Thus quality improvement relies, in part, on improvement of nursing education. Nursing students need to be included in the evaluation of nursing education and changes. As a student, you can help meet this need by providing course feedback and participating in curriculum committees when requested. Nursing education leaders should always review content and improve curriculum, but must have methods to do this in a timely, effective manner. When accreditation surveyors come to schools of nursing, they talk to students to get their feedback.

> What is needed by nursing today is to uphold the true spirit of innovation and overhaul traditional pedagogies to reform the way the nursing workforce is educated. This call to action will be accomplished through new pedagogies that are most effective in helping students learn to practice in rapidly changing environments where short stays in acute care facilities are common and where complex care is being provided in a variety of settings. These new pedagogies must be research-based, pluralistic and responsive to the unpredictable nature of the contemporary healthcare system. (Ben-Zur, Yagi, & Spitzer, 1999, as stated in NLN, 2003, p. 2)

ACCREDITATION OF NURSING EDUCATION PROGRAMS

Accreditation is important in assessing and maintaining standards to better ensure effective programs for students that meet practice requirements. Potential nursing students may not be as aware of accreditation of the schools they are considering, but they should be.

Nursing Program Accreditation

Accreditation is a process in which an organization is assessed regarding how it meets established standards. Minimum standards are identified by an accrediting organization, and nursing schools incorporate these standards into their programs. The accrediting organization then reviews the school and its programs. This is supposedly a voluntary process, but in reality it is not; to be effective, a school of nursing must be accredited. Nursing education programs should be accredited by the recognized organizations that provide standards and accreditation for nursing programs. Attending a program that is not accredited can lead to complications in licensure, employment, and opportunities to continue on to higher degree programs. Currently, two organizations offer accreditation of nursing programs: NLN and ANCC through their accrediting services ACEN and CCNE.

Nursing Program Accreditation: How Does It Work?

What is accreditation, and how does it work? Accreditation is based on minimum standards that schools of nursing must meet to obtain accreditation. The process is complex and takes time. Schools of nursing must pay for the review. Schools may or may not receive initial accreditation, and when they do, programs may be required to make changes;

they may also later be found to not be in compliance with the expected standards and may lose accreditation. Accreditation is not a legal requirement, but state boards of nursing require this type of accreditation from the NLN or ANCC to maintain state accreditation. Some specialty organizations accredit specific graduate programs within a school, such as the American College of Nurse Midwifery and the American Association of Nurse Anesthetists. A school may choose which organization (ACEN or CCNE) accredits the program unless mandated by state agency or law; however, schools with diploma and associate degree programs can be accredited only by the ACEN. The state board of nursing in each state is involved in this requirement and in the state accreditation process. During the accreditation process, the review team assesses the schools for the following:

- Mission and vision
- Structure and governance
- Resources and physical facilities, including budget
- Faculty and faculty outcomes
- Curriculum and implementation
- Student support services
- Admissions process and other academic processes
- Policies and procedures
- Ongoing assessment process (continuous quality improvement, student and program outcomes)

After the school of nursing completes a self-study based on the accreditation standards established by the accrediting organization, the written self-study results are submitted to the accrediting organization. The next step in the accreditation process is the on-site survey at the school. Surveyors visit the school and view classes and clinical experiences/practicums, review documents, and meet with school administrative staff; if the school of nursing is part of a university, they also meet with university administrative staff. In addition, surveyors meet with faculty, students, and alumni. They typically remain at the school for several days. Students have an obligation to participate in this survey and provide feedback. The goal is maintenance of minimum standards to ensure an effective learning environment that supports student learning and meets the needs of the profession.

REGULATION

How are professional regulation and nursing regulation for practice licensure related? **Regulation** for practice or licensure is clear, though problematic in some cases. This type of regulation is based on state laws and regulations and leads to licensure. However, this is different from the professional regulation, in which the profession itself regulates its practice. State boards of nursing are not nursing professional organizations, but rather state government agencies. This distinction can make it difficult to make changes in a state's practice of nursing. Professional organizations do have an impact on practice through the standards they propose and other elements of support and data that they provide. "For effective nursing workforce planning to occur and be sustained, Boards of Nursing must collaborate with nursing education and practice to support the safe and effective evolution of nursing practice" (Damgaard, VanderWoude, & Hegge, 1999, as cited in Loquist, 2002, p. 34).

"In 1950, nursing became the first profession for which the same licensure exam, the State Board Test Pool (now called NCLEX), was used throughout the nation to license nurses. This increased the mobility for the registered nurse and resulted in a significant advantage for the relatively new profession of nursing" (Lundy, 2005, pp. 21–22). The major purpose of regulation is to protect the public, and it is based on the 10th Amendment of the U.S. Constitution, the states' rights amendment. Each state has the right to regulate professional practice, such as nursing practice, within its own state.

In general, the regulatory approach selected should be sufficient to ensure public protection.

The following criteria are still relevant today in providing a framework for professional licensure (NCSBN, 1996, pp. 8–9):

- *Risk of harm for the consumer.* The evaluation of a profession to determine whether unregulated practice endangers the public should focus on recognizable harm. That harm could result from the practices inherent in the nature of the profession, the characteristics of the clients/patients, the settings, or supervisory requirements, or a combination of these factors. Licensure is applied to a profession when the incompetent or unethical practice of that profession could cause greater risk of harm to the public unless there is a high level of accountability; at the other extreme, registration is appropriate for professions where such a high level of accountability is not needed.

- *Skill and training needed.* The more highly specialized the services of the professional, the greater the need for an approach that actively inquires about the education and competence of the professional.

- *Level of autonomy.* Licensure is indicated when the professional uses independent judgment and practices independently with little or no supervision. Registration is appropriate for individuals who do not use independent judgment and practice with supervision.

- *Scope of practice.* Unless there is a well-demarcated scope of practice for the profession that is distinguishable from other professions and definable in enforceable legal terms, there is neither basis nor need for licensure. This scope may overlap other professions in specific duties, functions, or therapeutic modalities.

- *Consumer expectation.* Consumers expect that those professions that have a potentially high impact on the consumer or on their physical, mental, or economic well-being will be subject to regulatory oversight. The costs of operating regulatory agencies and the restriction of practitioners who do not meet the minimum requirements are justified to protect the public from harm.

- *Alternative to regulation.* There are no alternatives to the selected regulatory approach that would adequately protect the public. It should also be the case that when it is determined that regulation of the profession is required, the least restrictive level of regulation consistent with public protection is implemented.

Eight guiding principles apply to nursing regulation: (1) protection of the public, (2) competence of all practitioners regulated by the board of nursing, (3) due process and ethical decision making, (4) shared accountability, (5) strategic collaboration, (6) evidence-based regulation, (7) response to the marketplace and healthcare environment, and (8) globalization of nursing (NCSBN, 2007).

Nurse Practice Acts

Each state has a **nurse practice act** that determines the nature of nursing practice within the state. The nurse practice act is a state law passed by the state legislative body. Nurse practice acts for each state can be found state government websites. Every nurse who has a license should be knowledgeable about the nurse practice act that governs practice in the state where the nurse practices under the RN license. Typically, nurse practice acts do the following for their state (Masters, 2005, p. 166):

- Define the authority of the board of nursing, its composition, and its powers
- Define nursing and boundaries of the scope of practice
- Identify types of licenses and titles
- State the requirements for licensure
- Protect titles
- Identify the grounds for disciplinary action

The most important function of the nurse practice act is to define the scope of practice for nurses in the state to protect public safety.

State Boards of Nursing

State boards of nursing implement the state's nurse practice act, which is the statutory law governing nursing practice within a state or territory, and recommend state regulations and changes to this act when appropriate. This board is part of state government, although how it fits into a state's governmental organization varies from state to state. RNs serve on state boards of nursing, and the governor typically selects board members who serve for a specific term of office. Licensed practical nurses (LPNs), laypersons, or consumers (non-nurses) may also have representation on the board. The primary purpose of the state board of nursing is to protect the health and safety of the public (citizens of the state). A board of nursing has an executive director who runs the business of the board, along with staff who work for the board (state). The size of the state has an impact on the size of the board of nursing and its staff. Boards are not only involved in setting standards and licensure of nurses (RNs and LPNs/ licensed vocational nurses [LVNs]), but also are responsible for monitoring nursing education (RN and LPN) programs in the state. Such a board serves a regulatory function; as part of this function, it can issue administrative rules or regulations consistent with state law to facilitate the enforcement of the nurse practice act.

The board of nursing in each state also reviews problems with licensure and is the agency that administers disciplinary actions. If a nurse fails to meet certain standards, participates in unacceptable practice, or has problems that interfere with safe practice, and any of these violations are reported to the board, the board can conduct an investigation and review and determine actions that might need to be taken. Examples of these issues are assault or causing harm to a patient; having a problem with illegal drugs or with alcohol (substance abuse); conviction of, or pleading guilty to, a felony (examples of felonies are murder, robbery, rape, and sexual battery); and having a psychiatric illness that is not managed effectively and interferes with safe functioning. A nurse may be reprimanded by the board or denied a license, may be subject to suspended or revoked licensure, or may face licensure restriction with stipulations (for example, the nurse must attend an alcohol treatment program to retain licensure).

The board must follow strict procedures when taking any disciplinary action, which must first begin with an official complaint to the board. Anyone can make a complaint to the board—another nurse, another healthcare professional, a healthcare organization, or a consumer. The state nursing practice act identifies the possible reasons for disciplinary action. Boards of nursing publish their disciplinary action decisions because they are part of the public record. When nurses obtain a license in another state, they are asked to report any disciplinary actions that have been taken by another state's board of nursing. Not reporting disciplinary board actions has serious consequences for obtaining (and losing) licensure. A key point is that licensure is a privilege, not a legal right. It is important to consider this point as a student because the same rules apply when getting the first license—even if a student graduates from a nursing program this does not mean they have a right to take the NCLEX exam or to be given a license.

National Council of State Boards of Nursing

The NCSBN is a not-for-profit organization that represents all of the boards of nursing in the 50 states, the District of Columbia, and four U.S. territories (American Samoa, Guam, Northern Mariana Islands, and Virgin Islands). Through this organization, all boards of nursing work together on issues related to the regulation of nursing practice that affect public health, safety, and welfare, including the development of licensing examinations in nursing. Although the NCSBN cannot dictate change to individual state boards of nursing, it can make recommendations, which often carry significant weight. Individual state boards of nursing, unlike the NCSBN, are part of, and report to, state government.

The NCSBN performs the following functions (NCSBN, 2013a):

- Develops the NCLEX-RN, NCLEX-PN, NNAAP, and MACE examinations
- Monitors trends in public policy, nursing practice, and education
- Promotes uniformity in relationship to the regulation of nursing practice
- Disseminates data related to the licensure of nurses
- Conducts research on nursing practice issues
- Serves as a forum for information exchange for members
- Provides opportunities for collaboration among its members and other nursing and healthcare organizations by maintaining the Nursys database, which coordinates national publicly available nurse licensure information

Licensure Requirements

Each state's board of nursing determines its state's licensure requirements; however, all require passage of the NCLEX-RN, which is a national exam. Other requirements include criminal background checks for initial licensure and **continuing education** (CE) for renewal, though the latter requirement varies from state to state. Many nurses hold licenses in several states or may be on inactive status in some states. An RN should always maintain one license, even if not practicing, to make it easier to return to practice. Fees are paid for the initial license and for license renewal. States in which a nurse is licensed notify the nurse when the license is up for renewal. It is the nurse's responsibility to complete the required forms and submit payment, and many states now do this electronically.

Examples of licensure requirements and renewal requirements, which vary from state to state, include the following:

- Fee (always required, though the amount varies and depends on whether the nurse has active or inactive licensure status)
- Passage of NCLEX (required for first licensure and then covered for renewals or change of license)
- CE contact hours within a specified time period (number of contact hours varies from state to state, and some states do not require any CE for licensure renewal)
- Criminal background check (required typically for initial licensure in a state)
- Active employment for a specific number of hours within a specified time period (varies from state to state)
- Number of hours of professional nursing activities (varies from state to state)

Ultimately, each RN is responsible for maintaining competency for safe practice. Any person who practices nursing without a valid license commits a minor misdemeanor. If licensed in one state, the nurse can typically do the following in another state in which the nurse is not licensed:

- Consult
- Teach as guest lecturer
- Conduct evaluation of care as part of an accreditation process

National Council Licensure Examination

The NCLEX is developed and administered through the NCSBN (2013a). There are two forms of the exam: NCLEX-RN for RN licensure and NCLEX-PN for practical nurse licensure. In each jurisdiction (state) in the United States and its territories, licensing authorities regulate entry into practice of nursing. To ensure public protection, each jurisdiction requires a candidate for licensure

to pass an examination that measures the competencies needed to perform safely and effectively as a newly licensed, entry-level RN (NCSBN, 2013a). Content relates to the following patient/client needs categories: safe effective care environment (management of care, safety, and infection control), health promotion and maintenance, psychosocial integrity, and physiological integrity (basic care and comfort, pharmacologic and parenteral therapies, reduction of risk potential, physiological adaptation).

The examination is offered online. Most of the questions are written at the cognitive level of application or higher, requiring the candidate to use problem-solving skills to select the best answer. The exam is a computerized adaptive test. In this type of exam, the computer adjusts questions to the individual candidate so that the exam is then highly individualized, offering challenging questions that are neither too easy nor too difficult. The NCLEX-RN has a range of questions, numbering from 75 to 265. The exam ends when the computer determines with 95% certainty that the person's ability is either below or above the passing standard. The exam can also end when the time runs out or there are no more questions. Because of these factors, all candidates do not receive the same number of questions. The exam includes the following types of questions:

- *Multiple-response items:* The candidate is required to select one or more responses.
- *Fill-in-the-blank items:* The candidate is required to type numbers in a calculation item.
- *Hot spot items:* The candidate identifies an area on a picture or graphic.
- *Chart/exhibit format:* The candidate is presented with a problem and then must read information in a chart/exhibit to answer the question.
- *Drag-and-drop items:* The candidate ranks, orders, or moves options to provide the correct answer.

If a candidate does not pass the exam, he or she may take the NCLEX again. Most schools of nursing provide some type of preparation (for example, throughout the nursing program, or near the end); some may recommend that students complete a prep course on their own. These prep courses require a fee and are of varying length. Many publications are also available to assist with NCLEX preparation. The exam preparation takes place every day in the nursing programs—in courses and in clinical practice.

How the Process Works

Students are asked by their school to complete an application for NCLEX in the final semester before graduation. This application is sent to the state board of nursing in the state where the student is seeking licensure. After a student completes the nursing program, the school must verify that the student has graduated. At this point, the student becomes an official NCLEX candidate. The student receives an authorization to test and exam instructions and information about scheduling the exam. The authorization to test is the nursing graduate's pass to take the exam, so it is important to keep it. Students then schedule their own exam within the given time frame.

On the scheduled date, the student goes to the designated exam site to take the computerized exam. Candidates are fingerprinted and photographed to ensure security for the exam. Testing sites are available in every state, and a candidate may take the exam in any state. Licensure, however, is awarded by the state in which the candidate has applied for licensure.

An exam session lasts a maximum of 6 hours, but because of the computerized adaptive test method, the amount of time that an individual candidate takes on the exam varies; that time does not affect passing or failing. Every candidate must answer a minimum of 75 questions. This means that the exam is completed when one of the following occurs: (1) results measure a level of competency above or below the standard, and a minimum of 75 questions have been answered; (2) the candidate completes the maximum number of 265 questions; or (3) the candidate has used the maximum time of 6 hours. Candidates are provided an orientation and a brief practice session prior to taking the exam.

Passing scores are the same for every state and are set by the NCSBN. Candidates are usually informed of their results within 4 weeks; the result is pass or fail, with no specific score provided. Schools of nursing receive composites of student results. Data on individual school pass rates are available on state board of nursing websites and open to the public. Results from the NCLEX are an important element in a school of nursing's evaluation/assessment process. The first-time pass rate is reviewed routinely and must be reported to the school's accreditation organization; in addition, the state board monitors these results.

Critical Current and Future Regulation Issues

Compact Licensure

There has been a growing need to find licensure methods that address the following situations: a nurse lives in one state but works in an adjacent state; a nurse works for a healthcare company in several states; and a nurse works in telehealth, by which care might be provided via technology in more than one state. To address these types of issues, the NCSBN created a new model for licensure called mutual recognition or compact licensure. Each state in a mutual recognition compact must enact legislation or regulation authorizing the nurse licensure compact and also adopt administrative rules and regulations for implementation of the compact. Each compact state must also appoint a nurse licensure compact administrator to facilitate the exchange of information between the states that relates to compact nurse licensure and regulation. Twenty-four states have adopted this model. Other states have decided that this model is unconstitutional in their states because it delegates authority for licensure decisions to other states. A list of current states offering this multistate licensure is available from NCSBN (https://www.ncsbn.org/nlc.htm).

The same type of licensure questions apply to advanced practice nurses. In 2002, the NCSBN Delegate Assembly approved the adoption of model language for a licensure compact for APRNs. Only those states that have adopted the RN and LPN/LVN licensure compact may implement a compact for APRNs. From 2004 to 2007, three states—Utah, Iowa, and Texas—passed legislation. These states are now working on the implementation regulations, which must be put into effect prior to implementation of the compact. The APRN compact offers states the mechanism for mutually recognizing APRN licenses and authority to practice (NCSBN, 2013b).

Mandatory Overtime

A critical concern in practice today is requiring nurses to work overtime. Employers make this decision, and it is called mandatory overtime. This policy impacts the quality of care and has affected staff satisfaction and burnout. Boards of nursing in other states have become involved in state legislative efforts related to mandatory overtime.

Although legislative and regulatory responses have provided nurses with additional support for creating safer work environments, each of these legislative responses has a significant effect on the numbers and types of nursing personnel that will be required for care delivery systems in the future as well as the cost of care. Clearly, there is concern at the state and national levels regarding the impact that fewer caregivers will have on the health and safety of patients (Loquist, 2002, p. 37).

As students and new graduates interview for their first positions, they should ask about mandatory overtime if they are not in a state that has a law to protect them from it. Research is now being done regarding sleep deprivation and its connection to the rising number of medical errors (Girard, 2003; Manfredini, Boari, & Manfredini, 2006; Montgomery, 2007; Sigurdson & Ayas, 2007). This area of research is fairly new, and researchers will need to continue to provide concrete evidence of the links among sleep deprivation, long work hours, and medical errors. The aviation industry has cut back the number of hours that flight crews can work

without sleep, and the number of hours that medical residents can work consecutively has been decreased because of concern about fatigue and errors.

Foreign Nursing Graduates: Entrance to Practice in the United States

The number of nurses from other countries coming to the United States to work and/or study has increased. Some nurses want to work here only temporarily; others want to stay permanently. This movement of nurses internationally typically increases during a shortage, and today there is a worldwide shortage and a lot of nursing migration (International Centre on Nurse Migration, 2007).

> The NCSBN recently passed a new position statement regarding international nurse immigration, reaffirming that foreign-educated nurses need to comply with standards of approved or comparable education, hold a verified valid and unencumbered state license, and be proficient in their written and spoken English language skills. There still is the ethical question of "poaching" nurses from one country to another that results in the reduction of a scarce national resource in this worldwide shortage. (NCSBN, 2001, as cited in Loquist, 2002, p. 37)

What do these nurses have to do to meet practice requirements in the United States? The Commission on Graduates of Foreign Nursing Schools (CGFNS, 2007) is an organization that assists these nurses in evaluating their credentials and verifies their education, registration, and licensure. This is an internationally recognized, immigration-neutral, nonprofit organization that protects the public by ensuring that these nurses are eligible and qualified to meet U.S. licensure and immigration requirements. These nurses must also take the English as a foreign language exam to ensure that their English language ability is at an acceptable level. This requirement also applies to students who want to enter

U.S. nursing programs. A nurse who is licensed in another country must successfully complete the NCLEX and meet the state licensure requirements where the nurse will practice. If the nurse wants to enter a graduate nursing program, the nurse needs to get a U.S. RN license for clinical work that would be done as part of the educational program. This is not required for a prelicensure program in nursing.

Global Regulatory Issues

With the development of the Internet, telehealth and global migration have been forcing nursing to confront changes related to interstate nursing practice. Globalization has had a similar impact on migration (Fernandez & Hebert, 2004). This migration phenomenon supports the need for an international credentialing of immigrant nurses to ensure public safety as defined by the International Council of Nurses (Schaefer, 1990).

> New models for practice will continue to emerge to manage change, care, and plan for the future. Electronic technologies provide an opportunity to develop a new identity for nursing practice. New regulatory requirements will emerge to meet the need of practitioners to ensure public safety. As a new paradigm for ensuring competencies and self-regulation in a global market evolves, the need to explore global licensure will emerge. The future belongs to those who will accept the challenge to make a difference in a global marketplace and take the necessary risks to make things happen. (Fernandez & Hebert, 2004, p. 132)

The Global Alliance for Leadership in Nursing Education (GANES, 2011) is a nursing organization that focuses on getting nurse educators from around the world to work together to develop and facilitate nursing education and research in order to improve care globally. These new efforts to recognize the need for international standards in nursing education and regulation represent a significant step; nursing has moved from a focus on individual hospitals, to the state level, to the national level, and now to a global level.

Landscape © f9photos/Shutterstock, Inc.

CONCLUSION

This chapter has described critical issues related to nursing education, accreditation of nursing education programs, and regulation and nursing practice. All these elements interact to better ensure quality patient care, from education to practice.

Landscape © f9photos/Shutterstock, Inc.

CHAPTER HIGHLIGHTS

1. The evolution of nursing education influences how nursing is taught.
2. There is a need to improve nursing education to better meet patient care needs.
3. Different levels of nursing prelicensure education have different competencies and expectations, yet nurses at all levels take the same licensure examination.
4. Accreditation of nursing programs ensures quality education.
5. Licensure and the regulation of nursing practice set standards and rules for nursing education.
6. Examples of critical concerns related to education, regulation, and practice are compact licensure, mandatory overtime, and global migration of nurses.

Landscape © f9photos/Shutterstock, Inc.

DISCUSSION QUESTIONS

1. Why do you think it is important that nursing now emphasizes education over training? Consider Donahue's definitions for education and training found in the chapter.

2. Compare and contrast the types of entry programs in nursing: diploma, ADN, BSN, and accelerated or direct entry programs.

3. Select one of the following graduate nursing programs (master's—any type; DNP or PhD) and find, through the Internet, two different universities that offer the program. Compare and contrast admission requirements and the curricula.

4. Visit the NCLEX website (https://www.ncsbn.org/nclex.htm). Review the "Candidates" section and describe the exam process and what happens on exam day. Go to https://www.ncsbn.org/1287.htm and review the current NCLEX-RN detailed test plan for candidates. Which type of information is included in the plan? How might this information help you, both now and closer to the time when you take the NCLEX?

5. Does your state participate in the nurse licensure compact? Visit https://www.ncsbn.org/158.htm to find out. Why might this be important to you when you become licensed in your state after graduation?

Landscape © f9photos/Shutterstock, Inc.

CRITICAL THINKING ACTIVITIES

1. Conduct a debate in class with one other classmate. Take the side of diploma, associate degree, or both levels of entry into practice, with the other classmate supporting the BSN as the entry into practice level. The class should then vote on the side that presents the best support for one of the perspectives. You will need to research your issue and present a substantiated rationale for your side of the issue.

2. Conduct a debate in class with one other classmate. Take the side supporting the PhD in nursing, with the other classmate supporting the DNP. The class should then vote on the side that presents the best support for one of the perspectives. You will need to research your issue and present a substantiated rationale for your side of the issue.

Circuit Board: ©Photos.com

ELECTRONIC Reflection Journal

The NLN published an article discussing the future of nursing education (by Heller, Oros, and Durney-Crowley; the article can be accessed at http://www.nln.org/nlnjournal/infotrends.htm). Ten trends are discussed in this article. Review the trends, which are all associated with healthcare delivery, and then consider their implications for nursing. In your self-reflection activity for this chapter, describe what you think about each one. Save this reflection and return to it at the end of your nursing program. Then save it and check it again in 5 and 10 years: Were the predictions right? What has changed?

Landscape © f9photos/Shutterstock, Inc.

LINKING TO THE INTERNET

- American Academy of Nurse Practitioners (AANP): http://www.aanp.org
- American Association of Colleges of Nursing (AACN): http://www.aacn.nche.edu
- American Association of Nurse Anesthetists (AANA): http://www.aana.com/
- American College of Nurse Midwives: http://www.midwife.org
- American Nurses Association (ANA): http://nursingworld.org
- Commission on Graduates of Foreign Nursing Schools (CGFNS): http://www.cgfns.org
- National Association of Clinical Nurse Specialists (NACNS): http://www.nacns.org
- National Council of State Boards of Nursing (NCSBN): http://www.ncsbn.org
- National Council of State Boards of Nursing, NCLEX Exam: https://www.ncsbn.org/nclex.htm
- National League for Nursing (NLN), National Council of State Boards of Nursing Residency Program: https://www.ncsbn.org/441.htm

CASE STUDIES

Landscape © f9photos/Shutterstock, Inc.

Case Study 1

The Student Nurses' Association (SNA) executive committee in your school is meeting to plan a program for the membership. A lively discussion is going on to select the topic. One board member mentions the need to have a program about nursing education accreditation because the school will have an accreditation survey visit next semester. The SNA chapter president speaks up and says, "Many of us are getting ready to take NCLEX, and we have many questions about licensure." Both of these topics are important topics. Consider the questions that follow.

Case Questions

1. Which topic would you choose and why?
2. If someone said to you, "Accreditation is the business of the faculty," what would you say?
3. Which type of content might you include in the content for a program on accreditation and a program on licensure for your membership?
4. What are the short-term and long-term issues related to licensure that would be important to consider by every nurse?

CASE STUDIES (CONTINUED)

Case Study 2

Nursing education and the profession in general have experienced a very long disagreement about the appropriate entry-level degree for nursing. This debate first emerged in 1965, as noted in this chapter. In addition, studies supporting the BSN as the entry-level degree have been identified by authors such as by Kutney-Lee, Sloane, and Aiken (2013). A response was made to this study by Cynthia Maskey, PhD, RN, CNE, in the March 2013 issue of *Health Affairs*. Dr. Maskey also is quoted on the N-OADN website, and she is an N-OADN board member. The following are her comments:

At a point in time when national nursing leaders in both education and practice are working together to support and recognize the contributions of nurses at all educational levels, Dr. Aiken and her colleagues are releasing a study that is focused on problems rather than solutions. True leaders in nursing are focused on the future by encouraging their nursing colleagues to practice to the full extent of their education to improve the care of patients. Nursing leaders assist their colleagues in education and practice to achieve higher levels of education through deliberative academic progression, as was set forth in the report from the Institute of Medicine referenced by Dr. Aiken and her colleagues. The authors' focus on nursing education level as the single variable related to surgical patient mortality is too simplistic within Pennsylvania's complex health care delivery system, but it is also divisive within the nursing community. This study—conducted in a single state using a retrospective design with the admitted underlying assumptions with only two data collection points and selected nursing variables—asks the reader to concur that the researchers chose an accurate research model and did not omit or were able to control for all other intervening variables. This reader is left with questions related to the variables of surgeon qualifications, patient comorbidities, and overall hospital quality standards, among others. This is a retrospective, two-panel study with many intervening variables for which no statistical procedures can control within the complexity of the health care environment.

This particular study design does not support the conclusion of causation between educational level and patient mortality and regretfully resurrects old debates at a time when nurse leaders needs to be focused on collaboration, innovation, and academic progression at all levels. It is antithetical to the spirit and intent of the Institute of Medicine report, which is to advance a highly proficient, well-educated nursing workforce from associate degree and baccalaureate programs, with the goal of exceptional patient outcomes. (National Organization for Associate Degree Nursing, 2013)

Go to the website for *Health Affairs* at http://content.healthaffairs.org/content/32/3/579/reply#healthaff_el_476350 to read the full debate.

Case Questions

After reading these articles, consider the following questions.

1. What is your view of the entry-level disagreement?
2. Does it surprise you that this issue is a cause for disagreement? If so, why does it surprise you?
3. What is your opinion of the response from the ADN perspective?
4. What are the possible negative results from such a disagreement in the profession?

Words of Wisdom

Joy R. O'Rourke, BSN, RN, Norman, Oklahoma

Nursing school taught me essential clinical skills to care for clients as an LPN. At this level of education, we are taught how to give quality health care. I decided to continue my education in an LPN-BSN program to learn in more depth about why things are done a certain way. I was delighted to learn this program focuses on holistic care as well as the leadership skills needed to work effectively as a team. It is imperative to function as a team when caring for members of the community. The healthcare field is constantly changing. We as nurses must strive to reach our full potential to keep up with these changes. Nursing is an exciting and rewarding field with new things to learn every day.

My Journey from LPN to BSN

Sherri Jones, LPN

New Directions/Geriatric Psychiatric Unit, McCurtain Memorial Hospital

Idabel, Oklahoma

Student in LPN-to-BSN Program

During LPN school, I felt at times if I could just survive the year, that was as far as I cared to excel in my nursing education. After my first year working as an LPN on a medical/surgical unit, I realized the importance of continuing to the RN level, but was uncertain whether to go for my AD [associate degree] or BSN. The University of Oklahoma College of Nursing LPN-BSN program allows me to obtain my BSN in about the same time frame as the local associate degree program. I believe the more credentialed a nurse is, the more employable, and the more amplified the nurse's voice becomes when areas in the workplace perhaps need to be changed/modified. It was not an easy decision, because most LPNs choose the local ADN program, and I was intimidated about stepping out on my own. (It did not help that a local college counselor tried to discourage me and told me, "You're flying by the seat of your pants.") Thanks to the kind words and encouragement from another LPN in this program, my decision was made, and I have absolutely loved the LPN-BSN program. The most awesome thing about being a nurse is the fact that going to work does not feel like a burden, but more like a privilege that has been entrusted to me. The only downside to nursing is the nursing shortage, which can affect quality of time spent in patient care.

Lessons Learned the Hard Way

Francene Weatherby, PhD, RNC

Professor

University of Oklahoma College of Nursing

Member of the Oklahoma Board of Nursing

1. **The license belongs to me (the nurse) to safeguard … not to the doctor or the supervisor or the RN.**

I've learned that this is a difficult concept for some people to acknowledge. New graduates, those individuals who are quick to try to shift responsibility to others, and those individuals who don't think critically but simply react reflexively to an order have particular difficulty with this idea.

Words of Wisdom *(continued)*

© Roobcio/Shutterstock, Inc.

Example: A new nurse practitioner, educated in Texas, took her first position in a hospital in Oklahoma. The nurse practitioner was told by a physician that she did not need a Drug Enforcement Agency number for prescribing narcotics. Since he was her supervising physician, he said his Drug Enforcement Agency number would cover her. She didn't bother to check Oklahoma law regarding prescriptive authority. As a result, this nurse was required to take a course in nursing jurisprudence, a course in critical thinking, and a course in roles and responsibilities in prescribing controlled and dangerous substances, and pay a fine; she also received a reprimand in her file at the board of nursing.

2. Use equipment as the manufacturer intended it to be used.

"Necessity is the mother of invention" is a great saying if you're out of buttermilk for your cake and substitute whole milk with a little vinegar because you have both of these on hand. Invention is not always good in a hospital setting.

Example: A nurse mistakenly attached a nasogastric tube feeding of Crucial to a patient's triple-lumen, peripherally inserted central venous catheter. When the supervisor asked how this could possibly happen when feeding tubing is specifically designed not to fit into vascular tubing, three important errors were discovered: (1) The nurse was hanging a feeding prepared by a second nurse. The second nurse could not find any feeding tubing, so to save time and avoid delaying the patient's feeding, she substituted IV tubing in the tube feeding setup. (2) The first nurse did not know what Crucial was. (3) The first nurse did not check the orders or ask for clarification, but simply went in and attached the tubing to patient. Thereafter, the patient died.

3. The function of the board of nursing is to protect the public, not to protect the nurse.

This is perhaps one of the most difficult lessons a nurse who is serving on the board of nursing has to learn. Too often after hearing a case, the "nurse's cap" takes over and the board member begins to rationalize the nurse's actions—maybe the shift was extremely busy, maybe there were lots of new admissions that night, maybe the staffing was short, or maybe there were two critical patients down the hall. We're all too familiar with the many possibilities. But the bottom line is that each and every patient deserves and must be assured of receiving the best possible nursing care. This is one of the major criteria of a profession—that the members regulate their own. The public trusts us to carry out this monitoring and take corrective actions when patient safety is violated. I don't think all nurses really appreciate this fact.

Example: A nurse was caring for a patient with diabetes in a long-term care facility. She obtained finger stick blood sugar readings as follows: at 8:30 p.m. it was 535; at 8:45 p.m. it was 539; and at 9:15 p.m.it was 542. At 9:30 p.m., she reported the patient's status to one of the oncoming nurses. At 10:30 p.m., the blood sugar reading was 39. An ambulance was called, the nursing director was notified, and the patient was taken to the hospital and later died of hypoglycemic shock. The nurse responded that the wrong time was noted on the chart because the clock on the wall was 1 hour off. She indicated she had given the patient orange juice and sugar but didn't have the patient's chart with her, so she didn't write it down. The nurse surrendered her license and received a fine.

(continues)

Words of Wisdom (*continued*)

© Roobcio/Shutterstock, Inc.

4. It's great to be a patient advocate, but advocacy has to be done according to protocol.

There's a right way to do things, and there's a wrong way to do things. All nursing students learn early in their nursing school days that an important role of the nurse is to be a patient advocate. No nurse would deny this critical role. However, how to go about being an advocate is not often made clear. It's important to remember that there is a chain of command in reporting to follow, and there are facility policies and procedures to which the nurse must adhere or go through the proper steps to change. In an effort to take action as quickly as possible on the patient's behalf, these steps are often brushed aside for the nobler goal. When something goes wrong in the process, the nurse often finds herself out on a limb with no legal defense.

Example: A nurse working in a nursing home discovered gross neglect regarding wound care a particular patient was receiving. She discussed this situation with her supervisor, who commented that he remembered a similar case when he was in nursing school. The solution in that case had been to irrigate the decubitus ulcer with hydrogen peroxide (a wound care practice no longer recommended).

After 2 days off, the nurse returned on the night shift to find the patient decubitus in even worse shape. She decided to irrigate the ulcer with hydrogen peroxide without a physician order and in the process found bits of old dressing deep within the wound. Outraged with this discovery, the nurse first called the physician to report the situation. Receiving no response from the doctor, she next called the patient's family and told them they needed to have the patient transferred to another facility right away. The daughter of the patient had the patient transferred in the middle of the night. The next morning, the physician was very disturbed the patient had been transferred and filed a complaint with the facility against the nurse for failing to follow facility protocol regarding patient transfer.

The facts and circumstances in all the previous examples have been changed and do not reflect exact cases heard by the board. Every case must be examined to determine what, if any, violation of the nursing practice act occurred and what discipline should or should not be imposed.

Landscape © f9photos/Shutterstock, Inc.

REFERENCES

Aiken, L., Clarke, S., Cheung, R., Sloane, D., & Silber, J. (2003). Educational levels of hospital nurses and surgical patient mortality. *Journal of the American Medical Association, 290*, 1617–1623.

Aiken, L. H., Sloane, D. M., Bruyneel, L., Van den Heede, K., Griffiths, P., Busse, R., ... Sermeus, W., for the RN4CAST consortium. (2014, February 15). Nurse staffing and edu-cation and hospital mortality in nine European countries: A retrospective observational study. *Lancet.* doi: 10.1016/S0140-6736(13)62631-8

American Association of Colleges of Nursing (AACN). (2004). AACN position statement on the practice doctorate in nursing. Retrieved from http://www.aacn.nche.edu/DNP/DNPPositionStatement.htm

American Association of Colleges of Nursing (AACN). (2005a, May 6). *AACN applauds decision of the AONE board to move registered nurse education to the baccalaureate level* (press release). Washington, DC: Author.

American Association of Colleges of Nursing (AACN). (2005b). Alliance for Nursing Accreditation statement on distance education policies. Retrieved from http://www.aacn.nche .edu/education/disstate.htm

American Association of Colleges of Nursing (AACN). (2005c). *Fact sheet: Articulation agreements among nursing education programs.* Washington, DC: Author.

American Association of Colleges of Nursing (AACN). (2006). *Essentials of doctoral education for advanced nursing practice.* Washington, DC: Author.

American Association of Colleges of Nursing (AACN). (2007). *White paper on the education and role for the clinical nurse leader.* Washington, DC: Author.

American Association of Colleges of Nursing (AACN). (2008). *The essentials of baccalaureate education for professional nursing practice.* Washington, DC: Author. Retrieved from http://www.aacn.nche.edu/Education/pdf/BaccEssentials98.pdf

American Association of Colleges of Nursing (AACN). (2011). *Essentials of masters education for nursing.* Washington, DC: Author.

American Association of Colleges of Nursing (AACN). (2013). FY2012–2014 strategic plan goals and objectives. Retrieved from http://www.aacn.nche.edu/about-aacn/ mission-values

American Association of Colleges of Nursing (AACN). (2014, January). Enrollment growth slows at U.S. nursing schools despite calls for a more highly educated workforce (press release). Retrieved from http://www.aacn.nche.edu/

American Association of Colleges of Nursing (AACN), American Organization of Nurse Executives (AONE), & National Organization for Associate Degree Nursing (N-OADN). (1995). *A model for differentiated nursing practice.* Washington, DC: Author.

American Nurses Association (ANA). (1965). Education for nursing. *American Journal of Nursing, 65*(12), 107–108.

American Nurses Association (ANA). (2010). *Nursing scope and standards of practice.* Silver Spring, MD: Author.

American Nurses Association. (ANA). (2011). ANA fact sheet. Retrieved from http://nursingworld.org/NursingbytheNumbersFactSheet.aspx

American Organization of Nurse Executives (AONE). (1990). *Current issues and perspectives of differentiated practice.* Chicago, IL: American Hospital Association.

Americans for Nursing Shortage Relief. (2007). *Assuring quality healthcare for the United States: Building and sustaining an infrastructure of qualified nurses for the nation* (consensus document). Arlington, VA: Author.

Benner, P., Sutphen, M., Leonard, V., & Day, L. (2010). *Educating nurses: A call for radical transformation.* San Francisco, CA: Jossey-Bass.

Ben-Zur, H., Yagi, D., & Spitzer, A. (1999). Evaluation of an innovative curriculum: Nursing education in the next century. *Journal of Advanced Nursing, 30,* 1432–1531.

Brown, E. (1948). *Nursing for the future: A report prepared for the National Nursing Council.* New York, NY: Russell Sage Foundation.

Commission on Graduates of Foreign Nursing Schools (CGFNS). (2007). CGFNS website. Retrieved from http:// www.cgfns.org/

Cronenwett, L., Dracup, K., Grey, M., McDauley, L., Meleis, A., & Salmon, M. (2011). The doctor of nursing practice: A national workforce perspective. *Nursing Outlook, 59*(1), 9–17.

Damgaard, G., VanderWoude, D., & Hegge, M. (1999). Perspectives from the prairie: The relationship between nursing regulation and South Dakota nursing work-force development. *Journal of Nursing Administration, 29*(11), 7–9, 14.

Donahue, M. (1983). Isabel Maitland Stewart's philosophy of education. *Nursing Research, 32,* 140–146.

Estabrooks, C., Midodzi, W., Cummings, G., Ricker, K., & Giovannetti, P. (2005). The impact of hospital nursing characteristics on 30-day mortality. *Nursing Research, 54*(2), 74–84.

Fernandez, R., & Hebert, G. (2004). Global licensure. New modalities of treatment and care require the development of new structures and systems to access care. *Nursing Administration Quarterly, 28,* 129–132.

Girard, N. J. (2003). Lack of sleep another safety risk factor (editorial—medical errors). *AORN Journal, 78,* 553–556.

Global Alliance for Leadership in Nursing Education (GANES). (2011). Welcome. Retrieved from http://www.ganes.info/ index.php

Goldmark, J. (1923). *Nursing and nursing education in the United States.* New York, NY: Macmillan.

Hutchins, G. (1994). Differentiated interdisciplinary practice. *Journal of Nursing Administration, 24*(6), 52–58.

Institute of Medicine (IOM). (2001). *Crossing the quality chasm: A new health system for the 21st century.* Washington, DC: National Academies Press.

Institute of Medicine (IOM). (2003). *Health professions education: A bridge to quality.* Washington, DC: National Academies Press.

Institute of Medicine (IOM). (2010). *The future of nursing: Leading change, advancing health.* Washington, DC: National Academies Press.

International Centre on Nurse Migration. (2007). ICNM website. Retrieved from http://www.intlnursemigration.org/

Knowles, M. (1975). *Self-directed learning: A guide for learners and teachers.* Chicago, IL: Follett.

Knowles, M. (1984). *Andagogy in action.* San Francisco, CA: Jossey-Bass.

Kutney-Lee, A., Sloane, D., & Aiken, L. (2013). An increase in the number of nurses with baccalaureate degrees is linking to lower rates to post surgery mortality. *Health Affairs 30*(3), 579–586.

Leighow, S. (1996). Backrubs vs Bach: Nursing and the entry-in-to-practice debate: 1946–1986. *Nursing History Review, 4,* 3–17.

Loquist, R. (2002). State boards of nursing respond to the nurse shortage. *Nursing Administration Quarterly, 26*(4), 33–39.

Lundy, K. (2005). A history of healthcare and nursing. In K. Masters (Ed.), *Role development in professional nursing practice* (Ch. 1). Sudbury, MA: Jones and Bartlett.

Manfredini, R., Boari, B., & Manfredini, F. (2006). Adverse events secondary to mistakes, excessive work hours, and sleep deprivation. *Archives of Internal Medicine, 166,* 1422–1433.

Masters, K. (2005). *Role development in professional nursing practice.* Sudbury, MA: Jones and Bartlett.

McHugh, M., & Lake, E. (2010). Nurse education, experience, and the hospital context. *Research in Nursing & Health, 33,* 276–287.

Montag, M. (1959). *Community college education for nursing: An experiment in technical education for nursing.* New York, NY: McGraw-Hill.

Montgomery, V. L. (2007). Effect of fatigue, workload, and environment on patient safety in the pediatric intensive care unit. *Pediatric Critical Care Medicine, 8*(suppl 2), S11–S16.

National Council of State Boards of Nursing (NCSBN). (1996). Why regulation paper: Public protection or professional self-preservation? Retrieved from https://www.ncsbn.org/why_regulation_paper.pdf

National Council of State Boards of Nursing (NCSBN). (2001). *Position statement: International Nurse Immigration.* Chicago, IL: Author.

National Council of State Boards of Nursing (NCSBN). (2005). Position paper: Clinical instruction in prelicensure nursing programs. Retrieved from http://www.ncsbn.org/pdfs/Final_Clinical_Instr_Pre_Nsg_programs.pdf

National Council of State Boards of Nursing (NCSBN). (2007). Guiding principles of nursing regulation. Retrieved from https://www.ncsbn.org/Guiding_Principles.pdf

National Council of State Boards of Nursing (NCSBN). (2013a). About NCSBN. Retrieved from https://www.ncsbn.org/about.htm

National Council of State Boards of Nursing (NCSBN). (2013b). APRN consensus model toolkit. Retrieved from https://www.ncsbn.org/2276.htm

National League for Nursing (NLN). (2003). *Position statement: Innovation in nursing education: A call to reform.* New York, NY: Author.

National League for Nursing (NLN). (2007a). Academy of Nursing Education. Retrieved from http://www.nln.org/excellence/academy/index.htm

National League for Nursing (NLN). (2007b, Summer). The National League for Nursing strategic plan for 2007–2012. *NLN Report, 1,* 1–12.

National League for Nursing (NLN). (2013a, June 25). NLN data show capacity shortages easing in nursing programs. Retrieved from http://www.nln.org/newsreleases/annual-survey_062513.htm

National League for Nursing (NLN). (2013b). Nursing programs. Retrieved from http://www.nln.org/researchgrants/slides/topic_nursing_programs.htm

National Organization for Associate Degree Nursing (N-OADN). (2013). N-OADN board member Cynthia Maskey, PhD, RN, CNE addresses *Health Affairs* (March 2013) article. Retrieved from https://www.noadn.org/news/n-oadn-responds-to-health-affairs-article.html

O'Shea, E. (2003). Self-directed learning in nurse education: A review of the literature. *Journal of Advanced Nursing, 43*(1), 62–70.

Reinert, B., & Fryback, P. (1997). Distance learning and nursing education. *Journal of Nursing Education, 36*(9), 421.

Rick, C. (2003). AONE's leadership exchange: Differentiated practice. Get beyond the fear factor. *Nursing Management, 34*(1), 11.

Schaefer, B. (1990). International credentials review: Crucial and complex. *Nursing Healthcare, 11,* 431–432.

Sigurdson, K., & Ayas, N.T. (2007). The public health and safety consequences of sleep disorders. *Canadian Journal of Physiology and Pharmacology, 85,* 179–183.

Tri-Council for Nursing. (2010). Tri-Council for Nursing issues new consensus policy statement on the educational advancement of registered nurses. Retrieved from http://www.tricouncilfornursing.org/

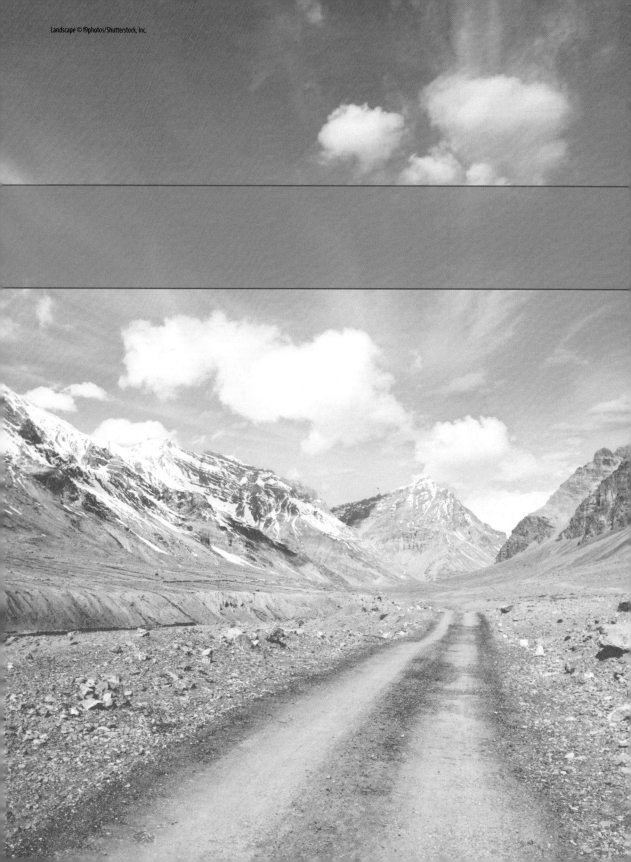

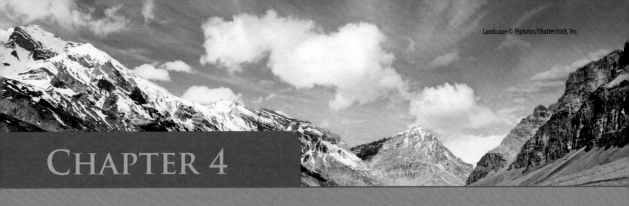

CHAPTER 4

Success in Your Nursing Education Program

CHAPTER OBJECTIVES

At the conclusion of this chapter, the learner will be able to:

- Discuss the differences in nursing education and other types of educational programs
- Describe the roles of the nursing student and faculty
- Assess one's own learning style
- Describe teaching–learning practices
- Apply tools for success in a nursing education program

- Explain the importance of lifelong learning
- Compare certification and credentialing
- Discuss the use of cooperative experience, internship/externship, and residency
- Examine the need for care of self and methods to support oneself as a student and as a nurse

KEY TERMS

Burnout	Internship/externship	Residency
Certification	Mentor	Simulation
Clinical experiences	Mentoring	Stress
Credentialing	Networking	Stress management
Compassion fatigue	Reality shock	Time management

INTRODUCTION

There is much work to do to become a professional nurse. The history of nursing indicates that the development of the profession and its education has been a long process. As you strive to reach your goal, you will find that the program of study is rigorous and not like other learning experiences you have had. This chapter focuses on each student and the experience of a nursing student—what it is and what you need to understand and do to be successful.

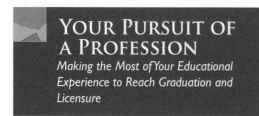

YOUR PURSUIT OF A PROFESSION
Making the Most of Your Educational Experience to Reach Graduation and Licensure

Beginning a nursing program is a serious decision. It means that you have chosen to become a professional RN. This text introduces you to the profession and provides an orientation to a variety of important material that will be covered in more depth in your future courses. One topic that needs to be addressed in the initial stages of your nursing education is how to make the most of the experience to reach your goal of graduation and licensure to practice as a professional RN and provide quality care. The following content discusses the roles of the student and faculty, tools for success, different teaching and learning practices used in nursing education,

opportunities to expand your experiences, and caring for self. This is all critical content—it may not be something you will be tested on, but the content provides some guidance to help you navigate through the nursing education process effectively. Nursing education will be different from other educational experiences that you have had. An important part of this experience is professional socialization, which is described as follows:

> [T]ransition into professional practice is characterized by the acquisition of the skills, knowledge, and behaviors needed to successfully function as a professional nurse. This process involves the new nurse's internalization of the values, attitudes, and goals that comprise his or her occupational identity. (Young, Stuenkel, & Bawel-Brinkley, 2008, p. 105)

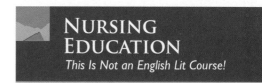

NURSING EDUCATION
This Is Not an English Lit Course!

Nursing education is different—different from other educational programs and courses. Students who enter a college- or university-based nursing program complete many courses in liberal arts and sciences as prerequisites to entering the full nursing curriculum. When they enter a nursing program, they arrive with certain expectations that are derived from their previous experiences. Students expect a didactic course similar to other courses they have taken, such as an English literature course. That is, they expect to go to the class, sit at their desk and listen, and then periodically turn in assignments and take exams. Recently, in some cases, students have taken some of these courses online.

Whether you take them in a face-to-face venue or online, nursing courses demand more. Much of the content relies on knowledge gained in previous courses and builds to subsequent courses. The expectation is that students will apply content from their previous courses to their current courses and to their clinical experiences. Learning becomes more of a continuum, as opposed to neat packages of content that can be filed away when a course ends. Understanding is more important than memorizing (though some memorization is required), and application of information becomes more important on exams and in practice.

In addition, many nursing courses include a clinical or practicum component, or they may have no didactic component and only a clinical focus. A student might think that these courses are equivalent to a chemistry lab, but this is not a fair comparison. A nursing clinical experience/practicum usually covers several hours per session and in some cases can require 8 to 12 hours several days each week. Students must prepare for these experiences and work these hours as students. Faculty are available to guide student learning, and in some situations, students are assigned to preceptors, who are nurses working in the healthcare organization. Students do their clinical work in a variety of clinical settings, such as hospitals, clinics, homes, and community settings. Such experiences are not equivalent to taking a 2-hour chemistry lab once a week. Some courses use a simulation laboratory, where students participate in a structured learning setting and practice skills and decision making in a simulated situation with faculty guidance.

As this description makes clear, nursing education is definitely not English lit! Nursing education is demanding and complex—but how did it get this way, and why is it this way?

ROLES OF THE STUDENT AND THE FACULTY

Non-nursing educational experiences are quite different from nursing educational experiences. Nursing education has two major components: didactic/theory- or content-focused experiences and clinical experiences. The latter is divided into laboratory or simulation experiences and experiences with patients in clinical settings. Throughout your nursing education, you need to assume a very active role in the learning process and to take responsibility for your own learning; this is not passive learning. Students who ask questions, read and critique, apply information even if it is risky, and are interested in working with others—not just patients and their families, but also fellow students and faculty—will be more successful. Students who wait to be told what to do and when to do it will not be as successful.

Nursing faculty facilitate student learning. This is done by developing course content and by using teaching–learning practices to assist the student in learning the required content and developing the required competencies. Faculty enhance learning situations in the simulation laboratory and in clinical settings by guiding students to practice and become competent in areas of care delivery. The best learning takes place when faculty and students work together and communicate about needs and expectations. Faculty members not only plan for a group of students, but also assess the learning needs of individual students and work with them to meet the course and program objectives or outcomes.

Becoming an RN involves more than just graduating from a nursing program. New graduates must pass the NCLEX, an examination that is not offered by the school of nursing but rather through the National Council of State Boards of Nursing and state boards of nursing. Throughout the nursing program, students may be offered opportunities to complete practice exams and receive feedback. In addition, course exam questions are typically written in the formats found in the NCLEX, such as application of knowledge questions rather than questions relating to memorized content. Becoming comfortable with this format is often difficult for new nursing students, because they are accustomed to taking exams in non-nursing courses that focus less on application and that do not build on knowledge gained from course to course. For example, in nursing you complete the anatomy and physiology course, and then you are expected to apply this information later when you take exams on clinical content. You learn about blood flow through the heart, and then, in conjunction with adult health content, you are expected to understand this content and apply it when providing care to a patient with a myocardial infarction (heart attack). Months or even a year may elapse between when you complete the anatomy and physiology course and when you take an adult health course or care for a patient with a myocardial infarction.

A critical key to success with faculty is communication: Ask questions, ask for explanation if confused, meet course requirements when due, and use the faculty as a resource to enhance learning.

STUDENT LEARNING STYLES

As you enter nursing courses, it is helpful for you to consider your own preferred learning style and to determine how your style might or might not be effective. If it is not effective, you may need to consider changes.

What does learning style mean? Learning style is a student's preferences for different types of learning and instructional activities. There are a variety of views of these styles. In doing a personal learning style self-assessment, you might apply Kolb's (1984) learning style inventory, which was further developed by Honey and Mumford (1986, 1992). Kolb described a continuum of four learning styles: (1) concrete experiences, (2) reflective observation, (3) abstract conceptualization, and (4) active experimentation. No person can be placed in only one style category, but most people have a predominant style (Kolb, 1984, as cited in Rassool & Rawaf, 2007, pp. 36–37):

- *Divergers*: Sensitive, imaginative, and people oriented; often enter professions such as nursing; excel in brainstorming sessions.
- *Assimilators*: Less focused on people and more interested in ideas and abstract concepts. Excel in organizing and presenting information; in formal education, prefer reading, lectures, exploring analytical models, and having time to think things through.
- *Convergers*: Solve problems and prefer technical tasks; less concerned with people and interpersonal aspects; often choose careers in technology. They excel in getting things done.
- *Accommodators*: People-oriented, active learners. Excel in concrete experience and active experimentation, and prefer to take a practical or experimental approach; attracted to new challenges and experiences; carry out plans.

Adapting Kolb's proposed styles, the following has been described as a variation by Rassool and Rawaf (2007):

- *Activists*: Having an experience. Focus on immediate experience; interested in here and now; like to initiate new challenges and be the center of attention.
- *Reflectors*: Reviewing the experience. Observers; prefer to analyze experiences before taking action; good listeners; cautious; tend to adopt a low profile.
- *Theorists*: Concluding from experience. Adopt a logical and rational approach to problem solving but need some structure with a clear purpose or goal; learning is

weakest when they do not understand the purpose, when activities are less structured, and when feelings are emphasized.

- *Pragmatists:* Planning the next steps. Like to try out new ideas and techniques to see if they work in practice; are practical and down to earth; like solving problems and making decisions.

Understanding your style can help you when you approach new content, read assignments, and participate in other learning activities. It can affect how easy or difficult the work may be for you. You may need to stretch—that is, to try to learn or do something that is challenging for you—and you may need to adapt your learning style.

TOOLS FOR SUCCESS

Organization and time management are very important tools for success in a nursing program. In the past, you may have gone to class for a few hours a day, but in nursing programs some courses meet once or several times a week for several hours. Some courses may be taught online, but require some attendance in a classroom setting—but maybe none. In addition, the clinical component of the program has a major impact on your schedule. You need to prepare for the clinical component and work this activity into your schedule to meet course requirements. Study skills and test-taking skills are critical. This educational experience will not be without some stress; thus, if you develop stress management skills to help you cope, you will find that the experience can be handled better. **Box 4-1** provides some links to websites with tools for student success.

Time Management

Time management is not difficult to define, but it is difficult to achieve. Learning how to manage time and requirements is also very important to effective nursing practice. Time management skills in

---

Box 4-1	Links for Student Success

Overcoming Procrastination:
http://ub-counseling.buffalo.edu/stressprocrast.shtml
Test-Taking Strategies:
http://www.d.umn.edu/kmc/student/loon/acad/strat/test_take.html
Tips and Strategies to Improve Your Test-Taking Skills:
http://www.collegetips.com/
Test-Taking Checklist:
http://www.d.umn.edu/kmc/student/loon/acad/strat/testcheck.html

---

school are not different from what is required for clinical work/practicum and after graduation in practice. **Figure 4-1** describes how to get started with time management.

There never is enough time, it seems, and no one can make more time, so it is best to figure out how to make the most of your available time. Everyone has felt unproductive or been guilty of squandering time. In simple terms, productivity is the ratio of inputs to outputs. What does a person put into a task or activity (resources such as time, energy, money, giving up doing something else, and so forth) that then leads to outcomes or results? For example, one student studies 12 hours for an exam and then gives up, going to a film with friends; another student studies 5 hours and goes to the same film. These two students put different levels of resources into exam preparation, and they get different results—the first student makes an A on the exam and the second a B. The second student then has to decide if it was worth it. Should more time be spent on studying for exams and the personal schedule arranged to allow for some fun, but after exams? Or is the B grade acceptable? The student with the A grade may decide too much time was spent on studying, was not

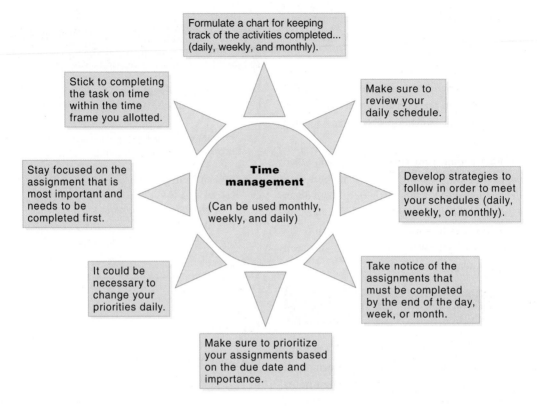

Figure 4-1 Getting Started With Time Management

Source: From Wilfong, D., Szolis, C., & Haus, C. (2007). *Nursing school success: Tools for constructing your future.* Sudbury, MA: Jones and Bartlett.

productive and could have been organized better to reduce study time. This more global perspective is certainly one aspect of time management, but time management also gets into the details of how one uses time to be efficient and effective, such as what the student with the A grade considered.

Time analysis is used to assess how one uses time. You might keep a log for a week and record all of your activities, including time spent on each activity and interruptions. If you commit to doing this, you need to be honest so that the data truly reflect your activities. After the data are collected, you then need to analyze the data using these questions:

- What were your activities, and how long did each take?
- Do you see a difference on certain days as to activities and time?

- What did you complete, and what did you not complete? Can you identify reasons for not completing a task or project?
- Did you set any priorities, and did you adhere to them?
- Which types of interruptions did you have? How many interruptions were really important and why?
- Did you procrastinate? Are there certain activities that you put off more than others? Why?
- Did you jump from one task to another?
- Look at your telephone calls, e-mails, texting, and so on. How did they affect your time management?
- Did you spend time getting ready to do a task, to communicate with others, and so on?

Was some of this required, or could it have been done more effectively?

- Did you take breaks? (Breaks are important.) How many breaks did you take, how long were they, and what did you do?
- Did you consult your calendar?
- Are there times during the day when you are more productive?

Nurses need to be able to plan their day's work and still be flexible because changes will occur. Ideally, they set priorities and follow through, evaluate how they use their time, and cut down on wasted time so that care can be delivered effectively and in a timely manner. They use communication effectively and prepare for procedures and other care delivery activities in an organized manner so that they are not running back and forth to get supplies and so on. They handle interruptions by determining what is important and what can wait. Your success in meeting these demands relates to your need to assess your own time management and learn time management skills.

Technology has made life easier and more organized in some respects, especially the use of computers, cell phones with multiple capabilities, tablets, e-mails, text messaging, and other communication media. However, these new resources can also interfere with time management. For example, you may stop what you are doing to answer an e-mail or a text message that just arrived, or you may spend so much time syncing all this technology that the work does not get done. Managing time today means managing personal technology, too.

Many people struggle with the same time management problems. Consider these examples and how they might apply to you:

- No planning—not using a calendar effectively or not using one
- Not setting goals and priorities, or having unclear goals and priorities
- Allowing too many interruptions
- Getting started without getting ready

- Inability to say, "No," often leading to over-commitment (the most common problem for many people)
- Inability to concentrate
- Insufficient rest, sleep, exercise, and unhealthy diet, making one feel perpetually tired
- High stress level
- Too much socializing when work needs to be done—not knowing how to find the right balance
- Ineffective use of communication tools, including overuse of e-mail, computer and Internet, cell phone, and so on
- Too much crisis management—waiting too long to act, so that then it is a crisis to get the work done
- Inability to break down large projects into small steps
- Wasting time—little tasks, procrastination

Other, more serious problems can have a major impact on time management. These difficulties arise when the student does not feel competent or does not know what is expected. Students often experience these problems, although they may not recognize them or want to admit them. Nevertheless, these feelings can lead to problems with time management as students struggle to feel better and/or try to figure out what they are supposed to do. If you experience one or both of these feelings, you need to talk to your faculty openly about your concerns. You are not expected to be perfect. The educational process is focused on helping you gradually build your competence. In some cases, perfectionism actually becomes a barrier to completing a task; you may fear that the task will not be completed perfectly, so you avoid the task or work on it longer than needed.

Benner (2001) described the experience of moving from novice to expert in nursing, which is a practice profession. Beginners or novices have no experience as nurses and, therefore, must gain clinical knowledge and expertise (competence) over time. A beginning student may enter a nursing program with some nursing care experience, such as nursing aide experience. That student may then be at a different novice level but still a novice. A graduate will not be an expert; this comes with time and experience. This change in status can be difficult for students who may have felt that they were competent in understanding the content after a course such as American history or introduction to sociology. Nursing competency, however, is developed over time. Each course and its content are relevant to subsequent courses. There is no neat packaging that allows one to say, "I have mastered all there is to know about nursing."

Another component of time management is setting clear goals and priorities. This helps to organize your time and focus your activities. You need to consider what is needed now and what is needed later. This is not always advice that is easy to follow; sometimes a student might prefer to work on a task that is not due for a while, avoiding work that needs to be done sooner. Sometimes writing down goals and priorities and putting them where they can be seen helps to center time management. Delegation plays a major role in health care and is related to time management. One of the key issues when prioritizing is determining who should complete the task. Perhaps someone else is a better choice to complete the task; in this case, the task may be delegated.

Tasks and activities can be dissected. Consider what the needs of the task are, when it is due, how long it will take, how critical it is, what impact it will have, and what the consequences will be if it is postponed or not completed. Large projects are best broken into smaller parts or steps. For example, the preparation of a major paper should be broken into a series of tasks, such as identifying the topic or problem, working with a team (if writing the paper is a team assignment), completing the research for the paper, writing the paper (which should begin with an outline), reviewing and editing, and polishing the final draft. Building in deadlines for the steps will help ensure that the final due date is met. Many large papers or projects in nursing courses cannot be

completed overnight. They may require active learning, such as interviews, assessments, and other types of activities. A presentation may need to be developed after the paper is written or a poster designed. Often this type of work is done with a team of students, which is important because nurses work on teams. Such group efforts take more time because team members have to learn to work together, develop a teamwork plan, and meet if necessary. Some team assignments are now done "virtually," through online activities in which students never physically meet at the same time. Getting prepared for the clinical experience/practicum is also a larger task that will be described later in this chapter. All this takes organization.

Some strategies for improving time management that you might consider include the following:

- Use a calendar or electronic method for a calendar; update it as needed.
- Decrease socializing at certain times to improve production.
- Limit use of your cell phone, text messaging, and e-mail during key times.
- Identify typical interruptions and control them.
- Anticipate—flexibility is necessary because something can happen that will disturb the plan.
- Determine the best time to read, study, prepare for an exam, write papers, and so on. Some people do better in early morning; others are more effective late at night. Know what works best for you.
- Work in blocks of time, minimizing interruptions.
- Develop methods for note taking and organizing learning materials to decrease the need to hunt for these materials.
- Conquer procrastination. Try dividing tasks into smaller parts to get a project done.
- Come prepared to class, clinical laboratory, and clinical settings. Preparation means that less time will be spent figuring out what needs to be done.

- Do not use electronic communication during class for non-class-related interaction.
- Do the right thing right, working effectively and efficiently.
- Develop a daily time management plan (see **Figure 4-2**).
- Remember that time management is not a static process, but rather a dynamic one; your time management needs will change.
- Organize your electronic course files so that they are easy to use.

Study Skills

Study skills are developed over time; however, this does not mean that these skills cannot always be improved. This is the time to review your study skills and determine what can be done to improve them. Typical components of study skills are reading, using class time effectively, preparing written assignments and team projects, and preparing for discussions and other in class learning activities, quizzes, and exams. In nursing, clinical preparation is also a key area.

Preparation

Students need to prepare for class, whether it is a face-to-face class, a seminar, or an online course. The first issue is what to prepare. The guide for this is the focus of the experience and its objectives/learning outcomes. Use the course syllabus and other course materials as a guide to the course and the expectations of students. The format—for example, a class session with 60 students versus a seminar with 10 students—also influences preparation. The latter is an experience in which the student will undoubtedly be expected to respond to questions and discuss issues. The larger class may vary; it could be a straight lecture, with little participation expected, or it could include participation requiring preparation. You need to be clear about the course expectations. If the course syllabus or other course materials do not provide clear explanations, you are responsible for asking about expectations or seeking clarification of confusing expectations. You then need to complete any work that is expected prior to the class or the learning experience to improve your learning.

DAILY TIME MANAGEMENT WORKSHEET

Primary Task	Projected Start Time	Projected Finish Time	Actual Time Taken to Complete Task

Secondary Task

Figure 4-2 Daily Time Management Worksheet

Source: From Wilfong, D., Szolis, C., & Haus, C. (2007). *Nursing school success: Tools for constructing your future.* Sudbury, MA: Jones and Bartlett.

Reading

There is much reading to do in a nursing program, ranging from textbooks and published articles to Internet resources and handout materials that faculty may provide. It is very easy to become overwhelmed by these materials. Explore the textbook(s) for the course from front to back. Sometimes students do not realize that a textbook has a valuable glossary or appendix that could help them. Review the table of contents to become familiar with the content. Some faculty may assign specific pages rather than entire chapters, so making note of the details of a reading assignment is critical. Review a chapter to become familiar with its structure. Typically, there are objectives and key terms; content divided into sections; additional elements, such as exhibits, figures, and boxed information; and finally the summary, learning activities, and references. Increasing numbers of textbooks have an affiliated website that offers additional information.

Some books are now published as e-books, which are highly interactive and can be downloaded to computers and tablets, smartphones, and so on. E-books typically enable you to highlight material, take notes, and search for content in the text. Often these books also have companion websites that provide additional student resources and learning activities. These trends are likely to continue.

Yes, this is all overwhelming, and where does one begin? Reading focuses on four goals:

- Learning information for recall is memorizing. This is important for some content, but if it is the only focus of reading, you will not be able to apply the information and build on learning.
- Comprehension of general principles, facts, and examples.
- Critical evaluation of the content. Ask questions and challenge the content. Does it make sense?
- Application of content, which is critical in nursing because nursing is a practice-oriented profession. For example, at some point you

will take a course that focuses on maternal–child content; later, you will be expected to apply that content in a clinical pediatric unit.

As noted in the previous section on time management, time is precious. The student who is trying to develop more effective reading skills should not waste time reading ineffectively, but rather should accomplish specific goals in a timely manner. The following are some tips to use in tackling a chapter that looks long and complex:

- Take a quick look at the chapter elements— objectives, terms, and major headers—and compare them with the course content expectations. Pay particular attention to the chapter outline, if there is one, and to the summary, conclusions, and/or key points at the end of the chapter.
- Read through the chapter not for details, but to get a general idea of the content.
- Go back and use a marker to highlight key concepts, terms, and ideas. Some students over-mark material, if this is done first. Using different colors for different levels of content may be useful for some students. You will need to go back and study the content; just highlighting is not studying.
- Note exhibits, figures, and boxes. (This is when it is important to check the reading assignment. Does it specify pages or content to read or ignore?)
- Some students make notes in the margins, highlight key points, and so on.
- E-books often provide features such as highlighting, the ability to add notes, and search capabilities.

Figures 4-3 and **4-4** illustrate two different formats for organizing notes from readings (if notes are taken). The format in Figure 4-3 can also be used to take notes in class.

Using Class Time Effectively

Attending any class can be a positive or negative learning experience. Preparation is important. In addition,

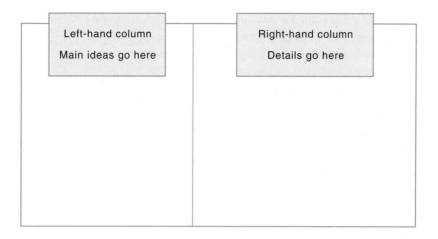

Figure 4-3 Taking Two-Column Notes

Source: From Wilfong, D., Szolis, C., & Haus, C. (2007). *Nursing school success: Tools for constructing your future.* Sudbury, MA: Jones and Bartlett.

how you approach the class is important. If you have trouble concentrating, sitting in the back of the room may not be the best approach. Sitting with friends can be helpful, but if it means you cannot concentrate, alternatives need to be considered. It is difficult to disconnect from other issues and problems, but class time is not the place to focus on them. One of the most common issues in class involves students who use class time to prepare for another class—working on assignments, studying for an exam, and so on. In the end, the learning experience on both ends is less effective. Students waste their time if they come to class without completing the reading, analyzing the content, or preparing assignments.

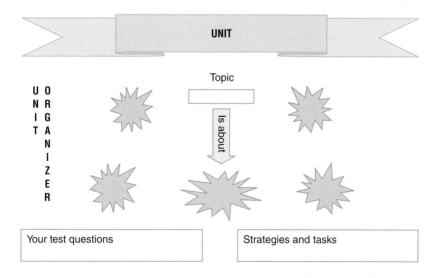

Figure 4-4 Unit Organizer

Source: From Wilfong, D., Szolis, C., & Haus, C. (2007). *Nursing school success: Tools for constructing your future.* Sudbury, MA: Jones and Bartlett.

Another element of preparation for class and other learning experiences involves bringing needed resources, such as the textbook, a notebook, assignments, and so on. In some schools, laptops and tablets may be used, so planning for access if the battery runs out is important. Learning will be compromised if a student uses electronic equipment such as a laptop, tablet, or smartphone for purposes that do not involve course content. Today, tablets are used more frequently in the classroom and for studying. Student options with tablets have expanded with the development of apps and pens for tablet writing. If you choose to use these options, research carefully what is available and how it might provide support for your learning. Make sure you know how to use the new options prior to using them in a course. The Internet includes a lot of information and reviews of apps.

If a course has face-to-face sessions, taking notes is important. Figures 4-3 and 4-4 illustrate two methods for organizing notes. It is critical to find a note-taking strategy that works for you. Some students may be visual learners, in which case they may draw figures, charts, concept maps, and so on to help them remember something—for example, using a tablet with a stylus pen to make sketch figures. Going back and reviewing notes soon after a class session will help you remember items that may need to be added and to recall information over the long term. As notes are taken in class, include comments from faculty that begin with "This is important," "You might want to remember this," and similar indicators of the material's importance. Questions that faculty might ask should be noted.

It is easy to get addicted to PowerPoint slide presentations and think that if you have these available in a handout, learning has taken place. In reality, this presentation content is only part of the content that nursing students are expected to learn. Students need to pay attention to content found in reading assignments, research, written assignments, and clinical experiences. Online courses also may include PowerPoint slide presentations, and some may have audio components.

Using the Internet

The Internet has become a critical tool in the world today. As students increasingly turn to the Internet to get information, it is important that reputable websites are used. Government sites are always appropriate sources, and professional organization sites also have valuable and appropriate information. Identify who sponsors the site. Bias is always a concern; for example, the site for a pharmaceutical company will inevitably praise that company's own products. Wikipedia is not considered a scholarly resource for references. When using a site, check when it was last updated. Sites that are not updated regularly have a greater chance of including outdated information.

In addition, the Internet is now used frequently for literature searches, usually through university libraries that offer online access to publications. Students need to learn about the resources available to them through their school libraries. It is important to properly attribute the source for content taken from the Internet for an assignment, using the correct citation format.

Preparing Written Assignments and Team Projects

The critical first step for any assignment is to understand the assignment—what is expected. What are the evaluation rubrics? You then complete the assignment based on those expectations. If the assignment describes specific areas to cover in a paper, this should be an important part of the outline for the paper—and these areas may even be used as key headers in the paper. If you have questions about the assignment, you should ask ahead of time.

For some assignments, students select their topics. If possible, selecting a topic similar to one used for a different assignment might save some time, but this does not mean that the student may submit an assignment that was done for another course. Plagiarism and submitting the same paper or assignment for more than one course are not acceptable. You need to be aware of your school's honor code.

Correct grammar, spelling, writing style, and citation format are critical for every written assignment. Nurses need to know how to communicate both orally and in written form.

Some assignments will require that you work with a team or group of students. Some students do not like these kinds of project, but the experiences provide a great opportunity to learn about working on teams, which is important in nursing. Teamwork requires clear communication among members and an understanding of the expectations for the work that the team needs to do. Effective teams spend time organizing their work and determining how they will communicate with one another. Conflicts may occur, and these need to be dealt with early. If the team must document its work and evaluate peer members, this must be done honestly, with appropriate feedback and comments about the work. Such evaluations are not easy to do.

To complete the team project successfully, the team must decide how to do the assignment, which might involve analysis of a case, writing a paper, developing a poster, a presentation or an educational program, or another type of activity. Having a clear plan of what needs to be done, by whom, and when will help guide the work and decrease conflict. Everyone is busy, and preventing conflicts and miscommunication will decrease the amount of time needed to do the work. If serious problems arise with communication or equality in workload that the team cannot resolve, faculty should be consulted for guidance.

Preparing for and Taking Quizzes and Exams

Quizzes and exams are inevitable parts of nursing education. Students who routinely prepare for them will experience less pressure at quiz or exam time—but this takes discipline. Building reviews into your study time, even if a review lasts for only a short period, does make a difference.

As is true for any aspect of a learning experience, knowing what is expected comes first during quiz and exam preparation. Which content will be covered in a specific quiz or exam? Which types of questions are expected, and how many? Exams in nursing typically use multiple-choice, true or false, essay, and some fill-in-the-blank questions, although the most common format is multiple choice. The first quiz or exam is always the hardest, as students get to know the faculty and the style of questions. Some faculty may provide a review guide, which should always be used.

Before a major exam, getting enough rest is an important aspect of preparation. Fatigue and sleep deprivation interfere with functioning—reading, thinking, managing time during the exam, clinical practice, and so on. Eating is also important. Students usually know how they respond if they eat too little or too much before an exam.

One aspect of nursing exams that seems to create problems for new students is the use of application questions. Preparing for a nursing exam by just memorizing facts will not lead to a positive result. You do need to know factual information, but you must also know how to use that information in examples.

Another common exam-taking problem is the inability to understand the multiple-choice question and its possible answers. Students may skip over words and think something is included in the question that is not. They may not be able to define all the words in the question and may not identify the key words. Reading the question and the choices carefully will make a difference. You should identify the key words and define them. If you do not know the answer to a question, you should narrow the choices by eliminating answers that you do understand or think might be wrong. Then, you should look for qualifiers such as "always," "all," "never," "every," and "none" because these may indicate that the answer is not correct. **Figure 4-5** describes a system for preparing for multiple-choice exams.

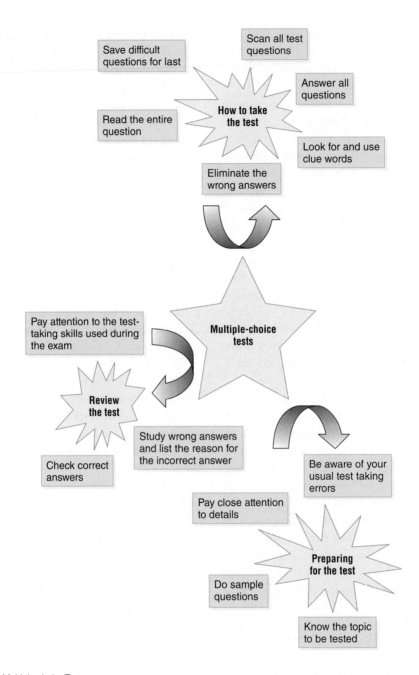

Figure 4-5 Multiple-choice Tests

Source: From Wilfong, D., Szolis, C., & Haus, C. (2007). *Nursing school success: Tools for constructing your future.* Sudbury, MA: Jones and Bartlett.

Essay questions require different preparation and skills. You need to have a greater in-depth understanding of the content to respond to an essay question. Some questions may ask for opinions. In all cases, it is important that your answer is clear and concise, provides rationales, includes content relevant to the question and to the material covered in the course, and presents the response in an organized manner. Sometimes the exam directions may provide guidelines as to the length of response expected, but in many cases, this must be judged according to what is required to answer the question. The amount of space provided on the exam may be a good indication. Grammar, spelling, and writing style are also important. Jotting down a quick outline will help in focusing your response and managing your time during the exam. It is important for you to review the essay response to make sure the question (or questions) has been answered. As is true for all types of exams, you must pace yourself based on the allotted time for essay questions. Spending a lot of time on questions that may be difficult is unwise. You can return to difficult questions and should keep this tactic in mind when managing time during the exam.

Study skills also include organizing. Retaining information from one course to another is important. Nursing education does not come in tidy little packages that one closes up and packs away before moving on to the next package. Instead, learning flows from one course to another, and students need to build on their knowledge and competencies and return to past information. Performance improvement and growth are the goals.

Networking and Mentoring

Professional nurses use networking and mentoring to develop themselves and to help peers. Consequently, you need to understand what these concepts are and begin to work toward using networking and mentoring.

Networking is a strategy that involves using any contact that might be helpful. Applying the networking strategy effectively is a skill that takes time to develop. Going to professional meetings offers opportunities to network. You can also begin to network in student organization activities, whether local, statewide, or national. Networking allows a person to meet and communicate with a wide variety of people, exchange ideas, explore new approaches, and obtain information that might be useful. Some of the networking skills that are important are meeting new people, approaching an admired person, learning how to start a conversation and keep it going, remembering names, asking for contact information, and sharing, because networking works both ways. Networking can take place anywhere: in school, in a work setting, at a professional meeting or during organizational activities, and in social situations. It can even happen online through the use of social networking media such as LinkedIn, Facebook, and Twitter.

Mentoring is a career development tool. A mentor–mentee relationship cannot be assigned or forced. A **mentor** is a role model and a career advisor. The mentee has to feel comfortable with the mentor and usually chooses the mentor. The mentor, of course, must agree to be part of this relationship. A mentorship can be short term or long term. It does take some time to develop the mentor–mentee relationship. Today, such a relationship could occur virtually.

When entering a nursing education program, you might think about acquiring a mentor, yet not know when a possible mentor might be met. Keep your eye out for possible future mentors. The mentor may be a nurse who works in an area where the student has clinical experience/practicum. New graduates can benefit from a mentorship relationship to help guide them in early career decisions; mentors can give them constructive feedback about their strengths and limitations and suggest improvement strategies. The mentor does not make decisions for the mentee, but rather serves as a sounding board to discuss options and allow the mentee to benefit from the mentor's expertise. In this way, the mentor acts as a guide and a teacher. An effective mentor has the following characteristics:

- Expert in an area related to the mentee's needs and interests
- Honest and trustworthy
- Professional
- Supportive
- Effective communicator
- Teacher and motivator
- Respected and influential
- Accessible

The mentor should not have a formal relationship, such as a supervisory or managerial relationship, with the mentee. Such a linkage could cause stress and not allow the mentor and mentee to communicate openly without concern about possible repercussions. However, there may come a time when a past supervisor becomes a mentor to a former employee.

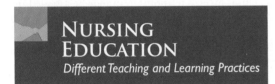

NURSING EDUCATION
Different Teaching and Learning Practices

As a new student begins a nursing program, it usually quickly becomes clear that nursing programs are different from past learning experiences. Competencies need to be developed to provide quality care to patients, families, communities, and populations. Nursing education not only uses traditional didactic learning experiences, which may be offered through face-to-face classes or seminars or online, but also depends greatly on practice in the clinical laboratory using simulation and in clinical settings with patients. What does this mean to you as a student?

Clinical Laboratory and Simulation Learning

Schools of nursing use a variety of methods for teaching clinical competencies. A competency is

an expected behavior that you must demonstrate. Two methods of developing clinical competencies that have become common in nursing education are the clinical laboratory (lab) and **simulation** learning, which is often combined with the lab experience. The simulation lab is a learning environment that is configured to look like a hospital or other type of clinical setting. It may take the form of a hospital room, a room with multiple beds, or a specialty room such as a procedure room or operating room. It contains the same equipment and supplies that are used in a healthcare setting, typically a hospital. Some schools have a simulation area that looks like a patient's home so that students can practice home care prior to an actual home care visit. The clinical lab is typically not configured to replicate a clinical setting in the same way that a simulation is, although it will have some of the same equipment. Some schools have only one type of lab—that is, a lab for using basic skills, with less opportunity for more complex learning in a simulated environment.

Students are assigned specific times in the lab as part of a course. Some didactic content might be delivered prior to the lab experience. Students are expected to come to the lab prepared (for example, having completed a reading assignment, viewed a video, or completed online learning activities). Preparation makes the lab time more effective, and well-prepared students will be able to practice applying what they have learned. To succeed in this setting, students need to be motivated and self-directed learners. (This is true for any learning experience in the nursing program.) Schools have different guidelines about dress and behavior in the lab. In some schools, the lab is treated as if it were an actual clinical setting/agency with certain dress and behavior expectations, such as wearing the school uniform or a lab coat and meeting all other uniform requirements related to appearance and professional behavior in the clinical setting.

What does the student learn in the lab? Most procedures and related competencies can be taught in a lab, such as health assessment, wound care, catheterization, medication administration, enema, general hygiene, and much more. Complex care may also be practiced in the lab setting using teams of students.

Simulation is an effective method to develop clinical competency. Practice is important, but guided practice is even more important, and ideally this should be risk free. Practicing on a real patient always carries a risk. It is not realistic to expect that a student will be able to provide care without some degree of harm potential the first time such care is given. For this reason, practicing in a setting without a real patient allows students to develop competence and gain self-confidence.

Simulation is "replication of clinical experiences in a safe environment as part of a student's education" (Finkelman & Kenner, 2012, p. 222). Levels of simulations vary, ranging from low fidelity to high fidelity. The difference between levels lies in how close the simulated scenario comes to reality (Jeffries & Rogers, 2007). Simulation also can involve task trainers for learning skills such as IV insertion, or it can entail the use of standardized patients (actors) who role play for the students in a safe practice environment simulating a clinical setting. Some simulation labs provide experiences for students in which they interact with an actor who is playing the role of patient, following a script and scenario.

Labs and simulation are used as part of the educational experiences of nursing students at all levels. Beginning students learn basic competencies in low-fidelity scenarios in which they practice skills and provide care in "a safe environment that allows them to make mistakes, learn from those mistakes, and develop confidence in their ability to approach patients and practice in the clinical setting" (Hovancsek, 2007, p. 4).

Simulation also allows faculty to design learning experiences that meet a variety of learning styles—visual, auditory, tactile, or kinesthetic—and give students time to incorporate their learning.

Time is devoted to discussing the care provided without concern for additional care that needs to be provided, as would occur in a clinical setting. This kind of debriefing is an important component of the simulation experience. During a simulation students may work alone, with faculty, and with other nursing students, as well as with other healthcare professions students in an interprofessional team. Faculty can better control the types of experiences in which students engage, whereas in the clinical setting it is not always easy to find a patient who needs a specific procedure or has certain complex care needs at one time. Simulation is an active learning method, which helps the student improve critical thinking/clinical reasoning and judgment (Billings & Halstead, 2005). Some schools are developing interprofessional simulation experiences that involve medical, pharmacy, respiratory therapy, and other healthcare professions students. These can be very important experiences that improve interprofessional teamwork over the long term.

Clinical Experiences

Clinical experiences or practicum is part of every nursing program. This experience occurs when students, with faculty supervision, provide care to patients. Such care may be provided to individual patients or to their families or significant others (e.g., providing care to a patient after surgery and teaching the family how to provide care after discharge), to communities (e.g., working with a school nurse in a community), or to groups of the population (e.g., developing a self-management education program for a group of patients with diabetes). Some nursing programs begin this experience early in the program and others later, but all include it as part of the nursing curriculum.

Typically, these practicums are conducted in blocks of time—for example, students are in clinical practice 2 days a week for 6 hours each day. Faculty may be present the entire time or may be available at the site or by telephone. The amount of supervision depends on the level and competency of the student, the type of setting, and the objectives of the experience. The clinical setting may also dictate the student–faculty ratio and supervision. The settings are highly variable—a hospital, clinic, physician's office, school, community health service, patient home, rehabilitation center, long-term care facility, senior center, child daycare center, or mental health center, among others. In some practicums, you may work with a group of students; in others, you may be alone. In the latter case, for example, you may be assigned to work with a school nurse.

Participating in clinical experiences (practicums) requires preparation. For many assigned experiences, you may need to go to the site of the clinical practicum before the clinical day begins (sometimes the day before) to obtain information about your patient(s) and to plan the care for the assigned time. This is done so that you are ready to provide care. You need to understand the patient's (or patients') history and problems, laboratory work, medications, procedures, and critical care issues, and plan care effectively. Often the student develops a written plan—perhaps in the form of a nursing care plan or a concept map—that is evaluated by the faculty. Students who arrive at clinical care settings unprepared will likely be unable to meet the requirements for that day.

Another important aspect of clinical experiences relates to professional responsibilities and appearance. When a nursing student is providing care, that student is representing the profession—a point pertinent to the content discussing the image of nursing. The student needs to meet the school's uniform requirement for the assigned experience, be clean, and meet safety requirements (such as appearance of hair) to decrease infection risk—for example, washing hands as required. Students who go to their clinical experience site and do not meet these requirements may be sent home. Making up clinical experiences is very difficult, and in some cases impossible, because it requires

reserving a clinical site again and securing faculty time, student time, and so on. Minimizing absences is critical; however, if the student is sick, the student should not care for patients. Schools have specific requirements related to illness and clinical experiences that should be followed. You should show up for every clinical experience dressed appropriately, prepared, and with any required equipment, such as a stethoscope. In addition, you need to be on time; set your alarm to allow plenty of preparation time, and plan for delays in traffic. All this relates to the practicing nurse: Employers expect nurses to come to work dressed as required, prepared, and on time.

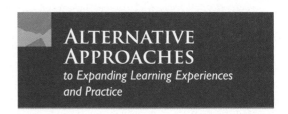

ALTERNATIVE APPROACHES
to Expanding Learning Experiences and Practice

When students approach their first nursing job after graduation, many experience **reality shock**. This is a shock reaction that occurs when an individual who has been educated in a nursing education system with one view of nursing encounters a different view of nursing in the practice setting (Kramer, 1985). New graduates do not have to experience reality shock. One measure that can prevent reality shock is developing better stress management techniques during the nursing education experience. This will not make the difference between your clinical experience and the real world of work completely disappear, but it will help the new graduate cope with this change in roles and views of what is happening in the healthcare delivery system. An increasing number of institutions are creating externship/internship and residency programs to guide new graduates through the first year of transition to graduate nursing status. Nursing, unlike medicine, pushes its "young" out of the nest without the safety net of a residency period (Goode, 2007).

Cooperative Experience

Some schools of nursing offer cooperative (co-op) experiences during the nursing program. These experiences are not common and vary in their design. Such a program might allow students (or even require students) to take a break from courses and work in healthcare settings. Students receive guidance in job searches, résumé development, interviews, and selecting the best experience. Some schools maintain lists of healthcare organizations that students often use. A co-op experience typically means the student is hired by the healthcare organization for several months and functions in an aide or assistant position supervised by RNs.

Nurse Internships/Externships

Students frequently want more clinical experiences in the summer, when many schools of nursing do not offer courses, and they also want to be employed. The nurse **internship/externship** is a program that offers this kind of opportunity for students. Students are often concerned about their first job as well; they wonder if they are ready. Nurse internships/externships are available in some communities as opportunities sponsored by hospitals (Beecroft, Kunzman, & Krozek, 2001). These programs are not usually associated with a school of nursing. They are short programs, such as 10 weeks, usually offered in the summer for students who will enter their senior year in the fall. There is great variation in the length of these programs, in what is offered to the student in the program, and in how much support the student receives in the program. The student is employed by the hospital and provided with orientation to the hospital, some content experiences, and preceptored and/or mentored experiences. Students need to investigate these programs and find out what each program offers and whether it meets their needs.

Nurse Residency Programs

Because of the nursing shortage and other job-related issues, such as staff burnout and concern about the level of new graduates' preparation and retention, some hospitals have developed nurse **residency** programs (Bowles & Candela, 2005; Casey, Fink, Krugman, & Propst, 2004; Halfer & Graf, 2006a, 2006b). After the nurse passes the licensure exam, the nurse residency program offers the new graduate a structured transition to professional nursing practice.

The American Association of Colleges of Nursing (AACN) conducted a pilot program to examine a national accreditation program and has developed standards for nurse residency programs. The National Council of State Boards of Nursing (NCSBN, 2011) also has worked on a pilot residency program known as Transition to Practice (TTP) in combination with its Taxonomy of Error, Root Cause Analysis, Practice-Responsibility (TERCAP) initiative. TTP and TERCAP are based on the five healthcare professions' core competencies and quality care definitions identified by the Institute of Medicine (IOM), which are an integral part of this text. (**Figure 4-6** describes the transition to practice model.) Both an IOM report (2011) and a recent nursing education report (Benner, Sutphen, Leonard, & Day, 2010) recommend residency programs as a standard part of nursing education, although at this time they are not required.

A nurse residency program is a special program that a nurse applies for after graduation, and it typically—and ideally—lasts a year (Goode & Williams, 2004). It serves as the nurse's first position as an RN. A nurse resident is employed by the hospital during the residency. The residency helps the new graduate with transition to practice in a structured program that provides content and learning activities, precepted experiences, mentoring, and gradual adjustment to higher levels of responsibility. These are paid positions, and typically the nurse resident must commit to working for the institution for a period of time after the residency. Such programs are proving to be helpful to new nurses and are decreasing turnover and improving staff retention. However, not all hospitals have residencies, and admission to these programs is competitive.

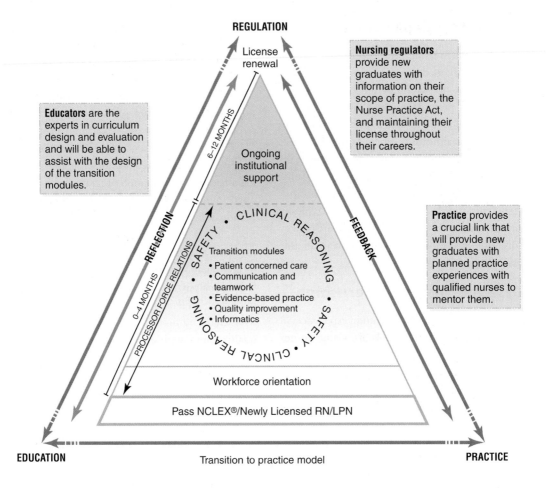

REGULATION

License renewal

Nursing regulators provide new graduates with information on their scope of practice, the Nurse Practice Act, and maintaining their license throughout their careers.

Educators are the experts in curriculum design and evaluation and will be able to assist with the design of the transition modules.

6–12 MONTHS

Ongoing institutional support

REFLECTION

FEEDBACK

SAFETY • CLINICAL REASONING

Practice provides a crucial link that will provide new graduates with planned practice experiences with qualified nurses to mentor them.

0–4 MONTHS

PROCESSOR FORCE RELATIONS

Transition modules
- Patient concerned care
- Communication and teamwork
- Evidence-based practice
- Quality improvement
- Informatics

SAFETY • CLINICAL REASONING

Workforce orientation

Pass NCLEX®/Newly Licensed RN/LPN

EDUCATION

Transition to practice model

PRACTICE

Figure 4-6 Transition to Practice Model

Source: National Council State Boards of Nursing. (n.d.) Transition to practice model. Retrieved from https://www.ncsbn.org/363.htm on April 23, 2011.

Some residency programs partner with schools of nursing—a relationship recommended by the AACN residency standards (AACN, 2011). In the first 6 years of the implementation of the AACN's residency program, the organization has established 62 sites in 30 states. (See http://www.aacn.nche.edu/education-resources/NRPParticipants.pdf for additional information about sites.) Students who are interested in this type of experience need to investigate these opportunities in their senior year. Only BSN graduates can participate in residency programs that follow the AACN residency model, but some other residency programs do not require a BSN and are open to ADN graduates. These programs usually encourage the new graduates to consider completing BSN.

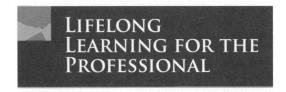

LIFELONG LEARNING FOR THE PROFESSIONAL

Lifelong learning is one of the major characteristics of a professional. This model of learning includes three major components:

- *Academic education:* The courses students take for academic credit—undergraduate and graduate—in an institution of higher learning that typically lead to a degree or completion of a certificate program. Nurses who return to school are pursuing lifelong learning goals.

- *Staff development education:* The systematic process of assessing and developing oneself to enhance performance or professional development—continued competence. Included in staff development are orientation (the process of introducing nursing staff to the organization and position), training required to do a job, and professional development.
- *Continuing education:* Systematic professional learning designed to augment knowledge, skills, and attitudes.

In 2010, the American Nurses Association (ANA) published updated *Nursing Professional Development: Scope and Standards of Practice.* The following is a summary description of the standards (ANA, 2010).

- Assessment of educational needs
- Identification of issues and trends that might require further education
- Outcomes identification for learning activities
- Planning of learning activities
- Implementation of learning activities including coordination of the activities, the learning and practice environment, and consultation with others to enhance the learning
- Evaluation of the learning activities
- Quality of nursing professional development practice
- Education of the professional development specialist
- Professional practice evaluation of the professional development specialist
- Collegiality to ensure partnerships to enhance learning activities
- Collaboration to facilitate learning
- Ethics
- Advocacy

- Research findings integrated into learning activities
- Resource utilization to most effectively provide learning activities
- Leadership

As a student you may wonder why this topic is important to you when you are just now entering nursing education. In fact, lifelong learning—particularly the need to recognize its importance to individual nurses, to the profession, to healthcare organizations, and to patient outcomes—begins when you enter a nursing education program. Students often have opportunities to participate in a variety of these learning activities even as students. Such activities are excellent opportunities to gain further knowledge and to better understand the importance of lifelong learning. You will also need to know the requirements for continuing education (CE) in the state(s) where you wish to apply for licensure. Lifelong learning must be driven by personal responsibility to improve even in regard to required practice components. Although professional organizations, regulatory agencies, and employers influence whether nurses participate in lifelong learning, successful lifelong learning is ultimately in the hands of the learner—that is, the nurse. The major report on nursing from the IOM (2011) includes the recommendation that the profession ensure that nurses engage in lifelong learning.

The natural assumption is that all nurses would want to get more education and stay current, but this is not necessarily the case. Required CE is a great motivator. Many states require CE if nurses are to maintain their licensure after the initial licensure is received. In these states, the state board of nursing designates the number of required CE credits for licensure renewal. States vary in terms of what is considered CE—short, structured CE programs; academic courses; attending conferences where educational content is presented; publishing; and so on. Nurses must follow their state's requirements. Another reason for obtaining CE is to meet certification requirements. The certification body determines the amount and type of required CE. If a nurse is licensed in more than one state, then the nurse must meet the CE requirements for all states in which he or she is licensed.

Sources for CE contact hours are highly variable. Credit can be obtained, for example, by attending a 1-hour or full-day educational offering, attending part or all of conference, reading an article in a professional journal and then taking an assessment quiz, and participating in an online program. Typically, a fee is charged unless the costs for the program are covered, such as by a grant to the sponsoring organization. Nurses do need to be careful and make sure that the program's credit is accepted by the organization requiring the CE. Organizations that approve and/or offer CE programs should be accredited programs. The American Nurses Credentialing Center (ANCC) accredits these programs, and state boards of nursing may have an accrediting process. Obtaining accreditation is voluntary, but the reality is that to get nurses to participate, accreditation is required: Nurses want to get CE from accredited programs that are guided by accepted standards. When a CE program is accredited through an organization such as ANCC, the consumer is assured that national standards of quality education have been applied (ANCC, 2007). It is assumed that CE has an impact on patient outcomes and quality care, but this relationship is not easy to prove in a consistent manner.

Nurses are responsible for maintaining their own CE activity records. In states where CE is required for relicensure, nurses may be required to produce documentation of these activities. In addition, nurses need to update their résumés to ensure that learning activities are included. In some cases, employers require documentation of CE. Nurses are usually required to document learning activities on an annual or biannual basis.

When nurses select learning programs, they should evaluate the following factors:

- Accreditation of the program
- Number of CE credits and related time commitment

- Schedule and location, including travel issues
- Cost (registration fee, parking and travel, housing, and meals)
- Qualifications of faculty
- Whether the program is based on adult learning principles (Is the program designed for the adult learner?)
- Identification of needs (What does the nurse need to gain? What are the personal or professional objectives? Does the course offer content to meet these objectives?)
- The program's learner objectives (Do they correlate with personal professional objectives?)
- Whether the program is based on current and relevant content
- Teaching methods
- Past experiences with the provider of the educational program (Quality programs attract nurses who return for other programs.)

A current issue in CE is the need for greater emphasis on interprofessional CE to increase the support for more interprofessional teamwork. The IOM (2010) addressed this issue in one of its reports. This report recommends that a national system be developed to support interprofessional CE:

The current system of continuing education for health professionals is not working. Continuing education for the professional health workforce needs to be reconsidered if the workforce is to provide high quality health care. A more comprehensive system of CE is needed, and CPD (Continuing Professional Development) provides a promising approach to improve the quality of learning. An independent public–private Continuing Professional Development Institute will be key to ensuring that the entire health care workforce is prepared to provide high quality, safe care. (IOM, 2010, p. 3)

In 2013, CE accreditor organizations for nursing, pharmacy, medicine, and other healthcare professions met together to discuss interprofessional continuing education (Accreditation Council for Continuing Medical Education, 2013). Participants in this meeting identified goals including creating standardized terminology and exploring a shared set of expectations and measures for interprofessional education in support of collaborative practice.

CERTIFICATION AND CREDENTIALING

Certification and credentialing are recognition systems that identify whether nurses meet certain requirements or standards. These recognitions may be required or voluntary, depending on the circumstances. Credentialing is typically required, whereas certification is often voluntary. To obtain certification or meet credentialing requirements, nurses must first be licensed as RNs.

Credentialing is a process that ensures practitioners such as RNs are qualified to perform as demonstrated by having licensure. Typically, it is used by healthcare organizations to check for licensure of healthcare professionals (such as nurses) and to monitor continued licensure. Nurses are required to show their current licensure to their employer, and the employer may then keep a copy of the license. Some states provide access to online checks of licensure status. Education, certification, and maintenance of malpractice insurance also may be reviewed, although this practice varies from one healthcare organization to another. The goal is to protect the public by ensuring that specific state requirements are met.

Certification is "a process by which a nongovernmental agency validates, based upon predetermined standards, an individual nurse's qualification and knowledge for practice in a defined functional or clinical area of nursing" (American Association of Critical Care Nurses, 2014, p. 4).

Certification is a method of recognizing expertise. It is done through an exam, recognition of completed education, and the description of clinical experience in a designated specialty area covered by the certification. Certification that might be given by a healthcare organization for accomplishing a specific goal, such as learning to perform cardiopulmonary resuscitation, is not the same type of certification that is awarded after meeting specific professional standards, a process that includes an exam. Pursuing this type of recognition is voluntary in that nurses are not required to have certification, although many employers acknowledge its importance, and some may require certification for certain positions—for example, for APRNs. This recognition is now available in most specialty areas. For example, the ANCC offers certification in multiple nursing specialties. After the nurse receives the initial certification, recertification is accomplished through demonstrating ongoing practice and through CE. Nurses may be certified in multiple areas as long as they meet the requirements for each area.

Cary (2001) identified the benefits of certification (although 25% of survey participants said that they received no benefit from certification):

- Certification recognized or publicized
- Full or partial reimbursement of costs
- Recognized as an expert in the field by colleagues
- Retention in position, one-time bonus
- Eligibility for a higher-level position
- Promoted to a higher-level position

Certification of nurse practitioners in the areas of adult, family, and adult–gerontology primary care is managed through the American Academy of Nurse Practitioners Certification Program (AAN-PCP). Other specialty nurse practitioner certifications are managed through different organizations.

Professional certification in nursing is a measure of distinctive nursing practice, and the benefits of certification are widely accepted. The rise of consumerism in the face of a compelling nursing shortage and the profession's movement to promote nursing as a more attractive career option has given further prominence to the value of certification in nursing. The value of certification is not just significant for nursing practice—focus on professional certification is also essential to meet multiple standards within the ANCC's Magnet Recognition Program for excellence in nursing services (ANCC, 2004, as cited in Shirey, 2005, p. 245).

The nursing profession has proposed a consensus model for regulation that includes licensure, accreditation, certification, and education to ensure greater consistency and clarity. This model reflects ongoing concern about the need for uniformity in educational requirements for and regulations related to APRNs. The consensus model will be fully implemented by 2015 (ANCC, 2013; NCSBN, 2013).

 # CARING FOR SELF

Caring for others is clearly the focus of nursing, but the process of caring for others can be a drain on the nurse. Students quickly discover that they are very tired after a long day in their clinical sessions. This fatigue is caused by the number of hours and the pace of clinical experiences, but stress also has an impact. When you graduate and practice, you may find that the stress does not disappear; indeed, in some cases, it may increase, particularly during early years of practice. Nurses often feel that they must be perfect. They may feel guilty when they cannot do everything they think they should be doing, both at work with patients and in their personal lives. There is still much to learn about nursing, working with others, pacing oneself, and figuring out the best way to mesh a career with a personal life—finding a balance and accepting that nursing is not a career of perfection. All nurses need to be aware of the potential for **burnout**, which is a "syndrome manifested by emotional exhaustion, depersonalization, and reduced personal accomplishments; it commonly occurs in professions like nursing" (Garrett & McDaniel, 2001, p. 92). A work–life balance is "a state where the needs and

requirements of work are weighed together to create an equitable share of time that allows for work to be completed and a professional's private life to get attention" (Heckerson & Laser, 2006, p. 27).

Learning how you routinely respond to **stress** and developing coping skills to manage stress can have a major impact and, it is hoped, prevent burnout later. Symptoms such as headaches, abdominal complaints, anxiety, irritability, anger, isolation, and depression can indicate a high level of stress. A review of anatomy and physiology explains how stress affects the body. When you experience stress, two hormones—adrenaline and cortisol—trigger the body to react and put the nervous, endocrine, cardiovascular, and immune systems on a state of alert. This is actually helpful because it helps you to cope with the stress, but the problem occurs when these stress responses happen frequently and over a period of months or years. Stress can be felt from a real or imagined threat, and the stressed person feels powerless. Exposure to constant or frequent stress can lead to chronic stress, which can have an overall impact on a person's health.

The best time to begin **stress management** is now, while you are still a student. Strategies for coping with stress can be found in a great variety of resources. **Box 4-2** identifies some websites that provide general

Box 4-2	Links to Help You Cope with Stress

Understanding and Dealing with Stress:
http://www.mtstcil.org/skills/stress-intro.html
Understanding Stress: Signs, Symptoms, Causes, and Effects:
http://helpguide.org/mental/stress_signs.htm
Eight Immediate Stress-Busters:
http://www.medicinenet.com/script/main/art.asp?articlekey=59875
Psych Central: Stress Busters:
http://psychcentral.com/blog/archives/2009/03/18/10-stress-busters/

information about stress. Following some guidelines can also help prevent and reduce stress:

- Set some goals to achieve a work–life balance.
- Use effective time management techniques and set priorities.
- Prepare ahead of time for assignments, quizzes, and exams.
- Ask questions when confused and ask for help—do not view this as a sign of weakness, but rather as strength.
- Take a break—a few minutes of rest can do wonders.
- Get an appropriate amount of exercise and sleep and eat a healthy diet. (Watch excessive use of caffeine.)
- Practice self-assertion.
- When you worry, focus on what is happening rather than what might happen.
- When you approach a problem, view it as an opportunity.
- Use humor.
- Set aside some quiet time to just think—even a short period can be productive.
- Care for self.

As noted earlier, when nurses take their first nursing jobs after graduation, many experience reality shock. One measure that can help prevent this reaction is to develop effective stress management techniques during your nursing education experience. This will not make the difference between your clinical experience and the real world of work disappear, but it will help you as a new graduate cope with this change in roles and views of what is happening in the healthcare delivery system. As described earlier in this chapter, many institutions are creating internship/externship and residency programs to guide new graduates through the first year of transition to graduate nursing status.

Two experiences that many nurses have after they practice for a while are burnout and compassion fatigue. These are the costs of caring, and they are similar but have some major differences. *Burnout* occurs when assertiveness–goal achievement intentions are not met, and **compassion fatigue** occurs when rescue-caretaking strategies are not successful (Boyle, 2011). Both lead to physical and emotional responses and impact quality of care and staff retention. Burnout is often discussed as part of an unhealthy work environment that is stressful and may be characterized by disruptive or incivil staff behavior. The nurse may reach the point of not wanting to go to work, having difficulty completing work, and having difficulty working with others. Compassion fatigue is the feeling of emotion that ensues when a person is moved by the distress or suffering of another (Boyle, 2011; Hooper, Craig, Janvrin, Wetsel, & Reimels, 2010; Schantz, 2007). Compassion is necessary for effective caring, but long-term coping with exposure to the distress (both physical and emotional) of others can lead to compassion fatigue or a state of psychic exhaustion. It is in the interpersonal connection with patients and families that nursing provides its best care, but this context carries risks for the nurse over time. Burnout is a reactional response to work stressors such as staffing, workload, managerial style, staff behavior, and so on, and occurs gradually; in contrast, compassion fatigue is relational, related to caring for others, and has a sudden onset (Boyle, 2011). This topic is included here because it relates to stress management, a set of skills that students need to develop while in school and continue to use throughout their career.

Interventions for burnout and compassion fatigue fall into three categories (Boyle, 2011). First, maintaining a healthy work–life balance is critical, nurturing self when you can. Second, you need to understand the sources of burnout and compassion fatigue. For example, compassion fatigue is often associated with basic communication skills—how do you effectively communicate with patients and families under stress without experiencing fatigue yourself? Third, work setting interventions are often helpful. For example, on-site counseling, support groups for staff, debriefing, on-site exercise, space to take a break, and so on, are important in preventing and reducing burnout and compassion fatigue.

Landscape © f9photos/Shutterstock, Inc.

CONCLUSION

This chapter has focused on the student and the learning process. Nursing education differs from other types of education programs and requires extensive experiences in labs, in simulation, and in clinical settings. Students are encouraged to assess their learning styles and methods used to successfully meet the education outcomes. Long-term education is an important part of any profession, but especially nursing. Caring for self is important both as a student and as a practicing nurse.

Landscape © f9photos/Shutterstock, Inc.

CHAPTER HIGHLIGHTS

1. The educational experience in nursing differs in important ways from educational experiences in other areas.

2. Students and faculty have active roles in the education process, whether in the classroom setting, online, or in lab/simulation/clinical experiences.

3. Students need to understand their learning style and then use this information to improve their learning methods.

4. Tools for success—such as reading methods, taking quizzes and exams, preparing written assignments, and so on—can make a difference in student performance.

5. Nurses need to be lifelong learners.

6. Certification and credentialing are methods used to assess competency, but they do not ensure competency.

7. Students use cooperative experiences to expand their learning experiences during their education program. Internships/externships may also be part of a student's education program, but are more formalized summer programs. Residencies are formal programs, used after completion of a nursing program and obtaining licensure, to provide a gradual integration into nursing.

8. Taking care of self is critical both as a student and a practicing nurse.

Landscape © f9photos/Shutterstock, Inc.

DISCUSSION QUESTIONS

1. Why is stress management important to you as a student nurse and to practicing nurses?

2. What is the purpose of a nurse residency program? Search on the Internet for information about specific nurse residency programs. How do they differ from one another? How are they similar?

3. Participate in a team discussion in class and share tools for success. You might discover some new tools to help you be more successful in your studies.

Landscape © f9photos/Shutterstock, Inc.

CRITICAL THINKING ACTIVITIES

1. Consider the learning styles described in this chapter. Where do you fit in? Why do you think the style(s) applies to you? What impact do you think the style(s) you identified will have on your own learning in the nursing program? Are there changes you need to work on?

2. Develop a study plan for yourself that incorporates information about tools for success.

Include an assessment of how you use your time.

3. Review your school's philosophy and curriculum. What are the key themes in this information? Do you think that the themes and content are relevant to nursing practice, and if so, why? Do you think anything important is missing, and if so, what is it?

ELECTRONIC *Reflection Journal*

Circuit Board: ©Photos.com

During your clinical experiences, observe how nurses use their time. Describe what you observe: Is the nurse effective? Which methods does the nurse use? How might you learn from this observation? Keep track of your time management when in clinical sessions and periodically comment on it in your Electronic Reflection Journal.

Landscape © f9photos/Shutterstock, Inc.

LINKING TO THE INTERNET

- Current certifications: http://www.nursecredentialing.org/certification.aspx#specialty
- American Nurses Credentialing Center: http://www.nursecredentialing.org/certification.aspx
- American Association of Colleges of Nursing, Nurse Residency Program: http://www.aacn.nche.edu/ccne-accreditation/new-applicant-process/nurse-residency

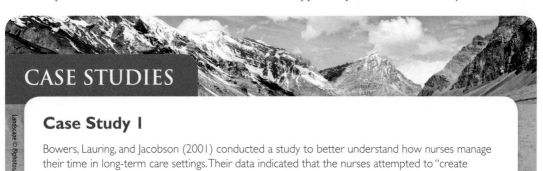

CASE STUDIES

Case Study 1

Bowers, Lauring, and Jacobson (2001) conducted a study to better understand how nurses manage their time in long-term care settings. Their data indicated that the nurses attempted to "create

(continues)

Landscape © f9photos/Shutterstock, Inc.

CASE STUDIES (CONTINUED)

new time" when time was short. As a student, you will be confronted with issues of time when you begin your clinical experience and then throughout your career as a nurse. Consider the following information from this study:

Longevity	Increasing the pace of work has consequences, such as less time to really talk to patients. This also results in an increased focus on technical or visible and urgent tasks and less focus on surveillance and follow-up. For nurses, this means increased frustration and lower morale.
Working faster	Combining or bundling tasks is done to complete work more quickly and to reduce interruptions. This can lead to errors when tasks are bundled together that may not fit well, and the nurse cannot focus.
Changing sequence of tasks	The order of some tasks may be changed in an attempt to create more time. You will fall behind by doing something just in case there is an interruption later.
Communicating inaccessibility	Minimizing some activities or eliminating them altogether to get more time typically relates to communication with patients and families. The message is "I don't have time for this."
Converting wasted times	Find ways to use wasted time or downtime; this can be helpful if done right—for example, doing a quick assessment of a patient while waiting for the patient to take oral medications.
Negotiating "actual time"	Nurses tried to maximize their "actual work time" by coming in early, skipping lunch and breaks, and so on.

Source: Bowers, B., Lauring, C., & Jacobson, N. (2001). How nurses manage time and work in long-term care. *Journal of Advanced Nursing, 33*(4), 484–491.

Case Questions

1. Consider your own schedule for a week. How would these strategies apply to your own personal methods for handling your time? How would they affect your time management, both positively and negatively?
2. Keep this list, and when you begin your clinical experience, consider whether you are using these strategies to create more time. Can time really be created? How might you solve this problem?

Case Study 2

A nursing student is completing her first year and meets with her advisor. The discussion is a difficult one. Her advisor tells the student that she is passing, but in several courses she is just barely passing. The student is defensive and says that no one said she had to make all A's. The advisor agrees with her that this is not the expectation; however, some of the student's grades are borderline and more importantly her performance in clinical sessions has been weak. The advisor tells the student that she needs to improve. The student leaves the meeting discouraged.

Case Questions

1. What more could the advisor have done in this meeting?
2. What does the student need to do? Describe steps the student might take (consider the content in this chapter).

Words of Wisdom

© Roobcio/Shutterstock, Inc.

Jamie White, MSN, RN

Staff Nurse, Neonatal Intensive Care Unit, University of Oklahoma Medical Center, Oklahoma City, Oklahoma

What would have made the transition to your first nursing job easier?

Transition to my job was very easy. What made it this way was working in the unit for a year and a half as a nurse partner and clerk prior to graduation. If you already know the basics of the unit, then transition is much easier.

What things were included in your education that was most helpful? Least helpful?

The most helpful educational tool was the group/team work. Nursing is all about being a member of a team and relying on others to help you perform your job more efficiently. The other helpful experience was how nursing school changes your mind-set of school and work. Nursing is ever changing, and so is nursing school. I remember being stressed out my first semester due to the ever-changing environment and no clear line. Now, I understand why it's that way—because nursing is that way. I cannot tell you the least helpful, only because for everything I thought at the time had no purpose, I found the purpose when I entered the field.

What advice would you give entering students?

My advice would be to come into nursing if you truly want to touch people's lives. Nursing is full of frustrations and politics, but if you are in it for the love of people, then you will do fine. The best feeling I get is to hand a family their sick infant for the first time and to see the hope and love that is expressed.

Landscape © f9photos/Shutterstock, Inc.

REFERENCES

Accreditation Council for Continuing Medical Education. (2013). CE accreditors meeting focuses on interprofessional education. Retrieved from http://www.accme.org/news-publications/highlights/ce-accreditors-meeting-focuses-interprofessional-education

American Association of Colleges of Nursing (AACN). (2011). Nurse residency. Retrieved from http://www.aacn.nche.edu/ccne-accreditation/standards-procedures-resources/nurse-residency

American Association of Critical Care Nurses, Certification Corporation. (2014). Certification exam policy handbook. Retrieved from http://www.aacn.org/wd/certifications/docs/cert-policy-hndbk.pdf

American Nurses Association (ANA). (2010). *Scope and standards of practice for nursing professional development.* Silver Spring, MD: Author.

American Nurses Credentialing Center (ANCC). (2004). *Magnet recognition program recognizing excellence in nursing service: Application manual 2005.* Washington, DC: Author.

American Nurses Credentialing Center (ANCC). (2007). ANCC Credentialing Center: Primary accreditation. Retrieved http://www.nursecredentialing.org/Accreditation/Primary-Accreditation.aspx

American Nurses Credentialing Center (ANCC). (2013). APRN consensus model. Retrieved from http://www.nursecredentialing.org/Certification/APRNCorner

Beecroft, P., Kunzman, L., & Krozek, C. (2001). RN internship: Outcomes of a one-year pilot program. *Journal of Nursing Administration, 31*(12), 575–582.

Benner, P. (2001). *From novice to expert* (commemorative ed.). Upper Saddle River, NJ: Prentice Hall Health.

Benner, P., Sutphen, P., Leonard, V., & Day, L. (2010). *Educating nurses: A call for radical transformation.* San Francisco, CA: Jossey-Bass.

Billings, D., & Halstead, J. (2005). *Teaching in nursing: A guide for faculty* (2nd ed.). Philadelphia, PA: Saunders.

Bowers, B., Lauring, C., & Jacobson, N. (2001). How nurses manage time and work in long-term care. *Journal of Advanced Nursing, 33,* 484–491.

Bowles, C., & Candela, L. (2005). First job experiences of recent RN graduates. *Journal of Nursing Administration, 35*(3), 130–137.

Boyle, D. (2011, January). Countering compassion fatigue: A requisite nursing agenda. *OJIN, 16.* Retrieved from http://www .nursingworld.org/MainMenuCategories/ANAMarketplace/ ANAPeriodicals/OJIN/TableofContents/Vol-16-2011/ No1-Jan-2011/Countering-Compassion-Fatigue.html

Cary, A. (2001). Certified registered nurses: Results of the study of the certified workforce. *American Journal of Nursing, 10*(1), 44–52.

Casey, K., Fink, R., Krugman, M., & Propst, J. (2004). The graduate nurse experience. *Journal of Nursing Administration, 34*(6), 303–311.

Finkelman, A., & Kenner, C. (2012). *Teaching IOM: Implications of the Institute of Medicine reports for nursing education* (3rd ed.). Silver Spring, MD: American Nurses Association.

Garrett, D., & McDaniel, A. (2001). A new look at nurse burnout. *Journal of Nursing Administration, 31,* 91–96.

Goode, C. (2007, July). Report given at the American Academy of Nursing Workforce Commission Committee on Preparation of the Nursing Workforce, Chicago, IL.

Goode, C., & Williams, C. (2004). Post-baccalaureate nurse residency program. *Journal of Nursing Administration, 34*(2), 71–77.

Halfer, D., & Graf, E. (2006a). Graduate nurse experience. *Journal of Nursing Administration, 34*(6), 303–311.

Halfer, D., & Graf, E. (2006b). Graduate nurse perceptions of the work experience. *Nursing Economics, 24,* 150–155.

Heckerson, E., & Laser, C. (2006). Just breathe! The critical importance of maintaining a work–life balance. *Nurse Leader, 4*(12), 26–28.

Honey, P., & Mumford, A. (1986). *The manual of learning styles.* Maidenhead, UK: Peter Honey.

Honey, P., & Mumford, A. (1992). *The manual of learning styles* (3rd ed.). Maidenhead, UK: Peter Honey.

Hooper, C., Craig, J., Janvrin, D. R., Wetsel, M. A., & Reimels, E. (2010). Compassion satisfaction, burnout and compassion fatigue among emergency room nurses compared with nurses in other selected inpatient specialties. *Journal of Emergency Nursing, 36*(5), 420–427.

Hovancsek, M. (2007). Using simulation in nursing education. In P. Jeffries (Ed.), *Simulation in nursing education* (pp. 1–9). New York, NY: National League for Nursing.

Institute of Medicine (IOM). (2010). *Redesigning continuing education in the health professions.* Washington, DC: National Academies Press.

Institute of Medicine (IOM). (2011). *The future of nursing: Leading change, advancing health.* Washington, DC: National Academies Press.

Jeffries, P., & Rogers, K. (2007). Evaluating simulations. In P. Jeffries (Ed.), *Simulation in nursing education* (pp. 87–103). New York, NY: National League for Nursing.

Kolb, D. (1984). *Experiential learning: Experience as the source of learning and development.* Toronto, ON: Prentice Hall.

Kramer, M. (1985). Why does reality shock continue? In J. McCloskey & H. Grace (Eds.), *Current issues in nursing* (pp. 891–903). Boston, MA: Blackwell Scientific.

National Council of State Boards of Nursing (NCSBN). (2011). TERCAP. Retrieved from https://www.ncsbn.org/441.htm

National Council of State Boards of Nursing (NCSBN). (2013). Campaign for consensus. Retrieved from https://www .ncsbn.org/2567.htm

Rassool, G., & Rawaf, S. (2007). Learning style preference of undergraduate nursing students. *Nursing Standard, 32*(21), 35–41.

Schantz, M. (2007). Compassion: A concept analysis. *Nursing Forum, 42*(2), 48–55.

Shirey, M. (2005). Celebrating certification in nursing. Forces of magnetism in action. *Nursing Administration Quarterly, 29,* 245–253.

Young, M., Stuenkel, D., & Bawel-Brinkley, K. (2008). Strategies for easing the role transition of graduate nurses. *Journal for Nurses in Staff Development, 24*(3), 105–110.

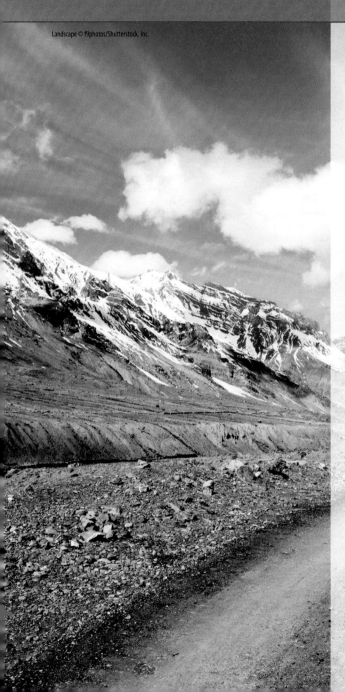

SECTION 2

The Healthcare Context

Section II sets the stage for the student. The healthcare environment the student now enters is complex. The Health Policy and Political Action: Critical Actions for Nurses *chapter introduces these topics and considers how they relate to the nursing profession.* The Ethics and Legal Issues *chapter moves to these related topics as they impact practice. With this background, the* Health Promotion, Disease Prevention, and Illness: A Community Perspective *chapter describes the importance of the public/community focus on healthcare delivery. The last chapter in this section,* The Healthcare Delivery System: Focus on Acute Care, *examines one type of healthcare organization, the acute care hospital, in depth as an exemplar of how healthcare organizations function and how nurses are involved in these organizations.*

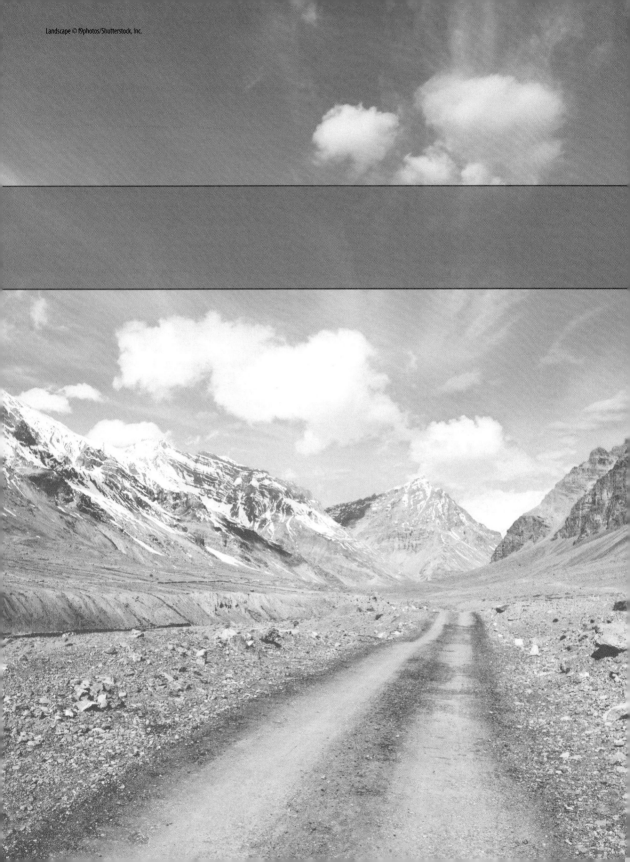

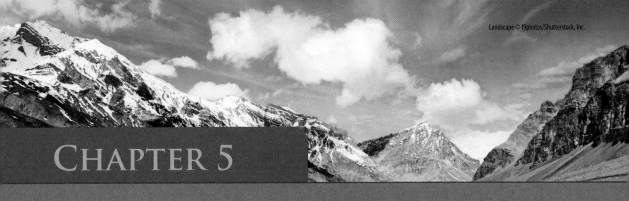

Landscape © f9photos/Shutterstock, Inc.

CHAPTER 5

Health Policy and Political Action: Critical Actions for Nurses

CHAPTER OBJECTIVES

At the conclusion of this chapter, the learner will be able to:

- Discuss the importance of health policies
- Define policy
- Describe the policy-making process
- Examine critical health policy issues and their impact on nurses and nursing
- Describe the political process
- Discuss the importance of the political process to nurses and nursing
- Explain the role of nurses in the political process
- Summarize the relationship between health policies and the political process
- Analyze the impact of the Patient Protection and Affordable Care Act of 2010

CHAPTER OUTLINE

INTRODUCTION

This chapter introduces content about health policy and the political process. Both have a major impact on nurses, nursing care, and healthcare delivery. When nurses participate in the policy process, they are acting as advocates for patients, as Abood explained:

> Nurses are well aware that today's healthcare system is in trouble and in need of change. The experiences of many nurses practicing in the real world of healthcare are motivating them to take on some form of an advocacy role in order to influence change in policies, laws, or regulations that govern the larger healthcare system. This type of advocacy necessitates stepping beyond their own practice setting and into the less familiar world of policy and politics, a world in which many nurses do not feel prepared to participate effectively. (Abood, 2007, p. 3)

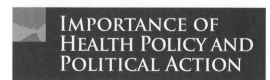

IMPORTANCE OF HEALTH POLICY AND POLITICAL ACTION

Why is it important for nurses to have knowledge about health policy? Every day, health policy impacts health delivery through means such as reimbursement policies, decisions made about how and where care might be provided and to whom, and decisions about whether someone receives care when it is needed. Understanding healthcare policy requires the nurse to step back and see the broader picture while understanding how such policy influences individual care. Political action is part of recognizing the need for health policy, developing policy, and implementing policy, including financing policy decisions. Nurses offer the following resources to health policy making:

- Expertise
- Understanding of consumer needs
- Experience in assisting patients in making healthcare decisions
- A link to healthcare professionals and organizations
- Understanding of the healthcare system
- Understanding of interprofessional care

Definitions

A **policy** is a course of action that affects a large number of people and is inspired by a specific need to achieve certain outcomes. The best approach to understanding health policy is to describe the difference between public policy and private policy. **Public policy** is "policy made at the legislative, executive, and judicial branches of federal, state, and local levels of government that affects individual and institutional behaviors under the government's respective jurisdiction. Public policy includes all policies that come from government at all levels" (Magill, 1984, as cited in Block, 2008, p. 7). Policy is a method for finding solutions to problems, but not all solutions are policies. Many solutions have nothing to do with government. There are two main types of public policies: (1) regulatory policies (e.g., registered nurse [RN] licensure that regulates practice) and (2) allocative policies, which involve money distribution. Allocative policies provide benefits for some at the expense of others to ensure that certain public objectives are met. Often the decision relates to funding of certain healthcare programs but not others. Health policy is policy that focuses on health and health-related issues. Examples of policies that have had national impact are those prohibiting smoking in public places (initiated through the legislative branch) and abortion rulings made by the U.S. Supreme Court (initiated through the **judicial branch**). **Private policy** is made by nongovernmental organizations.

This chapter focuses on public policy related to health because this is the most important type of health policy. Health policies include the following (Longest, 1998, as cited in Block, 2008, p. 6):

- Health-related decisions made by legislators that then become laws
- Rules and regulations designed to implement legislation and laws or that are used to operate government and its health-related programs
- Judicial decisions related to health that have an impact on how health care is delivered, reimbursed, and so on

Policy planning is developing a plan to change the value system or laws and regulations. It is considered broad health planning because it typically affects a large portion of the population.

Policy: Relevance to the Nation's Health and to Nursing

Policy has an impact on all aspects of health and healthcare delivery, such as how care is delivered, who receives care, which types of services are received, how reimbursement is doled out, and which types of providers and organizations provide health care. Policy affects nursing in similar areas.

Each of the areas in **Figure 5-1** relates to individual nurses and to the profession. Roles and standards are found in state laws and rules/regulations. Boards of nursing and each state's nurse practice act set professional expectations and identify what a nurse does. Federal laws and rules/regulations related to Medicare and Medicaid address issues such as reimbursement for advanced practice nurses (APRNs). How nursing care is provided and which care is provided are influenced by Medicare, Medicaid, nurse practice acts, and other laws and rules/regulations made by federal, state, and local governments. Health is influenced by federal policy decisions related to Medicare reimbursement for preventive services, the Department of Health and Human Services (HHS), and its agencies' rules and regulations. An agency for which rules and regulations are very important is the Food and Drug Administration (FDA), which manages the drug approval process in the United States. State laws, such as those passed in California and other states limiting or eliminating mandatory overtime, may determine staffing levels. Access to care is often influenced by policy, particularly that related to reimbursement policy and limits set on which services can be provided and by whom. This is particularly

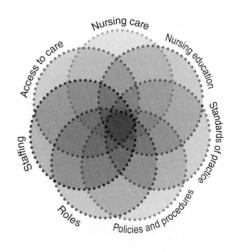

Figure 5-1 Healthcare Policy: Impact on Health Care and Nursing

relevant to Medicare, Medicaid, and state employee health insurance. Individual organizations have their own policies and procedures, but often these are influenced by public policy. Public policy also has an impact on nursing education through laws and rules/regulations—for example, through funding for faculty and scholarships, funding to develop or expand schools of nursing and their programs, evaluation standards through state boards of nursing, and much more. Nursing research is also influenced by policy—funding for research primarily comes through government sources, and legislation designates funding for government research.

Nurses are experts in health care, and in that role they can make valuable contributions to the healthcare policy-making process. Nurses' expertise and knowledge about health and healthcare delivery are important resources for policy makers. Nurses also have a long history of serving as consumer advocates for their patients and patients' families. Advocacy means to speak for or be persuasive for another's needs. This does not mean that the nurse takes over for the patient. When nurses are involved in policy development, for example, they are acting as advocates. Nurses may get involved in policy making both as individuals and as representatives of the nursing profession, such as by representing a nursing organization. Each of these forms of advocacy is an example of nursing leadership.

Collaboration is very important for effective policy development and implementation. The goal of health policy should be the provision of better health care for citizens. When nurses advocate for professional issues such as pay, work schedules, the need for more nurses, and so forth, they also influence healthcare delivery. If there are not enough nurses because pay is low, then care is compromised. If there are not enough nurses because few are entering the profession or because schools do not have the funds to increase enrollment or not enough qualified faculty, this compromises care. In other cases, nurses advocate directly for healthcare delivery issues, such as by calling for reimbursement for

hospice care or by supporting mental health parity legislation to improve access to care for people with serious mental illness.

General Descriptors of U.S. Health Policy

U.S. health policy can be described by the following long-standing characteristics, which have an impact on the types of policies that are enacted and the effectiveness of the policies (Shi & Singh, 2013). First, whereas most other countries have national, government-run healthcare systems, the United States does not. Instead, the private insurance sector is the dominant player in the U.S. system. The issue of a universal right to health care has been a contentious one for some time. Government does have an important role in the U.S. healthcare system, but it is not the major role. This stance reflects Americans' view that the government's role should be limited.

The second characteristic is the approach taken to achieve healthcare policy, which has been, and continues to be, fragmented and incremental. This approach does not look at the whole system and how its components work or do not work together effectively; parts are not connected to constitute a whole. Coordination between state and federal policies, and even between the branches of the government, is also limited. The system is further complicated by the wide array of reimbursement sources.

The third characteristic is the role of the states. States have a significant role in policy in the United States, and health policies vary from state to state. In some cases, there is a shared role with the federal government—for example, with the Medicaid program.

The last important characteristic is the role of the president (head of the executive branch of government), which can be significant. How does the president influence healthcare policy? Consider President Bill Clinton and his initiative to review the quality of health care in the United States. Clinton established a commission to start this process.

Although this commission no longer exists, it set the direction for extensive reviews and recommendations that have been identified by the Institute of Medicine (IOM). Clinton also pushed to get the Health Insurance Portability and Accountability Act (HIPAA) and the State Children's Health Insurance Program (S-CHIP) passed. Both laws resulted from the work of this healthcare commission. The work of this commission was supposed to be part of a major healthcare reform initiative that did not succeed at the time of the Clinton administration. Its goal was to make major changes in healthcare reimbursement, but this did not happen. Some significant policies did emerge from these efforts, such as the two previously mentioned laws and the IOM quality initiative. The issue of healthcare reform was not seriously addressed again until the Obama administration, which pushed for passage of the Patient Protection and Affordable Care Act of 2010.

Some legislative efforts are diluted over time or cancelled. The most recent example is S-CHIP. In 2007, Congress tried to expand this program, but President George W. Bush vetoed the bill. S-CHIP was established to provide states with matching funds from the federal government that would enable states to extend health insurance for children from families with incomes too high to meet Medicaid criteria but not high enough to purchase health insurance. Matching funds are one method used by the government to fund programs. With this method, the federal government pays for half, and the states pay for the other half (or some other configuration of sharing costs). Medicaid is funded with matching funds, whereas the only the federal government funds Medicare. The issue of S-CHIP came up again when the legislation was expiring, which opened it up for cancellation or renewal with or without changes. S-CHIP has been an effective program; it has provided reimbursement for needed care for many children, improved access to care and preventive care, and improved the health status of children. Congress and the administration disagreed over expansion and funding of this program,

and this dispute reached a stalemate during the Bush administration. When President Obama took office, the first bill he signed was one that continued the expansion of this program. This is an example of how legislation can be passed by one administration, vetoed by another administration, and then taken up again by yet another administration.

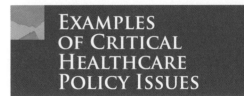

EXAMPLES OF CRITICAL HEALTHCARE POLICY ISSUES

Many healthcare policy issues are of concern to local communities, states, and the federal government. **Exhibit 5-1** highlights some of these issues, which are often of particular concern to nurses, nursing, and healthcare delivery in general. How policy is developed or whether policy related to each of these issues is developed at all may vary. Examining some of these issues in more depth provides a better understanding of the complexity of health policy issues. The examples of policy issues related to nursing covered in this section are not the only healthcare policy issues, but they illustrate the types that can be considered health policy issues.

Cost of Health Care

The cost of health care in the United States is rising steadily. There is no doubt that better drugs, treatment, and technology are available today to improve health and meet treatment needs for many problems; unfortunately, these new preventive and treatment interventions typically have increased costs. Defensive medicine, in which the physician and other healthcare providers order tests and procedures to protect themselves from lawsuits, also increases costs. Insurance coverage has expanded, and beneficiaries of coverage expect to get care when they feel they need it. In turn, cost containment and cost-effectiveness have become increasingly important.

> **Exhibit 5-1**   Potential Policy Issues
>
> - Access to care
> - Acute and chronic illness
> - Advanced practice nursing
> - Aging
> - Changing practice patterns and the physician
> - Diagnosis-related groups related to reimbursement
> - Disparities in health care
> - Diversity in healthcare workforce
> - Health promotion and prevention
> - Healthcare commercialization and industrial complex
> - Healthcare consumerism
> - Healthcare role changes
> - Immigration: impact on care and providers
> - International health issues
> - Managed care
> - Mental health parity
> - Minority health
> - Move from acute care to increased use of ambulatory care
> - Nursing education
> - Poverty and health
> - Public health
> - Quality care
> - Reimbursement
> - Restructuring and reengineering
> - Rural health care
> - Uninsured and underinsured

- The cost of prescription drugs would decrease.
- Billions of dollars in administrative costs would be saved.
- Competition could focus on quality, safety, and patient satisfaction.
- Resources would be redirected toward patients.

The healthcare reform of 2010 did not establish universal healthcare coverage in the United States, though it did provide insurance coverage through Medicaid for more people who could not afford insurance and other methods for people to enroll in healthcare insurance. It also established requirements for health insurance for the U.S. population as a whole.

Healthcare Quality

Healthcare quality is a hot topic in health care today. Following President Clinton's establishment of the Advisory Commission on Consumer Protection and Quality in Healthcare (1996–1998), a whole area of policy development was opened up: How can healthcare quality be improved? What needs to be done to accomplish this? This focus led to the federal government's request for the Institute of Medicine (IOM) to further assess health care in the United States, resulting in major reports and recommendations related to quality, safety, and other important topics.

Disparities in Health Care

The IOM reports on diversity in health care, and disparities and the Sullivan report on healthcare workforce diversity (IOM, 2002, 2004; Sullivan and Commission on Diversity in the Healthcare Workforce, 2004) drew attention to a critical policy concern—namely, inequality in access to and services received in the U.S. healthcare system. Nurses need more knowledge about culture and health needs, health literacy, the ways in which different groups respond to care, and healthcare disparities (IOM, 2002, 2004). How does this impact health

Health policy often focuses on reimbursement, control of costs, and greater control of provider decisions to reduce costs. The last of these measures has not proved popular with consumers/patients.

For a long time, a critical issue has been whether the United States should move to a universal (national) healthcare system. Coffey (2001) discussed universal health coverage and identified five reasons why it should be of interest to nurses:

- Insuring everyone under one national health program would spread the insurance risk over the entire population.

policy? Does it mean that certain groups may not get the same services (disparities)? If so, what needs to change?

Consumers

There is increasing interest in the role of consumers in health care. Today, consumers are more informed about health and healthcare services than members of previous generations were. An example of a law that focuses on health is the Health Insurance Portability and Accountability Act of 1996 (HIPAA). The major focus of this law addresses the issue of carrying health insurance from one employer to another, but it also includes expectations regarding privacy of patient information, which is now a critical factor considered by healthcare providers in daily practice.

Commercialization of Health Care

The organization of healthcare delivery systems has been changing into a series of multipronged systems. These multiple organizations generally form a corporate model. Such corporations may exist in a local community, statewide, or even nationally. In fact, some of the large healthcare corporations also have hospitals in other countries. This change has had an impact on policies related to financing health care and quality concerns.

Reimbursement for Nursing Care

Reimbursement of nursing care must be viewed from two perspectives. The first view considers reimbursement methods for nursing care services, particularly inpatient services. There has not been much progress in this area. Hospitals still do not clearly identify the specific costs of nursing care in a manner that directly impacts reimbursement. The second view involves reimbursement for specific individual provider services instead of reimbursement for an organization provider, such as a hospital. Physicians are reimbursed for their services. There have been major changes in how APRNs are reimbursed; thus this situation is improving but continues to need improvement. For example, if an APRN provides care in a clinic or a private practice, the question arises: How is the APRN reimbursed for the care? Will the patient's health insurance pay for these services? Some services are covered by federal government plans, but there is great variation in reimbursement from nongovernment plans. The healthcare reform of 2010 and other initiatives such as those identified in the IOM report, *The Future of Nursing: Leading Change, Advancing Health* (2010), have supported greater use of APRNs. To make this work, reimbursement practices will also need to support use of APRNs.

Immigration and the Nursing Workforce

Immigration of nurses to the United States has an impact of international healthcare delivery. This is an important policy issue, but one that is not yet resolved. Important considerations in this area include regulations (visas to enter the United States and work; licensure), level of language expertise, quality of education, orientation and training needs, and potential limits on immigration of RNs. Some of the issues need to be addressed by laws, rules and regulations related, and state boards of nursing.

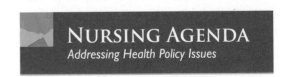

In 2005, the American Nurses Association (ANA) published a revision of its healthcare agenda. This agenda highlighted the problem with the healthcare system as one of a patchwork approach to healthcare reform and to policy development. The system is fragmented and expensive, and this has not changed over the last few decades. The ANA (2005) agenda states:

> ANA remains committed to the principle that all persons are entitled to ready access to affordable, quality health care services. Nursing, as the pivotal health care profession, is well positioned to advocate on behalf of and in concert with individuals, families and communities who are in desperate need of a well financed, functional and coordinated health care system that provides safe, quality care. Indeed, all of us stand to benefit from such a system. Accessible, affordable, and quality health care will positively contribute to our individual health, the strength of society, our national well-being, and overall productivity. (p. 4)

This view of the healthcare system was also described in the IOM report, *Crossing the Quality Chasm* (2001).

The ANA identifies key issues that it will focus on during each congressional session. For example, for the 113th congressional session, this organization targeted a number of issues that were directly related to the profession, such as advanced practice and safe staffing, as well as issues related to health care in general, such as mental health care, quality of care, gun violence, and Medicare and Medicaid.

Access to care means that care should be affordable for, available to, and acceptable to a great variety of patients. Quality of care remains a problem in the United States. The ANA supports the recommendations of the IOM *Quality Chasm* report series, which states that all care should be safe, effective, timely, patient centered, efficient, and equitable. "ANA believes that the development and implementation of health policies that reflect these aims, and are based on effectiveness and outcomes research, will ultimately save money" (ANA, 2005, p. 7). The organization's agenda also addresses the critical nature of the nursing workforce and the need for an "adequate supply of well-educated, well-distributed, and well utilized registered nurses" (ANA, 2005, p. 10). The agenda concludes:

> The need for fundamental reform of the U.S. health care system is more necessary today than in 1991 (date of previous ANA agenda). Bold action is called for to create a healthcare system that is responsive to the needs of consumers and provides equal access to safe, high-quality care for every citizen and resident in a cost-effective manner. Working together—policy makers, industry leaders, providers, and consumers—we can build an affordable health care system that meets the needs of everyone. (p. 12)

The ANA agenda is an example of how a professional organization speaks for the profession, delineates issues that need to be addressed through policies, commits to collaborating with others to accomplish the agenda, and advocates for patients through such statements and lobbying efforts. Individual nurses and nursing students should participate in this the process.

THE POLICY-MAKING PROCESS

Health policy is developed at the local, state, and federal levels of government, but the two most common levels are state and federal. At the state level, the typical broad focus areas are public health and safety (e.g., immunization, water safety, and so forth); care for those who cannot afford it; purchasing care through state insurance, such as for state employees; regulation (e.g., RN licensure); and resource allocation (e.g., funding for care services). At the federal level, there are many different needs and policy makers. The focus areas are much the same as at the state level but apply to the nation as a whole.

Federal legislation is an important source of health policy. Prior to the healthcare reform legislation of 2010, the two laws that had the greatest impact on U.S. health care were the **Social Security Act of 1935** and the **Public Health Act of 1944**. The Social Security Act established the Medicare and Medicaid programs, the two major government-run healthcare reimbursement programs. These laws also provided funding for nursing education through subsequent amendments to the law. The Public Health Act (1944) consolidated all existing public health legislation into one law, and it, too, has been amended over the years. Some of the programs and issues addressed in this law are health services for migratory workers; establishment of the National Institutes of Health; nurse training funding acts; prevention and primary care services; rural health clinics; communicable disease control; and family planning services. An amendment to this law established *Healthy People* in 1990 and its subsequent extensions (its current iteration is *Healthy People 2020*).

The policy-making process is described in **Figure 5-2**. The first step is to recognize that an issue might require a policy. The suggestion of the need for a policy can come from a variety of sources, including professional organizations, consumers/citizens, government agencies, and lawmakers.

The second step is not to develop a policy but rather to learn more about the issue. This investigation may reveal that there is no need for a policy. There may be, and often is, disagreement about the need and there also may be disagreement about how to resolve it if the need exists. Information and data are collected to get a clearer perspective on the issue, from sources such as experts, consumers, professionals, relevant literature (such as professional literature), and research.

Using this information, policy makers then identify possible solutions. They should not consider just one solution, because only under rare circumstances is a single solution possible. During this process, policy makers consider the costs and benefits of each potential solution. Costs are more than financial—a cost might be that some people will not receive a service, whereas others will. What impact will this have on both groups? After the cost–benefit analysis is done, a solution is selected, and the policy is developed.

It is at this time that implementation begins, although how a policy might be implemented must be considered as the solution is selected and policy developed. Perhaps implementation is very complex, which in turn will impact the policy. For example, if a policy decision is made that all U.S. citizens should receive healthcare insurance, the policy statement is very simple; however, when

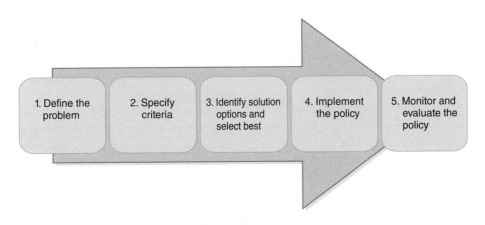

1. Define the problem   2. Specify criteria   3. Identify solution options and select best   4. Implement the policy   5. Monitor and evaluate the policy

Figure 5-2 The Policy-Making Process

implementation is considered, this policy would be very complicated to implement. How would this be done? Who would administer it? Which funds would be used to pay for this system? What would happen to current employer coverage? Would all services be provided? How much decision-making power would the consumer have? How would providers be paid, and which providers would be paid? Many more questions could be asked. Policy development must include an implementation plan. Social, economic, legal, and ethical forces influence policy implementation. The best policy can fail if the implementation plan is not reasonable and feasible. As will be discussed in the next section on the political process, the policy often is legislation (law). In such a case, implementation of the policy is largely determined by rules and regulations.

Coalition building is important in gaining support for a new policy. As will be discussed in the next section on the political process, gaining support is especially important in getting laws passed. Regarding a healthcare issue, some groups that might be included in coalition building are healthcare providers (e.g., medical doctors, nurses, pharmacists); healthcare organizations, particularly hospitals; professional organizations (e.g., the ANA, the American Medical Association, the American Hospital Association, The Joint Commission, the American Association of Colleges of Nursing, the National League for Nursing); state organizations; elected officials; business leaders; third-party payers; and pharmaceutical industry representatives. Members of a coalition that support a policy may offer funding to support the effort, act as expert witnesses, develop written information in support of the policy, and work to get others to support the policy; some, such as lawmakers, may be in a position to actually vote on the policy.

After a policy is approved and implemented, it should be monitored and its outcomes evaluated. This may lead to future changes or to the determination that a policy is not effective. The process may then begin again.

THE POLITICAL PROCESS

Politics is "the process of influencing the authoritative allocation of scarce resources" (Kalisch & Kalisch, 1982, p. 31). Typically, nurses participate in the policy-making process by using or participating in the political process. Public policy should meet the needs of the public, but matters in reality are more complex than this. Politics influences policy development and implementation, and sometimes politics interferes with the effectiveness of policy development and implementation. Political feasibility must be considered because this aspect can mean the difference between a successful policy and an unsuccessful policy. Political support, usually from multiple groups, is critical. Most major policy changes or new policies are made through the legislative process. This process can be correlated with the policy-making process.

Steps 1–4 of the policy-making process depicted in Figure 5-2 are similar to the legislative process steps. Once the policy is developed in the form of a proposed law, the legislative process merges with the policy-making process. The legislative process varies from state to state, but all states have a legislative process that is similar to the federal process. When a federal bill is written and then introduced in Congress, in addition to its title it is given an identifier includes either H.R. (House of Representatives) or S. (Senate) plus a number—for example, H.R. 102. The bill is then assigned to a committee or subcommittee by the leadership of the Senate or House, depending on where the bill begins its long process to approval through a final vote. In the committee, the bill may figuratively die, meaning that nothing is done with it. Conversely, if there is some support for the bill, the committee or the subcommittee will assess the content. This might include holding hearings on the bill for extensive discussion, often with witnesses. Amendments may be added. If the bill began in a subcommittee, it can be sent on to a full committee, and then progress to the full House or

Senate. If it began in a committee, it may go straight to the full House or Senate.

When the bill gets to the full House, it first goes to the rules committee. There, decisions are made about debate on the bill, such as the length of debate. These decisions can have an impact on the successful passage of the bill. The Senate does not have a rules committee, and senators can add amendments and filibuster or delay a vote on the bill. There is more flexibility in the Senate than in the House. The leader in the Senate (majority leader) and the House leader have a great deal of power over the legislative process. A bill cannot be passed only in the House or only in the Senate and become law; rather, *both* the House and the Senate must pass the bill. Sometimes a bill is introduced at the same time in both the House and the Senate, allowing the approval process to proceed in both simultaneously. Decisions may then need to be made to reconcile differences in the two bills. If this is the case, a conference committee composed of both representatives and senators work to make those decisions. The altered bill must then go back for votes in both the House and the Senate.

If both houses of Congress pass the bill, then the bill goes to the president for signature. At this time, the bill moves from the **legislative branch** of government to the **executive branch**. **Figure 5-3** identifies the branches of government.

The president has 10 days to decide whether to sign the bill into law. If the president waits longer than 10 days or Congress is no longer in session, the bill automatically becomes law just as if the

president had signed it. In some cases, it is made public, either before the bill comes to the president or soon after, that the president is vetoing a bill. This decision typically is an important political dialogue. In such a case, Congress may decide not to pursue the bill any further, or Congress may decide to bring the bill back for another vote to try to override the president's veto. This effort may or may not be successful, but it is often highly politicized situation. Depending on the number of votes, at this point the bill could either become law or die.

If the president signs the bill or if Congress overrides a presidential veto, the bill goes to the regulatory agency that would have jurisdiction over that particular law. For example, a health law would typically go to the Department of Health and Human Services (HHS). If the law relates to Medicare, it would go to the Centers for Medicare and Medicaid Services (CMS), an agency within the HHS. It is at this point that a very important step in the process occurs: Rules are written for the law that state specifically how the law will be implemented. These rules can make a significant difference in the effectiveness of the law. At specific steps in the regulatory development process, the public, including healthcare professionals, can participate by providing input. It is important that this input be given.

Once the final rules are approved, the law is implemented. There may be a date that the law ends, or "sunsets." If so, the law may expire, or it may be reintroduced into the legislative process.

Not all interested parties accept a policy, and efforts may be made to defeat a policy. Because of the various viewpoints on the same issue, there are often competing interests (Abood, 2007). In addition, partisan issues—that is, Democrat versus Republican—may affect the policy development process. "Decision-makers rely mainly on the political process as a way to find a course of action that is acceptable to the various individuals with conflicting proposals, demands, and values.... . Throughout our daily lives, politics determines who gets what, when, and how" (Abood, 2007, p. 3).

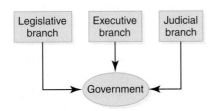

Figure 5-3 The Branches of the Federal Government in the United States

Nurses' Role in the Political Process: Impact on Healthcare Policy

Nurses bring a unique perspective to healthcare policy development because of their education, training, professional values and ethics, advocacy skills, and experiential background. Significant progress has occurred over the years toward advancing nursing's presence, role, and influence in the development of healthcare policy. However, more nurses need to learn how to identify issues strategically; work with decision makers; understand who holds the power in the workplace, communities, and state- and federal-level organizations; and understand who controls the resources for healthcare services (Ferguson, 2001, p. 546).

Nurses have expertise; understand consumer needs, the healthcare system, and interprofessional care; and have an appreciation of the care process. Although nursing has gained political power, it is still weaker than it should be. Put simply, given the large number of nurses in the United States, the nursing profession should have more influential power. Each nurse is a potential voter and, therefore, has potential influence over who will be elected and which legislative decisions are made. However, nursing as a profession has struggled with organizing, and this weakness has diluted the political power of nurses in the United States. At the most basic level, nurses have experienced serious problems defining the nursing profession. The use of multiple entry levels, licensure issues, and multiple titles confuses the public and other healthcare professionals. Policy makers do not understand the various nursing roles and titles, which in turn makes it difficult for nurses to speak with one voice.

Nurses need to develop political competence. Political competence involves the ability to use opportunities, including networking, highlighting nursing expertise, using powerful persuasion, demonstrating a commitment to working with others, thinking strategically, and persevering. It means being aware of the rules of the game and recognizing that the other side needs something. Sometimes giving up one viewpoint or action may lead to more effective results. Collective strength can be powerful, so finding partners makes a difference. Nurses can network to find those partners. Sometimes partners may be found in the least likely groups.

A policy is a tool for change, and nurses are very adept at working with change—something they do in practice on a daily basis. This capability should help nurses develop political competence. "Successful advocacy depends on having the power, the will, the time, and the energy, along with the political skills needed to 'play the game' in the legislative area" (Abood, 2007, p. 3). How can nurses have an impact on healthcare policy?

Getting into the Political System and Making It Work for Nursing

Lobbying

Lobbying is a critical part of the U.S. political process, and nurses are involved in lobbying. A **lobbyist** is a person who represents a specific interest or interest group that tries to influence policy making. The First Amendment to the U.S. Constitution gives citizens the right to lobby—to assemble and to petition the government for redress of grievances. Lobbyists try to influence legislators—the decision makers—as well as public opinion. They often collaborate via coalitions and work with other interest groups to gain more support for a specific interest. Lobbyists particularly want to make contact with legislative staff. The legislative staff assume a major role in getting data about an issue; formulating solutions that may become bills and, if those bills are passed, become laws; and communicating with elected representatives, their bosses, to accept a particular approach or solution. Nurses who visit state and federal representatives typically meet with legislative staff.

Professional organizations hire staff to be lobbyists at both state and federal levels. The ANA, the National League for Nursing, the American

---

Box 5-1 — Important Federal Government Departments and Agencies

Agency for Healthcare Research and Quality (AHRQ): http://www.ahrq.gov
Centers for Medicare and Medicaid Services (CMS): http://www.cms.hhs.gov
Centers for Disease Control and Prevention (CDC): http://www.cdc.gov
U.S. Consumer Product Safety Commission (CPSC): http://www.cpsc.gov
U.S. Department of Health and Human Services (HHS): http://www.hhs.gov
U.S. Food and Drug Administration (FDA): http://www.fda.gov
National Institute for Occupational Safety and Health (NIOSH): http://www.cdc.gov/NIOSH
National Institutes of Health (NIH): http://www.nih.gov
Occupational Safety and Health Administration (OSHA): http://www.osha.gov
Department of Veterans Affairs (VA): http://www.va.gov

Association of Colleges of Nursing, and other nursing organizations, for example, all have lobbyists in Washington, D.C. **Box 5-1** identifies the federal government agencies monitored by the ANA.

Committees

At both the state and federal levels of government, the legislative branches are highly dependent on committees. Legislative work mainly occurs within committees. There are committees on both sides of the federal legislative body, the House and the Senate. The various healthcare-related committees in the U.S. Congress are identified in **Exhibit 5-2**.

Within the House and the Senate, committees have representatives from both major parties, Democrat and Republican. The party with the majority in the House and in the Senate decides who will chair committees and who will serve on each committee. To effectively influence legislation, it is important to understand which committee will be involved in the legislation and who is on the committee. What are the chair's and the committee members' views

---

Exhibit 5-2 — U.S. Congressional Committees with Jurisdiction Over Health Matters

U.S. House of Representatives

House Appropriations Committee
House Commerce Committee
House Commerce Committee Subcommittee on Health and Environment
House Ways and Means Committee
House Ways and Means Committee Subcommittee on Health

U.S. Senate

Senate Appropriations Committee
Health, Education, Labor and Pensions Committee
Health, Education, Labor and Pensions Committee Subcommittee on Public Health
Senate Finance Committee
Senate Finance Committee Subcommittee on Health Care

on the issue? How can they be persuaded? Knowing this information can help in the development of a more effective strategy to influence the course of policy or to prevent it from progressing.

Political Action Committee

Political action committees (PACs) are very important in the political process. A PAC is a private group, whose size can vary, that works to get someone elected or defeated. PACs represent a specific issue or group. The Federal Election Campaign Act covers PACs and defines a PAC as an organization that receives contributions or makes expenditures of at least $1000 for the purpose of influencing an election. Other rules about PAC operations are also identified.

Why would nurses need to know about PACs? The nursing profession has its own PACs, such as the ANA PAC. The ANA considers political action to be a core mission activity, and the PAC is critical to success on Capitol Hill (Conant & Jackson, 2007). The PAC is a form of political advocacy that focuses on supporting candidates who support nursing issues. This organization endorses candidates, makes minimal campaign donations, and campaigns for candidates. The decision to support a candidate is not based on the candidate's party, but rather on whether the candidate supports issues important to nursing. In the end, this empowers the PAC members—in this case, nurses. The ANA PAC's overall goal is to improve the healthcare system in the United States. Any nurse can join this PAC by making a contribution to it. Nurses work in the PAC to get the desired results.

Working to Get the Message Across: Grassroots Advocacy

Many nurses communicate directly with legislators about specific issues of concern. One method of doing so is through written communication. In the past, this was primarily done through letter writing, but now it is easier, and preferred by legislators, to use e-mail for this purpose. E-mail is more efficient, and it allows nurses to respond quickly to a request to communicate their views. This request may come from a nursing organization, as a result of a personal recognition that something is going on that impacts health care and nursing, or from a colleague.

In written communication to legislators, it is important to state what the issue is, provide the bill number (if the correspondence is related to a pending bill), succinctly state one's position, and provide a brief rationale. The letter or e-mail should include one's full name, credentials, employment location, and contact information. To be more effective, the best contact is the nurse's elected representatives.

Another method of communication is to call elected representatives' offices. Before making the call, the nurse should prepare a brief statement that addresses the specific issue.

A third method of communication is to visit elected representatives' offices. This could be an elected official's local office or office in the state capital or in Washington, D.C. As mentioned earlier, the nurse probably will meet with the legislative staff, preferably staff responsible for health issues. This is not a step down, because staff members play a major role in the process. Make an appointment if possible and be on time. The meeting may be short or long. Be engaging, and let the staff or representative/senator know what you do as a nurse, where you work, and what your nursing and healthcare concerns are. Be prepared to discuss both the topic and the activities of the representative—legislation and other interests. Give specifics and stories that support facts and avoid generalities. Come prepared with facts and present them concisely. Provide useful information. Students, for example, might discuss the need for scholarships and financial aid monies, providing examples of how this support helps students to meet career goals and provide more nurses. Follow-up is important; send a thank-you note with a reminder of the discussion.

All these examples demonstrate leadership by the nurses who participate in these efforts to advocate for health care. **Exhibit 5-3** identifies some tips for making such grassroots efforts more effective.

Nursing organizations are involved in policy development through lobbying, through members and officers serving as expert witnesses to government groups and agencies, and through publishing information about issues in both professional and lay literature. Radio and television journalists may interview nurses. These activities place nurses directly in the policy-making process and also improve nurses' public image as experts and consumer advocates.

The ANA has established an initiative related to policy (Patton, 2007). This organization holds several conferences that focus on a specific policy issue. The purposes of these conferences are to increase nurses' inclusion at the policy-making table,

disseminate information, and educate nurses about policy making. The first policy conference was held in June 2007, and its focus was nursing care in life, death, and disaster (related to the Hurricane Katrina disaster). Rebecca Patton, a past president of the ANA, stated, "With your input, ANA will develop guidance dedicated to reconciling the professional, legal, and regulatory conflicts that can occur during such difficult times" (Patton, 2007, p. 22). To increase its ability to influence policy, the ANA invited representatives from the Centers for Disease Control and Prevention, Public Health Emergency Preparedness (an HHS agency), the U.S. Public Health Service, the National Bioterrorism Hospital Preparedness program, and the Agency for Healthcare Research and Quality (AHRQ), all of whom attended.

Exhibit 5-3   Grassroots Tips

Letter or E-Mail Communication with Legislators or Staff

- Make sure your topic is clear.
- Do not assume anything.
- Get the facts.
- Be brief and concise.
- Find a local focus.
- Make it personal.
- Identify that you are a nurse and include your credentials—for example, "I am a registered nurse who works at Hospital Y in Middletown, Missouri."
- Include your contact information.

Phone Calls to Legislators or Staff

- Where can you find the telephone numbers?
  - State: Call the state legislative body, get a directory, or visit your state government's website.
  - Federal: Call (202) 224-3121, or visit websites (http://www.house.gov, http://www.senate.gov).
- Prepare what you will say before you call; consider the comments made about written communication.

- Be sure to communicate up front what you are calling about.

Visiting Members of Congress or State Legislature

- You can visit when a representative is in the home district.
- You can visit the state capital or Washington, D.C.
- You should make an appointment.
- Follow all guides mentioned for other methods of contact. Time will be short, so you need to be prepared.
- Do not be disappointed if you meet with a staff person. Staff are very important and give the representative the information to make decisions, and in some cases are very involved in the decision making.
- Be ready to answer questions; prepare for this possibility.
- Be on time, but recognize that you may have to wait.
- Dress professionally.
- Enjoy yourself and be proud that you are a professional and an expert.

The American Association of Colleges of Nursing (AACN) holds student policy summits to inform students about involvement in Capitol Hill visits and policy work. Student participants then make visits to Capitol Hill with school of nursing deans and directors. Information is provided for all who make these visits so that they are prepared with the facts.

Nurses in Government

Some nurses seek election to government positions at local, state, and federal levels. Others serve as staff in health-related government agencies. Nurses who serve in government positions use their nursing expertise, and this provides many opportunities for nurses to be more visible at all levels of the government—legislative, administrative, and judicial. However, there needs to be greater representation of nurses in these positions.

There are numerous opportunities for nurses to gain some experience in the area of government practice. For example, fellowships—many of which are short term—at the federal and state levels provide opportunities for nurses to learn more about politics and the legislative process and to interact with people who work in government. This is a great way to learn more about health policy. Graduate programs that focus on health policy provide formal academic experiences that can lead to a career in the health policy field. Running for office at any level requires political support, finances, and guidance from those experienced in the world of politics and campaigning. If you choose to pursue this path, be aware that it takes time to build up support for a campaign. There are also positions for nurses at all levels of government, which provide great opportunities to use nursing expertise and to participate in health policy development and implementation.

Nurses can also serve in high-level government positions. For example, in 2013, Marilyn Tavenner, MHA, BSN, RN, was confirmed as the new administrator of the Centers for Medicare and Medicaid Services, which is part of the Department of Health and Human Services. This is an extremely important position providing oversight for the federal government's (and the nation's) largest entitlement program.

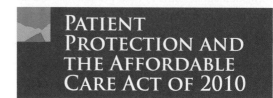

PATIENT PROTECTION AND THE AFFORDABLE CARE ACT OF 2010

Over the years, there have been many attempts to reform the U.S. healthcare delivery system. Most of these efforts have failed. Political issues have typically limited progress in this area—healthcare delivery is a critical political issue because it affects taxes and is a very expensive business. The 2008 presidential election brought healthcare reform to the forefront again. As was true with other efforts, nursing organizations got involved and spoke out about proposed changes. It was very important that nursing do this because healthcare reform would definitely have an impact on nursing, and it has proven to have an impact during its implementation.

In 2010, Congress passed significant legislation, known as the Patient Protection and Affordable Care Act, that reformed healthcare insurance coverage in the United States and that was signed into law by President Obama. Although universal healthcare coverage was not included in the final bill owing to a lack of political support, more people in the United States will have health insurance coverage under this law.

The healthcare delivery system is experiencing some changes as a result of the various reform efforts. Nurses are assuming new roles—for example, as advanced practice nurses, nurse managers, clinical nurse leaders, and clinical nurse specialists. How they are used in hospitals varies. In some cases, nurses with these advanced degrees are eligible for admitting privileges, meaning that they can admit their patients to the hospital from private practice or clinics. This is not the norm, but it does occur. Healthcare reform and other critical sources such as the IOM report, *The Future of Nursing* (2010), emphasize the need to expand use of APRNs in primary care. The United States is currently experiencing a lack of primary care providers, and with the changes in healthcare reform increasing the number of people who have health insurance coverage, there will be even greater demand for these providers.

Emergency services have been experiencing changes because of problems with how they are used by patients. Some patients use the emergency department as their private physician, coming in for services that are not acute or of an emergency nature. This has a major impact on the flow of patients into and out of the emergency department. The result may be long waits to see healthcare providers in the emergency department, making it difficult to admit more patients for emergency services. In some cases, the temporary diversion of patients to other emergency departments becomes necessary to deal with the backup. Another type of problem occurs when patients are not discharged in a timely manner from inpatient units, leaving hospitals with no beds for new patients. Emergency department patients who need to be admitted for inpatient treatment must then wait in the emergency department, sometimes for days.

The large number of patients who cannot pay for services and have no insurance coverage causes major financial problems for hospitals. In some situations, this may lead to the closing of units and fewer beds (decreasing the size of the hospital), termination of staff, and, in extreme cases, the closing of hospitals. Patient access to care has become a major problem in some communities. Access is more than just the ability to get an appointment; it involves the availability of services at times convenient for the patient (time of day and day of week), transportation to and from the care facility, reimbursement for care, and receipt of the right type of care, such as from a specialist. An increase in U.S. citizens with insurance coverage through the Affordable Care Act will have an impact on both these services and the ability to cover costs.

Healthcare reform continues to have an impact on nursing education, nursing practice, regulation of nursing, and professional roles. Nursing leadership will be required to help implement the laws effectively. There are already efforts to diminish the effects of these laws through the court system and part of the Affordable Care Act has been declared unconstitutional, so the long-term impact of the 2010 healthcare reform remains unknown. The provisions do not all go into effect at one time, which means the final results will not be determined for some time.

Landscape © f9photos/Shutterstock, Inc.

CONCLUSION

Nurses and students can and do play a critical role in policy making at the local, state, and federal levels of government. Through this role, they demonstrate leadership, expertise, advocacy, and the ability to collaborate with others to meet identified outcomes. Sometimes nurses are successful in getting the policy that they feel is needed for patients and for nursing, and sometimes they are not. The key to policy making is to come back and try again, but first to learn from the previous experience to improve the effort.

CHAPTER HIGHLIGHTS

1. Healthcare policy directly impacts nurses and nursing.
2. Nurses participate in policy making by sharing their expertise, serving on policy-making committees, working with consumers to get their needs known, and serving in elected offices.
3. A policy is a course of action that affects a large number of people and that is inspired by a specific need to achieve certain outcomes.
4. Policies are associated with roles and standards; specific laws and related programs such as Medicare and Medicaid; delineation of reimbursement requirements for services; staffing levels; access to care; policies and procedures; and nursing education.
5. Critical healthcare policy issues relevant to nursing are the nursing shortage and staffing, the cost of health care, healthcare quality disparities in health care, consumer issues, commercialization of health care, reimbursement

for nursing care, and immigration and the nursing workforce.
6. The policy-making process and the political process are connected, and it is important that nurses understand these processes in their advocacy efforts on behalf of consumers and for better health care.
7. Methods that nurses use when involved in the policy-making and political processes are lobbying, interacting with legislative committees, serving on PACs, participating in grassroots advocacy, working with elected officials who are nurses, and serving as elected officials.
8. In 2010, the U.S. Congress passed significant healthcare reform laws that will increase the number of citizens with health insurance, but the final result is still not universal healthcare coverage. This reform will impact nursing education, practice, regulation, and roles nurses assume.

DISCUSSION QUESTIONS

1. Why is policy important to nursing?
2. Describe the relationship between the policy-making process and the political process.
3. Discuss the roles of nurses in the policy-making process.
4. Why is advocacy a critical part of policy making?
5. Describe the political process.
6. Discuss the methods that nurses use to get involved in the policy-making process and the political process.

CRITICAL THINKING ACTIVITIES

1. Select one of the following topics and search the Internet to learn more about the issue. Why would this issue be of interest to nursing? Why would this be a healthcare policy issue? Has anything been done to initiate legislation on this issue? Teams of students can work on an issue and then share their work.

Landscape © f9photos/Shutterstock, Inc.

CRITICAL THINKING ACTIVITIES (CONTINUED)

a. Rural health care
b. Mental health parity
c. Aging and long-term care
d. Healthcare unions
e. Home care
f. Emergency room diversions

2. Visit the ANA's *Health Care Reform Headquarters* webpage (http://www.rnaction.org/site/PageServer?pagename=nstat_take_action_healthcare_reform) and review the content provided on healthcare reform and other policy issues. Look at the list of resources and select one to review. What does this resource provide nurses? Look at the Toolkit. Here you will find a list of current legislative/policy. What are they? Select one and examine the issue. Discuss your findings with your classmates.

3. Form a debate team that will address the following questions: How would you support or not support universal health care in the United States? How does healthcare reform affect this problem? The team should base its viewpoint on facts and relevant resources. Present the debate in class or online. Viewers (students who are not on the debate team) should vote for the viewpoint that they think is most persuasive.

4. Visit the U.S. House of Representatives (http://www.house.gov) and U.S. Senate (http://www.senate.gov) websites and see if you can identify which representatives and senators are RNs. Explore their websites and learn about the legislation that they have sponsored.

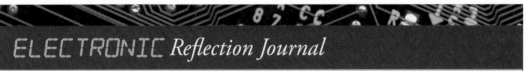

ELECTRONIC *Reflection Journal*

Circuit Board: ©Photos.com

Describe your personal view of nurses getting involved in politics. Would you get involved? Why or why not?

Landscape © f9photos/Shutterstock, Inc.

LINKING TO THE INTERNET

- American Nurses Association Health Care Policy:
  http://www.nursingworld.org/MainMenuCategories/Policy-Advocacy/Positions-and-Resolutions
- American Association of Colleges of Nursing Student Summit:
  http://www.aacn.nche.edu/government-affairs/student-policy-summit
- American Nurses Association:
  http://www.rnaction.org/site/PageServer?pagename=nstat_take_action_presidential_resource_center&ct=1

(continues)

LINKING TO THE INTERNET (CONTINUED)

- NLN Government Affairs: http://www.nln.org/governmentaffairs/index?.htm
- American Association of Colleges of Nursing:
  http://www.aacn.nche.edu/Government/npb.htm (Provides information about some of the organization's views)
- Kaiser Foundation: Health Policy Facts: http://facts.kff.org/
- Association of Women's Health, Obstetric and Neonatal Nurses: Health Policy & Legislation:
  https://www.awhonn.org/awhonn/section.by.state.do;jsessionid=A738259D67D6ADFEEC8905
  BF73DD8BD8?state=California&name=Legislation
- American Association of Colleges of Nursing: Overview of the *Patient Protection and Affordable Care Act*, Public Law No: 111-148; Nursing Education and Practice Provisions:
  http://www.aacn.nche.edu/government-affairs/HCRreview.pdf
- Federal Policy Agenda: http://www.aacn.nche.edu/government-affairs?/legislative-goals
- American Association of Colleges of Nursing: Supported Current Legislation:
  http://www.aacn.nche.edu/government-affairs/support-legislation
- National Association of Pediatric Nurse Practitioners: Advocacy:
  http://www.napnap.org/NAPNAPAdvocacy?.aspx
- American Psychiatric Nurses Association: Legislation:
  http://www.apna.org/i4a/pages/index?.cfm?pageid=4275&redirect=1
- Mandatory overtime:
  http://www.nursingworld.org/MainMenuCategories/Policy-Advocacy/State/Legislative-Agenda-Reports/MandatoryOvertime http://www.aacn.org/WD/Practice/Content/PublicPolicy/
  mandatoryovertime.pcms?menu=Practice
- National Council State Boards of Nursing: Policy and Legislative Affairs:
  https://www.ncsbn.org/government.htm

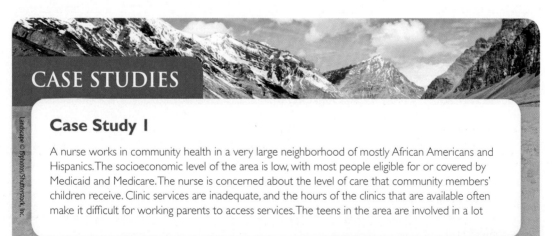

CASE STUDIES

Case Study 1

A nurse works in community health in a very large neighborhood of mostly African Americans and Hispanics. The socioeconomic level of the area is low, with most people eligible for or covered by Medicaid and Medicare. The nurse is concerned about the level of care that community members' children receive. Clinic services are inadequate, and the hours of the clinics that are available often make it difficult for working parents to access services. The teens in the area are involved in a lot

CASE STUDIES (CONTINUED)

of drug activity and have little to do after school. The community has one urban high school, one middle school, and one elementary school. There are two small daycare centers for preschoolers run by the city. The nurse is motivated to tackle some of these problems, but she is not sure how to go about it.

Case Questions

1. Do these problems have health policy relevance? Why or why not?
2. Which steps do you think the nurse should take in light of what you have learned about health policy in this chapter? Be specific regarding stakeholders, strategies, and political issues to consider.

Case Study 2

You have joined a nursing specialty organization. After you join, you decide you want to be active by volunteering for the Legislative Committee. At the first meeting you attend, the major topic is the upcoming state elections.

Case Questions

1. How should the committee prepare for the elections?
2. If you are going to visit a candidate, what might you do to prepare and which type of questions might you ask?
3. Which types of election activities might the committee recommend to the organization membership?

Words of Wisdom

Jennie Chin Hansen, MS, RN, FAAN

President, AARP; Senior Fellow, Center for the Health Professions, University of California, San Francisco; and part-time faculty member, San Francisco State University School of Nursing

Jennie Chin Hansen is a nurse who recognizes the importance of health policy and the nurse's role in it. She is an example of a nurse who has become a leader in non-nursing settings and organizations. She served as the American Association of Retired Persons president for the 2008–2010 biennium and in many of positions in this organization. One of her major contributions to improving health care was her role as executive director of On Lok, Inc., a nonprofit family of organizations in San Francisco that provides integrated and comprehensive primary and long-term care and community-based services. On Lok was the prototype for the Program of All-Inclusive Care for the Elderly, which was signed into federal law in 1997, making this Medicare/Medicaid program available in all

(continues)

Words of Wisdom (*continued*)

50 states. Hansen has also held government and other policy-making organization leadership roles, including as commissioner of the Medicare Payment Advisory Commission and board member of the National Academy of Social Insurance and of the Robert Wood Johnson Executive Nurse Fellows Program. She has won many awards and recognitions for work and is a good example of someone who has used her nursing background to impact healthcare delivery.

These are her words of wisdom:

We start our care in nursing focusing on a safe, evidence-based, and compassionate commitment to the patient and family. This is at the core of our professional practice. Over time, though, we learn through our experience how important critical systems thinking and cultural anthropology is for nurses to incorporate in order to assure we deliver on the goal of the best and most appropriate care for individual patients and society at large. We have an opportunity and obligation to contribute to the development, implementation, and evaluation of safe systems and cultures of caring and competence. We are fortunate to have the framing of issues and suggested tools that come from the rigorous work of the IOM studies. As the largest and most trusted health professional workforce in America, we have a wonderful chance to make a great and significant difference to health care in our country.

Student Perspective
Evan Skinner
Senior, the University of Oklahoma College of Nursing

Globalization, advances in technology, and labor standards are representatives of a dynamic landscape in which we all live. The constant modification of our world forces humans to struggle to maintain balance. Nurses are not exempt from the shifting sands of change; we are subject to the turbulent uncertainties of life, and we must competently encounter each challenge and adapt. Therefore, it is incumbent upon nurses to adopt what the military refers to as "situational awareness." This means that one is to remain vigilant and be knowledgeable of current events. Of that which we must be observant, legislative actions take priority. It is vital that nurses become politically active to promote and preserve the integrity and legacy of the profession of nursing. Alterations in public policy have the potential to have a profound impact on our scope of practice, opportunity for advancement, and work schedules. Awareness and activism within the political realm permit the informed nurse to protect the foundation of our profession against insult and promote its prosperity. Political activism, then, should not be considered merely an additional chore, but a duty.

Landscape © f9photos/Shutterstock, Inc.

REFERENCES

Abood, S. (2007). Influencing healthcare in the legislative arena. *Online Journal of Issues in Nursing, 12*(1), 3.

American Nurses Association (ANA). (2005). *ANA's health care agenda—2005.* Silver Spring, MD: Author.

Block, L. (2008). Health policy: What it is and how it works. In C. Harrington & C. Estes (Eds.), *Health policy* (5th ed., pp. 4–14). Sudbury, MA: Jones and Bartlett.

Coffey, J. (2001). Universal health coverage. *American Journal of Nursing, 101*(2), 11.

Conant, R., & Jackson, C. (2007, March). Brief overview of ANA political action committee. *American Nurse Today,* p. 24.

Ferguson, S. (2001). An activist looks at nursing's role in health policy development. *Journal of Obstetric, Gynecologic, and Neonatal Nursing, 30,* 546–551.

Institute of Medicine (IOM). (2001). *Crossing the quality chasm.* Washington, DC: National Academies Press.

Institute of Medicine (IOM). (2002). *Unequal treatment: Confronting racial and ethnic disparities in health care.* Washington, DC: National Academies Press.

Institute of Medicine (IOM). (2004). *Health literacy: A prescription to end confusion.* Washington, DC: National Academies Press.

Institute of Medicine. (IOM). (2010). *The future of nursing: Leading change, advancing health.* Washington, DC: National Academies Press.

Kalisch, B. J., & Kalisch, P. (1982). *Politics of nursing.* Philadelphia, PA: Lippincott.

Patton, R. (2007, March). From your ANA president: Taking a seat at ANA's policy-making table. *American Nurse Today,* p. 22.

Shi, L., & Singh, D. (2013). *Delivering health care in America.* Gaithersburg, MD: Aspen.

Sullivan, L., & Commission on Diversity in the Healthcare Workforce. (2004). *Missing persons: Minorities in the health professions.* A report of the Sullivan Commission on diversity in the healthcare workforce. Retrieved from http://www.aacn.nche.edu/Media/pdf/SullivanReport.pdf

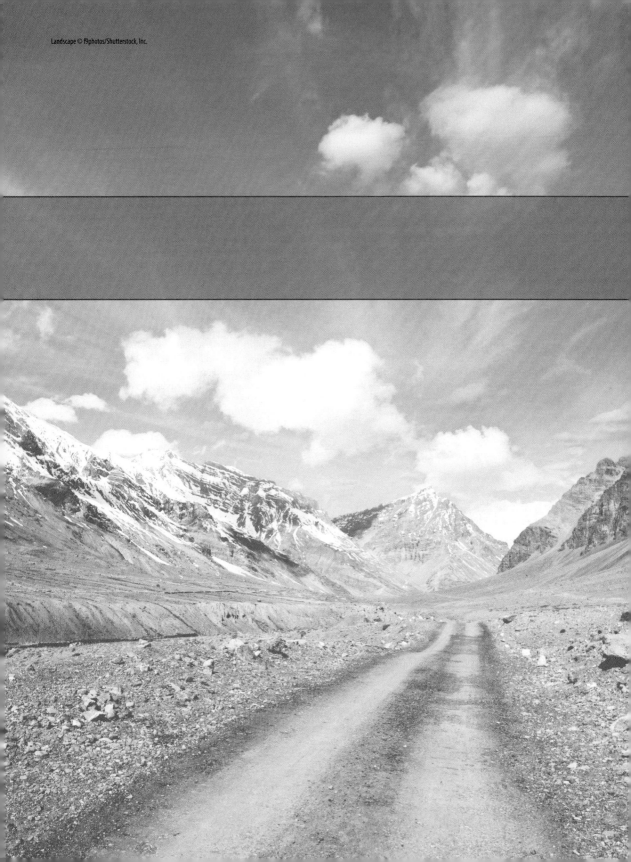

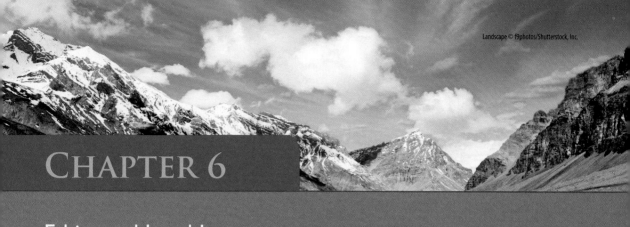

Landscape © f9photos/Shutterstock, Inc.

CHAPTER 6

Ethics and Legal Issues

CHAPTER OBJECTIVES

At the conclusion of this chapter, the learner will be able to:

- Apply ethical principles to decision making
- Discuss the importance of ethics to the nursing profession and its professional recognition
- Summarize current ethical issues
- Define major legal terms

- Discuss the relevance of legal issues to nursing practice
- Explain how malpractice relates to nursing practice
- Discuss examples of ethical and legal issues

CHAPTER OUTLINE

KEY TERMS

Advance directives	Ethical principles	Malpractice
Breach of duty	Ethics	Medical power of attorney
Confidentiality	Informed consent	Negligence
Do not resuscitate	Legal issues	Organizational ethics
Ethical decision making	Living will	Professional ethics

INTRODUCTION

The content in this chapter addresses ethics and legal issues in nursing. As a profession, nursing has ethical responsibilities. In the practice of nursing, legal and ethical issues often arise, and the nurse must understand them and take appropriate steps to address them. Ethics and legal issues involve professionalism, practice concerns, health policy, reimbursement issues, and the organizations that provide health care.

ETHICS AND ETHICAL PRINCIPLES

Definitions

The first question that could be asked in this type of content is *what is ethics?* It is easy to confuse ethics with morals. Morals refer to an individual's code of acceptable behavior, and they shape one's values that are influenced by cultural factors and experiences. **Ethics** refers to a standardized code or guide to behaviors. Morals are learned through growth and development, whereas ethics typically is learned through a more organized system, such as a standardized ethics code developed by a professional group. Ethics deals with the rightness and wrongness of behavior. Bioethics relates to decisions and behavior related to life-and-death issues. The latter sometimes

comes in conflict with a patient's morals, values, and ethics and a nurse's personal morals, values, and ethics. There may also be conflict between a nurse's and an organization's approach to morals, values, and ethics. Health policy also involves ethical decision making, particularly when cost–benefit analysis is used.

Ethical Principles

Four **ethical principles** are used in nursing and healthcare delivery; they are highlighted in **Figure 6-1**. Ethics is a difficult area, and these principles help guide nurses when confronted with ethical issues. Throughout this chapter, the term *patient* will be used, but in the case of a minor or a person who is under

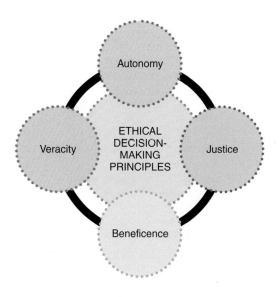

Figure 6-1 Ethical Decision-Making Principles

legal guardianship or power of attorney, *patient* refers to the family or the guardian, who makes the decisions in such cases. The four principles are autonomy, beneficence, justice, and veracity:

- *Autonomy* focuses on the patient's right to make decisions about matters that impact the patient. This means that if the patient wants to be involved in the treatment decisions, the patient makes the final decisions about treatment. To do so, patients need complete and open information or informed consent. The nurse's role is to provide information to better ensure that others, such as the physician, inform the patient, and then to support the patient's decision. Supporting the patient's decision is not always easy, because the nurse may think that the patient is making the wrong decision. It is not the role of the nurse to argue with the patient, but rather to act as the patient's advocate, respecting the patient's choice. The nurse can discuss the decision with the patient and ensure that the patient recognizes the potential consequences of decisions.
- *Beneficence* relates to doing something good and caring for the patient. This principle encompasses more than just physical care—it involves awareness of the patient's situation and needs. In the case of nurses, this also means doing no harm and safeguarding the patient, or nonmaleficence.
- *Justice* is about treating people fairly—for example, when deciding which patients receive treatment and which patients do not. There are more concerns about justice in health care today because of problems with disparity (e.g., some people are not getting care when they need it).
- *Veracity* means truth. For example, which information is the patient given during the informed consent process? Trust plays a major role in this principle. Veracity can be a difficult principle to apply because sometimes

a family member may request that the patient not be fully informed. Such a request is in direct conflict with ethical practices and patient-centered care. Some believe that if another principle is involved, it might be considered first, before veracity comes into play. For example, if it is believed that the truth would cause more harm, does beneficence outweigh justice? In any ethical dilemma, it is important to remember that no two situations are the same.

Other principles have been suggested that are applicable in today's healthcare delivery system—for instance, advocacy, caring, stewardship (management of finite resources), respect, honesty, and confidentiality (Koloroutis & Thorstenson, 1999).

Ethical Decision Making

Ethical decision making is about ethical dilemmas. An ethical dilemma occurs when a person is forced to choose between two or more alternatives, none of which is ideal. Typically, strong emotions are tied to the issue and the alternative solutions, and there is no way to say that one is better than the other. If an ethical dilemma arises and the nurse is involved in the care, the nurse should participate in the decision making. If the nurse is not involved in the issue, then the nurse should not step in.

Once the ethical dilemma is recognized, the next step is assessment to get facts. What are the medical facts, including information about treatment? What are the psychosocial facts? What does the patient want? Which values are involved, and what is the conflict? Getting this information requires talking to others, including the patient and—if the patient approves—to the family, significant others, and other healthcare providers. Neither the nurse nor the physician makes the decision about sharing of information with family or significant others, nor do they make the final decision about treatment unless the patient is in an emergency situation and cannot speak for himself or herself. The treatment team provides recommendations to the patient. Sometimes it is the nurse who thinks that the treatment team does not recognize the presence of an ethical dilemma; in this case, the nurse discusses this observation with the team.

After the assessment is concluded, the information is used to develop a plan to address the dilemma. This requires looking at the choices, goals, and parties involved. Options need to be prioritized.

Key to all of this is patient involvement, if the patient is able and willing to participate in the decision-making process. The decision must be one that the patient accepts. During implementation, the nurse must be the patient's advocate even if the nurse does not agree with the patient's final decision.

Professional Ethics and Nursing Practice

Ethics is a part of any profession, and in nursing, **professional ethics** is part of daily practice. Benner, Sutphen, Leonard, and Day (2010) emphasize that nursing education needs to focus more on ethical comportment. Students need to develop skills to respond ethically to errors and to make ethical decisions. "Nurses need the skill of ethical reflection to discern moral dilemmas and injustices created by inept or incompetent health care, by an inequitable healthcare delivery system, or by the competing claims of family members or other members of the healthcare team" (Benner et al., 2010, p. 28). It is not easy to find the right perspective on ethics in professional roles and in the care provided. Each nurse works to find this perspective and determine how it meshes with the nurse's personal views. This is the potential dilemma between the nurse's view of ethical behavior and the patient's.

American Nurses Association Code of Ethics

Professional organizations such as the American Nurses Association (ANA) and many of the specialty nursing organizations have developed a code of ethics with interpretative statements to help nurses understand the intent of the guiding principles. The ANA's *Guide to the Code of Ethics for Nurses: Interpretation and Application* (2010) is the primary source or guide for nurses when ethical issues are encountered. A nursing code of ethics was first discussed in the United States in 1896, and several editions of this code have been issued to ensure that the content and expectations stay current with practice and healthcare issues.

> The Code of Ethics reflects both constancy and change—constancy in the identification of the ethical virtues, values, ideals, and norms of the profession, and change in relation to both the interpretation of those virtues, values, ideals, and norms, and the growth of the profession itself. (ANA, 2010, p. xviii)

Obtaining a registered nurse license and entering the profession requires that nurses meet the professional roles and responsibilities identified by nursing. Ethics is a part of professionalism. Self-reflection, or the ability to look at a variety of possibilities and consider pros and cons, is also important. It is part of critical thinking and is particularly important when there does not seem to be one right answer, which is the case when an ethical dilemma is experienced. The ANA Code of Ethics provisions are described in **Exhibit 6-1**.

Reporting Incompetent, Unethical, or Illegal Practices

Each nurse has a responsibility to report incompetent, unethical, or illegal practices to the nurse's state board of nursing (ANA, 1994a). However, others can also report nurses, such as employers, consumers, and family members. Each state's nurse practice act (law) serves as the guide for the nurses in the state. This law should be familiar to all licensed nurses. Nurse practice acts vary from state to

Exhibit 6-1   Code of Ethics for Nurses

Provision 1

The nurse, in all professional relationships, practices with compassion and respect for the inherent dignity, worth, and uniqueness of every individual, unrestricted by considerations of social or economic status, personal attributes, or the nature of health problems.

Provision 2

The nurse's primary commitment is to the patient, whether an individual, family, group, or community.

Provision 3

The nurse promotes, advocates for, and strives to protect the health, safety, and rights of the patient.

Provision 4

The nurse is responsible and accountable for individual nursing practice and determines the appropriate delegation of tasks consistent with the nurse's obligation to provide optimum patient care.

Provision 5

The nurse owes the same duties to self as to others, including the responsibility to preserve integrity and safety, to maintain competence, and to continue personal and professional growth.

Provision 6

The nurse participates in establishing, maintaining, and improving healthcare environments and conditions of employment conducive to the provision of quality health care and consistent with the values of the profession through individual and collective action.

Provision 7

The nurse participates in the advancement of the profession through contributions to practice, education, administration, and knowledge development.

Provision 8

The nurse collaborates with other health professionals and the public in promoting community, national, and international efforts to meet health needs.

Provision 9

The profession of nursing, as represented by associations and their members, is responsible for articulating nursing values, for maintaining the integrity of the profession and its practice, and for shaping social policy.

Source: Fowler, M. (Ed.). (2010). *Guide to the code of ethics for nurses: Interpretation and application.* Silver Springs, MD: American Nurses Association. Reprinted with permission.

state because each act is considered part of a state's law and is not administered at the federal level.

State boards have specific processes and procedures that must be followed regarding making and handling complaints. The source of a complaint remains private. This confidentiality is intended to protect the person who reports the complaint as well as to eliminate fear of reprisal that would limit reporting of complaints. Among the common complaints brought to state board are using illicit drugs or alcohol while practicing, stealing drugs from a healthcare organization, committing a serious error

that might demonstrate incompetence, and falsifying records. It is important to remember that a complaint or an initiative by the board to investigate a nurse does not mean that the nurse is guilty. A legal process that gives the nurse rights to defend himself or herself must be followed.

Any nurse who is informed of a board of nursing complaint or recognizes that such a complaint might be filed should consult with an attorney. This legal advisor should not be the same attorney who represents the nurse's employer; rather, the nurse should retain the services of a personal attorney.

Dealing with disciplinary actions is a major responsibility of boards of nursing. The media, legislators, and policy makers are interested in disciplinary actions that the boards take. A board of nursing has to find a balance between protecting the public and protecting the individual nurse's right to practice and the nurse's right to due process.

In some situations, such as when a nurse is accused of drug abuse, the state board of nursing may offer the option of entering an alternative program. These programs are not treatment programs but rather monitoring programs. However, they do give nurses who meet specified criteria the opportunity to maintain their licensure and practice. The nurse must agree to enter a nondisciplinary program that provides identification and treatment support; agree to monitoring upon return to practice; and often agree to submit to regular drug testing. The risk of public knowledge about a drug problem may compel a nurse to accept the alternative program. Compliance with treatment and aftercare recommendations is also required. Return to practice or continuation of practice is not guaranteed, and the nurse is carefully monitored to ensure public safety.

CURRENT ETHICAL ISSUES

Rationing Care: Who Can Access Care When Needed

The United States rations care, albeit not formally. Rationing is the systematic allocation of resources, typically limited resources. In this case, the limited resources are funds to pay for care. Some people receive care, and others do not. Insurers do not cover all care; instead, they determine which care will be provided based on criteria that they identify.

Other forms of healthcare rationing also exist. For example, organ transplantation is a form of rationing—in both the allocation of funds to perform transplants and the allocation of limited organs.

Patients are put into a database to receive organ donations, and the order in which patients receive a transplant depends on specified criteria.

Oregon developed a rationing system for Medicaid by identifying the types of treatment that the state would cover, but this approach was not successful. This is an example of a situation in which the ethical principle of justice might be applied, because rationing, or allocation of resources, is related to equity. It appears to be more acceptable to say "resource allocation" than "rationing," but in the end, resource allocation and rationing are similar.

Healthcare Fraud and Abuse

Healthcare fraud and abuse are not especially uncommon. Fraud is a legal term that means a person deliberately deceived another for personal gain. Fraud also has a nonlegal definition, but the focus here is on fraud that involves breaking the law. In health care, it usually involves money and reimbursement. For example, a patient may be charged for care that the patient did not receive or may be charged more than the usual fee.

In 2013, the federal government recovered more than $4.3 billion from fraud-associated federal healthcare programs; it has recovered $19.2 billion over the last five years for fraud related to government-funded health care, including care covered by Medicare (Department of Health and Human Services [HHS], 2014). This is a lot of money that could have been used to provide health care. Recovering it is a positive step; however, the magnitude of the collections makes a sad statement about the level of healthcare fraud in the United States. Such actions have led to many legal cases and convictions.

Because of this ongoing major loss of monies, the Affordable Care Act of 2010 includes provisions to increase monitoring and enforcement of laws to prevent fraud (Office of the Inspector General, 2011). In March 2011, the Centers for Medicare and Medicaid Services (CMS) began an ambitious project to revalidate all 1.5 million

Medicare enrolled providers and suppliers under the Affordable Care Act screening requirements. As of September 2013, more than 535,000 providers were subject to the new screening requirements, and more than 225,000 lost the ability to bill Medicare due to the Affordable Care Act requirements and other proactive initiatives. Since the passage of the Affordable Care Act, CMS has also revoked 14,663 providers' and suppliers' ability to bill the Medicare program. These providers were removed from the program because they had felony convictions, were not operational at the address CMS had on file, or were not in compliance with CMS rules (HHS, 2014).

Fraud may be committed by physicians, pharmacists, nurses, and other healthcare providers; medical equipment companies; and healthcare organizations. **Exhibit 6-2** identifies examples of Medicaid fraud schemes. Areas of health care in which fraud is most prevalent include psychiatric care, home care, long-term care, and large corporate healthcare organizations.

Ethics and Research

Research is an area in which complex concerns about ethics and legal issues arise. Research has a history of ethical problems. Some key examples of situations in which research participants were abused include the Nazi medical experiments in World War II; the Tuskegee Syphilis Study, in which African American men with syphilis were not treated so that researchers could observe the course of the disease (1932–1972); and the Willowbrook Study, in which residents of an institution for mentally retarded children were deliberately infected with hepatitis (mid-1950s to the early 1970s). In the late 1970s, recognition of these major abuses led to reforms and the creation of legal guidelines that now must be followed by all healthcare researchers. The Belmont Report (National Commission for the Protection of Human Subjects of Biomedical and Behavioral Research, 1978) identified the key concerns and the need for greater attention to ethical principles in conducting and reporting research. **Exhibit 6-3** contains an excerpt from the Belmont Report's introduction.

Participation in research must include **informed consent**, and there are rules regarding how this consent must be obtained. The National Institutes of Health (NIH) is a key resource for information about consent. Some of the information that must be revealed includes the nature and purpose of an intervention; potential risks, discomforts, and benefits to the patient; alternative treatments; compensation if injury occurs; compensation for participating; and a clear statement that the participant may withdraw at any time without any negative

---

Exhibit 6-2   Examples of Medicaid Fraud Schemes

- Billing for "phantom patients"
- Billing for medical goods or services that were not provided
- Billing for more hours than there are in a day
- Paying a "kickback" in exchange for a referral for medical goods or services
- Concealing ownership in a related company
- Using false credentials
- Double-billing for healthcare goods or services not provided

Source: Modified from Department of Health and Human Services, Centers for Medicare and Medicaid Services. (2013). Common Medicaid rip-offs and tips to prevent fraud. Retrieved from http://www.cms.gov/Medicare-Medicaid-Coordination/Fraud-Prevention/FraudAbuseforConsumers/Ripoffs_and_Tips.html

> **Exhibit 6-3   The Belmont Report**
>
> On September 30, 1978, the National Commission for the Protection of Human Subjects of Biomedical and Behavioral Research submitted its report entitled "The Belmont Report: Ethical Principles and Guidelines for the Protection of Human Subjects of Research." The Report, named after the Belmont Conference Center at the Smithsonian Institution where the discussions that resulted in its formulation were begun, sets forth the basic ethical principles underlying the acceptable conduct of research involving human subjects. Those principles—respect for persons, beneficence, and justice—are now accepted as the three quintessential requirements for the ethical conduct of research involving human subjects.
>
> - Respect for persons involves recognition of the personal dignity and autonomy of individuals, and special protection of those persons with diminished autonomy.
> - Beneficence entails an obligation to protect persons from harm by maximizing anticipated benefits and minimizing possible risks of harm.
> - Justice requires that the benefits and burdens of research be distributed fairly.
>
> The Report also describes how these principles apply to the conduct of research. Specifically, the principle of respect for persons underlies the need to obtain informed consent; the principle of beneficence underlies the need to engage in a risk–benefit analysis and to minimize risks; and the principle of justice requires that subjects be fairly selected. As was mandated by the congressional charge to the Commission, the Report also provides a distinction between "practice" and "research." The text of the Belmont Report is thus divided into two sections: (1) boundaries between practice and research; and (2) basic ethical principles.
>
> *Source:* Department of Health and Human Services. *Institutional review board guidebook.* Retrieved from http://www.hhs.gov/ohrp/archive/irb/irb_guidebook.htm

impact on the patient. The institutional review board (IRB) is an organization's committee or department that ensures that the research process meets ethical and legal requirements in protecting participants in biomedical or behavioral research. Hospitals, universities, and other organizations that conduct research have IRBs. The following passage describes the differences between practice and research, which they can sometimes be confused in healthcare delivery:

> While recognizing that the distinction between research and therapy is often blurred, practice is described as interventions that are designed solely to enhance the well-being of an individual patient or client and that have a reasonable expectation of success. The purpose of medical or behavioral practice is to provide diagnosis, preventive treatment, or therapy to

particular individuals. The Commission distinguishes research as designating an activity designed to test a hypothesis, permit conclusions to be drawn, and thereby to develop or contribute to generalizable knowledge (expressed, for example, in theories, principles, and statements of relationships). Research is usually described in a formal protocol that sets forth an objective and a set of procedures designed to reach that objective. The Report recognizes that "experimental" procedures do not necessarily constitute research, and that research and practice may occur simultaneously. It suggests that the safety and effectiveness of such "experimental" procedures should be investigated early, and that institutional oversight mechanisms, such as medical practice committees, can ensure that this need is met by requiring that "major innovation[s] be incorporated into a formal research project. (HHS, 1993)

In healthcare research, subjects may be exposed to multiple risks, typically classified as physical, psychological, social, and economic risks (Levine, 1986, p. 42; HHS, 1993).

Physical Harms

Medical research often involves exposure to minor pain, discomfort, or injury from invasive medical procedures or harm from possible side effects of drugs. All of these should be considered risks for purposes of IRB review. Some of the adverse effects that result from medical procedures or drugs can be permanent, but most are transient. Procedures commonly used in medical research usually result in no more than minor discomfort (e.g., temporary dizziness, the pain associated with venipuncture).

Some medical research is designed only to measure more carefully the effects of therapeutic or diagnostic procedures applied in the course of caring for an illness. This research may not involve any significant risks beyond those presented by medically indicated interventions. Research designed to evaluate new drugs or procedures might present more than minimal risk and sometimes can cause serious or disabling injuries.

Psychological Harms

Participation in research may result in undesired changes in thought processes and emotion (e.g., episodes of depression, confusion, or hallucination resulting from drugs; feelings of stress, guilt, and loss of self-esteem). These changes may be transitory, recurrent, or permanent. Most psychological risks are minimal or transitory, but IRBs should be aware that some research has the potential for causing serious psychological harm. Stress and feelings of guilt or embarrassment may occur simply from thinking or talking about one's own behavior or attitudes on sensitive topics such as drug use, sexual preferences, selfishness, and violence. These feelings may

be aroused when the subject is being interviewed or filling out a questionnaire. Stress may also be induced when the researchers manipulate the subjects' environment—as when emergencies or fake assaults are staged to observe how passersby respond. More frequently, however, IRBs will confront the possibility of psychological harm when reviewing behavioral research that involves an element of deception, particularly if the deception includes false feedback to the subjects about their own performance.

Invasion of privacy is a risk of a somewhat different character. In the research context, it usually involves either covert observation or participant observation of behavior that the subjects consider private. The IRB must decide the following about the study: (1) Is the invasion of privacy involved acceptable in light of the subjects' reasonable expectations of privacy in the situation under study? and (2) Is the research question of sufficient importance to justify the intrusion? The IRB should also consider whether the research design could be modified so that the study can be conducted without invading the privacy of the subjects.

Breach of confidentiality is sometimes confused with invasion of privacy, but it is really a different problem. Invasion of privacy concerns access to a person's body or behavior without consent; breach of confidentiality concerns safeguarding information that has been given voluntarily by one person to another. Some research requires the use of a subject's hospital, school, or employment records. Access to such records for legitimate research purposes is generally acceptable, as long as the researcher protects the confidentiality of that information. The IRB must be aware, however, that a breach of confidentiality may result in psychological harm to individuals (in the form of embarrassment, guilt, stress, and so forth) or in social harm.

Social and Economic Harms

Some invasions of privacy and breaches of confidentiality may result in embarrassment within one's business or social group, loss of employment, or criminal prosecution. Areas of particular sensitivity are information regarding alcohol or drug abuse, mental illness, illegal activities, and sexual behavior. Some social and behavioral research may yield information about individuals that could label or stigmatize the subjects (e.g., as actual or potential delinquents or schizophrenics). Confidentiality safeguards must be effective in these instances. The fact that a person has participated in HIV-related drug trials or has been hospitalized for treatment of mental illness could adversely affect present or future employment, political campaigns, and standing in the community. A researcher's plans to contact these individuals for follow-up studies should be reviewed with care. Participation in research may result in additional actual costs to individuals. Any anticipated costs to research participants should be described to prospective subjects during the consent process.

Nurses should be concerned about these issues for two reasons. First, nurses conduct research, and they must follow the same rules as anyone else who uses human subjects or even animal subjects. Second, nurses assist in data collection and work in areas where research is ongoing. In these situations, the nurse must continue to act as the patient advocate and ensure that the patient's rights are upheld.

Some student projects such as capstones are also reviewed to see whether an IRB is needed for the project. Faculty work with students to determine if the IRB Committee should make the decision about the need to complete the IRB written requirements.

Knowledge and application of the ethical principles related to research need to be part of practice whenever nurses are directly or indirectly involved in research. **Exhibit 6-4** identifies key points of the Code of Federal Regulations related to research.

Organizational Ethics

In the late 1990s and early 2000s, there were serious breaches of **organizational ethics**. A major stimulus to address this problem occurred in 1994, when it was recognized that the federal government lost 10% of its total healthcare expenditures to fraud, equivalent to $100 billion (U.S. House of Representatives, 1994). Because of increasing corporate healthcare fraud and abuse of patients, the CMS, through legislation, now requires that any healthcare organization that is reimbursed through Medicare or Medicaid meet certain compliance conditions to better ensure it maintains appropriate organizational ethics. As it is rare that a hospital does not receive this type of reimbursement to cover

---

Exhibit 6-4   Code of Federal Regulations

- Risks to subjects are minimized.
- The risks to subjects are reasonable in relation to anticipated benefits.
- The selection of subjects is equitable.
- Informed consent must be sought from potential subjects or their legal guardians.
- Informed consent must be properly documented.
- When appropriate, research plans monitor data collection to ensure subject safety.
- When appropriate, privacy of subjects and confidentiality of data are maintained.
- Safeguards must be in place when subjects are vulnerable to coercion.

Source: From Schmidt, N. A., & Brown, J. M. (2015). *Evidence-based practice for nurses: Appraisal and applications of research.* Burlington, MA: Jones & Bartlett Learning.

care provided to Medicare or Medicaid enrollees, this mandate applies to the majority of hospitals. Organizations must identify a compliance officer who audits and monitors actions taken to detect, correct, and prevent fraud. Staff must know how to report concerns related to ethical behavior and potential fraud, and they must be provided with education about these critical issues. The federal government has established these requirements because it does not want patients abused. In addition, the government is concerned about the major loss of funds that has occurred because of fraud, such as paying for care that was not given, paying more than the typical rate, paying for patients who did not receive care, and so forth.

Whistle-blowing can be part of fraud and abuse situations. This action occurs when a person who works for an organization that is committing fraud and abuse reports these activities to legal authorities, sharing extensive information that would be difficult for the authorities to obtain on their own. The False Claims Act, a very old law, protects whistle-blowers. This law was passed during the Civil War and amended in 1982 to further shield whistle-blowers. Whistle-blowers are protected from being sued and from being fired for reporting the organization or staff within the organization. If the federal government pursues the case and recovers funds, the whistle-blower is given a portion of the funds. Anyone can be a whistle-blower, but the person must have information that could not be obtained otherwise or information that was not public knowledge (such as that reported in a newspaper). This type of legal action is complicated and very difficult to resolve.

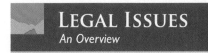

LEGAL ISSUES
An Overview

Legal issues are a part of each nurse's practice. Each state board of nursing identifies situations for which licensure could be denied. You can search

your state board of nursing's website for this information. Licensure itself is a legal issue that is implemented through the legal system. The nurse practice act in each state is a state law. Legal concerns are also directly related to practice. The following are some examples of nursing-related legal issues:

- When the nurse administers a narcotic medication, specific procedures must be followed to ensure that the medication is received only by the patient per healthcare provider order, and that the drug supply is monitored (counted) to make sure the amounts are correct. If there are errors, it could mean that a criminal act occurred—someone took the drug with no right to do so.
- Restraining a patient without a physician's order can be considered assault and battery.
- Falsifying medical records can have adverse legal consequences.
- Accessing an electronic medical record for a patient who is not in a specific nurse's care can be questioned.
- Inadequate supervision of patients that leads to falls or a suicide can have legal consequences.

Critical Terminology

The nurse may encounter the following legal terms as part of his or her practice:

- *Assault*: The threat or use of force on another individual that causes the person to feel reasonable apprehension about imminent harmful or offensive contact. An example is threatening to medicate a patient if the patient does not comply with treatment. This type of threat is not uncommon in behavioral or psychiatric care but should not be made.
- *Battery*: The actual intentional striking of someone, with intent to harm, or in a rude and insolent manner even if the injury is slight. An example of battery is conducting a procedure, such as starting an intravenous

line, without asking the patient. If this is an emergency situation and the patient's life is at risk or if there is risk of serious damage and the patient is not able to provide consent, the event would not be considered battery.

- *Civil law*: Law of private rights.
- *Criminal law*: Those statutes that deal with crimes against the public and members of the public, with penalties and all the procedures connected with charging, trying, sentencing, and imprisoning defendants convicted of crimes.
- *Doctrine of* res *ipsa loquitur*: A doctrine of law that a person is presumed to be negligent if he, she, or an organization/employer had exclusive control of whatever caused the injury, even though there is no specific evidence of an act of negligence, and without negligence, the accident would not have happened.
- *Emancipation*: A child is a minor, and therefore under the control of his or her parent(s)/guardian(s), until the child attains the age of majority (18 years), at which point he or she is considered to be an adult. In special circumstances, a minor can be freed from control by the minor's parent/guardian and given the rights of an adult before turning 18. In most states, the three circumstances under which a minor becomes emancipated are (1) enlisting in the military (which requires parent/guardian consent), (2) marrying (requires parent/guardian consent), and (3) obtaining a court order from a judge (parent/guardian consent not required). A minor can also petition the court for this status if financial independence can be proven and the parents or guardian agree. An emancipated minor is legally able to do everything an adult can do, with the exception of actions that are specifically prohibited if one has not reached the age of 18 (such as buying tobacco). From a healthcare perspective, emancipated minors can sue and be sued in their own name, enter into contracts, and seek or decline medical care.

- *Expert witness*: A person with specific expertise and knowledge who can provide testimony to prove the standard of care. A nurse may serve as an expert witness for nursing care but not for medical care issues. Typically, the nurse is also a specialist in the specific area of care addressed in the legal case. For example, for a case involving the death of a newborn in a neonatal intensive care unit, the expert witness might be a neonatal nurse.
- *False imprisonment*: Confinement of a person against his or her will. This can happen in health care—for example, when a patient wants to leave the hospital and is retained (an exception is when a patient is legally committed for medical reasons); when a patient is threatened or his or her clothes are taken away to prevent the patient from leaving; or when restraints are used without written consent or a sufficient emergency reason.
- *Good Samaritan laws*: Laws that protect a healthcare professional from being sued when providing emergency care outside a healthcare setting. The provider must provide the care in the same manner that an ordinary, reasonable, and prudent professional would in similar circumstances, including following practice standards. An example is a nurse stopping on the highway to assist an accident victim and following the expected standard for providing care to a person with a severe burn to maintain respiratory status under emergency conditions.
- *Malpractice*: An act or continuing conduct of a professional that does not meet the standard of professional competence and results in provable damages to the patient.
- *Negligence*: Failure to exercise the care toward others that a reasonable or prudent person would under the circumstances; an unintentional tort.

- *Proximate cause*: A cause that is legally sufficient to result in liability.
- *Respondent superior*: A principal (employer) responsible for the actions of his, her, or its agent (employee) in the course of employment. This doctrine allows someone—for example, a patient—to sue the employee who is accused of making an error that resulted in harm. The patient also may sue the employer, the hospital, because the employer is responsible for supervising the staff member. For example, if a nurse administers the wrong medication, and the patient experiences complications, the nurse can be sued for the action, and the hospital also can be sued for not providing the appropriate education regarding medications and medication administration, for not ensuring that the nurse received the education, and/or for not providing proper supervision. Typically, in such legal actions, multiple persons and organizations may be sued.
- *Standards of practice*: Minimum guidelines identified by the profession (local, state, national) and healthcare organization policies and procedures. Expert opinion, literature, and research also may be used as standards. Standards are used in legal situations to assess negligence malpractice actions.
- *Statutory law*: The body of law derived from statutes rather than constitutional or judicial decisions.
- *Tort*: A civil wrong for which a remedy may be obtained in the form of damages. An example of a tort that is most relevant to nurses and other healthcare providers is negligence, an unintentional tort.

Malpractice: Why Should This Concern You?

Negligence does occur in nursing—medication errors, not adequately providing for patient access to a call light when the patient needs help, a lack of assessment of risk for falls and failure to prevent falls, failure to institute appropriate interventions when required, and so on. Another example of negligence would be failure to communicate information that affects care, which encompasses situations such as not documenting care provided or response to care; not contacting the physician with information that would inform the physician of the need for a change in treatment; and failing to document lack of monitoring, changes in status, assessment of wound sites or skin status, or malfunctioning intravenous equipment. Negligence also includes inadequate patient teaching, inadequate monitoring and maintenance of medical equipment, lack of identification of an allergy or not following known information about allergies, failure to obtain informed consent, and failure to report another staff member to supervisory staff for negligence or problems with practice. All these examples can lead to malpractice suits.

Malpractice is an act or continuing conduct of a professional that does not meet the standard of professional competence and results in provable damages to the patient. Anyone can sue if an attorney can be found to support the suit; however, winning a lawsuit is not so easy. Often lawsuits are settled outside of court to prevent publicity; in such a case, even if the patient would not have been able to win the lawsuit, the patient may still receive payment of damages.

For a patient or family to be successful with a malpractice lawsuit, all of the following criteria have to be met:

1. The nurse (as person being sued) must have a duty to the patient or a patient–nurse professional relationship. The nurse must have provided care to the patient or been involved in the patient's care.
2. The duty must have been breached. This is called negligence, or the failure to exercise the care toward others that a reasonable or prudent person would under the circumstances. Any of

the following could be used as proof: a nurse practice act, professional standards, healthcare organization policies and procedures, expert witnesses (registered nurses, preferably in same specialty as the nurse sued), accreditation and licensure standards, professional literature, and research.

3. The **breach of duty** must be the proximate (foreseeable) cause, or the cause that is legally sufficient to result in liability harm to the patient. There must be evidence that the breach of duty (what the nurse is accused of having done or not done, based on what a reasonable or prudent person would do given the circumstances, such as what other nurses would have done in a similar situation) led directly to the harm that the patient is claiming. There might be other causes of the harm to the patient that have nothing do with the breach of duty.

4. Damages or injury to the patient must have occurred. What were the damages or injury? Are they temporary or permanent? What impact do they have on the patient's life? These questions and many more will be asked about the damages and injury. If the lawsuit is won, this information is also used to assist in determining the amount of damages that will be awarded, although the plaintiff (person suing) will identify an amount when the suit is brought.

These four malpractice elements are illustrated in **Figure 6-2**.

The plaintiff's attorney must prove that each of these elements exists before the judge or the jury agrees that all elements are present and that the plaintiff should be awarded damages. The nurse's attorney will defend the nurse by proving that one or more elements do not exist. If even one element is lacking, malpractice cannot be proved.

Malpractice lawsuits are very expensive and have affected both healthcare practice and costs of care. This is particularly true for medical

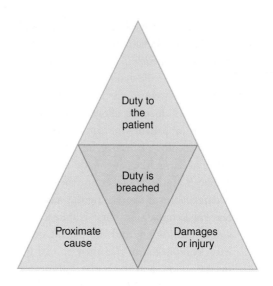

Figure 6-2 Elements of Malpractice

malpractice. The cases are very expensive to bring and defend, and awards are often very high when the case is won by the plaintiff. As mentioned earlier, even if the case is not won in the courtroom by the healthcare provider, a settlement may still be made to stop the legal process. Collectively, these issues have prompted many healthcare providers to practice "defensive medicine," in which physicians prescribe excessive diagnostic testing and other procedures to protect themselves. This approach increases the costs of care, and if testing or procedures are invasive, it can increase patient risk. Malpractice concerns also increase medical costs because physicians, other healthcare providers, and healthcare organizations must carry malpractice insurance to help cover their legal costs for any malpractice suits; these costs are then passed on to customers through patient service charges, increasing overall healthcare costs.

There are pros and cons to nurses carrying professional liability insurance. Such policies are not expensive for nurses, but the nurse needs to be clear about what the policy offers. A question could be asked as to why nurses would be sued when typically they do not have high levels of personal funds; however, they are sued. Often the nurse is included in a group that is being sued—for example, the physician(s), the hospital, specific staff in the hospital (or other type of healthcare organization), and others. When a nurse is sued, the nurse should not rely on the nurse's employer's attorneys to provide a defense; instead, the nurse needs an attorney who represents only the interests of the nurse. Professional liability insurance covers these fees.

As soon as a nurse learns of a possible lawsuit, the nurse should contact an attorney for advice. If the nurse has liability insurance, the nurse would contact the insurer for legal advice, and the insurer may assign an attorney to the case. In addition, the nurse should recognize that after the conclusion of a lawsuit in which the nurse and the nurse's employer are sued, the employer may then sue the nurse to reclaim damages to cover the nurse's employer's expenses for the lawsuit. Nurses must make informed decisions about whether they would rather have their employer's attorney defend them or seek out the services of an attorney who is covered under their own policy, which for some malpractice policies is required, or a personal attorney. In some instances, if the nurse has a personal attorney or an attorney from the nurse's malpractice policy, the institutional legal team will not assist the nurse.

There are also differences in the types of malpractice insurance that can be obtained. Two of the most common types are (1) claims-made coverage, which covers only those incidents that occur and that are reported during the policy's effective period, and (2) occurrence coverage, which provides protection for an incident that took place while the policy was in effect even if the claim was not filed until after the policy terminated. When accepting a job, the nurse should explore the pros and cons of carrying personal professional malpractice/liability insurance.

Nursing students are responsible for their own actions and can be held liable for them. Students are not practicing under the license of their faculty (Guido, 2001). Because of this, students must never accept assignments or do procedures for which they are not prepared. It is also critical that students discuss these situations with faculty rather than acting without guidance.

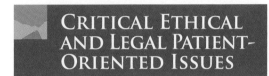

CRITICAL ETHICAL AND LEGAL PATIENT-ORIENTED ISSUES

Confidentiality and Informed Consent

Confidentiality is an issue that is relevant to practice every day. Nurses have the responsibility to keep patient information confidential except as required to communicate in the care process and with team members. Patient-centered care also implies that patients have the right to determine who sees their information, and this decision must be honored. It is important to remember that patient information should not be discussed in public areas (e.g., elevators, cafeteria, hallways) or any place where the information might be overheard by persons who have no right to hear the information. You will encounter patients who are part of your personal life; however, you must remember that what is known about the patient is private. Nurses who work in the community and make phone calls to and about patients using mobile phones in public places can easily forget that their conversations can be overheard.

The Health Insurance Portability and Accountability Act (HIPAA, 1996) has had a major impact on information technology and patient information. Nurses are required to follow this law to protect patient privacy. Patients are informed about HIPAA when they enter a hospital, visit another type of healthcare facility for care, or receive outpatient care.

It is important to remember that patients drive patient privacy. For example, nurses should not assume that patients want family members to have access to the patient's health information. Instead, patients have to be explicitly asked who can be told about any health information. As a student and as a nurse, you will have access to patient information for only those patients to whom you are directly providing care. You must have a reason related to healthcare provision to access patient information. If you do not adhere to these rules, then you are in violation of HIPAA. Be aware that patients can and do make HIPAA-related complaints to state boards and to educational institutions, in the case of students, about students or staff who do not uphold privacy rules/HIPAA.

Another legal concern related to confidentiality is consent. Consent occurs when the patient agrees to treatment, and it may be given either orally or in written form. Whenever possible, consent should be informed consent and documented in writing. The patient's physician or other independent healthcare practitioner is required by law to explain or disclose information about the medical problem and treatment or procedure so that the patient can have informed choice. The patient has the right to refuse the treatment. Failure to obtain informed consent puts the practitioner at risk for negligence.

The requirement to obtain informed consent applies to many nurses. An advanced practice nurse, for instance, has to get informed consent for treatments and procedures. By comparison, the nurse who is not an advanced practice nurse (nurse practitioner) does not have to get informed consent for every nursing intervention. Moreover, this nurse would not be the staff member who obtains patient consent for treatment or procedures. In some cases, the nurse may ask a patient to sign a written consent form, but in doing so, it is assumed that the patient's physician or other healthcare provider has explained the information to the patient. If the patient indicates that this conversation has not occurred, the nurse must talk with the physician or other healthcare provider involved and cannot have the patient sign the form until the patient and the physician have discussed the specific treatment or procedure. If a nurse is directly involved in getting the informed consent and fails to do so, the nurse is at risk for negligence.

A second type of consent is consent implied by law. This consent is applicable only in emergency situations, when a patient may not be able to give informed consent. Healthcare providers can provide care if the patient's life is at risk or if major damage or injury to the patient is likely. In this case, the assumption is that the patient would most likely give consent if the patient could, based on what a reasonable person would do. Nurses who work in the emergency department encounter this type of consent situation.

Advance Directives, Living Wills, Medical Powers of Attorney, and Do-Not-Resuscitate Orders

Advance directives are now part of the healthcare system. This type of legal document allows a person to describe personal medical care preferences. Often these documents describe the person's wishes related to end-of-life needs ahead of time, in which case the document is called a **living will**. Patients have the right to develop this plan, and healthcare providers must follow it.

Interventions that are typically covered in advance directives include (1) use of life-sustaining equipment, such as a ventilator, respirator, or dialysis; (2) artificial hydration and nutrition (tube feeding); (3) **do-not-resuscitate** (DNR) or allow-a-natural-death (AND) orders; (4) withholding of food and fluids; (5) palliative care; and (6) organ or tissue donation. The DNR and the AND directive either are forms of advance directives or may be part of an extensive advance directive. Such an order means that there should be no resuscitation if the patient's condition indicates need for resuscitation. A physician may write a DNR/AND order without an advance directive, but the physician must follow hospital policy and procedures. It is highly advisable that this situation be discussed with the patient, if the patient is able to comprehend, and with the family. The nurse may be present for this discussion but would not make this type of decision. If there are concerns about how it should be handled, the nurse needs to consult the nursing supervisor/manager. If the organization has an ethics committee, the nurse may consult with the committee.

Because state requirements vary, it is advised that patients ask physicians if they will uphold the patient's decisions about health care. Any advance directives should be part of the patient's medical record and easily accessible to the healthcare provider. Be aware that end-of-life issues are never simple.

A **medical power of attorney** document, a type of advance directive, designates an individual who has the right to speak for another person if that person cannot do so in matters related to health care. Another name for this document is durable power of attorney for health care or a healthcare agent or proxy. If a person does not designate a medical power of attorney and the person is married, the spouse can make the decisions if the sick spouse is unable to do so. If there is no spouse, the decision would be made by adult children or parents. People should speak with those who will be their medical powers of attorney about which types of care are preferred and how aggressive that care should be. The proxy or agent is not forced to follow the patient's instructions if they are not written in a legal document; if there is no written document, a sick person should trust that the proxy or agent will follow the guide discussed.

The decision not to receive "aggressive medical treatment" is not the same as withholding all medical care. A patient can still receive antibiotics, nutrition, pain medication, radiation therapy, and other interventions when the goal of treatment becomes comfort rather than cure. This is called palliative care, and its primary focus is helping the patient remain as comfortable as possible. Patients can change their minds and ask to resume more aggressive treatment. If the type of treatment a patient would like to receive changes, however, it is important to be aware that such a decision may raise insurance issues that will need to be explored with the patient's healthcare plan. Any changes in the type of treatment a patient wants to receive should be reflected in the patient's living will. (National Cancer Institute, 2000)

A link at end of the chapter can be accessed to review the National Institute of Nursing's research on palliative care.

Organ Transplantation

As mentioned earlier, organ transplantation is a form of resource allocation. Specific criteria are developed for each type of organ donation, and potential recipients are categorized according to the criteria to determine who might receive a donation and in what order. Organ transplantation registries are a critical component of this process. Nevertheless, it is not always so clear as to who should get a transplant. Many factors are considered—such as age, other illnesses, what the person might be able to contribute, whether the person is single or married, whether the person has children, comorbidities (other illnesses) such as substance abuse, and ability to comply with follow-up treatment—and some of these factors complicate the decision-making process. Organ transplantation is expensive and may not be covered, or only partially covered, by health insurance. The patient will need lifetime specialized care, which is also costly.

Of course, organ donation must occur first so that organ transplantation is possible. Some people designate their willingness to be organ donors while they are healthy—for example, on their driver's license. However, when the time comes to actually honor this request, family members may be reluctant to consent to it. Other people may not have identified themselves as organ donors when healthy, but then something happens that makes them eligible to be organ donors, such as an accident. This situation is even more complex, ethically and procedurally. Healthcare providers do ask for organ donations, and hospitals have policies and procedures that describe what needs to be done. It is difficult to approach family members and say that loved ones are no longer able to sustain themselves, and then to ask for an organ donation at the same time. With organ donations and transplants, time is a critical element to maintain organ viability. Nurses do not ask for the donation but may assist the physician in this most difficult discussion. Later, family members or the patient (if responsive) may want to discuss it further with the nurse.

Assisted Suicide

Assisted suicide is a complex ethical and legal issue, but the nurse's role is very clear: The nurse cannot participate in helping a person end his or her life. In 1997, Oregon passed the first state law pertaining to assisted suicide, the Death with Dignity Act, which allowed terminally ill citizens of Oregon to end their lives through voluntary self-administration of lethal medications prescribed by a physician for this purpose. The law describes who can be involved and the procedure or steps that must be taken. Two physicians must be involved in the decision. As of 2014, three states (Oregon, Vermont, and Washington) have legalized physician-assisted suicide by passing legislation, and one state (Montana) has legalized physician-assisted suicide owing to a court ruling. In other states, this act is considered to be illegal. Some countries other than the United States allow assisted suicides.

The American Nurses Association (ANA) believes that the nurse should not participate in assisted suicide. Such an act is in violation of the *Code for Nurses with Interpretive Statements (Code for Nurses)* and the ethical traditions of the profession. Nurses, individually and collectively, have an obligation to provide comprehensive and compassionate end-of-life care which includes the promotion of comfort and the relief of pain, and at times, forgoing life-sustaining treatments. (ANA, 1994b, p. 1)

The ANA has also issued a position statement on the withdrawal of nutrition and hydration (ANA, 2011). This statement indicates that the patient or the patient's surrogate should make this decision, and the nurse should provide expert end-of-life nursing care.

Social Media and Ethical and Legal Issues: A New Concern

Social media or the use of networking web-based instruments or sites such as Facebook, Myspace, LinkedIn, Instagram, Google+, Flickr, and Twitter has presented nurses with new ethical and legal issues. There have been times when such sites such as CaringBridge.org have assisted families in sending information out to friends and relatives when there is a hospitalization, yet sometimes these types of sites are problematic. This is a gray area today, as Saver (2011) points out. Nurses have been fired for sending photos or discussing patient information on Facebook. In the spring of 2011, a student nurse was dismissed from a nursing program when the student's photos related to a patient's care were posted on Facebook. After a legal process, the student was readmitted to the school.

Many healthcare organizations have established their own policies on the use of social media that must be followed by students and staff. A link at the end of the chapter connects to the National Council of State Boards of Nursing (NCSBN) social media guidelines, which support the ANA's principles for using social media.

The ANA Code of Ethics emphasizes the protection of confidentiality of patient information by nurses. HIPAA also protects patient information, and educational and healthcare institutional policies outline the legal issues related to discussion or sharing of protected information. A simple rule of thumb is this: When in doubt, do not post (Saver, 2011).

Landscape © f9photos/Shutterstock, Inc.

CONCLUSION

This chapter presented introductory information about the ethical and legal issues in nursing. Nurses deal daily with ethical concerns about their patients and encounter numerous issues that could lead to potential legal concerns. A healthcare professional cannot avoid either ethics or legal issues. A nurse cares for patients, families, and communities, and in doing so the nurse must consider how that care impacts the feelings and rights of others. From the time a nurse achieves licensure, the nurse operates under a legal system through the nurse practice act and other laws and regulations.

Landscape © f9photos/Shutterstock, Inc.

CHAPTER HIGHLIGHTS

1. Ethics is concerned with a code of behaviors, whereas bioethics relates to life-and-death decisions.

2. Ethical dilemmas arise when there is conflict among the nurse's, profession's, organization's, and patient's codes for decision making.

3. Principles of ethical behavior fall into four areas: autonomy, beneficence, justice, and veracity.

4. A professional code of ethics guides an entire discipline and is generally set at the national level.

5. State boards of nursing outline the expectations of nurses within their jurisdiction.

6. Reporting unethical, immoral, and unsafe actions is part of a nurse's ethical responsibility to protect the public from harm.

7. Some of the ethical issues in today's healthcare delivery involve scarcity of resources and resource allocation, or rationing of services.

8. Healthcare fraud and abuse involve deliberate deceptive activities to steal funds.

9. Research activities require stringent considerations of ethical principles, such as protection of the public from physical, psychological, social, and economic harm, and informed consent for the research protocol offered in language that is understandable to the research subject.

10. An emancipated minor is one who is afforded all the rights of an adult unless expressly prohibited by state or federal law.

11. Organizational ethics refers to an institution's ethical expectations of itself as an organization and its employees and the patient's rights.

12. Malpractice and negligence charges can be filed against a nurse. The nurse must understand both of these concepts.

13. A nurse must consider the pros and cons of and the differences in institutional and personal professional liability insurance coverage.

DISCUSSION QUESTIONS

1. Describe malpractice and how it applies to nursing care.
2. What is the IRB?
3. Explain the potential harms in research that IRBs are concerned about.
4. How does ethical decision making apply to nursing students?
5. Explain how the profession of nursing incorporates ethics into practice and the profession.
6. Discuss one example of an ethical issue and how the ethical principles apply to this issue.

CRITICAL THINKING ACTIVITIES

1. Visit your state board of nursing website and find information about making complaints to the board. Review the information. What do you think about it?
2. Visit https://www.ncsbn.org/3771.htm, the website for the National Council of State Boards of Nursing, and select one of the topics under the Discipline heading. Summarize the topic and discuss why it is relevant to you as a student, and why it would be relevant to you as a nurse.
3. Select one of the following topics: confidentiality and informed consent, advance directives, living wills, DNR orders, or organ donation. Explain what it is in language that consumers could understand. What makes the issue you selected an ethical and/or legal issue?

ELECTRONIC *Reflection Journal*

Describe an experience you have had in your clinical sessions that presented an ethical dilemma for you. Why was it difficult for you? What did you do to cope with it? What will you do if you experience a similar situation in the future?

LINKING TO THE INTERNET

- Department of Health and Human Services Office for Human Research Protections: http://www.hhs.gov/ohrp/
- U.S. National Institutes of Health, National Cancer Institute: Introduction to Clinical Trials: http://www.cancer.gov/clinicaltrials

Landscape © f9photos/Shutterstock, Inc.

LINKING TO THE INTERNET (CONTINUED)

- American Association of Legal Nurse Consultants: http://www.aalnc.org/
- American Nurses Association: Ethics and Standards:
  http://nursingworld.org/MainMenuCategories/ThePracticeofProfessionalNursing/NursingStandards
- National Council of State Boards of Nursing on Social Media Use: https://www.ncsbn.org/2930.htm
- National Institute of Nursing Research Palliative Care:
  http://www.ninr.nih.gov/newsandinformation/newsandnotes/conversationsmatter-patients#
  .U2pOhsfTaCI

CASE STUDIES

Case Study 1

A 5-day-old premature baby was believed to require a blood transfusion because of increasing anemia. The parents were Jehovah's Witnesses and did not wish to have blood or blood products given to the baby. A court order was obtained with the parents' knowledge, and the blood was given. However, the physician on call the next night did not think he needed to obtain the court's consent for an additional blood transfusion because it had been granted for the earlier transfusion. The blood was ordered, and the nurse was asked to hang the blood. The nurse refused for ethical and legal reasons.

Case Questions

1. What might be the ethical and legal reasons for a nurse to refuse to follow the physician's orders?
2. Which steps should the nurse take?
3. How do you think the nurse should respond to the parents?

Case Study 2

Following the death of a patient who had received the wrong medication, the hospital, the physician, and the nurse who administered the medication were sued by the patient's family. The nurse is very concerned and agrees to legal representation from the hospital attorneys. Weeks go by before she hears from the attorney. The nurse has malpractice insurance, but she is unsure what to do about it. She is frustrated and talks to a friend who is also a nurse. She tells her friend that she feels like she should call the patient's family. The following are questions that come up.

Case Questions

1. Is it wise for the nurse to not have her own legal representation? If not, why?
2. What should the nurse do about her malpractice coverage?
3. What does the plaintiff (patient's family) have to prove?
4. Why should the nurse not call the patient's family?

Words of Wisdom

Pamela Holtzclaw Williams, JD, MS, RN

A competent nurse applies ethical values in all nursing practice; the need for application does not simply kick in only when there are controversies, conflicts, or disagreements regarding what is right or wrong. Ethical values are learned norms of professional behavior applicable in all nursing roles and activities. These values must be part of the professional culture and present in classwork, but especially evident in applied reality settings such as student clinical experiences. After formal education, graduation, and immersion in the clinical setting, the new nurse benefits from reinforcement of these values through continuing education formats. Employers and nursing professional organizations should strive to provide ethics mentorship for nurses as a worthwhile goal.

Landscape © f9photos/Shutterstock, Inc.

REFERENCES

American Nurses Association (ANA). (1994a). *Guidelines on reporting incompetent, unethical or illegal practice*. Silver Spring, MD: Author.

American Nurses Association (ANA). (1994b). *Position statement: Assisted suicide*. Silver Spring, MD: Author.

American Nurses Association (ANA). (2010). *Guide to the code of ethics for nurses: Interpretation and application*. Silver Spring, MD: Author.

American Nurses Association (ANA). (2011). *Position statement: Forgoing nutrition and hydration*. Silver Spring, MD: Author.

Benner, P., Sutphen, M., Leonard, V., & Day, L. (2010). *Educating nurses: A call for radical transformation*. San Francisco, CA: Jossey-Bass.

Guido, G. (2001). *Legal and ethical issues in nursing*. Upper Saddle River, NJ: Prentice Hall.

Health Care Portability and Accountability Act of 1996 (HIPAA), Pub. L. No. 104-191, 110 Stat. 1998 (1996).

Koloroutis, M., & Thorstenson, T. (1999). An ethics framework for organizational change. *Nursing Administrative Quarterly, 23*(2), 9–18.

Levine, R. (1986). *Ethics and regulation of clinical research* (2nd ed.). Baltimore, MD: Urban and Schwarzenberg.

National Cancer Institute. (2000). Fact sheet: Advance directives. Retrieved from http://www.cancer.gov/search/results

National Commission for the Protection of Human Subjects of Biomedical and Behavioral Research. (1978). *The Belmont report: Ethical principles and guidelines for the protection of human subjects of research*. Washington, DC: Author.

Office of the Inspector General. (2011). Health care fraud and abuse control program report. Retrieved from http://www.oig.hhs.gov/publications/hcfac.asp

Saver, C. (2011). *How social media affects the work of nurse leaders*. Presentation at the Institute for Nursing Healthcare Leadership, Boston, MA.

U.S. Department of Health and Human Services (HHS). (1993). Protecting human research subjects: Institutional Review Board guidebook. Retrieved from http://www.hhs.gov/ohrp/archive/irb/irb_guidebook.htm

U.S. Department of Health and Human Services (HHS). (2014, January 26). Departments of Justice and Health and Human Services announce record-breaking recoveries resulting from joint efforts to combat healthcare fraud. Retrieved from http://www.hhs.gov/news/press/2014pres/02/20140226a.html

U.S. House of Representatives. (1994, July 19). *Deceit that sickens America: Healthcare fraud and its innocent victims*. Hearings before the Subcommittee on Crime and Criminal Justice of the Committee on the Judiciary House of Representatives, one hundred and third Congress, second session. Washington, DC: U.S. Government Printing Office.

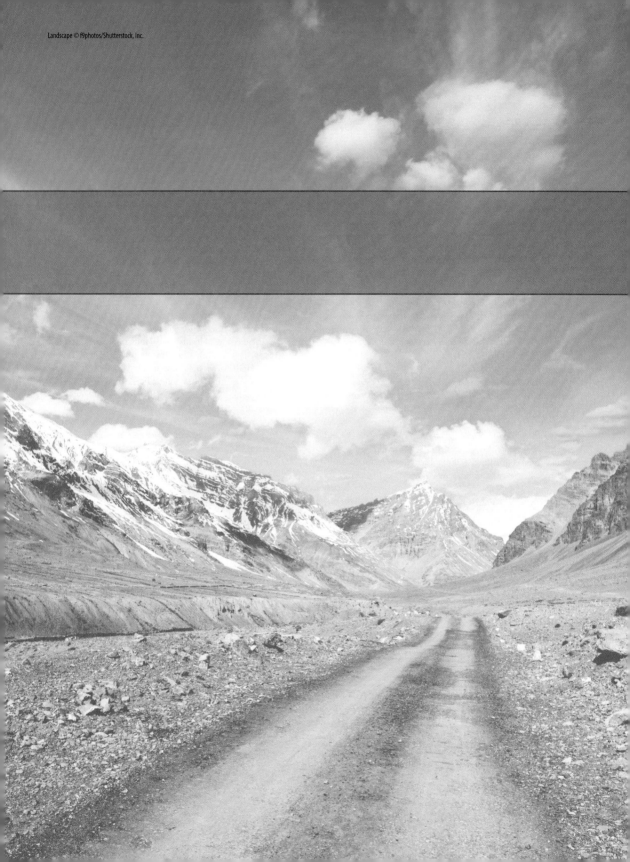

CHAPTER 7

Health Promotion, Disease Prevention, and Illness: A Community Perspective

CHAPTER OBJECTIVES

At the conclusion of this chapter, the learner will be able to:

- Discuss the national initiative to improve the United States' health: *Healthy People 2020.*
- Describe public/community health, expansion of the U.S. healthcare system, and healthcare reform
- Discuss the continuum of care and continuity of care and its relationship to the individual, family, and community across the life span, as well as healthcare disparities
- Define health promotion and disease prevention
- Explain the importance of stress, coping, and resilience to health promotion, disease prevention, and illness
- Explain the relevance of vulnerable populations to the healthcare system

- Examine the problem of increasing chronic disease in the United States
- Discuss examples of public/health services: community preparedness, migrant and immigrant health issues, home health care, rehabilitation, extended care, long-term care, elder care, hospice and palliative care, case management, occupational health care, and alternative and complementary medicine
- Discuss the relevance of genetics and public/community health
- Discuss critical global healthcare concerns and nursing's role in improving global health

CHAPTER OUTLINE

KEY TERMS

Acute care	Family	Occupational health care
Caregiver	Health	Palliative care
Case management	Healthcare disparity	Primary care
Collaboration	Health promotion	Rehabilitation
Community	Healthy community	Resilience
Continuum of care	*Healthy People 2020*	Secondary caregiver
Coordination	Home care	Stress
Coping	Hospice	Stress management
Disease prevention	Illness	Tertiary care
Extended care	Long-term care	Wraparound services

INTRODUCTION

This chapter provides an introduction to public/community health, health promotion and disease prevention, the continuum of care, healthcare disparities, the importance of chronic disease, and delivery of care in a variety of settings in the community. Nursing programs provide clinical experiences for students in many of the settings and situations discussed in this chapter, and students will learn about public/community health in more depth in public/community health courses. Where do patients receive care? Who are the patients? How are health and illness viewed by patients and by nurses, and what impact does this view have on healthcare delivery? Nurses need an understanding of these critical public/community health issues.

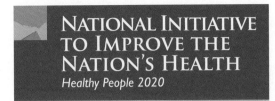

NATIONAL INITIATIVE TO IMPROVE THE NATION'S HEALTH
Healthy People 2020

Healthy People 2020 (U.S. Department of Health and Human Services [HHS], 2010) is a national prevention initiative that focuses on improving the health of Americans by providing a comprehensive set of disease prevention and health promotion goals and objectives with target dates.

> *Healthy People* is used as a tool for strategic management by the federal government, states, communities, and many other public- and private-sector partners. Its comprehensive set of objectives and targets is used to measure progress for health issues in specific populations, and serves as (1) a foundation for prevention and wellness activities across various sectors and within the federal government, and (2) a model for measurement at the state and local levels. (HHS, 2010)

These goals and objectives are used by the Department of Health and Human Services and other health agencies (federal, state, and local) to develop programs that promote health and prevent disease and illness; they are also used to evaluate outcomes. The ultimate measure of success of this health improvement initiative is the health status of the target population.

There have been five editions of *Healthy People* (1979, 1990, 2000, 2010, and 2020). The vision and the major goals that should be reached by 2020 include the following:

Vision

A society in which all people live long, healthy lives.

Mission

Healthy People 2020 strives to:

- Identify nationwide health improvement priorities

- Increase public awareness and understanding of the determinants of health, disease, and disability and the opportunities for progress
- Provide measurable objectives and goals that are applicable at the national, state, and local levels
- Engage multiple sectors to take actions to strengthen policies and improve practices that are driven by the best available evidence and knowledge
- Identify critical research, evaluation, and data collection needs

Overarching Goals

- Attain high-quality, longer lives free of preventable disease, disability, injury, and premature death
- Achieve health equity, eliminate disparities, and improve the health of all groups
- Create social and physical environments that promote good health for all
- Promote quality of life, healthy development, and healthy behaviors across all life stages

Figure 7-1 presents *Healthy People 2020* in the form of a graphic model. The model emphasizes critical determinants for a society in which all people live long, healthy lives. These determinants are the physical environment, the social environment, individual behavior, biology and genetics, and health services. All of the determinants impact health outcomes, and the determinants of health interact with one another. The determinants need to be monitored and evaluated to improve health status of individuals, families, and communities. According to *Healthy People*, health status is determined by measuring birth and death rates, life expectancy, quality of life, morbidity from specific diseases, risk factors, use of ambulatory care and inpatient care, accessibility of health providers and facilities, financing of health care, health insurance coverage, and other factors. Access to health care is critical. This is a complex area, and all of the elements included in this area affect the health

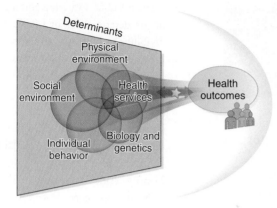

Overarching goals:

- Attain high quality, longer lives free of preventable disease, disability, injury, and premature death.
- Achieve health equity, eliminate disparities, and improve the health of all groups.
- Create social and physical environments that promote good health for all.
- Promote quality of life, healthy development, and healthy behaviors across all life stages.

Figure 7-1 Healthy People 2020

Source: From U.S. Department of Health and Human Services. (2010). *Healthy People 2020.* Washington, DC: U.S. Government Printing Office. Retrieved from http://www.healthypeople.gov

status of individuals and communities. For example, when the causes of death in the United States are examined, there typically is not one single factor or behavior that determines outcomes, but rather multiple factors—such as genetics, lifestyle, gender, and race/ethnic factors; poverty level, education, injury, violence, and other factors in the environment; and the unavailability or inaccessibility of quality health services—play intertwined roles that lead to death.

Healthy People 2020 focuses on topics that are tracked and monitored to assess outcomes. **Exhibit 7-1** describes these topics (which are similar to the priority areas of care identified by the Institute of Medicine [IOM]) and identifies their related indicators and objectives.

A **community** is defined as "people and the relationships that emerge among them as they develop and use in common some agencies and institutions and share a physical environment" (Williams, 2006, p. 3). The *Healthy People 2020* initiative describes a **healthy community** as one that embraces the belief that health is more than merely an absence of disease; a healthy community includes those elements that enable people to maintain a high quality of life and productivity. A healthy community has the following characteristics:

It is safe; provides both treatment and prevention services to all community members; has the infrastructure (roads, schools, playgrounds, and other services) to meet needs; and is a healthy environment (regarding issues of pollution, for example). Educational and community-based programs need to focus on preventing disease and injury, promoting and improving health, and enhancing the quality of life. According to *Healthy People 2020,* to provide broad access, programs should be located in schools, workplaces, healthcare facilities, and community sites. Such programs typically include the following topics:

- Chronic diseases
- Injury and violence prevention
- Mental illness/behavioral health
- Unintended pregnancy
- Oral health
- Tobacco use
- Substance abuse
- Nutrition and obesity prevention
- Physical activity

One method that a community might use to develop a healthy community is called "MAP-IT," which is an approach recommended by *Healthy People* to work with community members in planning

Exhibit 7-1	*Healthy People* Topics, Indicators, and Objectives

Topic	Indicators	Objectives
Access to care	Proportion of the population with access to healthcare services	1. Increase the proportion of persons with health insurance. 2. Increase the proportion of persons with a usual primary care provider. 3. (Developmental) Increase the proportion of persons who receive appropriate evidence-based clinical preventive services.
Healthy behaviors	Proportion of the population engaged in healthy behaviors	4. Increase the proportion of adults who meet current federal physical activity guidelines for aerobic physical activity and for muscle-strengthening activity. 5. Reduce the proportion of children and adolescents who are considered obese. 6. Reduce consumption of calories from solid fats and added sugars in the population aged 2 years and older. 7. Increase the proportion of adults who get sufficient sleep.
Chronic disease	Prevalence and mortality of chronic disease	8. Reduce deaths from coronary heart disease. 9. Reduce the proportion of persons in the population with hypertension. 10. Reduce the overall cancer death rate.
Environmental determinants	Proportion of the population experiencing a healthy physical environment	11. Reduce the number of days on which the air quality index exceeds 100.
Social determinants	Proportion of the population experiencing a healthy social environment	12. (Developmental) Improve the health literacy of the population. 13. (Developmental) Increase the proportion of children who are ready for school in all five domains of healthy development: physical development, social–emotional development, approaches to learning, language, and cognitive development. 14. Increase educational achievement of adolescents and young adults.
Injury	Proportion of the population that experiences injury	15. Reduce fatal and nonfatal injuries.
Mental health	Proportion of the population experiencing positive mental health	16. Reduce the proportion of persons who experience major depressive episodes.
Maternal and infant health	Proportion of healthy births	17. Reduce low birth weight and very low birth weight.

(continues)

Exhibit 7-1 *(continued)*

Responsible sexual behavior	Proportion of the population engaged in responsible sexual behavior	**18.** Reduce pregnancy rates among adolescent females. **19.** Increase the proportion of sexually active persons who use condoms.
Substance abuse	Proportion of the population engaged in substance abuse	**20.** Reduce past-month use of illicit substances. **21.** Reduce the proportion of persons who engage in binge drinking of alcoholic beverages.
Tobacco	Proportion of the population using tobacco	**22.** Reduce tobacco use by adults. **23.** Reduce the initiation of tobacco use among children, adolescents, and young adults.
Quality of care	Proportion of the population receiving quality healthcare services	**24.** Reduce central line–associated bloodstream infections.

Source: Data from U.S. Department of Health and Human Services. (2010). *Healthy People 2020.* Retrieved from http://www.healthypeople.gov

what needs to be done to improve the community's health. The MAP-IT steps follow:

M Mobilize individuals and organizations that care about the health of the community into a coalition.

A Assess the areas of greatest need in the community, as well as the resources and other strengths that planners can tap into to address those areas.

P Plan the approach. Community leaders/members start with a vision of where they want to be as a community; they then add strategies and action steps to help them achieve that vision.

I Implement a plan using concrete action steps that can be monitored and will make a difference.

T Track progress over time.

The *Healthy People 2020* initiative not only provides a 10-year plan to improve health care in the United States, but also monitors progress periodically to determine if the goals and objectives are being met. Data on current outcomes can be found on the *Healthy People* website (http://www.healthypeople.gov). When the 10-year time period is completed, all outcomes are evaluated, and this information and data are then used to develop the goals and objectives for the next 10 years.

Healthy People even has had an impact on curricula in schools of nursing. "In 2006, 91% of Council on Education for Public Health (CEPH) accredited schools of public health, CEPH accredited academic programs, and schools of nursing (with a public health or community health component) integrated the Core Competencies for Public Health Professionals into curricula. The Healthy People 2020 target for this integration is 94%" (HHS, 2013). Schools of nursing have long had public/community health content, but now there is more emphasis on it, with *Healthy People* content being explicitly included.

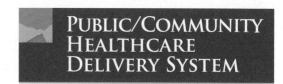

PUBLIC/COMMUNITY HEALTHCARE DELIVERY SYSTEM

Structure and Function of the Public/Community Healthcare Delivery System

Public health plays a critical role in improving and maintaining the health of individuals, families, and communities. Public health includes issues related to the public health workforce, financing and economics, structure and performance, and information and technology. It is a complicated endeavor, requiring multiple services to meet needs of populations and communities (Robert Wood Johnson Foundation [RWJF], 2012). There is a great need to address multiple complex health problems in communities, such as violence, including domestic, child, and elder abuse; substance abuse and alcohol dependency; tobacco use; injuries; automobile accidents; environmental factors such as air and water quality; food safety and consequent health issues; and communicable diseases. Public health has recently become more important with the increasing concern about disaster management and terrorism. Communities need to develop effective plans to provide healthcare services in major crisis situations. All these concerns require more than just care for individuals who are experiencing these problems.

Public health incorporates three functions:

1. *Assessment:* Assess and diagnose the status of the community's health and identify the needs for services using epidemiology, surveillance, research, and evaluation.

2. *Policy development:* Some problems require changes in laws, programs for prevention and treatment, and reimbursement for these services. There is a great need for strategic plans and interventions, and appropriate evaluation of outcomes needs to be developed through the government and its agencies at all levels (local, state, and federal).

3. *Assurance:* Ensure universal access to care when it is needed and to health promotion and prevention of disease and illness through community-wide health services.

The public/community healthcare delivery system is complex and can be viewed from the perspectives of the federal, state, and local levels. The U.S. Department of Health and Human Services (HHS), along with the Centers for Disease Control and Prevention (CDC), Food and Drug Administration (FDA), and the Public Health Service (PHS), all have major responsibilities in ensuring the health of the nation. States and local areas vary as to how their public/community healthcare delivery systems are organized and the types of services they provide; however, services typically include immunizations, environmental health issues (water, air, sanitation), transportation safety, food safety, maintenance of licensure for healthcare providers (such as physicians, nurses, hospitals, long-term care facilities, and others), clinic systems, disaster planning, school health through public schools, and much more. Each state has a public health department or division, and typically counties and other local entities also have their own public/community health services. It is important that all three levels of government public health services collaborate and communicate to ensure effective community/public health services; however, this is not always the case. There is hope that with the healthcare reform of 2010, there will be greater opportunity to develop a more coordinated healthcare system that includes public/community health delivery, although the Affordable Care Act focuses primarily on healthcare reimbursement.

Nurses are very active in all types of public/community services, serving in administrative and planning roles at the federal, state, and local levels; assessing service needs; providing services in clinics and other state and local healthcare facilities; providing immunizations; working toward tuberculosis control; providing human immunodeficiency virus (HIV)/acquired immunodeficiency syndrome (AIDS) care and prevention; developing and implementing health promotion and disease prevention; providing home care and hospice care; working as school nurses and occupational health nurses; conducting research in areas of public/community health; participating in epidemiology activities; and other roles. When students take public/community health courses, they learn more about this critical area of health care and the roles of nurses and other members of the public/community health team.

Continuum of Care

The **continuum of care** is an important concept in nursing and health care. In 2004, The Joint Commission (then called the Joint Commission on Accreditation of Healthcare Organizations) defined the continuum of care as "matching an individual's ongoing needs with the appropriate level and type of medical, psychological, health, or social care or service within an organization or across multiple organizations" (p. 317). The goal of the continuum of care is to decrease fragmented care and costs. The continuum includes health promotion, disease and illness prevention, ambulatory care, acute care, **tertiary care**, home health care, long-term care, and hospice and palliative care. In the current healthcare delivery system, patients receive care in a variety of settings from a variety of healthcare providers, and they move back and forth along the continuum. The continuum is a view of health care that describes a range of services in a variety of settings so that a patient might receive care at different stages of health and illness.

Continuity of Care

"Continuity of care is the degree to which a series of discrete events is experienced as coherent and connected and consistent with the patient's medical needs and personal context" (Haggerty, Reid, Freeman, Starfield, Adair, & McKendry, 2003, p. 1219). This definition was developed after a multidisciplinary review of continuity of care literature to determine how different healthcare professionals viewed the concept. It was noted that continuity of care is different from other views of care because it focuses on care over time and on individual patients.

The review also identified three types of continuity of care. Each is emphasized at different times and is dependent on the care setting.

1. *Informational continuity*: Information is very important in health care, across the continuum of care and with continuity of care. This type of continuity focuses on information that is needed to link care from one provider and setting to another. Such information includes medical information and the patient's preferences, values, and context.

2. *Management continuity*: When patients have complex and chronic problems, management of several providers becomes critical to ensure that all providers are aware of what each is doing and that all are working toward the same outcomes. This requires sharing information and plans and demonstrating flexibility to ensure quality, safe care. A common problem that occurs in these situations is that one provider does not know which medications the other provider has prescribed. Often a home health nurse discovers this lack of coordination when the nurse reviews all the medications (medication reconciliation) a patient is taking that may have been prescribed by different physicians or other providers. Serious medication errors can result from this problem. As more care is provided in the community, there will be increased risk associated with managing clinical problems unless there is improved structure and communication within the community.

3. *Relational continuity*: This type of continuity concerns the needs of patients to build relationships with providers, particularly a **primary care** provider in the community. The primary care provider often serves as the entry point into the healthcare system, and if used by the patient, should coordinate the patient's overall care and make referrals to specialists when necessary. This was the goal of the primary care provider position when it was designed by managed care, but it has not proved completely successful for all patients. Relational continuity emphasizes the need for providers to be familiar with the patient and the patient's history so that when the patient becomes ill, there is someone who has a relationship with the patient and can easily access past medical information.

Nurses are very involved in continuity of care when they transfer and coordinate care over time and focus on consistency of care. Typically, this is done through discharge planning. Nurses who work in the community especially need to recognize the importance of continuity of care and integrate this into planning for individuals, families, and populations within the community.

> Staff nurses feel responsible for their patients to get well, recover, or return to baseline prior to hospital discharge; yet in the new reality, patients' recovery may involve several settings across the continuum of care. Staff nurses must create fluid nursing environments and provide the appropriate nursing activities at the right time along this continuum, even if it requires discarding traditional care regimens they believe are fundamental. (Dingel-Stewart & LaCosta, 2004, p. 214)

Individual, Family, and Community Health

The usual assumption is to consider the patient as an individual, and most patients are individuals. There are, however, other views of the patient. The family, the community, and specific populations, such as patients with specific chronic diseases, may also be viewed as patients. In public/community health, there is greater emphasis on the health of families, populations, and communities.

A **family** is defined as "two or more individuals who depend on one another for emotional, physical, and/or financial support. Members of a family are self-defined" (Kaakinen, Hanson, & Birenbaum, 2006, p. 322). Functional families are considered healthy families in which there is a state of bio/psycho/socio/cultural/spiritual well-being. A healthy family provides autonomy and is responsive to individual members within the family. In contrast, dysfunctional families have poor communication and relationships

with one another and do not provide support to family members.

Nurses work with families in many ways along the continuum of care. The family itself may be the patient, or the nurse may be involved with a family because of one family member's illness. For example, the home health nurse caring for a patient who has uncontrolled diabetes and is recovering from surgery and who lives with her daughter and family must be aware of family dynamics, needs, caregiver strain, and other health issues that can impact the identified patient's care and outcomes such as dietary changes.

Family members may also be caregivers. A **caregiver** is someone who provides care to another person. He or she is a nonprofessional healthcare provider. Because many insurance plans provide limited or no coverage for home care, families often need to serve as caregivers for short-term or long-term needs of family members. This is not easy to do when family members work and have other obligations. Serving as a caregiver for a family member on a long-term basis can lead to caregiver psychological, physical, social, and financial problems. The majority of caregivers are women; men are more likely to be cared for by their wives than the reverse because men have a shorter life expectancy (Schumacher, Beck, & Marren, 2006). Caregiver strain is something that the nurse needs to assess periodically to ensure that the caregiver(s), and therefore the family, receive the support needed. Primary caregivers provide the majority of daily aspects of care, and **secondary caregivers** help with intermittent activities (shopping, transportation, home repairs, getting bills paid, emergency support, and so on). Both types of caregiving can put a strain on the caregiver, but primary caregivers are at greater risk.

Nurses offer services in communities as part of community health, and they may focus on an entire community or a specific population that lives in the community. A population is "a collection of people who share one or more personal or environmental characteristics" (Williams, 2006, p. 4). Examples of populations within a community include children, the elderly, those with a chronic disease, and the homeless. A nurse might work in school health, assess needs of the elderly in the home, develop programs to screen for diabetes in people in the community who might be at risk, manage a clinic for the homeless, or develop and implement a community disaster preparedness plan. There are many other ways that a nurse might work with different populations within a community.

Access to Care

Access to care is, of course, the first step in receiving care, and it is not a simple process for many people; for some, there are major barriers. Access to care is a critical public/community health issue at federal, state, and local levels. Many people think of access as solely the ability to physically get to a destination, but access to care actually involves many factors:

- Ability to pay for care, either by insurance or personally
- Transportation to get to care
- Hours of operation at the clinical site
- Waiting time to get an appointment
- Long waits at the time of appointment to see a physician or other healthcare provider
- Ability to get an appointment
- Availability of type of healthcare provider needed
- Ability of the patient and provider to communicate and make use of accommodations for language, hearing, and sight
- Timeliness of laboratory tests
- Handicap provisions at the healthcare site
- Childcare provisions to go to the appointment
- Cultural barriers
- Inadequate information or lack of information
- Lack of provider time (rushed)
- Insurer not covering care

- Provider not accepting patient's insurance coverage
- Inadequate transportation choices, schedules, and cost

As this list suggests, access is a complex issue, particularly for vulnerable populations.

Access to care has a major impact on the continuum of care. Can the patient get the care that is needed when it is needed? Where is the best location for care? When patients experience barriers to access, they may neglect routine care and put off getting care when it is needed. These patients may then need more complex care and use the safety net, which are services that cover patients who cannot pay for care or who have other access barrier problems. Examples of safety net sites include free clinics, academic medical centers, and emergency rooms. This type of care may (or may not) meet the patient's immediate need, and it does not support an effective continuum of care and continuity of care. Patients who fall into the safety net often get lost in the system, and their outcomes may not be positive. *Healthy People 2020* includes a goal that focuses on this concern (HHS, 2010). The goal is to achieve health equity, eliminate disparities, and improve the health of all groups.

One approach to improving access to healthcare services is to offer comprehensive and wraparound services. Comprehensive services are best described as "one-stop shopping," in that the patient can go to one place and receive multiple services. These services are typically offered in convenient locations such as neighborhoods, schools, or work sites. Health promotion and illness prevention can also be built into these services. Recognizing that social and economic problems have a major impact on a person's health and access to services needed, **wraparound services** can be combined with comprehensive services when the healthcare sites also offer social and economic services. Such wraparound services might include access to a social worker to assist patients with getting food and housing, job issues, and reimbursement for health care.

Another critical factor that has the most impact on access to care is the ability to pay for care, typically with some type of insurance. The Affordable Care Act of 2010 (ACA) primarily addresses this issue, although its implementation does not mean all citizens will have insurance. This law does not establish a universal healthcare system. If people do not obtain insurance—which is now easier to get, especially given that the law provides financial support to help some people cover the costs—they will have to pay penalties. This carrot-and-stick strategy represents a complex approach to the problem, and the full results of the ACA will not be known for some time. The start-up period for enrollment did not go well, with many technological problems being encountered. The overall goal is to reduce the number of uninsured in the United States. In 2012, the U.S. Census Bureau reported that 15.4% of the U.S. population (48 million people) had no insurance. This was a slight improvement from 2011, when the corresponding share was 15.8% (48.6 million people), but is not a significant difference. The ACA and its provisions should begin to bring this number down more in 2013 and beyond; however, it is important that the people who enroll in the new insurance options represent balanced needs, ideally with a lot of young, healthy people to offset the costs attributable to older, sicker enrollees who require more care. As of March 2014, more than 8 million people had signed up for insurance through state or federal exchanges established under the ACA.

Unfortunately, providing insurance coverage does not always equate to ensuring access to care. For example, in Massachusetts, the first state to attempt to implement healthcare coverage similar to the ACA coverage, there are many people in need of services, especially in rural communities, but not enough primary care providers—either physicians or nurses—to render the care. This situation is being addressed through increased numbers of physician assistant programs as well as increased academic practice partnerships to boost nursing school enrollments such as in nurse practitioner programs.

Accountable care organizations (ACOs) are another outgrowth of the healthcare reform and the ACA. These organizations attempt to contain healthcare costs by fostering care coordination across disciplines and providing for integrated care delivery. An example of one such ACO is Kaiser Permanente, in which the insurer, physician groups, and healthcare institutions work together to provide integrated services from acute care to community-based care (Accountable Care Facts, 2014).

Across the Life Span

Patients may enter the healthcare system for a variety of needs and services, and they may enter at any point in the life span. This span includes:

- Conception
- Birth
- Infancy
- Childhood
- Adolescence
- Young adulthood
- Middle adulthood
- Older adulthood
- End of life

Each of these periods of the life span includes specific health concerns and needs, as well as potential disease and illness risks. In addition, social and psychological experiences impact health and wellness. These experiences include situations such as the death of a loved one, change in or loss of a job, beginning school, moving, marriage, birth of a child, divorce, the need to care for a family member who is ill, retirement, and other stressful situations. The federal government collects data about health and illness across the life span. **Exhibit 7-2** provides a list of the leading causes of death that impact public/community health status.

Healthcare Disparities

Healthcare disparities have become even more important in the last 10 years. The Institute of

---

Exhibit 7-2   Leading Causes of Death in the United States, Preliminary Data for 2011

- Diseases of heart
- Malignant neoplasms
- Chronic lower respiratory diseases
- Stroke (cerebrovascular diseases)
- Accidents (unintentional injuries)
- Alzheimer's disease
- Diabetes mellitus
- Nephritis, nephrotic syndrome, and nephrosis
- Influenza and pneumonia
- Intentional self-harm (suicide)

Source: Modified from Centers for Disease Control and Prevention. (2011). Leading causes of death. Retrieved from http://www.cdc.gov/nchs/fastats/lcod.htm

---

Medicine has issued reports with supporting data demonstrating that the U.S. healthcare system has severe problems with health/healthcare disparities (IOM, 2002). A health disparity is an inequality or gap that exists between two or more groups. Health disparities are believed to be the result of the complex interaction of personal, economic, societal, and environmental factors. *Healthy People 2020* considers measures of race/ethnicity, gender, physical and mental ability, and geography to be among these factors (HHS, 2010). According to the 2012 national disparities report, "Unfortunately, Americans too often do not receive care they need, or they receive care that causes harm. Care can be delivered too late or without full consideration of a patient's preferences and values. Many times, our system of health care distributes services inefficiently and unevenly across populations. Some Americans receive worse care than others. These disparities may occur for a variety of reasons, including differences in access to care, social determinants, provider biases, poor provider–patient communication, and poor health literacy" (Agency for Healthcare Research and Quality, 2012). The disparities report is typically two years behind the current year, but you can examine the most current disparities report by using the link at the end of the chapter.

Health Promotion and Disease Prevention

The American Hospital Association (AHA) developed an initiative in 2010 that describes a road map for improving America's healthcare system. It focuses on wellness rather than acute care. The goals of this initiative (Health for Life: Better Health. Better Healthcare) are as follows (AHA, 2010):

- Focus on wellness—across the life span and for all types of needs
- Most efficient affordable care
- Highest quality care-team effort including patients and families
- Best information, including functionality to access information when needed using electronic methods in an effective manner
- Health coverage for all; paid by all—this is a shared responsibility (individuals, business, insurers, and governments)

Disease prevention and health promotion can be easily confused, but they are different and related. One schema for understanding health promotion and prevention was developed by Leavell and Clark (1965):

1. Health promotion (primary prevention)

2. Specific protection (primary prevention)
3. Early diagnosis and treatment (secondary prevention)
4. Disability limitation (secondary prevention)
5. Restoration and rehabilitation (tertiary prevention)

Health Promotion

Health promotion focuses on changing lifestyle to maximize health and is an important part of primary prevention. This is very difficult to accomplish for most people. In 2006, the National Prevention Summit addressed disease prevention, health preparedness, and health promotion and featured innovative programs that are making a difference in communities across the country to build a healthier country (Office of Disease Prevention and Health Promotion, 2006). These programs focused on healthy lifestyle choices—eating a nutritious diet, being physically active, making healthy choices, and getting preventive screenings—to help prevent major health threats and burdens such as diabetes, asthma, cancer, heart disease, and stroke. One special emphasis was the prevention of childhood overweight and obesity, which have become major problems since 2006 and can lead to long-term chronic diseases such as diabetes (CDC, 2011b). Another emphasis was on preparing for public health emergencies, such as influenza, biochemical hazards, and natural disasters. The need for this preparation continues in all communities.

Many models describe how health promotion might be effective. Pender's health promotion model (Pender, Murdaugh, & Parsons, 2006) is a nursing model that has been used in many studies about health promotion. This model does not include fear or threat as a motivator to make people change their behaviors, and it can be used across the life span. Pender's health promotion model includes individual characteristics and experiences; that is, it emphasizes that each person is unique. The following aspects of health promotion have an impact on health and should be considered:

- *Prior related behavior:* The frequency of the same or similar behavior in the past is the best predictor of behavior.
- *Personal factors:* Biological (examples: age, weight, pubertal status, and strength), psychological (examples: self-esteem, coping style, and self-motivation), and sociocultural (examples: race, ethnicity, education, and socioeconomic status) factors may influence the cognitions, affects, and health behavior that are the focus.
- *Behavior-specific cognitions and affects:* These cognitions and affects are very important because nursing interventions can change them, which can in turn move a person toward health-promoting behaviors.
- *Perceived benefits of action:* Whether a person will be active in participating in changing behavior is highly dependent on whether the person sees any benefit in doing so—that is, whether there are perceived benefits. It is important to determine whether perceived barriers are real. If perceived barriers to success are felt by a person, it is much more difficult for that person to change a behavior to a health-promoting behavior.
- *Perceived self-efficacy:* Self-efficacy relates to whether a person feels that it is possible to do what is needed. It does not mean that the person has the competency to do this, but rather centers on whether the person feels that he or she could actually do what needs to be done.
- *Activity-related affect:* Emotions tied to actions are important to recognize, because they can determine whether a person repeats a behavior. Did the person feel good about what he or she did? Did it make the person anxious?
- *Interpersonal influences:* A person is influenced by others—family, friends, coworkers, peers, healthcare providers, and so on. This influence—what it might be and how

it might be felt—may or may not be reality based, but it still can influence a person's behavior and the person's ability to change to health-promoting behavior.

- *Situational influences:* A situation or context can influence a person's behavior. If a person smokes and is told that all smoking must take place outside the building in a designated area regardless of the weather, this situation or context may influence a change in behavior.
- *Commitment to a plan of action:* Is a person committed to a specific plan to change to health-promoting behavior? Commitment is not enough; strategies must be laid out that will enable the person to reach the desired outcomes.
- *Immediate competing demands and preferences:* What might interfere with a person changing to health-promoting behavior? Will the family be supportive? Are there other actions that must take precedence (for example, work over exercise)? Each person has alternative behaviors that compete with what the person needs to do to change to a healthier lifestyle.
- *Health-promoting behavior:* This is the outcome, and from this, a person reaches positive health outcomes.

In any context, the social determinants of health impact an individual's health status. The World Health Organization (WHO, 2011) defines the social determinants of health as geographic region and condition of birth and life, work environment, age, and the health care that is available and accessible. Health is always influenced by access to care—a factor that may be related to an understanding of healthy habits or how to use available health resources, socioeconomic status, and resources that are allocated by governments for the populace (WHO, 2011).

Disease Prevention

Disease prevention focuses on interventions to stop the development of disease, but it also includes treatment to prevent disease from progressing further and leading to complications. The major levels of prevention are primary, secondary, and tertiary.

Primary prevention includes interventions that are used to maintain health before illness occurs. Health promotion is a critical component of primary prevention. Examples are teaching people (children and adults) about healthy diets before they become obese and encouraging adequate exercise (education about health and healthy lifestyles is an important intervention at this level).

Secondary prevention occurs when a person is asymptomatic but after disease has begun. The focus here is on preventing further complications. Examples are breast cancer screening using mammography and blood pressure screening to diagnose hypertension.

Tertiary prevention occurs when there is disability and the need to maintain or, if possible, improve functioning. Examples would be teaching a person with diabetes how to administer insulin and manage the disease or referring a stroke patient for rehabilitation or providing long-term home care.

Healthcare reform through the ACA mostly focuses on reimbursement for health care, but the law also includes provisions related to the need for greater services to prevent illness and promote health (though this is not the strength of the legislation). An example is the requirement that insurers pay for certain healthcare screening as part of their covered services; some of these screening services must not be charged to the patient. However, this provision is easy to misunderstand. If the screening is for diagnosis purposes, then it is not free. For example, if a woman notices she has a lump in her breast and has a mammogram to determine if there is a problem, this test would not be covered; in contrast, if she was having a routine annual mammogram (with no notice of a potential problem), then the screening would be free. Over the long term, this law will increase the quality of life for many and reduce healthcare costs, but how much improvement and what will improve remain to be determined.

In 2011, the Office of the Surgeon General initiated the National Prevention Strategy, which aims to guide the United States in improving the health and well-being of its population. The strategy prioritizes prevention by integrating recommendations and actions across multiple settings to improve health and save lives (HHS, Office of the Surgeon General, 2013). The initiative includes actions that public and private partners can take to help Americans stay healthy and fit and improve the nation's prosperity. It outlines four strategic directions that, collectively, are fundamental to improving the nation's health:

1. *Building healthy and safe community environments*: Prevention of disease starts in communities and at home, not just in the physician's office.
2. *Expanding quality preventive services in both clinical and community settings*: When people receive preventive care, such as immunizations and cancer screenings, they have better health and lower healthcare costs.
3. *Empowering people to make healthy choices*: When people have access to actionable and easy-to-understand information and resources, they are empowered to make healthier choices.
4. *Eliminating health disparities*: By eliminating disparities in achieving and maintaining health, the goal is to improve quality of life for all Americans.

Several initiatives related to health promotion and disease prevention are identified in this chapter, and they are all connected. For example, *Healthy People*, healthcare reform/Affordable Care Act, and the National Prevention Strategy all focus on both individuals and their communities. Another theme that runs through these initiatives is the need to decrease health disparities—an issue noted in the Surgeon General's strategy, the IOM reports on health care, healthcare reform, and *Healthy People 2020*.

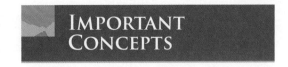

IMPORTANT CONCEPTS

Patient as Focus of Care and Member of the Healthcare Team

The patient is always the focus of care, even when the larger community is considered. Patients should be viewed as members of the healthcare team and should be involved in decision making about their own care. Patient-centered care means that the patient is the center of that care—receiving the care—and must be involved in care decisions. This point does not just apply to individual patients. In public or community health, the patient may be an individual, family, population, or the community, and all should be part of assessment, planning and decision making. If this does not happen, the public/community health efforts are at risk for failure.

Vulnerable Populations

A vulnerable population is a group of persons who are at risk for developing health problems. They need careful assessment and monitoring to identify problems early so that complications can be prevented. Typically, complex factors increase risk, such as economic, ethnic, social, and communication factors. There may also be problems related to diet, housing, safety, and transportation. These populations often have problems accessing care when they need it. Such vulnerable populations include children, the elderly, people with chronic disease, immigrants, illegal aliens, migrant workers, people who live in rural areas, homeless people, the seriously mentally ill, victims of abuse and violence, pregnant adolescents, and people who are HIV positive.

Poverty is an important concern with many of these populations. In 2014, the U.S. Census Bureau announced that in 2012, 46 million people lived in poverty in the United States. Poverty guidelines

Table 7-1	2014 Department of Health and Human Services Poverty Guidelines		
Persons in Family	**48 Contiguous States and Washington, D.C.**	**Alaska**	**Hawaii**
1	$11,670	$14,580	$13,420
2	15,730	19,660	18,090
3	19,790	24,740	22,760
4	23,850	29,820	27,430
5	27,910	34,900	32,100
6	31,970	39,980	36,770
7	36,030	45,060	41,440
8	40,090	50,140	46,110
For families/households with more than 8 persons, add	4060	5080	4670

Note: The poverty guideline figures shown are *not* the figures that the Census Bureau uses to calculate the number of poor persons. The figures that the Census Bureau uses are the poverty thresholds.

Source: Reproduced from *Federal Register.* (2014, January 22). Annual update of the HHS poverty guidelines. Retrieved from https://www.federalregister.gov/articles/2014/01/22/2014-01303/annual-update-of-the-hhs-poverty-guidelines

are determined by the federal government based on the income of a family of a specific size, as noted in **Table 7-1**, and these guidelines change annually. Poverty guidelines are important because financial eligibility for certain federal programs is based on poverty levels; to receive specific services, a person must not have an income higher than the poverty level.

Health and Illness

Health and wellness are terms that tend to be used interchangeably. But what does health mean? There is no simple response to this question. A simple definition of **health**, albeit one that is not complete, is to be structurally and functionally whole. Absence of this state is **illness**.

The World Health Organization defines health as "a state of complete well-being, physical, social, and mental, and not merely the absence of disease or infirmity" (WHO, 2006). This is a common definition and one that is often quoted. WHO addresses health and illness from a global perspective. Its constitution identifies the following principles:

- Health is not merely the absence of disease or infirmity.
- The enjoyment of the highest attainable standard of health is one of the fundamental rights of every human being without distinction of race, religion, political belief, or economic or social condition.
- The health of all peoples is fundamental to the attainment of peace and security and is dependent upon the fullest cooperation of individuals and states.
- The achievement of any state in the promotion and protection of health is of value to all.
- Unequal development in different countries in the promotion of health and control of disease, especially communicable disease, is a common danger.

- Healthy development of the child is of basic importance; the ability to live harmoniously in a changing total environment is essential to such development.
- The extension to all peoples of the benefits of medical, psychological, and related knowledge is essential to the fullest attainment of health.
- Informed opinion and active cooperation on the part of the public are of the utmost importance in the improvement of the health of the people.
- Governments have a responsibility for the health of their peoples that can be fulfilled only by the provision of adequate health and social measures.

Effective definitions of health should be applicable to all—to those who are well; to those with illness or disease that can be treated; and to those with acquired or genetic impairments that result in a chronic disease or disability. The definition has to be applied to individuals, families, communities, and nations (RWJF, 2000). The determinants of health or factors that have an impact on health are physical, mental, social, and spiritual. Stress and socioeconomic factors are also very important.

Disease and illness are terms that are often used interchangeably. Disease is an indication of a physiological dysfunction or pathological reaction. Other terms related to health and illness are distributive and episodic care. "Distributive care refers to health maintenance and disease prevention or primary prevention" (Pizzuti, 2006, p. 594). "Episodic care refers to the curative and restorative aspects of practice, or secondary and tertiary prevention" (Pizzuti, 2006, p. 594). A nurse in a clinic changing a dressing on a patient who has a leg ulcer is an example of someone providing episodic care. If during the visit, the nurse provides information about weight reduction, this is an example of distributive care.

Life expectancy for Americans has reached an all-time high of 78.7 years, according to data published in 2012. U.S. mortality statistics released by the CDC and updated data from 2010 indicate that life expectancy is 76.5 years for men, which is an increase of 5 years from 2007 data (HHS, 2012). Women have a life expectancy of 81.3 years, an increase from 77 years in 2007. In 2011, the United States ranked 26 out of 36 Organization for Economic Cooperation and Development (OECD) member countries in terms of life expectancy; thus, on a global scale, the United States is not doing well on this measure (OECD, 2013). Differences in mortality between the Black and White populations persist in the United States, with White women having the highest life expectancy. As of 2014, the infant mortality rate in the country was 6.17 deaths per 1000 live births, which reflects very little change since 2007 (Central Intelligence Agency [CIA], 2014).

Stress, Coping, Adaptation, and Resilience

Stress is a complex experience, which is felt internally. It makes a person feel a loss or threat of a loss. Stress is present in all parts of life, and it plays a role in health and illness. Stress can lead to health problems, or it can have an impact on current health status. For example, a patient with a cardiac problem can experience more symptoms when experiencing high levels of stress. Patients who have socioeconomic problems may not have an adequate diet because of lack of money, or they may experience sleep problems because they work two jobs—all factors that increase stress. Not all persons who experience stress experience negative outcomes. Communities may also experience stress—for example, stress caused by economic problems, lack of critical healthcare services, increase in violence, or inadequate education for children.

The most effective intervention for stress is **stress management**. Eliminating stress completely is not possible, but helping individuals, families, vulnerable populations, and communities better cope with stress is an important goal in improving health and developing health-promoting behaviors. Effective **coping** can reduce the negative impact of stress and, in many cases, prevent a person, family, or community from experiencing stress. This might be done through identifying stressors or stimuli that cause a person (family, community) to experience stress. Stressors can be biological, sociological, psychological, spiritual, or environmental. Self-assessment to identify stressors is critical to improving coping. Stress management interventions might include relaxation techniques, humor, better sleep, healthy diet, exercise, music, and use of assertiveness. Community-oriented interventions might include reducing violence by providing places for teen after-school activities; increasing access to community clinics; increasing jobs; improving transportation to areas where healthcare services are available; providing parenting classes, or increasing exercise classes and social activities in community centers.

Resilience, or the ability to cope with stress, is an important factor. Adaptation to situations is also important. The same principles of stress apply to everyone, including patients—individuals, families, and communities.

Acute Illness

Acute illness is typically self-limiting and occurs in a short period of time. Cure is the focus for care. Some of the care for acute illness takes place in the hospital, commonly referred to as the **acute care** setting, but today, more care is taking place in the home or community through primary care and ambulatory services. Examples of acute illness are an infectious disease such as the flu or pneumonia, a broken leg, appendicitis, and a urinary tract infection.

The curative model has long been viewed as the best approach to health; however, this model has come under criticism (RWJF, 2000). Yes, cure is a good goal, but is this a view that really can be

applied to the complex area of health? There are other important goals, as noted by the RWJF:

- Restoring functional capacity
- Relieving suffering
- Preventing illness, injury, and untimely death
- Promoting health
- Caring for those who cannot be cured

These additional goals expand what can be done to help those who need it. Cure is not always possible. Moreover, with the increase in the number of people with chronic diseases and the growing elderly population, cure is becoming less important from the patient's daily perspective, and there is more focus on functioning at the best possible level. The curative model focuses more on the biological approach, which relies on a hierarchical system of decision making in which physicians make diagnoses. Nursing is more involved in additional functions, although the nurse certainly participates in providing care that is directed at cure, such as surgery to repair a fractured hip. The hip can be repaired, but the patient typically has other needs after this surgery that are tied to the additional functions. The patient will need help gaining functional capacity, and he or she may never regain full capacity. The patient may require help with promotion of health if the cause of the fracture was osteoporosis (e.g., lifestyle changes related to diet, vitamins, and exercise). These factors need to be taken into account in follow-up care in the community.

Greater Emphasis on Chronic Disease

Another factor that supports including patient-centered care as a healthcare professions' core competency is the growing number of patients with chronic diseases. The IOM has identified priority areas of care, along with the need to move away from a disease- and clinician-focused approach to one that includes the patient; this emphasis moves the patient to the center, while recognizing that the priority areas may change over time as care improves in some areas and needs increase in other ones (IOM, 2003). In the United States, the total number of persons with chronic diseases has increased, as has the number of people with more than one chronic disease. The following data related to this problem support the strong need to focus on chronic disease (CDC, 2011a):

- Each year, 7 out of 10 deaths among Americans are from chronic diseases. Heart disease, cancer, and stroke account for more than 50% of all deaths each year.
- In 2005, 133 million Americans—almost one out of every two adults—had at least one chronic disease.
- Obesity has become a major health concern. One in every three adults is obese, and almost one in five youth between the ages of 6 and 19 is obese (body mass index at or greater than the 95th percentile of the CDC growth chart).
- One fourth of people with chronic conditions have one or more daily activity limitations.
- Arthritis is the most common cause of disability, with nearly 19 million Americans reporting activity limitations from this disease.
- Diabetes continues to be the leading cause of kidney failure, nontraumatic lower-extremity amputations, and blindness among adults.
- Nearly half of Americans aged 20–74 have some type of chronic condition.

Data reported in 2013 indicate that approximately 133 million Americans (45% of the total population) have chronic illnesses. By 2020, this number is projected to increase to 157 million, with 81 million having multiple conditions (National Health Council, 2013).

One reason that the United States has these problems with chronic disease is that there is better treatment today, so people with chronic diseases live longer; consequently, there are more people with chronic disease. A second reason is that the United States still needs to improve care provided for chronic disease, particularly for patients with multiple chronic illnesses. Chronic disease is a serious problem not only in the United States, but also worldwide.

It can be difficult for a healthcare provider to understand the need for a change when caring for patients with chronic diseases. If the nurse typically cares for patients with sudden-onset illnesses or with injuries for which the cure model is the focus, it may be difficult for the nurse to appreciate the differences in care for chronic diseases and needs of these patients. Chronic diseases are diseases for which there is no effective cure; in turn, their treatment focuses on control of symptoms, support, psychosocial issues, and if possible, prevention of deterioration and improved quality of life. Examples of chronic diseases include heart disease, diabetes, stroke, hypertension, rheumatoid arthritis, obesity, and even cancer (cancer survivors live with the long-term effects of the cancer and/or the treatment). Chronic diseases are the leading cause of death worldwide, killing more than 36 million people in 2008. Cardiovascular diseases were responsible for 48% of these deaths, cancers 21%, chronic respiratory diseases 12%, and diabetes 3% (WHO, 2011).

As with adults, chronic illness and disease prevention in children are major health considerations. According to the CDC (2010), about 7.1 million children have asthma; 14% of all children in the United States take medications for more than 3 months; 8% of all U.S. children have a learning disability, and 8% have no health insurance coverage (although the ACA is expected to mitigate some of this insurance coverage problem). Childhood obesity is on the rise, increasing the incidence of diabetes, hypertension, and other related complications. Obesity rates have increased 13.1% in 30 years (CDC, 2011b).

Eliopoulos (2001) identified the following key goals for chronic care:

- Maintain or improve self-care capacity
- Manage the disease effectively
- Boost the body's healing abilities

- Prevent complications
- Delay deterioration and decline
- Achieve highest possible quality of life
- Die with comfort, peace, and dignity

Because of the increased recognition of chronic disease, innovations in interventions and services for patients with chronic diseases have increased. Examples from the government payment perspective are important. For example, the Centers for Medicare and Medicaid Services (CMS) is using innovative trial models of care to promote care **coordination**, such as using medical homes. Under this model, patients receive transitional care, care coordination, and comprehensive care management services. Self-management and health literacy are important to consider when planning services for patients with chronic illness to ensure a comprehensive public/community health program. Methods for delivering care for chronic disease have improved, though much more needs to be done. For example, greater use of disease management, which is another systematic approach to managing a chronic disease, has affected care for chronic illnesses. Typically, interventions used in disease management have been tested with large groups; thus they may be more effective than interventions tested in studies with a narrower scope. Disease management emphasizes interprofessional teams with expertise in the specific disease; use of evidence-based clinical guidelines; clear descriptions of interventions and procedures, and recommended timelines; patient support and education; and measurement of outcomes. Nurses assume important roles in disease management; specifically, they may be on the team or lead the team. Insurers, hospitals, and other healthcare providers develop and sponsor disease management programs. The major goals are to assist patients in maintaining the best quality of life possible and to prevent complications that might lead to deterioration and increased costs of care.

Disease management programs also emphasize prevention, although it is important to emphasize prevention throughout the healthcare system and particularly in community care—not just in special focused programs. Examples of prevention services include tobacco cessation counseling, screening (breast cancer, colorectal cancer, prostate cancer, diabetes, hypertension, hearing, vision, cholesterol, and so on), and immunizations. Prevention is not always successful. Some of the barriers to its success are related to availability and use of previous services (Peters & Elster, 2002):

- Lack of reimbursement for these services
- Lack of time for services
- Lack of access for populations who need these services
- Inadequate consumer education to support need
- Uncertainty as to effectiveness (from both consumer and provider perspectives)
- Failure to assure empowerment of patients, which leads to effective self-management

Patients with chronic illness need support, as well as information, to become effective managers of their own health. To meet these needs, it is essential for them to have the following resources:

- Basic information about their disease and an understanding of self-management skills
- Ongoing support from members of the practice team, family, friends, and community as part of the self-management process
- Providers who are sensitive to the roles that families, caregivers, and communities assume in different cultures

In general, better patient outcomes are achieved through use of evidence-based techniques that emphasize patient activation or empowerment, collaborative goal setting, and problem-solving skills. The provider team can use standardized assessments of patient self-management needs and activities to enhance their ability to support patients. Such assessments include questions about self-management knowledge, skills, confidence, supports, and barriers (Institute for Healthcare Improvement, 2011).

In 2012, the Institute of Medicine (IOM) published a report titled *Living Well with Chronic Illness: A*

Call for Public Action. The existence of a publication such as this from the IOM indicates that there is greater interest in chronic illness and meeting the needs of people with these illnesses. The IOM, for its part, describes this issue as a major public health problem:

> The concept of living well reflects the best achievable state of health that encompasses all dimensions of physical, mental, and social well-being. Living well is shaped by the physical, social, and cultural surroundings and by the effects of chronic illness—not only on the affected individual, but also on family members, friends, and caregivers. In this way, progress toward living well can be achieved through the combined efforts of both individuals and society to reduce disability and improve functioning and quality of life, regardless of each unique individual's current health status or specific chronic illness diagnosis. (IOM, 2012)

Medical Home Model

The medical home model is a multidimensional solution for planned, clinically integrated care to meet the complex care needs of people with chronic disease; its elements include organizing care around patients, working in teams, and coordinating and tracking care over time (National Committee for Quality Assurance, 2013). The focus is on interprofessional primary care teams. **Figure 7-2** depicts the chronic care model, which includes two major delivery focus areas: (1) the community needs to have resources and health policies that support care for chronic diseases and (2) the health system needs to have healthcare organizations that support self-management and recognize that the patient is the source of control; have a delivery system design that identifies clear roles for staff in relation to chronic disease care; supply decision support, with integration of evidence-based guidelines into daily practice; and feature clinical information systems to ensure rapid exchange of information and reminder

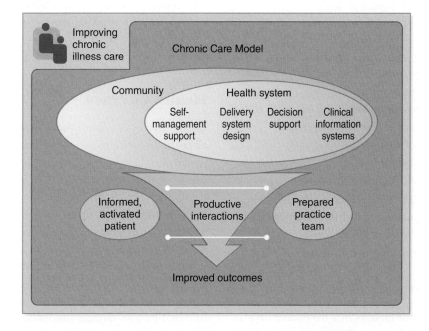

Figure 7-2 Chronic Care Model

Source: Reproduced from Wagner, E. H. (1998). Chronic disease management: What will it take to improve care for chronic illness? *Effective Clinical Practice, 1,* 2-4. Figure 1.

and feedback systems. If all of these elements are in place and effective, the results should be productive interactions with an informed, active patient and a prepared, proactive care team. The ultimate result should then be improved outcomes. The medical home model reinforces the need to have a healthcare team that is patient centered and places greater emphasis on care in the community.

Four major medical associations (Academy of Family Physicians, Academy of Pediatrics, American College of Physicians, and American Osteopathic Association) have identified several key principles of the patient-centered medical home:

- *Personal physician (provider)*: Each patient has an ongoing relationship.
- *Physician-directed medical practice*: The personal physician leads the team.
- *Whole-person orientation*: The personal physician provides all of a patient's healthcare needs or refers the patient to appropriate specialists for all stages of life; for acute and chronic care; for preventive services; and for end-of-life care.
- *Coordination of care*: Care is coordinated and/or integrated.
- *Quality and safety*: Quality and safety are critical elements of all care.
- *Enhanced access.*
- *Payment*: The amount of payment is appropriate to the value of the services.

The Joint Commission includes advanced practice nurses in its standards for ambulatory care/medical homes. This is a significant change, although there is still disagreement among healthcare professionals over the role of the advanced practice nurse in medical homes (American Nurses Association [ANA], 2011).

Self-Management

Self-management requires that the patient have access to health information (IOM, 2003). Electronic personal health records are useful in facilitating self-management (Mitchell & Begoray, 2010). For example, this record can be used to help patients manage their health through individualized care plans, graphing and recording of symptoms, passive biofeedback, individualized instructive or motivational feedback, aids to assist in decision making about health care, and reminders. Security, privacy, and confidentiality are all critical factors in the use of electronic personal health records.

It is important that when these systems are used, the system is able to adjust or meet the health literacy needs of the patient. One definition of health literacy is "the extent to which an individual is able to access and accurately interpret and evaluate health information" (Mitchell & Begoray, 2010). Effective health literacy improves self-management and engages the patient in the process. Three key supporting interventions to better ensure health literacy are as follows (Sand-Jecklin, Murray, Summers, & Watson, 2010):

1. Identify patients at risk for lack of understanding and not acting on health information.
2. Communicate health information and instructions in a way that promotes patient understanding.
3. Check for patient understanding.

Health Literacy

Health literacy is a factor that has implications in all healthcare settings and for all patients. As mentioned elsewhere in this text, diversity is a key element of patient-centered care, but it is important to explicitly recognize it in terms of its relevance to public/community health as well. Patient education, whether from the perspective of individual patients, families, populations, or communities, is influenced by the relevant patient's health literacy or "the degree to which individuals have the capacity to obtain, process and understand basic information and services needed to make appropriate decisions regarding their health" (IOM, 2004, p. 2).

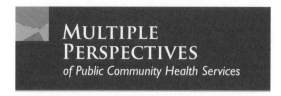

MULTIPLE PERSPECTIVES
of Public Community Health Services

Community Emergency Preparedness

Communities may be confronted with numerous challenges—natural disasters (e.g., fires, floods, severe winter weather, hurricanes, and tornados), infectious diseases, excessive violence, and potential attacks such as bioterrorism—that could lead to major community health needs and safety concerns. The Agency for Health Research and Quality (AHRQ) has developed resources for public health emergency preparedness; more on this topic can be found at the agency's website (http://www.ahrq .gov/prep/). Community planning for such events is critical to better ensure the health and safety of the community.

In the last few years, there have been major weather-related disasters in the United States, such as in New Orleans, Oklahoma, and the East Coast, as well as tragic violence that has harmed a large number of children and adults. Communities are now more alert to the need for planning for these situations. Nurses are involved both in this planning and in working during the crisis period to help others, either in their regular positions or on specific

disaster teams that respond to the needs. For example, school nurses should participate in planning as part of emergency preparation. **Box 7-1** identifies some critical links that provide more information on this important topic.

Managing Population Health

There is greater emphasis today on learning how to effectively manage population health to reduce costs and improve outcomes. The first step is to identify the target population (Larkin, 2010). The second step is to assess the health status and needs of the population and then to use interventions and prevention to improve the population's health. This approach can have an impact on overall health care.

What might represent a population? With the increase in number of persons with chronic diseases, focusing on a population with a specific chronic disease, such as arthritis or diabetes, can be useful. Coordinating services across a continuum of care and tracking data about outcomes are important aspects of managing population health within a community. The Patient Protection and Affordable Care Act of 2010 includes many provisions that emphasize community and population health. For example, the law calls for increased funding for community health centers, development of medical homes and community-based transition grant programs, incentives to reduce readmission rates, outcome measures for chronic diseases and wellness and prevention

Box 7-1	Sources for Information About Emergency Preparedness

- http://www.ready.gov/
- http://www.fema.gov/
- http://emergency.cdc.gov/preparedness/
- http://www.nursingworld.org/MainMenuCategories/ANAMarketplace/ANAPeriodicals/OJIN/ TableofContents/Volume112006/No3Sept06/Overview.aspx
- http://nursingworld.org/MainMenuCategories/HealthcareandPolicyIssues/DPR.aspx

programs, development of employer wellness programs, and requiring nonprofit hospitals to conduct comprehensive needs assessments every three years and report to the Internal Revenue Service the activities they pursue to address the identified needs.

Migrant and Immigrant Issues

In 2011, the American Nurses Association published a policy brief on immigrant health care, *Nursing Beyond Borders: Access to Health Care for Documented and Undocumented Immigrants Living in the United States* (Trossman, 2011). Access to healthcare services for these two populations is weak. Even though this is a complex political issue, it is still important for nurses to understand the needs of these two populations and provide care to them. These populations do not increase healthcare expenditures; in fact, their expenditures are lower than most adult citizens and they visit the emergency department less often than U.S. citizens. Many of them are employed, but they do not get health insurance coverage. However, they often work in hazardous jobs, such as agriculture and construction, increasing their risk for injuries and illness. There have been increased efforts on the federal level to pass new immigration legislation.

Home Health Care

The amount of care provided in the home has increased in the United States. As part of efforts to control costs, patients are being discharged earlier and earlier from the hospital. At this point, many patients are not fully recovered or ready to care for themselves. **Home care** provides healthcare services in the home. These services can vary as to the type of services, the amount of time that the care provider is in the home, the number of visits per week, and the length of services (e.g., provided for three months). In addition, there is variation in the type of healthcare provider needed: a home health aide who provides assistance with activities of daily living services (bathing, ambulation, simple care, light housekeeping, food preparation); a registered nurse who assesses the patient, develops the care plan, monitors progress, assesses the home environment for safety, and provides more complex care; a physical therapist who helps the patient with exercises to gain strength; or a social worker who assists with obtaining other services that the patient may need such, as Meals on Wheels, payment for healthcare services, and so on. Telehealth is used in some home care situations; with this service, health information is sent from one site to another by electronic communication. Given the growing number of persons with chronic disease and the aging population, it is expected that home health care will continue to grow as a community health service.

Rehabilitation

Rehabilitation is part of tertiary prevention. The goal of rehabilitation interventions is to attain and retain the best possible level of functioning for a person who has an illness or disability that is permanent and irreversible. Rehabilitation can take place in the hospital, in an extended care or long-term care facility, in an ambulatory care facility, or in the home. Rehabilitation therapists assist the patient. The nurse may be the healthcare provider who identifies the need for rehabilitation, or the nurse may be involved by following the rehabilitation plan. A patient may require a specialized therapist, such as a physical therapist, an occupational therapist, a speech-language pathologist, or a vocational therapist. Patients may need to learn how to complete activities of daily living, such as taking care of personal hygiene and dressing; ambulating safely with or without assistive devices such as a walker, cane, or wheelchair; learning basic life skills, such as cooking or driving with a disability; and learning new job skills. Some patients recover more fully than others. Examples of patients who may require rehabilitation are those who have suffered a stroke or severe burns, and those who have experienced a major automobile accident or a work-related accident, such as a serious fall or being cut, impaled, or crushed by equipment.

Extended Care, Long-Term Care, and Elder Care

The U.S. population is aging, and the need for services to meet this population is growing. Gerontological nursing is an important specialty that focuses on care of the elder population in all settings; however, the most important **extended care** settings involve care in the home. This includes skilled nursing or intermediate-care and **long-term care** in which patients can receive a range of services, from housing, meals, and activities to routine personal care, rehabilitation, and specialized treatment. There is great need within the community for more elder-care services, such as adult day care (a facility where elders may go during the day for socializing and activities), home health, senior centers, and retirement and assisted-living facilities (these can vary from single rooms to independent living situations with support services as needed).

Older adults can experience health problems in all body systems and psychologically. They may also experience social problems, with losses of spouse and friends and lessened ability to be mobile, and they may become isolated. Financial problems are not uncommon, and these problems impact food, housing, social activities, transportation, and access to medical care.

Hospice and Palliative Care

Hospice care is a philosophy of care for the terminally ill tha t involves supporting the quality of one's life as long as possible. It is not a place, though it can be—for example, a freestanding building in which hospice service is provided. Hospice care can also be provided in the patient's home or in a special unit in an acute care hospital. This philosophy of care includes active participation of the patient and family in all care decisions. Specially trained staff, including physicians, nurses, social workers, and often spiritual professionals as well as other healthcare providers as needed, support the patient and family during the critical last stages of life. **Palliative care** focuses on alleviating symptoms and meeting the special needs of the terminally ill patient and the family. A place designated for patients to come and receive palliative care may be referred to as a hospice, or care providers in this area of care may provide palliative care at the patient's home. There is strong support for more nursing leadership and provision of palliative care by nurses. The *Future of Nursing* report (IOM, 2010) identifies nurses as the ideal providers of palliative care.

Case Management

Case management is a system that aims to get the right services to the patient at the right time and avoid fragmented and unnecessary care that can be costly (Finkelman, 2011). It facilitates effective care delivery and outcomes for patients. Case management requires **collaboration** or cooperative effort among healthcare providers and other sources of resources that the patient may require. Coordination is required to organize care so that it is available when needed. Communication is also critical because the case manager must work with many people to get the care required. Case managers frequently do all their work on the telephone and never actually see the patient or family. They are typically employees of an insurance company, a government agency, or a healthcare organization, particularly acute care settings (hospitals). Because one of the employer concerns is cost-effective care delivery, case managers need to have extensive knowledge about reimbursement and understand how to manage the care services in a manner that controls costs. Case managers, who may be nurses or social workers, work directly with patients (clients) and their families to assess needs, direct the patient to care when needed, and monitor progress. Hospitals may also use case managers to assist with complex patient needs. Case management is a growing area of care delivery that has proved effective in helping patients get the care they need in an often complex and confusing healthcare system.

Occupational Health Care

Occupational health care may seem a strange topic, but nurses are very active in this setting providing health promotion, disease and illness prevention, and treatment services. Occupational health care also involves looking at risks of illness and injury associated with the work environment. This healthcare service is considered part of public/community health. Providing these services at the work site makes it easier for employees to obtain the services with less concern about getting to appointments during work hours. Many employers have found it to be beneficial to provide these services on site for employees, often reducing their potential health risks and providing prompt treatment. All of this can reduce employer health insurance costs and increase work productivity; however, employee privacy continues to be an issue.

Employers may provide a variety of health promotion and prevention services, such as exercise classes or even gym access, stress management resources and classes, diet and weight-loss classes, smoking cessation programs, immunizations, weight management services, and other types of opportunities for employees to maintain a healthy lifestyle. Employers may also consider factors such as the food, and related nutritional factors, served in the cafeteria; environmental health issues; walking areas for employees during breaks; equipment to prevent back injuries; air quality at work; noise; and so on.

Complementary and Alternative Therapies or Integrative Medicine

The National Center for Complementary and Alternative Medicine (NCCAM, 2011) describes complementary and alternative medicine (CAM) as a group of diverse medical and healthcare systems, practices, and products that are not presently considered part of conventional medicine. Conventional medicine is medicine typically practiced by holders of medical doctor or doctor of osteopathy degrees and by allied health professionals, such as registered nurses, physical therapists, and psychologists. Some healthcare providers practice both CAM and conventional medicine. Although some scientific evidence exists regarding some CAM therapies, for most, there are key questions that have yet to be answered through well-designed scientific studies—questions such as whether these therapies are safe and whether they work for the diseases or medical conditions for which they are used. The list of what is considered CAM changes continually, as therapies that are proved to be safe and effective are adopted by conventional health care and as new approaches to health care emerge. Patients typically seek out these interventions in their communities. For example, in San Francisco, California, groups of senior citizens participate in tai chi in the parks.

Many of these interventions are not new, but their use has increased in recent years. However, many of these CAM interventions still have a long way to go before they become part of conventional medicine. Examples of these interventions are acupuncture, acupressure, massage, light energy, botanical treatment, Reiki, tai chi, and the use of a variety of herbs and other supplements, such as garlic, shark cartilage, and ginseng. With the creation of NCCAM, there is now an organized system for clinical trials to gather data about the use of CAM and outcomes. Nurses may provide some CAM interventions in their practice, and some insurers cover these services. As more data are obtained to support their efficacy, there will probably be more inclusion of these interventions in care, and they will gain greater reimbursement coverage.

GENETICS
Rapid Change with Major Impact on Community Health

The U.S. Department of Energy and the National Institutes of Health funded the Human Genome Project, which began in 1990 and was completed in 2003. This project focused on mapping all the loci of the 20,000 to 25,000 genes that make up the human body. The implications of this project are many. We have learned that the interaction of the genetic makeup of an individual and the environment (genomics) often determines whether the person will be healthy or ill for the majority of his or her life. The benefits of this research include the following:

- Improved diagnosis of disease
- Earlier detection of genetic predispositions to disease
- Rational drug design
- Gene therapy and control systems for drugs
- Pharmacogenomics/custom drugs (Human Genome Project, 2007)

When this information is used in combination with a family history tool to gather information about diseases in the family, a very thorough risk assessment can be completed (HHS, 2007). If this risk assessment is used in health promotion, the health professional can explain to patients and families not only their risk of a disease because of their genetic profile, but also the interactions between the environment and the person's genomic risk. With the knowledge of how a person's genes interact with drugs, better pain medications may be designed to address individuals. We now have the ability in some cases to fix a bad gene because we know its location. The technology to diagnose diseases and conditions even prenatally is becoming available, giving us the tools to allow a fetus to continue to grow normally instead of having major anomalies at birth. The possibilities are endless for disease prevention and management.

We are just at the beginning of a new frontier of health care and related nursing care. The essentials for genetics competencies have already been written for nursing curricula (Consensus Panel, 2008). These are just as critical as the other competencies regarding nursing processes that lead to better patient outcomes and safe care.

GLOBAL HEALTHCARE CONCERNS AND INTERNATIONAL NURSING

WHO is the major international health organization. Its goals focus on (1) development to decrease poverty; (2) fostering health security—for example, decreasing infectious diseases incidence and epidemics; (3) strengthening the health systems needed for people to provide health care; (4) using research, evidence-based practice, and information to support care decisions; (5) building partnerships to ensure stronger care systems; and (6) improving performance (WHO, 2008).

In September 2000, leaders from 189 nations agreed on a vision for the future: a world with less poverty, hunger, and disease; greater survival prospects for mothers and their infants; better-educated children; equal opportunities for women; and a healthier environment—a world in which developed and developing countries work in partnership for the betterment of all. This vision took the shape of eight millennium development goals, which provide a framework for development planning for countries around the world, and time-bound targets by which progress can be measured (WHO, 2008). The WHO millennium development goals are as follows:

- Eradicate extreme poverty and hunger
- Achieve universal primary education
- Promote gender equality and empower women

- Reduce child mortality
- Improve maternal health
- Combat HIV/AIDS, malaria, and other infectious diseases
- Ensure environmental sustainability
- Develop a global partnership for development

These goals are community focused and include some concerns that on the surface may not appear to be health related; however, they are all health related. The WHO Constitution states, "The enjoyment of the highest attainable standard of health is one of the fundamental rights of every human being" (WHO, 2008).

The International Council of Nurses (ICN) is also involved in global health by providing a voice for nursing throughout the world. Its stated mission is

> to represent nursing worldwide, advancing the profession and influencing health policy. ICN's Strategic Intent is to enhance the health of individuals, populations, and societies by: championing the contribution and image of nurses worldwide; advocating for nurses at all levels; advancing the nursing profession; and influencing health, social, economic and education policy. (ICN, 2014).

Both this organization and WHO focus on the health of individuals, families, and communities.

Landscape © f9photos/Shutterstock, Inc.

CONCLUSION

This chapter introduced content about public/community health as a critical component of the U.S. healthcare delivery system. Concepts related to health and illness were highlighted to provide a framework in which health care is delivered to facilitate a better understanding of what patients experience. The continuum of care covers all aspects of health and wellness and delivery of healthcare services to those who experience illness or injury with the community.

Landscape © f9photos/Shutterstock, Inc.

CHAPTER HIGHLIGHTS

1. *Healthy People 2020*, coupled with the IOM reports on the quality of health care, require health professionals to understand the concepts of patient safety, quality of care, health outcomes, and health indices, as well as to address health disparities in everyday care in the community.

2. The focus of health care is changing to patient-centered care, with the patient in the key decision-making position. This applies to all types of healthcare settings in the community, across the life span and the continuum of care, to meet healthcare needs within the community and ensuring continuity of care.

3. Stress, coping, and resilience have an impact on health promotion, disease prevention, and illness.

4. Continuum of care means that nursing care must be provided in the home, community, and acute care settings.

5. Vulnerable populations are groups of people who are at risk for developing health problems. Examples include children, the elderly, people with chronic diseases, the homeless, and others.

Landscape © f9photos/Shutterstock, Inc.

CHAPTER HIGHLIGHTS (CONTINUED)

6. Important concepts to consider in public/community health care are disease prevention, health promotion, life span, vulnerable populations, health and illness, acute illness, chronic disease, self-management, health literacy, continuity of care, and continuum of care.

7. Critical public/community services include community emergency preparedness, migrant and immigrant care, occupational health care, home care, hospice and palliative care, rehabilitation, extended care, long-term care, elder care, case management, complementary and alternative care, and managing population health.

8. The Human Genome Project changed our knowledge of disease risk factors, identification, and management. It also brought greater recognition of the role that genomics plays in disease prevention, health promotion, and care management, and as part of critical public/community health concerns.

9. WHO focuses its attention on global health issues, and the International Council of Nurses represents the nursing profession's global interests.

Landscape © f9photos/Shutterstock, Inc.

DISCUSSION QUESTIONS

1. Why is *Healthy People 2020* an important national health initiative?
2. Why is public/community health a critical concern today?
3. Discuss the various views of health and illness presented in this chapter.
4. Analyze the chronic disease model and its relevance to nursing in the community.
5. How does the life span impact the continuum of care in the community?
6. Compare and contrast acute illness and chronic disease related to public/community care.
7. Why are global health issues important considerations for healthcare providers in the United States?

Landscape © f9photos/Shutterstock, Inc.

CRITICAL THINKING ACTIVITIES

1. Go to the Take the First Step to Prevention page at the Centers for Disease Control and Prevention's website (http://wonder.cdc.gov/data2010/HU.htm). Search for your state and review the most current data. Select a specific health indicator, and look at the national data and then data from your own state. How do they compare? Search for data focused on a specific population.

2. Visit the National Center for Health Statistics' website (http://www.cdc.gov/nchs/). Search for current data related to births/natality, infant health, child health, adolescent health, men's health, women's health, and older people's health.

(continues)

Landscape © f9photos/Shutterstock, Inc.

CRITICAL THINKING ACTIVITIES (CONTINUED)

3. Visit http://www.ahrq.gov/clinic/pocketgd.htm to review the current version of the *U.S. Guide to Clinical Preventive Services*. How might you use this information if you were planning services for a community health center?

4. Visit these WHO sites:
   a. Global Health Observatory (http://www.who.int/gho/mortality_burden_disease/life_tables/life_tables/en/)
   b. Mortality Database (http://www.who.int/healthinfo/mortality_data/en/)
   c. Global Health Estimates (http://www.who.int/healthinfo/global_burden_disease/en/index.html) What can you learn about global life expectancy, mortality, and the burden of disease? How does the United States compare with other countries?

5. Select one of the vulnerable populations and discuss issues that would have an impact on the health and illness for that population. Consider issues such as health promotion, disease prevention, and access to care.

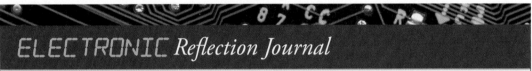

ELECTRONIC *Reflection Journal*

Circuit Board: ©Photos.com

Use your journal to describe your own perspective on health and illness, and explain how this has influenced you as a nursing student compared to your views before becoming a nursing student.

Landscape © f9photos/Shutterstock, Inc.

LINKING TO THE INTERNET

- Agency for Healthcare Research and Quality, National Healthcare Disparities Report: http://www.ahrq.gov/research/findings/nhqrdr/nhdr12/index.html
- Agency for Healthcare Research and Quality, Patient-Centered Medical Homes: http://www.pcmh.ahrq.gov/portal/server.pt/community/pcmh__home/1483
- Centers for Disease Control and Prevention: Chronic Disease: http://www.cdc.gov/chronicdisease/index.htm
- Community Guide: http://www.thecommunityguide.org
- Consumer e-health tools: http://www.cms.gov/ehealth/?gclid=CJP62LLIuLwCFawWMgodJHkAIw
- Department of Health and Human Services: Poverty Guidelines, Research, and Measurements: http://aspe.hhs.gov/poverty/
- U.S. Department of Health and Human Services: http://healthfinder.gov

Landscape © f9photos/Shutterstock, Inc.

LINKING TO THE INTERNET (CONTINUED)

- *Healthy People 2020,* Educational and Community-Based Programs: http://www.healthypeople.gov/2020/topicsobjectives2020/objectiveslist.aspx?topicId=11
- Implementing *Healthy People 2020*: MAP-IT: http://www.healthypeople.gov/2020/implement/mapit.aspx
- International Council of Nurses: http://www.icn.ch/
- U.S. federal poverty guidelines: http://aspe.hhs.gov/poverty/13poverty.cfm
- U.S. Preventive Services Task Force: http://www.uspreventiveservicestaskforce.org
- World Health Organization: http://www.who.org
- National Prevention Strategy: America's Plan for Better Health and Wellness: http://www.surgeongeneral.gov/initiatives/prevention/strategy/
- Healthcare Reform and Healthcare Prevention and Promotion: http://www.preventioninstitute.org/index.php?option=com_content&view=article&id=95&Itemid=186, http://www.healthcare.gov/law/features/rights/preventive-care/index.html
- Institute of Medicine Report: *Living Well with Chronic Illness*: http://www.iom.edu/reports/2012/living-well-with-chronic-illness.aspx

Landscape © f9photos/Shutterstock, Inc.

CASE STUDIES

Case Study 1

Imagine that you are a member of an interprofessional team in a rural community in your state. The team is looking into improving the health status of the community. The community has a high rate of cancer (particularly breast and lung); accidents (farm related); alcohol abuse, particularly among teens; and obesity (adults, but with increasing weight gain in children). The interprofessional team is composed of two registered nurses (one who works in the local hospital, and you, the only school nurse in the area), one physician in private practice, the local hospital administrator, the mayor of the largest town in the area, a psychologist in practice, and a clergyman.

Case Questions

1. Describe how you think the team should approach these problems based on what you have learned in this chapter.
2. How might you apply information about *Healthy People 2020* in this case?

(continues)

CASE STUDIES (CONTINUED)

Case Study 2

Health literacy has been a long-time problem in health care. Data from a recent community survey completed for a moderate-size city indicate that health literacy problems are increasing and that minority populations have increased in the last five years. Chronic illnesses in these populations have also increased, such as diabetes and hypertension. Clinics and home health agencies have reported an increase in medication errors for patients who are taking medications at home. Many of these errors appear to be due to poor understanding of medication directions and ability to read these directions either in written patient directions or reading medication containers.

Case Questions

1. Given the data provided, identify the key problems and related settings.
2. Research additional information on health literacy and its impact on quality of care.
3. Describe three interventions to address the issues in this community.

Words of Wisdom

Tina M. Marrelli, MSN, MA, RN
Former President, Marrelli and Associates, Inc.; Editor, *Home Healthcare Nurse*

The patient's home can be, and should be, the healthcare setting of choice for numerous reasons. Some of the easy-to-understand reasons include lower costs, the general absence of causative virulent agents that can be found within hospital walls, patient choice, and the patient being a true equal partner in care and care planning. A more important reason might be the safety considerations of being in one's own home—because there is only one patient, there is less room for medication or other treatment errors being provided to the wrong patient. However, the most important reasons for home being the best site for care come from patients and families themselves. This includes such seemingly simple things as no one (e.g., as opposed to the hospital or nursing home) telling patients what to wear (e.g., a hospital gown), how old their visitors can be, what time to eat, during which times visitors may visit, and numerous other reasons. When you add the fact that older adult patients in particular know their environment the best, that situation further supports safety—patients know every inch of their house, what they can or cannot navigate safely, and how things work for themselves and their families. It is not surprising that patients who experience problems such as mentation problems, falls, and other safety concerns in an inpatient setting do not experience these problematic symptoms when within the confines of their own home space.

There is no better place for health education and promotion to occur—the education/intervention is one to one; it is truly individualized; families/friends are involved; and the patient is in charge. The nurse and other team members are truly guests in any patient's home, and this dynamic alone provides a special situation that I believe further enhances the therapeutic relationship.

REFERENCES

Accountable Care Facts. (2014). Top 10 questions on ACOs and health care delivery reform. Retrieved from http://www.accountablecarefacts.org/

Agency for Healthcare Research and Quality (AHRQ). (2012). Highlights from the national healthcare quality and disparities report. Retrieved from http://www.ahrq.gov/research/findings/nhqrdr/nhdr12/highlights.html

American Hospital Association. (2010). *Health for life: Better health. Better healthcare.* Chicago, IL: Author. Retrieved from http://www.aha.org

American Nurses Association (ANA). (2011, May 25). ANA applauds Joint Commission standards for "medical homes": Patients gain with decision to include nurse-led clinics. Retrieved from http://nursingworld.org/Especially?For?You/AdvancedPracticeNurses/APRN-News/Joint-Commission-Standards-for-Medical-Homes.aspx

Centers for Disease Control and Prevention (CDC). (2010). Summary health statistics for U.S. children: National health interview survey, 2009. Retrieved from http://www.cdc.gov/nchs/data/series/sr_10/sr10_247.pdf

Centers for Disease Control and Prevention (CDC). (2011a). Chronic disease prevention and health promotion. Retrieved from http://www.cdc.gov/chronicdisease/index.htm

Centers for Disease Control and Prevention (CDC). (2011b). Healthy youth! Health topic: Childhood obesity. Retrieved from http://www.cdc.gov/healthyyouth/obesity

Central Intelligence Agency. (CIA). (2014). Infant mortality rates. Retrieved from https://www.cia.gov/library/publications/the-world-factbook/rankorder/2091rank.html

Consensus Panel. (2008). Essential nursing competencies curricula guidelines for genetics and genomics, 2nd ed. Retrieved from http://www.genome.gov/Pages/Careers/HealthProfessionalEducation/geneticscompetency.pdf

Dingel-Stewart, S., & LaCosta, J. (2004). Light at the end of the tunnel: A vision for an empowered nursing profession across the continuum of care. *Nursing Administration Quarterly, 28,* 212–216.

Eliopoulos, C. (2001). *Gerontological nursing.* Philadelphia, PA: Lippincott.

Finkelman, A. (2011). *Case management for nurses.* Upper Saddle River, NJ: Pearson Education.

Haggerty, J., Reid, R. J., Freeman, G. K., Starfield, B. H., Adair, C. E., & McKendry, R. (2003). Continuity of care: A multidisciplinary review. *British Medical Journal, 327,* 1219–1221.

Human Genome Project. (2007). Potential benefits of Human Genome Project Research. Retrieved from http://www.ornl.gov/sci/techresources/Human_Genome/project/benefits.shtml

Institute for Healthcare Improvement (IHI). (2011). Self-management support of patients with chronic conditions. Retrieved from http://www.ihi.org/knowledge/Pages/Changes/SelfManagement.aspx

Institute of Medicine (IOM). (2002). *Unequal treatment: Confronting racial and ethnic disparities in health.* Washington, DC: National Academies Press.

Institute of Medicine (IOM). (2003). *Priority areas for national action: Transforming healthcare quality.* Washington, DC: National Academies Press.

Institute of Medicine (IOM). (2004). *Health literacy: A prescription to end confusion.* Washington, DC: National Academies Press.

Institute of Medicine (IOM). (2010). *The future of nursing: Leading change advancing health.* Washington, DC: National Academies Press.

Institute of Medicine (IOM). (2012). *Report brief: Living well with chronic illness: A call for public action.* Washington, DC: National Academies Press.

International Council of Nurses (ICN). ((2014)). Our mission, strategic intent, core values and priorities. Retrieved from http://www.icn.ch/about-icn/icns-mission/

Joint Commission on Accreditation of Healthcare Organizations. (2004). *Hospital accreditation standards.* Oakbrook Terrace, IL: Author.

Kaakinen, J., Hanson, M., & Birenbaum, L. (2006). Family development and family nursing assessment. In M. Stanhope & J. Lancaster (Eds.), *Foundations of nursing in the community* (pp. 321–340). St. Louis, MO: Mosby.

Larkin, H. (2010, October). Managing population health. *H&HN, 28–32.*

Leavell, H., & Clark, A. (1965). *Preventive medicine for doctors in the community.* New York, NY: McGraw-Hill.

Mitchell, B., & Begoray, D. (2010). Electronic personal health records that promote self-management in chronic illness. *Online Journal of Issues in Nursing, 15*(3). Retrieved from http://www.nursingworld.org/MainMenuCategories/ANAMarketplace/ANAPeriodicals/OJIN/TableofContents/Vol152010/No3-Sept-2010/Articles-Previously-Topic/Electronic-Personal-Health-Records-and-Chronic-Illness.html

National Center for Complementary and Alternative Medicine (NCCAM). (2011). What is complementary and alternative medicine? Retrieved from http://nccam.nih.gov/health/whatiscam/

National Committee for Quality Assurance (NCQA). (2013). Patient-centered medical home. Retrieved from http://www.ncqa.org/tabid/631/Default.aspx

National Health Council. (2013). About chronic diseases. Retrieved from http://www.nationalhealthcouncil.org/NHC_Files/Pdf_Files/AboutChronicDisease.pdf

Office of Disease Prevention and Health Promotion. (2006). National Prevention Summit: Prevention, preparedness, and promotion. Retrieved from odphp.osophs.dhhs.gov/pubs/prevrpt/Volume21/Iss2-3Vol21.pdf

Organization for Economic Cooperation and Development (OECD). 2013. Health at a glance 2013: OECD indicators. Retrieved from http://gallery.mailchimp.com/de-3259be81e52e95191ab7806/files/HAG2013.pdf

Pender, N., Murdaugh, C., & Parsons, M. (2006). *Health promotion in nursing practice*. Upper Saddle River, NJ: Pearson Education.

Peters, K., & Elster, A. (2002). *Roadmaps for clinical practice. A primer on population-based medicine*. Chicago, IL: American Medical Association.

Pizzuti, D. (2006). The nurse in home health and hospice. In M. Stanhope & J. Lancaster (Eds.), *Foundations of nursing in the community* (pp. 587–609). St. Louis, MO: Mosby.

Robert Wood Johnson Foundation (RWJF). (2000). Definition of healthcare. Retrieved from http://www.rwjf.org/reports/grr/036111.htm

Robert Wood Johnson Foundation (RWJF). (2012). A national research agenda for public health services and systems. Retrieved from http://www.rwjf.org/en/research-publications/find-rwjf-research/2012/05/a-national-research-agenda-for-public-health-services-and-system.html

Sand-Jecklin, K., Murray, B., Summers, B., & Watson, J. (2010). Educating nursing students about health literacy: From the classroom to the bedside. *Online Journal of Issues in Nursing, 15*(13). Retrieved from http://www.nursingworld.org/MainMenuCategories/ANAMarketplace/ANAPeriodicals/OJIN/TableofContents/Vol152010/No3-Sept-2010/Articles-Previously-Topic/Educating-Nursing-Students-about-Health-Literacy.aspx

Schumacher, K., Beck, C., & Marren, J. (2006). Family caregivers: Caring for older adults, working with their families. *American Journal of Nursing, 106*(8), 40–48.

Trossman, S. (2011). New ANA policy brief: Aiming to help nurses better understand ramifications of immigrants' lack of access to healthcare services. *American Nurse Today, 6*(3), 34–36.

U.S. Department of Health and Human Services (HHS). (2007). U.S. Surgeon General's family initiative. Retrieved from http://www.hhs.gov/familyhistory/

U.S. Department of Health and Human Services (HHS). (2010). Healthy people 2020: MAP-IT. Retrieved from http://healthypeople.gov/2020/implement/MapIt.aspx

U.S. Department of Health and Human Services (HHS). (2012). Health, United States, 2012. Retrieved from http://www.cdc.gov/nchs/data/hus/hus12.pdf#018

U.S. Department of Health and Human Services (HHS). (2013). Healthy people, 2020: Topics and objectives). Retrieved from http://www.healthypeople.gov/2020/Topics-Objectives2020/nationalsnapshot.aspx?topicId=35

U.S. Department of Health and Human Services (HHS), Office of the Surgeon General. (2013). National Prevention Strategy. Retrieved from http://www.surgeongeneral.gov/initiatives/prevention/strategy/

Williams, C. (2006). Community-oriented nursing and community-based nursing. In M. Stanhope & J. Lancaster (Eds.), *Foundations of nursing in the community* (pp. 3–16). St. Louis, MO: Mosby.

World Health Organization (WHO). (2006). WHO Constitution. Retrieved from http://www.who.int/governance/eb/constitution/en/index.html

World Health Organization (WHO). (2008). Millennium development goals, 2008. Retrieved from http://millennium-indicators.un.org/unsd/mdg/Default.aspx

World Health Organization (WHO). (2011). Social determinants of health. Retrieved from http://www.who.int/social_determinants/en/

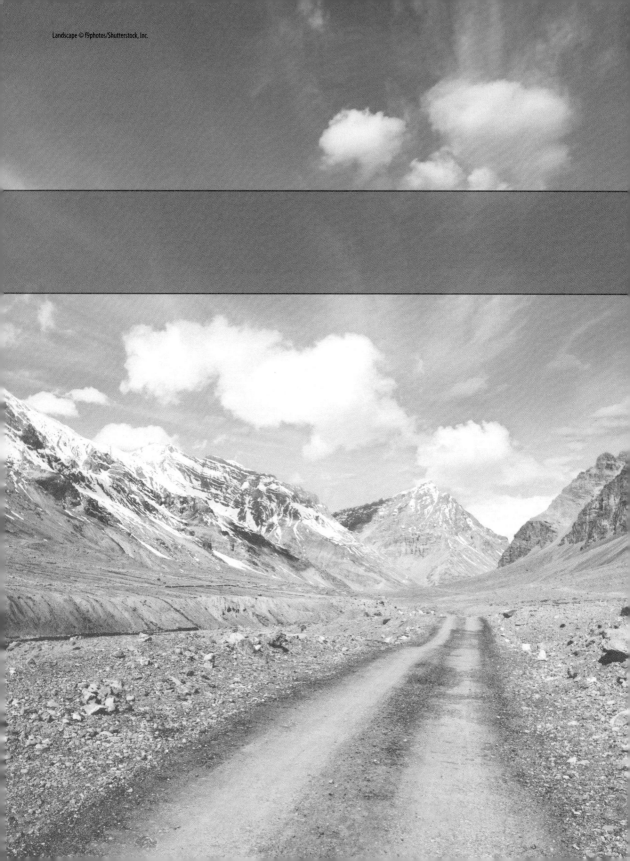

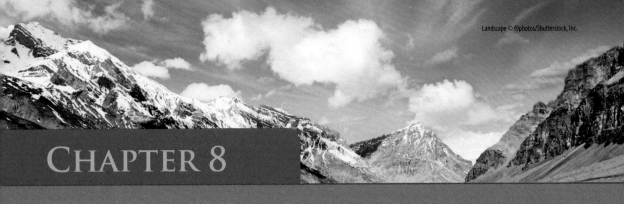

CHAPTER 8

The Healthcare Delivery System: Focus on Acute Care

CHAPTER OBJECTIVES

At the conclusion of this chapter, the learner will be able to:

- Discuss the corporatization of health care by comparing and contrasting for-profit and not-for-profit systems
- Compare and contrast the structure and process of an organization
- Identify the types of hospitals
- Identify the typical departments in a hospital and their services

- Describe the healthcare provider team and its relationship to nursing
- Discuss critical elements related to healthcare financial issues and reimbursement
- Explain the importance of organizational culture
- Discuss examples of changes in the healthcare delivery system
- Describe how nursing fits into the overall hospital organization and how it functions

CHAPTER OUTLINE

KEY TERMS

Annual limit	For-profit	Organizational culture
Copayment	Medicaid	Process
Corporatization	Medicare	Reimbursement
Deductible	Not-for-profit	Structure

INTRODUCTION

Healthcare delivery is a complex process and system. The total system includes a variety of types of healthcare provider organizations, such as acute care organizations (hospitals), ambulatory care centers (clinics), private provider offices, public/community health facilities, home care agencies, hospice agencies, extended care facilities, and so on. This chapter focuses on the largest type of healthcare organization: the acute care hospital. This does not mean that the others are not important; however, nursing students typically spend more of their clinical time in hospitals. Many of the organizational elements of a hospital are similar to those of other healthcare organizations but may vary depending on the organization and purpose. The content in this chapter explores current issues related to hospitals, hospital organization and function, and the hospital provider team, and provides an introduction to healthcare financial issues and nursing organization and functions within the hospital.

Many factors impact hospitals, leading them to change their services, collaborate with others in their communities, realign their organization with other organizations, close because of financial issues, and so forth. Among the factors that influence hospitals today are these:

- Increase in healthcare costs
- Shortage of healthcare staff (nurses and other providers)

- Increased number of uninsured and underinsured patients who are unable to pay for care
- Compromised access to care for some individuals, leading to disparities in healthcare services
- Advances in medical technology that can improve care but that may be costly and require special staff training, and that may not be accessible to those who cannot pay for them
- A greater use of informatics in documentation and for other healthcare informational purposes
- Growing diversity in patients and workforce—for example, the need for interpreter services and greater representation of ethnic groups in the healthcare workforce
- Increasing consumerism—more knowledgeable patients who demand more information and participation
- Hospital mergers and closings, altering access to services
- Shifting of beds and changing number of beds; changing specialty services (e.g., increasing the number of intensive care beds or eliminating obstetric services)
- Changes in patient demographics that require reassessment of which services and how those services are provided (e.g., increasing services for the elderly, immigrants, and single parents; expanding clinic hours to facilitate access; and so on)

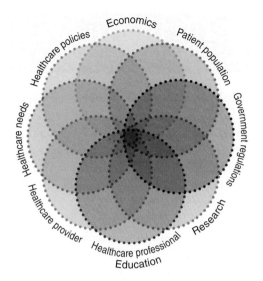

Figure 8-1 Influences on Healthcare Delivery

Examples of key influences on health care are highlighted in **Figure 8-1**. **Box 8-1** identifies examples of organizations that influence healthcare delivery.

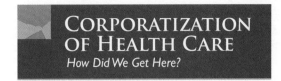

CORPORATIZATION OF HEALTH CARE
How Did We Get Here?

Using the term **corporatization** or *business* when referring to a hospital may seem strange; however, health care is a business—a very large business. It provides services to most of the population at some time during a person's life. Hospitals have a very large employee pool, providing jobs for many people—both professionals and nonprofessionals. Thus they represent one of the largest employment sectors. Within a community, healthcare organizations also usually own or lease a large amount of property, purchase a great number of supplies and equipment, and pay taxes—all activities that bring income into a community. Typically, healthcare leaders hold significant positions in the business community. Health care consumes the largest amount of federal and state dollars through healthcare reimbursement programs such as Medicare and Medicaid.

Box 8-1	Examples of Organizations Important to the Healthcare Delivery System

- National Association of Children's Hospitals and Related Institutions: http://www.childrenshospitals.org
- American Academy of Hospice and Palliative Medicine: http://www.aahpm.org
- American Association of Homes and Services for the Aging: http://www.leadingage.org
- American Association of Retired Persons: http://www.aarp.org
- American Health Care Association: http://www.ahcancal.org/Pages/Default.aspx
- American Hospital Association: http://www.aha.org/aha/about
- American Nurses Association: http://www.nursingworld.org
- Nursing Specialty Organizations: http://www.nursingcenter.com/library/JournalArticle.asp?Article_ID=623779
- American Public Health Association: http://www.apha.org
- Arthritis Foundation: http://www.arthritis.org
- American Diabetes Association: http://www.diabetes.org/?loc=404page
- The Joint Commission: http://www.-jointcommission.org
- National Association of Public Hospitals: http://www.naph.org
- National Committee on Quality Assurance: http://www.ncqa.org
- National Health Council: http://nationalhealthcouncil.org

For-Profit and Not-for-Profit Organizations: What Does This Mean?

The terms **for-profit** and **not-for-profit** can be confusing. The first critical point is that every hospital needs to make a profit, which means the healthcare organization needs to have money left over after expenses are paid. The distinguishing characteristic between for-profit and not-for-profit organizations is what is done with that profit. The assumption by most is that all hospitals are not-for-profit organizations, but this is not correct. Many large healthcare organizations are for-profit corporations. Some of their profit must go to their stockholders/shareholders or to their owners. However, even for-profit organizations must reinvest money into the hospital for maintenance, to expand space and renovate, to develop new services, to purchase equipment and supplies, and so on. Not-for-profit organizations do not have stockholders/shareholders, but these hospitals still need to make a profit for the same reasons that for-profit organizations need a profit.

Knowing whether the hospital you work for is a for-profit or not-for-profit organization can help you understand why and how decisions are made. For example, if a not-for-profit hospital is burdened with a high number of nonpaying patients, the hospital may eventually spend more than it is making and thus be "in the red" as its debt increases. When this happens, the hospital may cut staff, limit new equipment purchases, control use of supplies, fail to maintain equipment effectively, neglect facility maintenance needs and renovation, attempt to reconfigure services to attract paying patients, decrease staff education, and make other changes to improve the hospital's financial condition. A for-profit healthcare organization must always have funds to pay stockholders or owners, and this consideration can have an impact on the availability of money for other purposes that affect nurses and nursing.

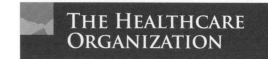

THE HEALTHCARE ORGANIZATION

Hospitals are one type of healthcare organization, and the largest. Other types of healthcare organizations are identified in **Exhibit 8-1**. All healthcare organization descriptions include information about the organization's structure and process and staff and organizational culture. Although the majority of registered nurses (RNs) work in hospitals, many work in other healthcare organizations, and the percentage working in hospitals has decreased over recent years. Nurses work in all of the healthcare settings identified in Exhibit 8-1. **Figure 8-2** provides data on employment settings of registered nurses.

The discussion here focuses on the acute care hospital as an example of a healthcare organization. How hospitals are organized does vary, but there are

Exhibit 8-1	Types of Healthcare Organizations

- Substance abuse treatment centers (inpatient and outpatient)
- School health clinics
- Diagnostic centers
- Ambulatory care surgical centers
- Dental offices and clinics
- Long-term care facilities
- Skilled nursing facilities
- Occupational health clinics
- Rehabilitation centers
- Acute care hospitals
- Physician offices
- Medical homes
- Advanced practice nurses practice sites
- Specialty hospitals (e.g., pediatric)
- Long-term care hospitals (e.g., psychiatric)
- Urgent care centers
- Home health agencies
- Hospice care
- Ambulatory care/clinics

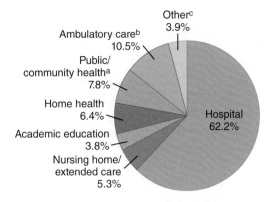

Other[c]
3.9%

Ambulatory care[b]
10.5%

Public/
community health[a]
7.8%

Home health
6.4%

Academic education
3.8%

Nursing home/
extended care
5.3%

Hospital
62.2%

Note: percentages do not add up to 100 because of the effect of rounding. Only RNs who provided setting information are included in the calculations used for this figure.
[a]Public/community health includes school and occupational health.
[b]Ambulatory care includes medical/physician practices, health centers, and clinics, and other types of non-hospital clinical settings.
[c]Other includes insurance, benefits, and utilizations review.

Figure 8-2 Employment Settings of Registered Nurses

Source: Reproduced from U.S. Department of Health and Human Services, Health Resources and Services Administration, (2010). *The registered nurse population. Findings from the 2008 National Sample Survey of Registered Nurses.* Washington, DC: Author.

some standard types of organizations. In the past, it was more common to have a single hospital operating as a single organization. Now, more hospitals have formed complex organizations consisting of multiple hospitals; in some cases, these systems also include other healthcare entities such as home care agencies, rehabilitation centers, long-term care facilities, and freestanding ambulatory care centers. Most of the reasons for this change in organizational structure are related to financial issues and the survival of the organization—to keep patients in the system, to increase services, and to expand the continuum of care. Some communities have seen multiple changes in their local hospitals, with some hospitals switching systems or trying to go it alone. The critical message is that hospitals are changing their overall organization, and it is not clear what the future holds.

Small hospitals with 100 or fewer beds and hospitals in rural areas are particularly vulnerable. They have difficulty filling beds and, therefore, often lose money. In addition, they must keep costly equipment current, purchase new equipment, and

maintain their equipment and physical facilities. These vulnerable hospitals also have problems recruiting RNs for their workforces because many RNs prefer to work in urban centers and in large, up-to-date hospitals. Schools of nursing in states with large rural areas are increasingly partnering with rural hospitals to improve enrollment from these areas and, they hope, increase the RN pool in these geographic regions. Such partnerships provide courses and clinical experiences in rural healthcare settings and may use distance education to facilitate the programs.

In 2013, the Institute of Medicine (IOM) published a report entitled *Best Care at Lower Cost: The Path to Continuously Learning Health Care in America*. This report describes the system in this way:

Health care in America presents a fundamental paradox. The past 50 years have seen an explosion in biomedical knowledge, dramatic innovation in therapies and surgical procedures, and management of conditions that previously were fatal, with ever more exciting clinical capabilities on the horizon. Yet, American health care is falling short on basic dimensions of quality, outcomes, costs, and equity. (IOM, 2013, p. 1)

The U.S. healthcare delivery system has an estimated $750 billion in wasted resources in the system. This money is lost, so it cannot be spent on improving healthcare outcomes. The IOM notes that the United States needs the best care at a lower cost, not a higher cost. Compared to other countries, the United States is paying more for less, resulting in poorer healthcare outcomes than are found in other industrialized nations. The complex U.S. healthcare delivery system has to manage costs while simultaneously ensuring quality, evidence-based care. Trying to achieve this balance will lead to more changes in the healthcare delivery system and impact nursing.

Structure and Process

One way to describe a hospital is to consider its structure and process. A hospital's **structure** is based on how the organization is configured, and the best source for a view of a hospital's structure is its organizational chart. **Figure 8-3** is an example of a hospital organizational chart, which displays the components of the hospital. The structure depicted in Figure 8-3 can be described as vertical. The chart identifies whom staff report to, or rather, who is a staff member's manager or supervisor. Organizations that focus more on this type of structure tend to be bureaucratic and highly centralized, and key persons in the organization make decisions. Bureaucratic organizations have the following characteristics:

- *Division of labor:* descriptions of jobs that include clearly defined tasks
- *Defined hierarchy:* clear description of the reporting relationships
- *Detailed rules and regulations:* greater emphasis on policies and procedures; expectation that these will be followed and will guide decision making
- *Impersonal relationships:* expectation that staff will do their jobs and that supervisors will ensure that jobs are done as expected

Organizational structure also includes the span of control or the number of staff managed by each supervisor or manager. The more staff a manager supervises, the more complex that supervision becomes.

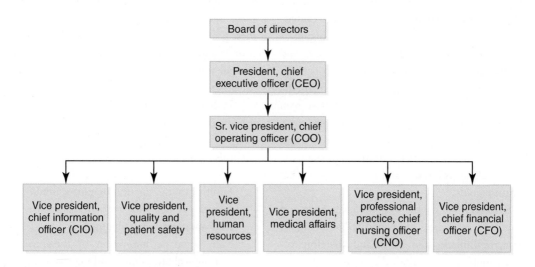

Figure 8-3 Example of a Hospital Organizational Chart

Although bureaucratic organizations are less common today, many hospitals still operate as these types of organizations, emphasizing a vertical structure that includes these elements, but is less rigid than the structure of formal bureaucratic organizations. Line authority, or chain of command, is very important, in that each staff member knows to whom to report, and it is expected that this order will be followed. A true bureaucratic organization does not expect or want much staff input regarding decisions.

A horizontal structure is decentralized, with emphasis being placed on departments or divisions; decisions are made closer to the staff who do the work. Departments or divisions focus on special functions such as nursing care, laboratory tests, and nutrition and patient food services—a scheme called departmentalization.

The matrix organization structure is newer and less clear than the traditional bureaucratic organization that is centered on departments. In a matrix organization, staff might be part of a functional department, such as nursing services, but if the nurse works in surgery, the nurse is also considered a staff member in the surgical services/department. This type of organization is considered flatter because decisions do not flow clearly from the top down.

Hospitals typically have hierarchical management levels. The top level consists of the board of trustees or board of directors. This board typically includes members of the community and community leaders who are not directly involved in health care. The board is responsible for developing the overall direction of the hospital and ensuring that the goals of the organization are met. The board hires the hospital's chief executive officer (CEO; also sometimes called the organization's president), and this person reports to the board. The CEO then hires the other major leaders for the hospital, such as the chief financial officer (CFO) and the nursing leader. The nursing leader may be called the chief nursing executive (CNE), the chief nursing officer (CNO), or, in some cases, the vice president for nursing or patient services. This last title may also reflect the person's oversight of other disciplines or ancillary services, such as occupational therapy, physical therapy, or nutrition. Often the board approves these hires. Because the board has ultimate responsibility for the budget, it has significant influence over matters that impact nurses, such as staffing and other resources important to nursing.

Process, the other dimension of organizations, focuses on how the organization functions. How would a staff member gain an understanding of a hospital's process? The hospital's vision, mission statement, and goals are a good place to begin to find out what is important to the organization and how the hospital describes itself and its functioning. Other sources of information relevant to process include policies and procedures, communication systems and expectations, decision-making processes, delegation process, implementation of coordination (teams), and evaluation methods (quality improvement). The key question is, *how does the work get done?*

Classification of Hospitals

Hospitals can be classified using a variety of descriptors. Following are some of these descriptors:

- *Ownership:* Is the hospital for-profit (investor owned), not-for-profit, part of a corporate system, faith based, or government (state, federal)? Government hospitals include Veterans Administration (VA) hospitals, military hospitals, state mental health hospitals, the National Institutes of Health Clinical Center, and Indian Health Service hospitals.
- *Public access:* How much access does the general community have to the hospital's services? Is it a community or private hospital?
- *Number of beds:* Bed size, or the number of beds, can vary widely from hospital to hospital.
- *Licensure:* Licensure of hospitals is done by each state's health department, which ensures that hospitals meet certain state standards. Licensure and accreditation are not the same. Licensure comes from a government agency.

Accreditation is a process to determine whether a hospital meets certain minimal standards; this process is voluntary and is provided by a nongovernmental organization. For hospitals to receive Medicare and Medicaid reimbursement—and this is an important source of income—they must be certified or given authority by the Centers for Medicare and Medicaid Services (CMS) to provide services to Medicare and Medicaid recipients. Meeting all these requirements and participating in the surveys take staff time, which is costly, but it is very important for the overall financial status of an institution. In addition, hospitals that do not meet these requirements cannot be used as sites for healthcare professional students' clinical practice experiences (nursing, medicine, and others).

- *Teaching:* A hospital is classified as a teaching hospital if it offers residency programs for physicians. The expansion of nurse residency programs may also become a method for classifying hospitals in the future, although this is not certain at this time and few hospitals have such programs.
- *Length of stay:* Length of stay refers to how long patients typically stay in a hospital, a measure given as a range or average length of stay. Fewer than 30 days is referred to as short stay, and more than 30 days is long term. Length of stay has been decreasing in the last 15 years because of decreasing reimbursement of hospital care and a greater push to provide more healthcare services outside the hospital. Reducing readmissions is important for all hospitals. The Institute for Healthcare Improvement (2014) recommends that hospitals use the following interventions to decrease the risk of readmission:
  - Focus on the person, not the condition.
  - Know your data.
  - Establish what success looks like.
  - Form a cross-continuum team.
  - Improve the discharge process.
  - Mobilize enhanced transitional care support for individuals at high risk for readmission.
  - Engage patients and families.
- *Multihospital system:* Since 1991, there has been growth in large hospital systems that include multiple hospitals. These systems often provide more than just acute care services; for example, they may offer hospice care, home care, long-term care, and other services. This partnering provides the hospitals with a continuum of services, from acute care to long-term care, to meet the needs of their patients. In a sense, the system does not lose the patient; the patient just goes on to a different part of the system for additional care needs and may return for other services if needs change. For example, suppose a patient has been in a hospital intensive care unit for complications related to chronic obstructive pulmonary disorder. The patient returns home after discharge and receives home care from the hospital's home care agency. One week after discharge, the home care nurse assesses the patient and decides that the patient needs to be rehospitalized because of pneumonia. The patient is then admitted to the same hospital.

Typical Departments in a Hospital

As was discussed in relation to the structure of organizations, hospitals are made up of departments, divisions, and/or services. This structure has existed for a long time. Students need to be familiar with these departments because nurses interact with all of them at some point in their practice, and they need to know how to coordinate care by using services from a variety of departments.

What are some of the departments found in an acute care hospital? Titles may vary from hospital to hospital, but the functions described here are typical and part of daily hospital operations:

- *Administration:* This is the leadership for the hospital, the central decision-making source—for example, the CEO or administrator, assistant administrators, financial services and budget staff, and often the CNO, chief nursing executive, or vice president for nursing or patient services.

- *Nursing:* This is the largest department in terms of employee numbers. Often it is called patient services, which is a title used by some hospitals since the early 1990s. This does not mean that patients receive only nursing care; many other departments are directly involved in patient care, such as laboratory, dietetic services, respiratory services, pharmacy, and others. However, nursing service is the 24/7 coordinator of patient care and provides the largest percentage of direct care to patients.

- *Medical staff:* Physicians who practice in a hospital, if not part of a training program such as a residency or fellowship, must be members of the medical staff. Their credentials are reviewed, and they are given admitting privileges. This is done to ensure that standards are met. A director or chief of medical staff leads the medical staff. Medical staff may or may not be employees of the hospital. If a college of medicine is partnered with the hospital, the organization can be more complex. For example, the dean of the college of medicine may hold a key administrative position in the hospital and the college of medicine chairs of departments may also hold positions in the hospital. This may be true for a dean of nursing as well.

- *Admission and discharge:* This department manages all aspects of admission and discharge for patients, including paperwork, reimbursement, patient room assignments, and, in some cases, assignment of physicians.

Case management may be part of this department or part of patient services.

- *Medical records:* Documentation is a critical part of all aspects of care. The medical records department provides oversight of documentation, whether hard-copy documentation or information in a computerized system. This complex function requires nursing input to ensure that nursing documentation needs are recognized and information is included.

- *Information management:* This department ensures that required information is collected, analyzed, monitored, and summarized. Its function is directly related to medical records and documentation.

- *Quality improvement:* This department is charged with ensuring that the hospital has a quality improvement program, implements it, evaluates its outcomes, and makes changes to improve care. Nurses often are staff in this department because they have much to offer with their experience and knowledge in providing and assessing quality care.

- *Infection control:* This function has become increasingly important with the greater need to provide services that decrease infection risk. Nurses are very active staff members in this department; they develop policies and procedures, monitor infection rates, and train staff.

- *Research and evidence-based practice (EBP):* Many hospitals, particularly academic medical centers, have research departments. Typically, this department is led by professionals in medicine, although nurses often participate in the studies and may lead nursing studies. The department's purpose is to conduct research studies. The nursing department may have its own nurse researchers. In some healthcare organizations, research and EBP are combined or there may be a separate EBP service or department. The EBP department is one of the newest in hospitals, and not all hospitals have this type of department. Some hospitals are incorporating the management of EBP—both medicine and nursing—into other departments, such as EBP for nursing. The EBP functions may be part of nursing or patient services, quality improvement, or evidence-based medicine related to medical staff organization.

- *In-service or staff development:* This is the department that implements orientation and education for staff.
- *Environmental services (housekeeping):* Staff from this department interact with nurses in the patient care areas to ensure that areas are clean for patients.

Other departments focus on specific health needs, such as pharmacy, respiratory therapy, clinical laboratory, infusion therapy, occupational therapy, radiology, physical therapy, and social services. Nurses get involved in all these services. Hospitals are typically organized around clinical areas (units, services, and, in some cases, departments) such as medicine, surgery, intensive care (medical intensive care unit [MICU], surgical intensive care unit [SICU], cardiac care unit [CCU], and neonatal intensive care unit [NICU]), post-anesthesia unit (PACU), labor and delivery (L&D), postpartum, nursery, gynecology, pediatrics, emergency department (ED), urgent care, psychiatric or behavioral health, ambulatory care, ambulatory care surgery, and dialysis. Clinical areas may also be specific to a specialty, such as medical units for the post-cardiac care unit, referred to as step-down units; oncology; or surgical units that focus on orthopedics, urology, and so on.

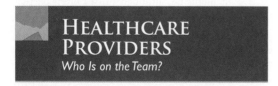

HEALTHCARE PROVIDERS
Who Is on the Team?

The hospital healthcare team is composed of a variety of healthcare providers, both professional and nonprofessional. All are important in the care process. In addition, many other staff are critical to the overall operation of a hospital, such as office support staff, dietary staff, housekeeping staff, facilities management and maintenance staff, patient transportation staff, medical records staff, communications (information technology) staff, equipment maintenance and repair staff, and many others. For our purposes, the focus is on the staff who provide care, either direct care or indirect care, to a patient. A staff member who provides direct care, such as a nurse, comes in contact with the patient. An indirect care provider might be someone who works in the lab to complete a lab test, but this provider may never actually see the patient. However, the work done in the lab is very important to the patient's care.

The group of providers who provide care to a patient is referred to as a team. They have a common purpose: providing patient care. Interprofessional teamwork is one of the five core competencies recommended by the IOM for all healthcare professionals. Nurses work with other nursing staff (RNs, licensed vocational nurses [LVNs]/licensed practical nurses [LPNs], and assistants on teams) to provide care; however, today there is also greater emphasis on the need for interprofessional teams in which nurses collaborate and coordinate with members of multiple disciplines, such as physicians, pharmacists, social workers, and many other members.

The following are some of the major team members and their functions. Not all patients require services from all these healthcare professionals; instead, services are based on individual patient needs.

- *Registered nurse (RN):* Nurses are the backbone of any acute care hospital. They work in a great variety of positions and departments, not just the nursing department. Nurses also work in medical records, quality improvement, infusion therapy, case management, staff development, radiology, and ambulatory care, among other departments. Some nurses are in management positions and do not provide direct care.

- *Advanced practice nurse (APRN):* A nurse practitioner is an RN with a master's degree in a specialty. In some states, an advanced practice nurse may provide some services independently of physician orders, such as prescribing certain medications and treatment procedures. APRNs may work in clinics but typically do not work in acute care units, although this situation is changing. In some states, APRNs may have admitting privileges along with their prescriptive authority (i.e., the right to prescribe medication). The future plan is that APRNs will get a doctor of nursing practice (DNP) degree instead of a master's degree. For example, nurse anesthesia/certified registered nurse anesthetist education programs are already changing to a DNP degree due to the mandate from the American Association of Nurse Anesthetists (AANA), their professional organization.
- *Clinical nurse specialist (CNS):* A CNS is an RN with a master's degree. This nurse is prepared to provide care in acute care settings and guides the care provided by other RNs. Examples of CNS specialties are cardiac care and behavioral health (psychiatry).
- *Doctor of nursing practice (DNP):* A DNP is an RN with a terminal doctoral practice degree. This nurse is prepared to carry out roles similar to the traditional APRN and CNS in addition to focusing at the systems level on evidence-based practice, quality improvement, leadership, and financing expertise.
- *Clinical nurse leader (CNL):* "The CNL role is a new position. This nurse has a master's degree and is a provider and a manager of care at the point of care to individuals and cohorts [groups of patients]. The CNL designs, implements, and evaluates client care by coordinating, delegating and supervising the care provided by the healthcare team, including licensed nurses, technicians, and

other health professionals" (American Association of Colleges of Nursing, 2007, p. 6).
- *Certified nurse–midwife (CNM):* A nurse–midwife has a master's degree and is prepared to provide women's health services and services to obstetric patients. In some states, certified nurse–midwives have admitting privileges. Their scope of practice may be regulated under either the medical or nursing practice act, depending on the state.
- *Certified registered nurse anesthetist (CRNA):* This nurse anesthetist has a master's degree and is prepared to provide services to patients requiring anesthesia.
- *Physician:* A physician has a medical degree and typically has a specialty such as surgery, medicine, pediatrics, or obstetrics and gynecology; some physicians may even have a subspecialty. For example, a physician with a specialty in internal medicine may subspecialize in rheumatology, dermatology, oncology, or neurology. A surgeon may subspecialize in orthopedics, oncology (and even more specifically in breast surgery), and so on. In a teaching hospital, which has medical students and residents, the typical team includes faculty/attending physician, the chief resident, residents, interns, and medical students. They are responsible for the medical aspects of patient care and have oversight of overall care requirements.
- *Physician's assistant (PA):* A physician's assistant is prepared to practice some aspects of medicine under the supervision of a physician. The PA conducts physical examinations, performs diagnostic workups, makes diagnoses, prevents and treats diseases, and may have some prescribing privileges. PAs do not have a licensure at this time, such as a physician or a nurse might have.
- *Licensed practical/vocational nurse (LPN/ LVN):* An LPN/LVN is a member of the nursing staff who has completed a one-year

nursing program and successfully passed the LPN/LVN licensing exam. These nurses are supervised by RNs and are important team members. The state board of nursing determines what care they may provide, although not all states use the LPN/LVN designations. It is important for RNs to know what LPNs/LVNs are allowed to do and to provide supervision for this care. RNs can delegate to LPNs/LVNs, but the reverse is not true.

- *Occupational therapist (OT):* Occupational therapists are not present in every hospital, but they provide important services for patients with rehabilitation needs because of impaired functioning, such as patients who have had a stroke or patients who have experienced a serious automobile accident. Another type of therapist who might be used, especially for patients who have had a stroke, is a speech-language pathologist. These types of therapists are found commonly in rehabilitation services but can be provided in all types of settings, such as in hospitals, in long-term care facilities, and in home care.

- *Patient care assistant or nursing assistant:* Patient care assistants or certified nursing assistants may have a variety of titles. They are nonprofessional nursing staff who have a short training period (typically a few months) that prepares them to provide direct care, such as assisting with activities of daily living (bathing, taking vital signs, and so on). They are supervised by RNs or in some cases by LPNs/LVNs and are important members of the team.

- *Pharmacist:* The pharmacist has completed professional education and ensures that pharmaceutical care is appropriate for patient needs. Given the growing concern about medication errors, pharmacists are highly important members of the team,

and nurses should work closely with them. Some hospitals have a centralized pharmacy department, with all pharmaceutical services coming from a central unit. Others have moved to include pharmacists as direct team members on units, providing an invaluable service at the point of care.

- *Physical therapist (PT):* Physical therapists provide musculoskeletal care to patients, such as assisting with teaching post-stroke patients how to walk, use crutches, or use other assistive devices. They also help design exercises to ensure or increase mobility.

- *Registered dietitian:* Dietitians work with patients to help resolve dietary and nutritional needs. Nurses work with dietitians as patient dietary needs are identified and implemented.

- *Respiratory therapist:* Respiratory therapists provide care to patients who have a variety of respiratory problems. They are trained to provide specific types of treatments, such as oxygen therapy, inhalation therapy, intermittent positive-pressure ventilators, and artificial mechanical ventilators. Respiratory therapists go to the patient's bedside for these treatments, and some respiratory therapists may be assigned to work solely in intensive care units, where there is great need for these treatments. Respiratory therapists are also part of the team that responds to codes when patients experience cardiac or respiratory arrests.

- *Social worker:* Social workers have professional degrees and assist patients and their families with such issues as reimbursement, discharge concerns, housing, transportation, and other social services. Nurses work with social workers to identify patient issues that need to be resolved in order to decrease stress on patients and families. A social worker may serve as a case manager, but case managers may also be RNs.

Two of the newest members of the healthcare team are the hospitalist and the intensivist. The hospitalist position usually is a doctor of medicine (MD), although APRNs and CNSs hold this position in some hospitals. The hospitalist is a generalist who coordinates the patient's care, serving as the primary provider while the patient is in the hospital. The patient's primary provider outside the hospital is not involved in the inpatient care, and the patient returns to that provider after discharge. This reduces the time that the primary care provider (internist, family practitioner, pediatrician) has to devote to inpatient care. Thus, the primary care provider (PCP) has more time to focus on the patient's outpatient needs. In addition, the hospitalist is more current with acute care and the treatment required. The intensivist is similar to the hospitalist, but this MD focuses on care of patients in intensive care, which is a more specialized area of care.

The hospitalist and intensivist positions were developed to increase coordination and continuity of care in the hospital. Both of these providers are paid by the hospital as hospital employees. A major disadvantage of this model of medical care is that the patient has no relationship with the hospitalist or the intensivist prior to hospitalization and will not have any contact after hospitalization. Some patients may not be satisfied with a nurse in this role. Patient choice is always an important factor to consider. Patients may want to see their own physician or see a physician instead of an APRN.

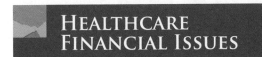

HEALTHCARE FINANCIAL ISSUES

Healthcare financial issues can be viewed from three perspectives. The first perspective is the macro view, or the status of healthcare finances viewed from a national or a state perspective. The second is the micro view, which focuses on a specific healthcare organization and its budget. Nurses are not usually involved in the development of budgets unless they are in a management position; however, it is important for nurses to understand what a budget is and why it is important. The third perspective focuses on payment of care and reimbursement.

The Nation's Health Care: Financial Status (Macro View)

The macro view is important because it encompasses the major financial support for the U.S. healthcare system. The United States spends a lot of money on health care, yet not everyone has been covered by insurance for their health care. Consequently, reimbursement issues play a major role in the status of health care and coverage of these expenses. **Figure 8-4** describes the nation's healthcare dollar—how much Medicare and Medicaid spent on different categories of services. **Figure 8-5** describes overall Medicare healthcare expenditures, and **Figure 8-6** provides information on Medicare benefit payments by type of service for 2012. These expenditures are changing, and they are increasing.

The Individual Healthcare Organization and Its Financial Needs (Micro View)

The hospital budget is used by every hospital to manage its financial issues. The budget is prepared for a specific time period, usually a year. In addition, a longer-term plan covering several years is prepared, although this plan must be adjusted over time because of changes in the organization's financial status. The budget describes the expected expenses, such as staff salaries and benefits, equipment, supplies, utilities, pharmaceutical needs, facility maintenance, dietary needs, administrative services, staff education, legal fees, insurance coverage, parking and security, and so on. The budget also describes the projected revenues, or money coming into the organization.

It is very important that nursing management participate in the budget process because the budget has a major impact on nurses and nursing care.

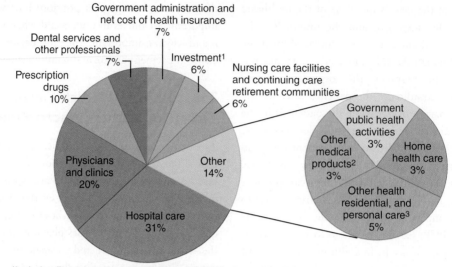

¹Includes Research (2%) and Structures and Equipment (4%).
²Includes Durable (1%) and Non-durable (2%) goods.
³Includes expenditures for residential care facilities, ambulance providers, medical care delivered in nontraditional settings (such as community centers, senior citizens centers, schools, and military field stations), and expenditures for Home and Community Waiver programs under Medicaid.
Note: Sum of pieces may not equal 100% due to rounding.

Figure 8-4 The Nation's Health Dollar, Calendar Year 2011, Where it Went

Source: Centers for Medicare & Medicaid Services, Office of the Actuary, National Health Statistics Group. Retrieved from http://www.cms.gov/Research-Statistics-Data-and-Systems/Statistics-Trends-and-Reports/NationalHealthExpendData/Downloads/PieChartSourcesExpenditures2011.pdf

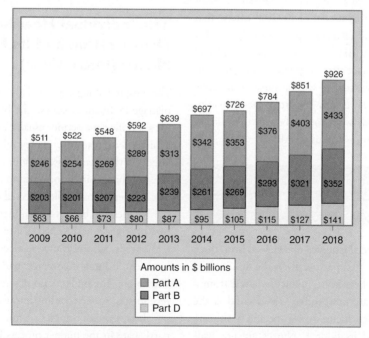

Figure 8-5 Overall Medicare Spending, 2009–2018

Source: 2009 Annual Report of the Boards of Trustees of the Federal Hospital Insurance and Federal Supplementary Medical Insurance Trust Funds. Retrieved from http://kaiserfamilyfoundation.files.wordpress.com/2013/01/7905.pdf

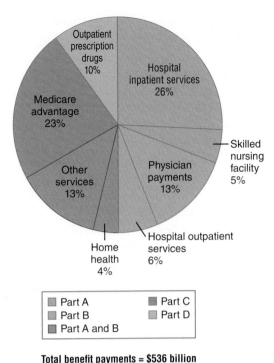

Total benefit payments = $536 billion

NOTE: Excludes administrative expenses and is net of recoveries. *Includes hospice, durable medical equipment, Part B drugs, outpatient dialysis, ambulance, lab services, and other services.

Figure 8-6 Medicare Benefit Payments

Source: The Henry J. Kaiser Family Foundation. Retrieved from http://kff.org/medicare/fact-sheet/medicare-spending-and-financing-fact-sheet/

The board of directors approves the final budget. After a budget is approved and implemented, it is important that budgetary data are monitored on a regular basis and that this information is shared with all managers. This monitoring is done to better ensure that the budget goals are met and to facilitate early recognition of budget issues that may require adjustment.

Reimbursement: Who Pays for Health Care?

Reimbursement is a critical topic in health care, and it is complex. It represents the third perspective on healthcare financial issues. Nursing students may wonder why this topic is relevant to them or even to nurses in general. Basically, reimbursement pays the patient's bill for services provided, and this payment in turn covers costs of care, such as staff salaries and benefits, drugs, medical supplies, physician fees, facility maintenance and upgrades, equipment, general supplies, and much more. These monies then provide healthcare providers with funds to pay their bills and for their services. So, for example, reimbursement dollars eventually become the dollars that pay staff their salaries. The healthcare delivery system is long past focusing on charity care.

Hospitals that do not bring in enough money to pay their bills are said to be operating "in the red," and this is not a good position for a hospital to be in. It means that the hospital cannot pay all its bills. Most hospitals are operating in the red, but how far in the red can make the difference between modernizing or filling staff positions or not doing so—and whether the hospital stays open for business. Some hospitals in this country have closed. Particularly hard hit have been hospitals in rural areas and small hospitals that are not able to compete for patients. Their closing has a major impact on access to care. Some patients may not have access to a local hospital for needed services, or even for emergency services. Some people may have to travel long distances for obstetric care or specialized care for children (pediatrics, neonatal care for newborns), mental health services, oncology (diagnosis and treatment), complex surgical procedures, and many other services.

The United States is experiencing a serious crisis in its safety net hospitals. These public hospitals serve those populations that have limited or no resources to pay for services. This does not mean that these hospitals do not or could not serve patients with excellent reimbursement; however, it is typically the case that the majority of their patients cannot provide sufficient reimbursement. These patients also tend to be more complex in terms of their care; many are vulnerable and have had limited preventive care. Some have chronic medical conditions that have not been treated. Other complications include socioeconomic problems, language issues, and immigrant status, all of which contribute to the need for complex healthcare treatment. It is clear that the safety net hospital system is not operating effectively and cannot meet the complex needs of vulnerable populations today (Dewan & Sack, 2008).

It is important for nurses to understand basic information about reimbursement. Patients today frequently worry about payment for care. Questions that arise are: Do patients have insurance coverage? How much of their care will be covered by insurance? Will they get the treatment they need from the providers they prefer? Experiencing an illness is difficult for any patient and the patient's family, and to add worry about payment for services to this stress can have an impact on a patient's health as well as the patient's response to the health problem. This stress can affect whether patients can follow treatment recommendations. Can the patient afford the medications, or would the costs compromise the patient's ability to buy food or pay rent? Can the patient afford to take a bus or taxicab to a doctor's appointment? Can the patient afford to take off work for an appointment? None of this is simple. One of the goals of healthcare reform (the Affordable Care Act of 2010) is to reduce the number of patients without insurance, thereby decreasing the problem of patients who cannot pay and, in turn, impacting the financial status of healthcare organizations; however, patients still have to pay co-payments and deductibles for their healthcare services.

The Third-Party Payer System

The U.S. healthcare delivery system is funded primarily through a third-party payer system (insurance) that is employer based, with healthcare services primarily paid by someone other than the patient. This means if your employer does not offer an insurance benefit, you must either purchase your own insurance, apply for Medicaid if you are eligible, apply for Medicare if you are eligible, or go without insurance. Under the Affordable Care Act, going without insurance means you have to pay a penalty. Examples of third-party payers include Blue Cross, Humana, Medicaid, and Medicare. The patient pays for part of the care, but the payment for most patients goes through another party, the insurer (the third-party payer). Typically, the patient or enrollee in the insurance policy is covered as part of a group, most likely through the enrollee's employer healthcare policies.

The 2010 healthcare reform legislation established insurance exchanges (at the federal level and in some states as well). An individual can buy personal health insurance through these exchanges when he or she does not have access to employer healthcare insurance (e.g., someone who is self-employed or whose employer does not provide insurance). The new legislation also provides some financial support and reduced costs for people who have to buy insurance through the exchanges, but they must meet certain criteria to obtain this support. The launch of this system was accompanied by numerous problems—particularly technological problems, but also issues related to the insurance plans and some people having to change coverage, which in some cases was more costly or required a change in providers. It is unclear what the long-term results of these changes will be, but they should ultimately reduce the number of people who do not have any insurance coverage. As of March 2012, more than 8 million people had enrolled in such healthcare coverage plans, including people who were younger and healthy, with no major health problems.

Fee-for-service is the most common reimbursement model in the United States. In this model, physicians or other providers, such as hospitals, bill separately for each patient encounter or service that they provide, rather than receiving a salary or a set payment per patient enrolled. The third-party payer actually pays the bills, but the enrollee usually has some payment responsibilities that vary from one policy to another. This is a complex area, so nurses, as consumers of health care and as healthcare providers, need to understand the basics. Enrollees (patients) may pay any or all of the following:

- *Deductible:* The **deductible** is the part of the bill that the patient must pay before the insurer will pay the bill for the services. After the patient pays that amount due per year, the patient pays no additional deductible for that year.
- *Copayment and coinsurance:* The **copayment** is the fixed amount that a patient may be required to pay per service (physician visit, lab test, prescription, and so on), and this amount can vary among insurance policies. It is typically a small amount—for example, $10 per physician visit.

Both the deductible and the copayment represent the patient's out-of-pocket expenses each year, in addition to the annual fee that the employee pays for the coverage. Employers also pay a portion of the annual insurance fee. Fees vary from policy to policy and from one employer to another. There had long been no requirement in the United States that every employer provide healthcare insurance coverage, although this has changed with the healthcare reform of 2010; now this requirement is based on how many employees the employer has.

Annual limits are also important. They mean that enrollees have a defined amount that they would have to pay—a maximum amount; and after that level is reached, they no longer have to contribute to the payment. For example, suppose the employee or enrollee has bills exceeding $5000, and the annual limit is $5000. This enrollee or patient would not have to pay any more for care that year after paying $5000; thereafter, the patient is 100% covered for care.

Employees may include their families on their employer insurance coverage. The healthcare reform legislation of 2010 now makes it a requirement that insurers allow families to include uninsured adult children up to age 26 on their insurance even if the adult child is no longer dependent on the parents. Typically, employees have to pay more per year for family insurance, and there may be different requirements for the family (e.g., a higher annual out-of-pocket limit) than for an individual.

Another critical element of reimbursement is preexisting conditions. A preexisting condition is a medical condition that a person has developed before the person applies for a particular health insurance policy; this condition could affect the person's (enrollee or employee) ability to get coverage or how much the enrollee has to pay for it. What is considered a preexisting condition? Differences in how policies answered in this question have long been a problem; however, the healthcare reform of 2010 has had an impact on the preexisting condition requirement in that insurers are no longer able to use a preexisting condition as a reason to deny insurance coverage.

Government Reimbursement of Healthcare Services

State and federal governments cover a large portion of the healthcare costs in the United States, but there is no universal coverage, meaning that not all citizens have healthcare coverage. The United States is one of the few industrialized countries that does not have universal coverage. The healthcare reform of 2010 does not support full universal healthcare coverage, although more people are now able to get coverage and all are required to have coverage or pay a penalty.

There are several types of government-sponsored reimbursement. The largest programs are Medicare and Medicaid, which are managed by the CMS, Department of Health and Human Services. In 1965, Title XVIII, an amendment to the Social Security Act, established **Medicare**. Medicare is the federal health insurance program for people aged 65 and older, persons with disabilities, and people with end-stage renal disease. Medicare had 49,435,610 beneficiaries in 2012, and this number increases each year. The need for Medicare coverage is growing because of the increase in the population older than age 65. Medicare covers hospital services (Part A) and physician and outpatient care (Part B), and it offers coverage for prescriptions. Enrollees have to pay a portion of costs for Part B and prescriptions. Part C (Medicare Advantage) covers Part A and B but through private insurance companies approved by Medicare. The healthcare reform of 2010 will impact this part over time. Part D provides prescription coverage. Medicare does not pay for long-term care but does cover some skilled nursing and home health care for specific conditions.

The CMS sets standards and monitors Medicare services and payment. Medicare covers many patients in acute care today. It is a very important part of the U.S. healthcare delivery system that supports older citizens and other populations; however, there is concern about financing this program in the future because of the increase in the number of citizens who will be 65 and older.

Medicaid, established in 1965 by Title XIX of the Social Security Act, is the federal/state program for certain categories of low-income people. Medicaid covers health and long-term care services for more than 51 million Americans, including children, the aged, the blind, disabled persons, and people who are eligible to receive federally assisted income maintenance payments. The number of people enrolled in Medicaid is increasing and will increase even further with the implementation of the healthcare reform of 2010, as more people are now eligible for Medicaid owing to changes in the program made by the Affordable Care Act. For example, it is estimated that enrollment nationally will increase by 27.4%, with state spending increasing by 1.4%, federal spending increasing by 22.1%, and overall spending increasing by 13.2% (StateFacts.Org, 2011). In June 2012, enrollment in Medicaid reached 54.1 million, as high unemployment rates caused many people to become eligible for this program owing to their low incomes; as economic conditions improved, however, a gradual

drop in Medicaid enrollment occurred. (Government data are typically one to two years behind the current year.)

Medicaid is tied to insurance coverage offered by the Affordable Care Act, although not all states opted to include expansion of Medicaid as a method for expanding insurance coverage as part of healthcare reform. The Medicaid program is funded by both federal funds and state funds, but each state sets its own guidelines and administers the state's Medicaid program. The federal poverty guidelines, which establish the annual income level for poverty defined by the federal government, are important in identifying people who meet coverage criteria for Medicaid reimbursement.

In an effort to improve care and reduce costs, in 2008 the CMS began to deny payment for certain preventable hospital-acquired conditions. The list of these conditions is changing as more evidence mounts to support the contention that certain problems are preventable (Kurtzman & Buerhaus, 2008). This is a critical decision because it means that hospitals will not be paid for these conditions when patients experience them. For example, suppose a patient who is covered by Medicare falls in the hospital and incurs an injury. Treatment for that injury may not be charged to Medicare and may not be charged to the patient. In 2011, a new rule was passed to include patients covered by Medicaid in the hospital-acquired complications (HAC) categories as of 2012, which means now there is a list of patient events or complications that Medicaid will not cover. The media links found at the end of the chapter provide more information about the current list of HACs and related issues.

Nurses can make a difference in preventing HACs, and they need to be involved in determining interventions to prevent these conditions or other "never" events. The current list of "never" events can be found at the CMS website. The CMS's goal is to stimulate hospitals to improve care—to decrease preventable hospital-acquired conditions—and this has begun to happen.

In spring of 2014, the Department of Health and Human Services announced that new preliminary data show an overall 9% decrease in hospital-acquired conditions nationally during 2011 and 2012. National reductions in adverse drug events, falls, infections, and other forms of hospital-induced harm are estimated to have prevented nearly 15,000 deaths in hospitals, avoided 560,000 patient injuries, and [avoided] approximately $4 billion in health spending over the same period. Hospital readmissions fall by 8% for Medicare beneficiaries. In 2010 there were 145 HACs per 1,000 discharges and in 2012 132 HACs per 1,000 discharges. (U.S Department of Health and Human Services, 2014)

Covered Medicaid services include inpatient care (excluding psychiatric or behavioral health); outpatient care with certain stipulations; laboratory and radiology services; care provided by certified pediatric and family nurse practitioners when licensed to practice under state law; nursing facility services (long-term care) for beneficiaries aged 21 and older; early and periodic screening, diagnosis, and treatment for children younger than age 21; family planning services and supplies; physician services; medical and surgical care; dentist services; home health for beneficiaries who are entitled to nursing facility services under the state's Medicaid plan; certified nurse–midwifery services; pregnancy-related services and services for other conditions that might complicate pregnancy; and 60 days' postpartum pregnancy-related services.

A second group of persons are also eligible for Medicaid: the medically needy. These are persons who have too much money (which may be in savings) to be eligible categorically for Medicaid but who require extensive care that would consume all their resources. Each state must include the following populations in this group: pregnant women through a 60-day postpartum period; children younger than the age of 18; certain newborns for 1 year; and certain protected blind persons. States may add others to this list. The federal government requires that each state cover, at a minimum, persons who qualify for Aid to Families with Dependent Children; all needy children younger than age 21; those who qualify for old-age assistance; those who qualify for Aid to the Blind; persons who are permanently or totally disabled; and those older than 65 who are on welfare.

The government also reimburses care through the following organizations and methods:

- *Military health care:* In this system, the government not only pays for the care but also is the provider of the care through military hospitals and other healthcare services. The military also covers care of dependents whose care may or may not be provided at a military facility.
- *U.S. Department of Veterans Affairs:* The VA provides services to veterans at VA facilities and covers the cost of these services. VA hospitals are found across the country and provide acute care; ambulatory care; and pharmaceutical services, rehabilitation, and specialty services. In some cases, the VA provides care at long-term care facilities. The VA does not cover healthcare services for families of veterans.
- *Federal Employees Health Benefit Program:* Federal employee reimbursement is mandated by law. More than 10 million federal employees, retirees, and their dependents are covered. Enrollees choose from a variety of healthcare insurance plans as part of the Federal Employees Health Benefit Program. This is just a reimbursement or insurance program; it does not provide healthcare services.
- *State insurance programs:* States offer health insurance to their state employees. Typically, the state government is the largest employer in a state and, therefore, the state's largest

insurer. State employees choose from a variety of plans and contribute to the coverage in the same way that non–state employees pay into their employer health programs.

The Uninsured and the Underinsured

The United States has a large population of people who are not insured or who are underinsured (i.e., they do not have enough insurance coverage to pay for their needs). As more Americans register for insurance as required by the Affordable Care Act, the number of uninsured will decrease, but the problem of uninsured will not be eliminated. Data revealing the scope of this problem include the following statistics (U.S. Census Bureau, 2011):

- In 2011, the percentage of people without health insurance decreased to 15.7%, down from 16.3% in 2010. The number of uninsured people also decreased to 48.6 million in 2011, down from 50.0 million in 2010.
- Both the percentage and the number of people with health insurance increased in 2011, to 84.3% and 260.2 million, respectively, up from 83.7% and 256.6 million in 2010.
- The percentage of people covered by private health insurance in 2011 was not statistically different from the percentage in 2010, at 63.9%. Likewise, the number of people covered by private health insurance in 2011 was not statistically different from the number in 2010, at 197.3 million.
- The percentage and the number of people covered by government health insurance increased to 32.2% and 99.5 million in 2011, respectively, up from 31.2% and 95.5 million in 2010.
- The percentage and the number of people covered by employment-based health insurance in 2011 were not statistically different from those data in 2010, at 55.1% and 170.1 million, respectively.

- The percentage and the number of people covered by Medicaid in 2011 increased to 16.5% and 50.8 million, respectively, up from 15.8% and 48.5 million in 2010. The percentage and the number of people covered by Medicare increased in 2011 to 15.2% and 46.9 million, respectively, up from 14.6% and 44.9 million in 2010.
- In 2011, 9.4% of children younger than age 18 (7.0 million) were without health insurance, a proportion not statistically different from the 2010 estimate. The uninsured rate for children in poverty, 13.8%, was higher than the corresponding rate for all children, 9.4%.
- The rate and the number of uninsured for non-Hispanic Whites decreased in 2011 to 11.1% and 21.7 million, respectively, down from 11.6% and 22.5 million in 2010. The uninsured rate and the number of uninsured for Blacks also decreased in 2011 to 19.5% and 7.7 million, respectively, down from 20.8% and 8.2 million in 2010.
- The percentage and the number of uninsured Hispanics in 2011 were not statistically different from the 2010 estimates, at 30.1% and 15.8 million, respectively.

Data such as the number of uninsured are always a few years behind the current year. Current data can be found at the U.S. Census Bureau website. These data will continue changing as more Americans get insurance coverage.

The uninsured and underinsured are in great need of healthcare services—preventive, ongoing, acute, and chronic care. They have complex needs related to housing, finances, food, transportation, and education. Discharge planning to meet these needs should include a thorough assessment of the patient's needs at home and a plan to ensure that patients receive the care they need post hospitalization. Complex and vulnerable populations need care and are at serious risk for not being able to access the care they need.

Through the development of the previously mentioned insurance exchanges, the Affordable Care Act has sought to ensure that citizens can more readily access information about health insurance, and all citizens are required to subscribe to insurance or receive either Medicare or Medicaid. This requirement became effective in 2014; persons who fail to have such healthcare insurance coverage must pay a penalty fee. The impact of this change is unknown—for example, how many people will opt to pay the penalty fee instead of purchasing insurance. A critical aspect of this system—and one that will affect the overall cost of the Affordable Care Act—is the need for healthy people, such as younger people, to sign up for coverage, as their payments into the system will balance out the demands on the system by enrollees who need more and higher-cost care. The percentage of the enrollees who fell into each group was not known immediately after the first open enrollment period ended, with conflicting reports emerging regarding how many young, healthy people enrolled for insurance.

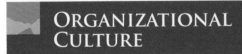

ORGANIZATIONAL CULTURE

Typically, culture refers to an individual person's culture, the culture of a group in a country, or a country's culture, but there is also **organizational culture**. Curtin described organizational culture in this way:

> There is in each institution an implicit, invisible, intrinsic, informal, and yet instantly recognizable welenschaung that is best described as "corporate culture." Like most important things, it is difficult to define or even describe. It is not "corporate climate," "organizational climate," or "corporate identity." The corporate culture embodies the organizational values that implicitly and explicitly specify norms,

shape attitudes, and guide the behaviors of the members of the organization. (Curtin, 2001, p. 219)

Organizational culture has an impact on nursing. First, the overall healthcare organization has a culture. Nursing within an organization also has a culture; the nursing department and even separate divisions or units may have different cultures. New staff members need to get to know the culture of the organizations that they are considering for employment. Students may be able to identify cultural issues in the units where they have practicum.

Two terms are often used to describe organizational culture: dissonant and consonant. Hospital leaders need to be aware of which label applies to their organization's culture. A dissonant culture means that the organization is not functioning effectively. Such organizations have the following characteristics (Jones & Redman, 2000, p. 605):

- Unclear individual staff and department expectations (Staff do not know what they should be doing and how they should be working.)
- Lack of consistent measurement of quality of service (Data from quality assessment lead to improvement, but a dysfunctional organization is not as interested in improvement or may not have effective processes to monitor quality.)
- Organized to serve the staff (providers of care) instead of serving the consumers (patients) (Consumers are less important, and thus services will not focus on consumer needs.)
- Limited concern for employee welfare (Employees are viewed only as workers and not as part of the team and not valued.)
- Limited education and training of staff (Educated staff members lead to better care and improvement, but the dysfunctional organization is not interested in improvement and better patient outcomes or has difficulty

providing education that is of benefit to the staff.)

- Frequent disagreements among staff that relate to control (turf battles) (This indicates a high stress level among staff and thus impacts effective functioning.)
- Lack of patient involvement in decision making (Lack of interest in consumers affects the type of product produced or the care provided and its quality.)
- Limited recognition of staff accomplishment (The organization does not value staff.)

The goal is to develop and maintain a consonant culture, or a functional and effective organization—one that would have the opposite of each of the characteristics of a dissonant organization.

There is increasing concern about staff bullying in the healthcare environment. Nurses participate in this by not supporting one another or by criticizing one another in extremely negative ways, which can even be cruel. New nurses have sometimes been targets of this type of behavior. This type of behavior has an impact on staff retention and quality care: When staff are frustrated, stressed, angry, and feel unsupported, it is more difficult to concentrate on work and in the end staff may leave such an environment.

People like to work in organizations that are effective, creative, and productive. How does an organization attain these characteristics? First, the hospital's formal framework lays the groundwork for an effective workplace. This includes the hospital's structure, chain of command, rules and regulations, and policies and procedures. The hospital's vision and mission statements are important. The vision statement describes the hospital's values and its view of the future, and it provides direction for the organization. The mission statement describes the hospital's purpose. Here is another way of understanding the difference between mission and vision: The mission describes the current state of the organization, and the vision is what the organization aspires to be. Hospitals also identify goals

and objectives that flow from the vision and mission statements. All these are part of the organization's process and are very important to the organization's culture. The vision, mission, goals, and objectives should not be filed away, but rather implemented in the hospital's process and in its structure.

It is not always easy to describe an organization's culture. The first response to an organization's culture takes the form of a gut feeling that a patient has when the patient enters the hospital and observes its physical appearance, how staff respond, the ease of finding one's way around, services set up for the consumer, and so on. The following are other considerations:

- The organization's structure and process
- Communication (types, effectiveness, who is included in communication, level of secrecy, information overload, timeliness of communication, and so on)
- Acceptance of new staff (who become members of the organization)
- Willingness of staff to listen to new ideas
- Inclusion of staff in decision making
- Morale
- Vacancies and turnover
- Acceptance of students (all types of healthcare professions)
- Positive feelings by patients about their care experiences
- Welcome feeling by visitors

Nurses usually know which hospitals are functional (consonant) organizations in the communities in which they live and practice. They share this information with colleagues, and this can have an impact on recruitment of new staff.

Workforce diversity and patient diversity both influence the hospital's culture. All the people who work in the organization and all the people who interact with the organization, such as the patients and their families, affect organization culture. Workforce diversity has become a critical issue in health care—specifically, there is need for greater diversity in all healthcare professions. Labor laws affect this diversity. Title VII of the Civil Rights Act of 1964 and Executive Order 11246 prohibit employer discrimination on the basis of race, color, religion, sex, or national origin. The Americans with Disabilities Act of 1990 prohibits discrimination as a result of disability, including mental illness, if the person can complete the job requirements. These federal laws apply to any hospital that receives federal funds such as Medicare or Medicaid reimbursement. On a practical level, this means nearly all hospitals are subject to these requirements, because few do not provide services to patients covered by these two payment systems or receive some other type of federal funding/payment. Language is another issue that is related to diversity: Hospitals need to have access to interpreters to communicate with patients if staff cannot do so.

Another aspect of the hospital's culture that is critical to its effectiveness and has become more widely recognized since 2001 is whether the environment is a healing environment. This is just as difficult to define or describe as organizational culture. Some of the factors considered when assessing the environment are (1) the privacy provided, (2) air quality, (3) noise levels, (4) views from windows, and (5) visual characteristics. The needs of patients can vary and, in turn, affect the type of healing environment needed. The elderly may require more safety measures to prevent falls, but if this is accomplished by restraining patients, the person's (patient, family) view of the environment may be impacted. Restraining a patient may prevent injury, but the patient may feel imprisoned. The elderly often have problems hearing and can tolerate more noise. Others may not be able to tolerate a lot of noise and may complain that they cannot sleep in the hospital. From a historical perspective, Florence Nightingale's view of care was associated with healing and the patient's need for fresh air, cleanliness, quiet, diet, and light. Other aspects of a healing environment include physical environment—use of color, sameness or variety, sense of warmth in furnishings, type of artwork on the walls, and so on. Some colors

are more peaceful than others. Put simply, is the architecture patient-centered?

Planetree is a nonprofit organization concerned with the environmental impact of the delivery system on health care. It is one example of a model of healing in health care. The focus in this model is on body, mind, and spirit, with active patient and family involvement. Hospitals that meet specific criteria can be designated as Planetree hospitals. This patient-centered healing environment model emphasizes the principles found in **Exhibit 8-2**.

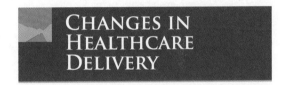

CHANGES IN HEALTHCARE DELIVERY

Historically, hospitals have experienced much change. In the past, hospitals had a significant role in nursing education, but their most important role—then and now—is the provision of healthcare services to their communities. What has been the history of hospitals? The reengineering of health care—that is, the redesigning of how care is provided and how the organization functions—has led to major changes in healthcare organizations. Many healthcare organizations have undergone some level of reengineering in the last decade. This might include remodeling, restructuring, developing new services, and improving processes and systems, or perhaps decreasing services. A major response to periods of healthcare worker shortages has been to redesign how work is done and by whom. If there are not enough providers, the organization needs to consider how people are working and how work processes and resources can be improved to be more effective. As hospitals change, many factors influence the need for change and how it occurs. Some of these factors were highlighted in Figure 8-1.

Change is inevitable in any organization today, but particularly in health care. Science and knowledge have driven some of this change, but there are other factors at work as well. Change is a process that is driven by forces that motivate a person or an organization to consider what needs altering. The key is to be clear about this need and to understand the *why* before taking the next steps. It is also important to consider whether staff are ready for the change. Staff can act as either barriers to or facilitators of change. Staff members are typically tired of changes and feel that there are too many. They often also feel left out of the decision process that leads to changes. In such a case, they may become critical of the change, or feel no commitment to the change. This attitude, in turn, becomes a major barrier to the change's success. For example, if the staff do not understand the need behind a decision to change a form in the medical record, it will be more difficult to train them in the use of the form, and it may be difficult to get them to even use the form or to use

it correctly. The complexity of the change and how frequently changes are made can lead to overload for staff. The goal is to have staff behind the change and committed to it; they will then be facilitators of change. Understanding resistance to change can help in preparing for the change and in developing any training that might be required. When changes are planned within a hospital, planners need to consider the impact that those changes may have on policies and procedures; accreditation and regulation requirements; financial issues; the structure of the organization; the ways in which staff do their work; patients, visitors, and students (e.g., nursing, medical, other); and much more.

The change process includes the following steps:

1. Identify the issue or problem/need for change and factors that influence the need for change

2. Gather information to better understand the need and possible solutions
3. Identify barriers to and support for the change
4. Describe solutions to solve a problem or to improve (change)
5. Decide which solution to implement
6. Prepare staff for the change (inform them of the change, the reasons for the change, what the change will be, the timeline, planning and implementation, and training staff if needed)
7. Implement the change (the solution)
8. Evaluate the results (including staff feedback)
9. Determine whether any adjustments are needed; ideally, include relevant staff early in the process to enhance staff commitment

In the United States, the major change in health care since 2005 has been the Affordable Care Act of 2010. This legislation will be implemented over an extended period, and it will take more time to understand more about the actual impact it will have on healthcare delivery in the United States.

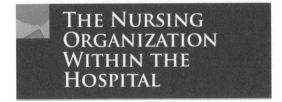

THE NURSING ORGANIZATION WITHIN THE HOSPITAL

RNs are members of the nation's largest healthcare profession, and they practice wherever people need nursing care. Common care sites are hospitals, homes, schools, workplaces, and community centers; less common areas include children's camps and homeless shelters. Figure 8-2 provides data on RN work settings. There has been a serious shortage of all types of nurses in the United States in recent years. Although that trend slowed down somewhat from 2009 to 2011, it is expected to pick up speed again. The shortage of nursing faculty continues to be a major, long-term problem.

Nurses assume critical roles in a variety of healthcare settings—a topic explored throughout this text. The focus in this chapter is on hospitals as one example of a healthcare organization. Nursing services may be organized differently in hospitals. The traditional nursing organization—which is still the most common type—is a nursing department. In this model, nursing staff (RNs, LPNs/LVNs, patient care assistants) are all part of the nursing department, which often includes unit support staff or a unit clerk (secretary and other titles) as well. The title for the unit clerk position varies, but this is the person or persons who help with administrative issues such as records, supplies, reception at the central desk area, and so on.

The second and newer organization model is a patient services department. In this case, the department focuses on the function of multiple patient services, not just nursing. Other patient care services might include medical records, respiratory therapy, infusion therapy, infection control, and so on. The configuration varies widely from one hospital to another. **Figure 8-7** and **Figure 8-8** show examples of this organization. **Figure 8-9** describes a hospital unit structure.

An RN is the designated leader in Figures 8-7 and 8-8, which illustrate two department models. An RN must be the leader of nursing services to meet The Joint Commission accreditation standards. The nurse leader title has changed over time. Director of nursing was the title most commonly used in the past, and some hospitals still use this title today. The traditional director of nursing (DON) just focused on nursing and had little, if any, input into the functioning of the hospital as a whole and no input into the budget. Today, even if the nurse leader is called a director of nursing, the DON has much more input into all aspects of the hospital administration and the budget. This is an important change. Given that nurses account for the largest percentage of hospital staff and provide most of the direct care, it is critical that nurses are represented by a nurse leader who is recognized in the organization as an important leader and can participate in major decision making. In the 1970s and 1980s, directors

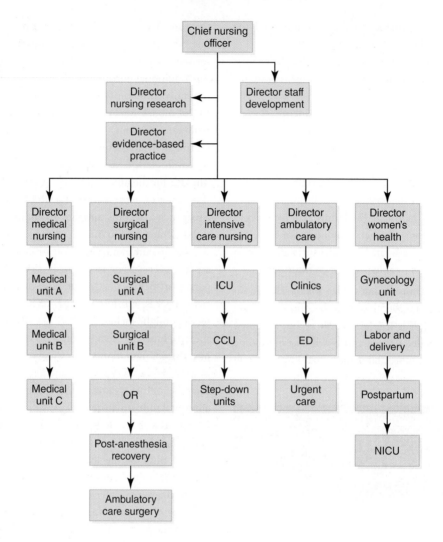

Figure 8-7 An Example: Nursing Department Organizational Chart

of nursing began to gain more power, and their titles began to change to vice president for nursing or patient services in recognition of their organization leadership role—but the focus was still on nursing. At this time, increasing numbers of nursing leaders began to complete graduate degrees. It was recognized that they were running large, complex departments that represented a significant portion of the overall hospital budget. Gradually, the vice

president of nursing (VPN) entered into the budget process as an equal partner. The next change was the evolution of the vice president of patient services position, in which the nurse leader was responsible for more than just nursing. This was a major shift, but the idea that a nurse could manage other healthcare disciplines changed very slowly.

As is true for all such information about hospitals, there is great variation from one hospital to

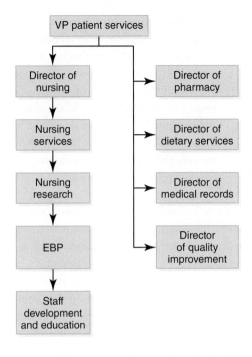

Figure 8-8 An Example: Patient Services Organizational Chart

another. The size of the hospital has an impact on how the nursing services are organized.

More nurses today are also taking positions in hospital administration that are not related to just nursing; a nurse could be the chief operating officer (COO) or chief executive officer (CEO), for example. This is a major shift, and there are not many nurses in these positions. Today, any nurse who serves in a nursing leadership position in a healthcare organization needs to be competent in administrative responsibilities such as planning, budgeting, staffing, communicating, coordinating, and public speaking, and must also demonstrate leadership. The nurse administrator must involve others in decision making and teamwork, and work with other healthcare professionals to support effective interprofessional teamwork.

The nursing organization or department includes a variety of nursing management staff. Typically, there are three levels of management:

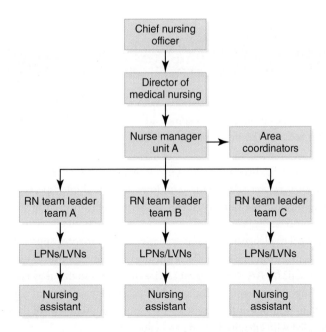

Figure 8-9 An Example: Medical Nursing Unit Organizational Chart

- *Upper level:* Responsible for establishing goals, objectives, and strategic plans for the organization. The director of nursing, vice president of nursing, and vice president of patient services positions are in upper-level management.
- *Middle level:* Supervise first-level managers. For example, there may be directors of specific types of services—director of women's health, director of surgical services, director of behavioral health, and so on. These directors supervise multiple units that have a common function or specialty, such as women's health (e.g., gynecology, obstetrics).
- *First level:* Managers who provide the day-to-day or operational direction for the nursing service and units. This group is composed of supervisors and managers. Titles for these managers vary. Some examples are nurse manager, head nurse (not used much today), nursing unit manager, and nursing or nurse

coordinator. These managers are critical to the effectiveness of any hospital because they deal with the daily functioning of patient care areas, quality and safety, staffing, budget implementation and use of resources, staff issues and morale, teamwork, coordination, and communication. They work with multiple disciplines to ensure that patients get the care they need. Nurse managers do not typically provide direct care.

Participation in nursing committees and interprofessional committees provides opportunities for nurses to be directly involved in decision making and have an impact on care delivery. Some of the committees typically found in hospitals are those that focus on policies and procedures, quality improvement, staffing, staff development and education, medical records and documentation, pharmacy, evidence-based practice, and research. Some committees are special task forces that address specific issues.

Landscape © f9photos/Shutterstock, Inc.

CONCLUSION

This chapter has focused on healthcare organizations, with acute care hospitals as the major example of a healthcare organization. Understanding how hospitals are structured and their processes (functions) helps the nurse practice in this setting. The departments and team members assume important roles in how the organization functions.

The U.S. healthcare system has been undergoing many changes. This will continue through the full implementation of the Affordable Care Act and its long-term impacts on multiple aspects of the healthcare delivery system, patients, and healthcare professionals. Nurses are very much involved in these changes and should participate in the change process.

Financing health care is a challenge because it is expensive, and a variety of approaches are used for covering costs through reimbursement. Reimbursement affects nursing care and responses to questions such as these: (1) Are there enough nursing staff? (2) Are there support services for nurses so that they are free to provide care? (3) Are the most up-to-date supplies and equipment available? (4) Is there an efficient computerized documentation system? (5) Is orientation sufficient for new staff? (6) Do nursing staff receive the training they need? (7) Are nurse managers provided with effective training and education?

CONCLUSION (CONTINUED)

Greater emphasis has been placed on shared governance in healthcare organizations because of the need for greater input from nurses regarding the hospital decision-making process. Although this chapter focuses on acute care hospitals, the United States has been moving toward changes in healthcare priorities that will affect all healthcare settings, as described in **Figure 8-10**.

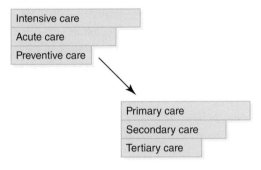

Figure 8-10 Need to Change Healthcare Priorities

CHAPTER HIGHLIGHTS

1. Healthcare delivery is a complex process and system that includes multiple delivery sites: acute care organizations (hospitals), ambulatory care clinics, private provider offices, community health facilities, home care agencies, hospice agencies, extended care facilities, and so on.

2. Many factors impact hospitals that cause changes in their services and how they collaborate with others, realign their organization with the external environment, or even close because of financial issues.

3. Health care is a business; it provides services to a population.

4. Healthcare entities may be for-profit or not-for-profit organizations depending on what they do with their revenues.

5. Healthcare organizations may differ depending on their structure and process. For example, a bureaucratic structure receives little input from staff as part of its decision-making processes.

6. Horizontal structure is decentralized, with an emphasis on departments or divisions; decisions are made closer to the staff who do the work.

7. The matrix organization structure is newer and less clear than the traditional bureaucratic organization centered on departments. A matrix organization is flatter (i.e., decisions do not flow from the top down).

8. The process of an organization focuses on how it functions.

(continues)

Landscape © f9photos/Shutterstock, Inc.

CHAPTER HIGHLIGHTS (CONTINUED)

9. Classification of hospitals varies greatly and may reflect a hospital's mission of teaching or research, for example. Hospitals may be public or private.

10. The hospital healthcare team is composed of a variety of healthcare providers, both professional and nonprofessional.

11. Hospitalists and intensivists are generally physicians who specialize in acute in-hospital care, although some hospitals use CNSs and APRNs in these roles.

12. Healthcare finances can be viewed from a macro, micro, or reimbursement perspective.

13. Medicare was established in 1965 by Title XVIII, which is an amendment to the Social Security Act. It is the federal health insurance program for people aged 65 and older, persons with disabilities, and people with end-stage renal disease.

14. Medicaid, established in 1965 by Title XIX of the Social Security Act, is the federal–state program for certain categories of low-income people, children, the disabled, blind persons, and so forth.

15. The number of uninsured and underinsured individuals has been growing in the United States, but implementation of the Affordable Care Act of 2010 should reduce this number.

16. Organizational culture reflects the mission, core values, and vision of the entity.

17. Healthcare delivery systems may be viewed as a healing environment.

18. Healthcare delivery has been reorganized or redesigned for many reasons. One of the major reasons has been the most recent shortage of healthcare workers. How work is done, and by whom, has had to change to cope with this shortage.

19. Healthcare reform through changes in healthcare reimbursement has been undertaken for a variety of reasons, not the least of which are access and health disparities issues.

20. Nursing within an organization is a critical component of healthcare delivery and is an essential ingredient in patient satisfaction.

Landscape © f9photos/Shutterstock, Inc.

DISCUSSION QUESTIONS

1. What is the difference between organizational structure and process? Identify examples for each.

2. If you were not a nursing student, which other healthcare team member would you want to be and why? Does this healthcare team member have something in common with nursing?

3. Compare and contrast the three financial perspectives—macro, micro, and reimbursement.

4. Describe ways to organize nursing services in a hospital, key roles of nursing services, and nursing services' relationship to other departments.

5. What does organizational culture mean, and why is it important?

6. What is your opinion of the health environment model? How do you think the designation of a Planetree hospital might impact nursing care?

Landscape © f9photos/Shutterstock, Inc.

CRITICAL THINKING ACTIVITIES

1. What is your reaction to the corporatization of health care?

2. Search the Internet for a hospital website. See if you can find information on that hospital's vision, mission, goals, and objectives. Many hospital websites include this information. After you find an example, review the information. How does this information apply to nursing?

3. Visit the website for the American Hospital Association (http://www.aha.org). What is the American Hospital Association? Click on "Issues" and select one issue to explore. What have you learned about the issue? Groups of students should select different issues to review and then share what they learned. Consider the implications for nursing.

4. Search the Internet for information about one type of healthcare team member to learn more about the profession.

5. Visit the Cover the Uninsured website (http://www.rwjf.org/coverage/product.jsp?id=72459&cid=xdr_ccs_001learn_about_your_state) and find your state. What can you learn about the uninsured and underinsured in your state?

6. Visit the consumer site for Medicare (http://medicare.gov). If you were a Medicare beneficiary, how helpful would this site be? Which information can you find? Click on Compare Hospitals in Your Area (www.hospitalcompare.hhs.gov/) and review hospitals in your area from the perspective of a consumer who is 70 years old and needs to have a hip replacement.

7. Find out which preventive services are covered by Medicare (http://www.medicare.gov/coverage/preventive-and-screening-services.html). What does the ombudsman do?

8. Visit http://www.whitehouse.gov/healthreform/healthcare-overview to get current information on the status of the implementation of the Affordable Care Act. Discuss the implications of what you find.

ELECTRONIC *Reflection Journal*

Circuit Board: ©Photos.com

Write a description of a healthcare organization where you have had a clinical experience. Consider the information in this chapter as you describe the organization. Reflect on its culture and how you felt while being in the organization. How do you think staff, patients, and families might feel? What could be improved in the organization based your experience?

Landscape © f9photos/Shutterstock, Inc.

LINKING TO THE INTERNET

- American Hospital Association: http://www.aha.org
- The Joint Commission: http://www.jointcommission.org
- Centers for Medicare and Medicare Services: http://www.cms.gov
- Planetree Healing Environments: http://www.planetree.org

(continues)

LINKING TO THE INTERNET (CONTINUED)

- CMS never events (HACs): http://psnet.ahrq.gov/primer.aspx?primerID=3
- The Never Events Collaborative: http://www.neverevents.org/
- Nursing Takes the Lead: Nurses Have a Big Role in Preventing "Never Events": http://confidenceconnected.com/connect/article/nursing_takes_the_lead_nurses_have_a_big_role_in_preventing_never_even/journals.lww.com/nursingmadeincrediblyeasy/Fulltext/2011/01000/Preventing_never_events__What_frontline_nurses.10.aspx
  http://www.news-medical.net/news/20090810/New-online-tool-to-help-nurses-prevent-the-10-Never-Events.aspx
- Affordable Care Act: https://www.healthcare.gov/
- U.S. Census Bureau: http://www.census.gov

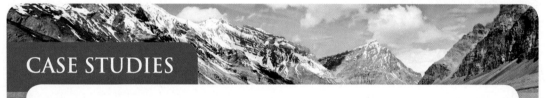

CASE STUDIES

Case Study 1

For this chapter, you will write your own case study. Describe a situation or series of events that occurred during your clinical experiences that demonstrates the culture of the organization/unit where you had that experience.

Discuss your views with your classmates in groups of four, using the questions that follow as a guide. After you have done this, explain two changes you would make in the organization or on the unit and justify your choices (relate this to chapter content).

Case Questions

1. What is the status of the unit's/organization's culture?
2. What needs to be improved? What is effective?
3. How does the culture impact nurses and nursing in the organization?

Case Study 2

You are a staff nurse on a surgical unit. The nurse manager has formed a task force to provide input on the budget for the unit. She asks you to serve on the task force. You tell her you do not feel competent because you have been a nurse for only one year, but she says she wants fresh input. Now, you find yourself at the first meeting. The chair opens the meeting with some questions. How would you respond to them?

CASE STUDIES (CONTINUED)

Case Questions

1. Which type of budget do we have for a unit?
2. What are the types of expenses we have?
3. If we find that some of these expenses have been increasing, what might we suggest to attempt to lower the expenses?
4. Why should staff get involved in unit budget planning?

Words of Wisdom

Kendra Coleman, BSN, RN
Graduate Student, University of Oklahoma College of Nursing
Nurse Manager, Labor and Delivery, St. John Medical Center, Tulsa, Oklahoma

Making the transition into management has definitely been a challenge. I have asked myself on more than one occasion, "Why did I want to get into management?" Then I would remind myself that my number one goal was to support the nursing staff and empower them to practice excellent nursing without the intimidation of physicians. At the same time, I had to show the physicians that we appreciate their business and wanted to do what was in the best interest of the patients. What I quickly learned was I must always be armed with the latest research to support our practice and display the recommendations of our professional organization as well as the board of nursing.

I was placed in a unique situation in that the previous manager stepped down to be a floor nurse on the unit (I am now her manager), and I had previously worked on this particular floor. So I knew most of the staff, but it was very important for me to connect with my team members and for them to see me in my new role. Over the first month, I sat down with each employee and laid out my expectations. It was very important for them to know that I had the same conversation with each person, and I would treat each of them the same and would hold each person accountable.

I earned the trust of people from whom I thought it would take a long time to earn. Nurses came to me with issues that they fully expected me to do something about. There were many regulatory issues that I had no clue about and had to quickly research them. I felt it was odd for people to ask me for permission to do certain things, especially since I am one of the youngest people on the unit. I still go out on the floor to help clean and move patients. I answer phones, and I am very visible on the floor. I think it is important to let the staff know that I am not out of touch with what they are going through, but at the same time they do not expect me to carry a full team. They have a certain respect for me that came overnight, one that still takes me by surprise at times.

(*continues*)

Words of Wisdom (*continued*)

Management is complicated. We must set boundaries, be professional, be knowledgeable, and support the staff. We must hold people accountable and establish a way for people to take ownership of their practice. When I have a rough day, I remind myself why I am in this position: to help empower the staff through information sharing, support, and presence.

Marietta Carter, RN, AND, OCN
RN-BSN student at the University of Oklahoma College of Nursing
Nurse Manager, Oncology Clinic, Valley View Regional Hospital, Ada, Oklahoma

Nursing leadership is one of the most rewarding and challenging jobs available to RNs. I was previously an assistant manager of the intensive care unit and home healthcare units and have been nurse manager of a hospital-based outpatient oncology clinic for almost 17 years. The main drawback of a leadership position is that your work is never really finished. It is extremely important to learn to prioritize and let go of the things that can wait until tomorrow. The best part of leadership is the opportunity to mentor new nurses and take them from a point of being scared to death and questioning every little care decision to be made, into a professional nurse who is knowledgeable and confidant in the care he or she provides.

Transformational leadership is the theory I mostly use, and I've always felt and seen, evidenced in practice, that the best leaders lead by example. Staff nurses develop respect for leaders who work right alongside them, and this method also allows the leader to impart skills and knowledge to the new nurse. A big challenge for nursing leaders today is leading through change, in a climate of almost daily changes in rules and regulations, policies, reimbursement, etc. The participative theory allows shared decision making to get staff involved in how changes will be managed. Shared governance and allowing for autonomous practice will almost always help to get the staff to buy in to new methods and policies.

REFERENCES

American Association of Colleges of Nursing. (2007). *White paper on the education and role of the clinical nurse leader.* Washington, DC: Author.

Curtin, L. (2001). Healing healthcare's organizational culture. *Seminars for Nurse Managers, 9*, 218–227.

Dewan, S., & Sack, K. (2008, January 8). A safety-net hospital falls into financial crisis. *The New York Times*, pp. A1, A18–A19.

Institute for Healthcare Improvement. (2014). Readmissions. Retrieved from http://www.ihi.org/Topics/Readmissions/Pages/default.aspx

Institute of Medicine (IOM). (2013). *Best care at lower cost: The path to continuously learning health care in America.* Washington, DC: National Academies Press.

Jones, K., & Redman, R. (2000). Organizational culture and work redesign: Experiences in three organizations. *Journal of Nursing Administration, 30*, 604–610.

Kurtzman, E., & Buerhaus, P. (2008). New Medicare payment rules: Danger opportunity for nursing? *AJN, 108*(6), 30–35.

StateFacts.org. (2011). Medicaid expansion to 133% of federal poverty level (FPL): Estimated increase in enrollment and spending relative to baseline by 2019. Retrieved from http://kff.org/statedata/

U.S. Census Bureau. (2011). Highlights health insurance coverage, 2011. Retrieved from http://www.census.gov/hhes/www/hlthins/data/incpovhlth/2011/highlights.html

U.S. Department of Health and Human Services. (2014). *Press release: New HHS data show quality improvements saved 15,000 lives and $4 billion in health spending.*

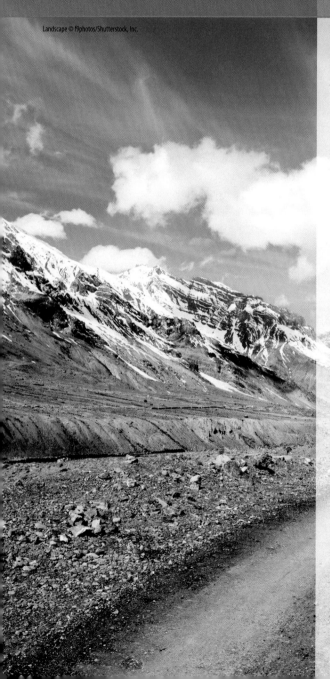

SECTION 3

Core Healthcare Professional Competencies

In its 2003 report, Health Professions Education, *the Institute of Medicine (IOM) identified core competencies for healthcare professionals. These competencies were based on the need to improve the quality of health care and the recognition that healthcare professional education was not including these five critical competencies. The IOM does not recommend that these be considered the only competencies required, but rather that they form the core competencies addressed during the education of all healthcare professionals: nurses, physicians, pharmacists, allied health professionals, and healthcare administrators. The five core competencies are summarized here:*

1. Provide patient-centered care: *Identify, respect, and care about patients' differences, values, preferences, and expressed needs; relieve pain and suffering; coordinate continuous care; listen to, clearly inform, communicate with, and educate patients; share decision making and management; and continuously advocate disease prevention, wellness, and promotion of healthy lifestyles, including a focus on population health.*

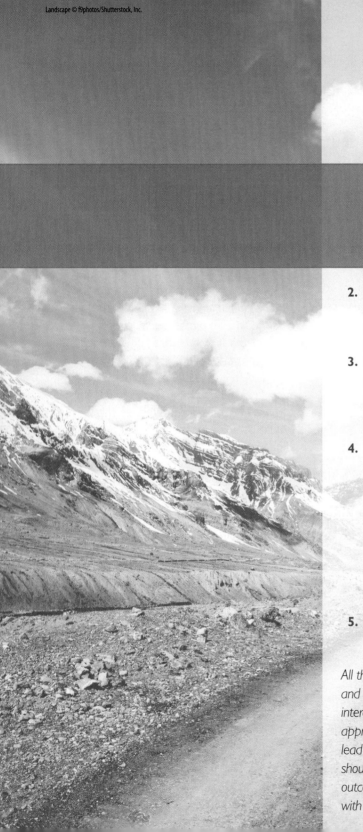

2. Work in interprofessional teams: *Cooperate, collaborate, communicate, and integrate care in teams to ensure that care is continuous and reliable.*

3. Employ evidence-based practice: *Integrate best research with clinical expertise and patient values for optimal care and participate in learning and research activities to the extent feasible.*

4. Apply quality improvement: *Identify errors and hazards in care; understand and implement basic safety design principles, such as standardization and simplification; continually understand and measure quality of care in terms of structure, process, and outcomes in relation to patient and community needs; and design and test interventions to change processes and systems of care, with the objective of improving quality.*

5. Utilize informatics: *Communicate, manage knowledge, mitigate error, and support decision making using information technology.*

All these competencies are interrelated, and all should be applied in most clinical interactions. This competency-based approach to healthcare education should lead to improved quality because educators should be able to gather data about outcomes that could then be associated with better patient care, the desired goal.

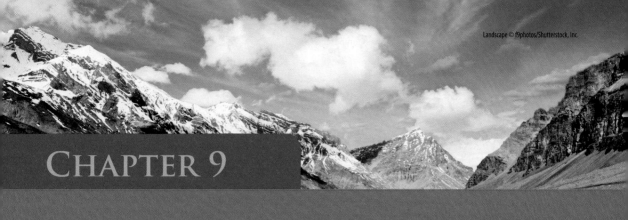

CHAPTER 9

Provide Patient-Centered Care

CHAPTER OBJECTIVES

At the conclusion of this chapter, the learner will be able to:

- Describe the Institute of Medicine competency: provide patient-centered care
- Apply examples of relevant nursing theories connected to patient-centered care
- Discuss the importance of consumerism in health care
- Explain the relationship of culture and diversity to health and healthcare delivery
- Examine disparities in health care

- Support the need for patient advocacy
- Summarize processes that nurses use to ensure better care coordination
- Describe the relationship of critical thinking/clinical reasoning and judgment to patient-centered care
- Explain the need for self-management of care
- Discuss the impact of the therapeutic use of self on the nurse–patient relationship

KEY TERMS

Bias	Disparities	Patient advocacy
Care coordination	Diversity	Patient-centered care
Care map	Ethnicity	Prejudice
Clinical judgment	Ethnocentrism	Race
Clinical reasoning	Health literacy	Self-management of care
Consumer/customer	Macro consumer	Stereotype
Critical thinking	Micro consumer	Therapeutic use of self
Culture	Nursing process	Unlicensed assistive personnel

INTRODUCTION

This chapter begins the discussion about the core competencies identified by the Institute of Medicine (IOM) for nurses and all healthcare professionals. The first core competency focuses on **patient-centered care**. The U.S. healthcare system is patient centered, but it is not at the level it should be. This content describes patient-centered care, relevant nursing theories, and consumerism in health care, cultural diversity and disparities, patient advocacy, care coordination to meet patient-centered care needs, self-management of care, and therapeutic use of self in the nurse–patient relationship. As you enter your nursing education program, it is assumed that you are in a nursing program because of your concern about patients; however, providing patient-centered care does not come naturally. It takes knowledge, time, critical thinking, clinical reasoning, and judgment to ensure that care is coordinated and that the implementation process focuses on patient-centered care. This all must be done during a time of many changes in health care. These changes include the following:

- The U.S. population is becoming older and more diverse.
- Preventive care and chronic care are increasingly joining curative and acute primary care as the focus of health care.
- Chronic disease management is becoming more prominent in many medical practices.
- More patients want active involvement in their health care.
- The financial mechanisms that support health care are changing.
- There is greater concern about the interrelationship of access, cost, quality, and outcomes.

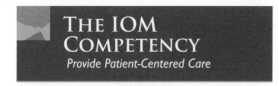

THE IOM COMPETENCY
Provide Patient-Centered Care

The IOM identified five key core competencies for all healthcare professionals, and this chapter focuses on the first core competency: provide patient-centered care. The IOM definition follows:

> Identify, respect, and care about patients' differences, values, preferences, and expressed needs; relieve pain and suffering; coordinate continuous care; listen to, clearly inform, communicate with, and educate patients; share decision making and management; and continuously advocate disease prevention, wellness, and promotion of healthy lifestyles, including a focus on population health. (IOM, 2003a, p. 4)

On the surface, this definition may seem simple, but it is not; patient-centered care includes multiple factors and activities—all aimed at making the patient the center of care. The content in this chapter focuses on the key elements of the core competency as illustrated in **Figure 9-1**.

Support of Patient-Centered Care

Why is patient-centered care included in the core competencies? What is the basis for emphasizing patient-centered care? **Figure 9-2** illustrates the relationship of the core competencies. Note that the major focus is *provide patient-centered care*. Evidence-based practice, quality improvement, and use of informatics all impact patient-centered care, and interprofessional teams encircle all and bring care to the patient.

Crossing the Quality Chasm: A New Health System for the 21st Century (IOM, 2001) describes

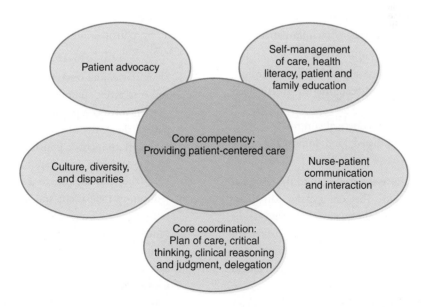

Figure 9-1 Providing Patient-Centered Care: Key Elements

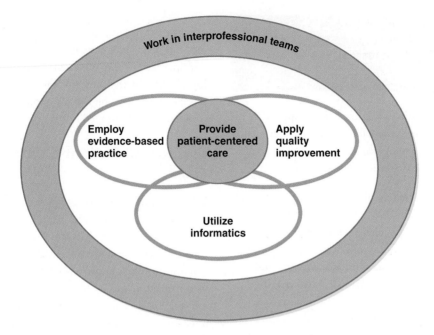

Figure 9-2 IOM Relationship Core Competencies

Source: Core Competencies for Interprofessional Collaborative Practice Report of an Expert Panel © 2011 American Association of Colleges of Nursing, American Association of Colleges of Osteopathic Medicine, American Association of Colleges of Pharmacy, American Dental Education Association, Association of American Medical Colleges, and Association of Schools of Public Health. From Interprofessional Education Collaborative Expert Panel. (2011). Core competencies for interprofessional collaborative practice: Report of an expert panel. Washington, D.C.: Interprofessional Education Collaborative., p. 14 (Figure 5).

10 rules for redesigning patient care and presents a vision of the U.S. healthcare delivery system. The first four rules specifically apply to patient-centered care, supporting the need to include patient-centered care in the core competencies:

1. Care is based on continuous health relationships.
2. Care is customized according to patient needs and values.
3. The patient is the source of control.
4. Knowledge is shared, and information flows freely.

The other six rules are not directly related to patient-centered care. They are a major part of the framework to improve the quality of care and are discussed in the *Apply Quality Improvement* chapter. Improving health care requires improved competencies in all healthcare professionals, beginning with providing patient-centered care.

The IOM identified patient-centered care as one of six domains of quality. This organization summarized

issues related to specific skills that are needed to ensure patient-centered care. A description of these skills provides additional information about what is meant by patient-centered care (IOM, 2003a, pp. 52–53):

- Share power and responsibility with patients and caregivers (family, significant others) (e.g., involve the patient in care, make the patient the center of care and decision making; work to increase patient understanding, acceptance, and cooperation; help caregivers as they provide care to a family member [education for patient and family]; support self-management; provide comfort and emotional support; manage pain and suffering; relieve anxiety; provide expert care to manage symptoms).
- Communicate with patients in a shared and fully open manner (e.g., patients have access to information, communication with

healthcare providers [including nurses], and use of technology to communicate).

- Take into account patients' individuality, emotional needs, values, and life issues (e.g., culture, religion, family, profession).
- Implement strategies to reach those who do not present for care on their own, including care strategies that support the broader community (e.g., underserved members of the community).
- Enhance prevention and health promotion (e.g., population focus, risk factors, health promotion, and prevention strategies).

As hospitals focus more on patient-centered care, the inevitable question is, How do we accomplish satisfactory patient- and family-centered care? Three key elements in a hospital organization make a major difference (Balik, Conway, Zipperer, & Watson, 2011, p. 3):

1. An integrated system is key to achieving the aim of an excellent patient and family experience of inpatient hospital care.
2. Leadership behavior at the executive, middle, and front-line levels is essential to achieving exceptional results.
3. The path to achieving excellence in the patient and family experience includes a group of dynamic, positively reinforcing actions rather than a linear set of activities.

Exhibit 9-1 describes the Institute for Health Improvement model for exceptional patient experience.

Exhibit 9-1   Patient-and Family-Centered Care at Various Levels

Level	Location	Examples
Environment	Community, region, state	Community groups Care coordination across organizational boundaries Accountable care organizations, medical homes Advanced care planning (e.g., medical orders for life-sustaining treatment) School and church programs Public health and other consumer campaigns
Organization	Health system, including hospital, nursing home, ambulatory care centers, and others	Patient experience surveys, patient complaints Patient and family councils, advisors, faculty Resource centers, patient portals Access to help and care around the clock Medication lists
Microsystem	Clinic, unit, emergency department	Parents, advisors, and advisory councils Open access, optimized flow Family participation in rounding
Individual experience of care	Bedside, exam room, in the home	Access to the patient record Shared care planning Smart patients ask questions (Partnership for Healthcare Excellence)

Source: Balik, B., Conway, J., Zipperer, L., & Watson, J. (2011). *Achieving an exceptional patient and family experience of inpatient hospital care*. IHI Innovation Series White Paper. Cambridge, MA: Institute for Healthcare Improvement. Available on IHI website: www.IHI.org

The primary drivers in this model are as follows (Balik, Conway, Zipperer, & Watson, 2011):

- *Leadership:* Governance and executive leaders demonstrate that *everything* in the culture is focused on patient- and family-centered care, which is practiced everywhere in the hospital—at the individual patient level; at the microsystem level; and across the organization, including governance.
- *Hearts and minds:* The hearts and minds of staff and providers are fully engaged through respectful partnerships with everyone in the organization and in a commitment to the shared values of patient- and family-centered care.
- *Respectful partnership:* Every care interaction is anchored in a respectful partnership, anticipating and responding to patient and family needs (e.g., physical comfort, emotional, informational, cultural, spiritual, and learning needs).
- *Reliable care:* Hospital systems deliver reliable, quality care around the clock.
- *Evidenced-based care:* The care team instills confidence by providing collaborative, evidence-based care.

Patient-centered or person-centered care is the key focus for all nurses. "This care alleviates vulnerability in all of its forms. That care should and must then be delivered at the right time, at the right level, in the right place, and so on. If care were on a compass, it would be true north and all other functions would stand in line to provide added value and service to that fact" (Hagenow, 2003, p. 204).

Levels of Patient-Centered Care

There are three levels of concern when discussing patient-centered care. The first relates directly to the identification of patient-centered care as the core healthcare professional competency, focusing on the care provided by an individual healthcare professional. What each healthcare professional, such as a nurse, must know and apply to provide patient-centered care will be discussed in this chapter. The second level focuses on the organizational level and the ways in which healthcare organizations situate themselves to be patient-centered organizations. The third level is the macro focus—how the healthcare system, as viewed from the local, state, and national perspectives, ensures that it is patient centered. Strategies to ensure the third level are primarily healthcare policy concerns.

There is consensus about the key attributes describing patient-centered care at the healthcare systems level. In a systematic review of nine models and frameworks used to define patient-centered care, the following six core elements were identified most frequently (Shaller, 2007):

1. Education and shared knowledge
2. Involvement of family and friends
3. Collaboration and team management
4. Sensitivity to nonmedical and spiritual dimensions of care
5. Respect for patient needs and preferences
6. Free flow and accessibility of information

The following factors contribute to reaching these six core elements and have an impact on patient-centered care at the organizational level (Shaller, 2007):

- Leadership, at the level of the chief executive officer and board of directors, sufficiently committed and engaged to unify and sustain the organization in a common mission
- A strategic vision clearly and constantly communicated to every member of the organization
- Involvement of patients and families at multiple levels, not only in the care process, but as full participants in key committees throughout the organization
- Care for the caregivers through a supportive work environment that engages employees in all aspects of process design and treats them with the same dignity and respect that they are expected to show patients and families

- Systematic measurement and feedback to continuously monitor the impact of specific interventions and change strategies
- Quality of the physical environment that provides a supportive and nurturing physical space and design for patients, families, and employees alike
- Supportive technology that engages patients and families directly in the process of care by facilitating information access and communication with their caregivers

An example of an approach to improve patient-centered care within healthcare organizations is the Planetree Institute initiative, "Putting Patients First." The Planetree Institute is a nonprofit membership organization that partners with hospitals and health centers to develop and implement patient-centered care in healing environments.

Since its founding as a nonprofit organization, Planetree has pioneered methods for personalizing, humanizing, and demystifying the healthcare experience for patients and their families. The Planetree model of care is a patient-centered, holistic approach to health care, promoting mental, emotional, spiritual, social, and physical healing. It empowers patients and families through the exchange of information and encourages healing partnerships with caregivers. It seeks to maximize positive healthcare outcomes by integrating optimal medical therapies and incorporating art and nature into the healing environment. (Planetree Institute, n.d.)

The Planetree Designation Program provides a structured, operational framework for evaluating the organizational systems and processes necessary to sustain organizational culture change. It converts the aspirational aim of becoming more "patient-centered" into something that is defined, attainable and measurable—a practical blueprint for that work by translating high-level concepts into actionable, attainable and sustainable practices. (Planetree Institute, n.d.)

In addition to focusing on services and relationships, the Planetree Model recognizes the importance of architectural and interior design in the healing process. "The physical environment is vital to healing and well-being. Each hospital and continuing care community is designed to incorporate the comforts of home, clearly valuing humans, not just technology. By removing architectural barriers, the design encourages patient and family involvement. An awareness of the symbolic messages communicated by the design is an essential part of planning. Spaces are provided for both solitude and social activities, including libraries, kitchens, lounges, activity rooms, chapels, gardens and overnight accommodation for families" (Planetree Institute, n.d.). This description of an environment organized to support patient-centered care is also an integral part of nursing. Nursing has long emphasized the importance of the environment, meaning the milieu in which a patient recovers, and its relationship to physical, emotional, and spiritual well-being. When nursing care is planned and implemented, these factors are often considered.

Does a Patient-Centered Healthcare System Exist in the United States?

Throughout its *Quality Chasm* reports, the IOM emphasizes the need for patient-centered care.

Research shows that orienting health care around the preferences and needs of patients has the potential to improve patients' satisfaction with care as well as their clinical outcomes. Yet, one of five American adults reports that they have trouble communicating with their doctors and one of 10 says that they were treated with disrespect during a healthcare visit. Patients often report that test results or medical records were not available at the time of a scheduled appointment or that they received conflicting information from their providers. (Commonwealth Fund, 2008)

Patients want to be partners in their care, but why? This approach offers benefits in the following areas:

- Provider–patient communication
- Patient educational materials about health concerns
- Self-management tools to help patients manage their illness or condition and make informed decisions
- Access to care (timely appointments, off-hours services, and so on) and use of information technology (e.g., automated patient reminders and patient access to electronic medical records)
- Continuity of care
- Posthospital follow-up and support
- Management of drug regimens and chronic conditions
- Access to reliable information about the quality of physicians and healthcare organizations, with the opportunity to give feedback

"Ensuring that all patients have a medical home would be an important first step toward creating a patient-centered care system" (Commonwealth Fund, 2008). People need a regular place to receive care and the opportunity to develop a relationship with healthcare providers.

A serious difficulty in developing and maintaining a patient-centered healthcare system is that much of what is described as patient-centered care is not reimbursable. For example, insurers do not cover care coordination; it is just considered a natural part of care delivery. However, this really does not account for the time that staff must spend on coordinating care, communicating with team members, and so on. In addition, alternative communication methods are not typically covered, such as communication with patients over the Internet or telephone. To really change the system, this critical issue of reimbursement must be addressed. As it is, insurers are telling providers that they need to be more productive and that they have less time to spend with patients; at the same time, insurers are also telling providers that they have to be more patient centered. Meeting the latter demand requires more—not less—time with patients. The nursing shortage (which has fluctuated over the last few years) also comes at a time when nurses are expected to provide patient-centered care, yet the shortage in some areas has had an impact on nurses' ability to provide this care—less time, more stress, more acutely ill patients requiring more time, not enough staff, and so on. This causes conflict and frustration.

The growing **diversity** of patients also demands more patient-centered care. Diversity is a key driver of change in healthcare delivery today. Along with the changes in diversity is the grave concern about disparities in health care, with some ethnic and culture populations receiving different care than others; as noted by the IOM (2003a), treatment is all too often unequal.

> The concept of patient-centered health care is beginning to take hold. Increasingly, patients expect physicians to be responsive to their needs and preferences, to provide them with access to their medical information, and to treat them as partners in care decisions. But despite being named one of the key components of quality health care by the Institute of Medicine, "patient-centeredness" has yet to become the norm in primary care. (Davis, Schoenbaum, & Audet, 2005, pp. 953–954)

How can this goal of patient-centered care be reached at the same time that insurance coverage, access to care, and quality of care are improved in the United States? In addition, as the IOM recommends, all healthcare professionals need to be competent in providing patient-centered care, or change will not occur across the continuum of care in all healthcare settings. The following attributes of patient-centered care indicate what needs to be done to reach this goal and relate to what staff need to be able to do (Davis et al., 2005, p. 954), with examples as to how they might be described:

1. Improved access to care (e.g., patients can easily make appointments; waiting times are short; off-hours service is available)

2. Greater patient engagement in care (e.g., patients have the option of being informed and engaged partners in their care; patients are given information on treatment plans; self-care and counseling assistance are provided)

3. Clinical information systems that support high-quality care, practice-based learning, and quality improvement (e.g., healthcare organizations maintain patient registries and monitor adherence to treatment; patients receive decision support and information on recommended treatments)

4. Care coordination (e.g., care is coordinated across the continuum and settings; systems are in place to prevent errors that occur when multiple healthcare providers are involved; posthospital follow-up and support are provided)

5. Integrated and comprehensive team care (e.g., there is a free flow of communication among physicians, nurses, and other health professionals)

6. Routine patient feedback to physician/healthcare providers (e.g., low-cost, Internet-based patient surveys are used to learn from patients and inform treatment plans)

7. Publicly available information (e.g., patients have accurate, standardized information on healthcare providers (physicians, hospitals) to help them choose where they will get their care)

Other experts and researchers have recommended the following strategies to improve patient-centered care: (1) share power and responsibility with patients and caregivers, and (2) engage in an ongoing discussion with patients to increase understanding, acceptance, cooperation, and identification of common goals and related care plans (Gerteis, Edgman-Levitan, Daley, & Delbanco, 1993; Halpern, Lee, Boulter, & Phillips, 2001; IOM, 2001; Lewin, Skea, Entwistle, Zwarenstein, & Dick, 2001; Pew Health Professions Commission, 1995; Stewart, 2001, as cited in IOM, 2003a, pp. 52–53).

To reach the goal of significantly improved patient-centered care within a healthcare organization requires redesigning care processes to improve care delivery. It requires partnerships among practitioners, patients, and patients' families as appropriate and even stronger partnerships between schools of nursing and clinical organizations to enable students to gain more experience (Finkelman & Kenner, 2012). Care decisions need to respect patients' values, needs, preferences, and cultural issues, incorporating active use of the patient input and making the patient a partner in all aspects of care delivery. The IOM reports on quality indicate that it is more common for the patient to have to adapt to the healthcare delivery system, rather than the system adapting to the patient's needs and preferences. This approach needs to change. Patients who are involved in their own care tend to have better outcomes. There is greater and greater access to information among healthcare providers, which in turn means that patients also have more access to information. Information provides more power and control—not just for healthcare providers, but for patients as well. This all leads to a growing need for greater patient empowerment, a topic discussed further in this chapter in the sections on consumerism and self-management. There is a great need to develop patient-centered models that focus on particular populations, such as persons with chronic illness, populations in rural areas, urban populations, minority groups, women, children, the elderly, persons with special needs, and patients at the end of life. Nurses assume major roles in these new models and will continue to be active as additional models are developed.

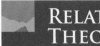

RELATED NURSING THEORIES

Examples of theories that are particularly relevant to the issue of patient-centered care are Watson's theory on caring, Orem's self-care theory, Leininger's cultural theory, Peplau's interpersonal theory, and some theories related to learning. Here we consider why these theories are relevant to this content:

- *Watson's theory on caring:* This theory focuses on caring. Patient-centered care includes an emphasis on caring—how the patient receives care, how the patient perceives care, and how nurses and other healthcare providers perceive their roles and implement care.
- *Orem's self-care theory:* This theory focuses on providing support and guidance to patients so that they can be actively involved in their own care. Self-management of care is part of patient-centered care and one of the overall priority areas of care identified by the IOM.
- *Leininger's cultural diversity theory:* This theory focuses on cultural issues and their importance in health and healthcare delivery. The IOM's definition of patient-centered care includes cultural aspects of care, and the IOM reports also discuss disparity in health care.
- *Peplau's interpersonal relations theory:* This theory emphasizes the importance of the nurse–patient relationship and communication. It is difficult to discuss or provide patient-centered care without considering the patient–provider relationship and communication.
- *Learning theories: Knowles's adult learning and the health belief model:* These two theories particularly relate to a patient-centered approach to patient education. Patient and family education about health and illness is a critical part of patient-centered care. This education emphasizes the active role of the

patient in the care delivery process and the patient as a decision maker—the center of care with greater emphasis on self-management. If a patient does not have adequate information and/or necessary skill to care for self, this diminishes patient-centered care.

The adult learning theory (Knowles, 1972) emphasizes that adult learners are different from younger learners—a factor that must be considered in any educational endeavor with adults. Patient education certainly includes children; however, there are more adult patients. Often adult education is approached in a paternalistic manner in which they are not treated as adult learners.

The health belief model is also referred to as the theory of reasoned action, which focuses on health promotion (Hochbaum, 1958). This model was developed to predict if a person would follow medical recommendations and to gain a better understanding of patient motivation. According to this model, a person's response to a health threat is based on the following factors (Masters, 2009, p. 173):

- The person's perception of the severity of the illness
- The person's perception of susceptibility to illness and its consequences
- The value of the treatment benefits (e.g., do the cost and side effect of treatment outweigh the consequences of the disease?)
- Barriers to treatment (e.g., expense, complexity of treatment, access to care)
- Costs of treatment in physical and emotional terms
- Cues that stimulate taking action toward treatment of illness (e.g., mass-media campaigns, pamphlets, advice from family or friends, and postcard reminders from healthcare providers)

By assessing these factors, nurses can develop a more effective patient education plan.

CONSUMERISM
How Does It Impact Health Care and Nursing?

Consumerism might seem a strange term to use in a nursing text. It is commonly encountered in business, particularly in advertising. However, consumerism in health care has become a very important concept, and it relates directly to patient-centered care. As far as nursing is concerned, nursing has long viewed the patient as an integral part of the nursing process, but what does this really mean, and has nursing grasped the concept of consumerism so that it is not only spoken about, but actually incorporated as a critical part of the implementation of nursing care? With the growing number of advanced practice nurses, many will be in their own practices or hold roles where consumerism is even more relevant to them.

Nursing speaks of patient advocacy, yet how patient advocacy is actively included in nursing care can vary widely. Patients, however, expect more and more to be active in their own care at all levels. They do not like it when they are ignored and left out of decision making. Families are also becoming much more assertive. Both patients and families are more concerned about quality and costs. The 1999 IOM report on safety led to greater recognition of the major safety problem in health care. When this report was published, the media widely shared the information in it via reports in newspapers, radio and television, and the Internet. The statistics in the report about the high level of errors were frightening and consequently woke up the public (consumers) to the need to be more vigilant.

Who Are the Consumers or Customers?

There are two major types of **consumers/customers** in health care. The **macro consumers** are the major purchasers of care: the government and insurers. They pay for care and, therefore, are consumers in that they have expectations of the product (the care delivered) and can influence that care. The **micro consumer** is the patient. Patient families and significant others, when the patient agrees that they have a role in the patient's care and/or decision-making process, are also micro consumers. Patients are turning more to nurses and asking questions about their health care and the healthcare delivery process. In the past, nurses knew little about reimbursement and the delivery process, but today's nurses need to be prepared to answer patient questions or to direct patients to resources for answers.

Customer-centered health care means that the nurse must be more aware of customer/patient needs, but this is not a simple process. Typically, one thinks of the statement, "The customer is always right"; however, in health care, this may not always be the case. The patient may not have all the information necessary to make an informed decision and may require the expertise of healthcare professionals to meet his or her needs. Nurses need to find a balance—meeting patient needs, including the patient, and respecting the patient's opinion. Customer service goals that are important in today's healthcare system and are related to nursing include the following (Leebov, 2008, pp. 21–23):

1. *Caring with compassion:* This is not a foreign concept for nurses. Nurses know that patients have multiple needs and often feel vulnerable in the healthcare setting and when they are sick.

2. *Making sure caring comes across:* It is easy to wonder why caring should even be discussed in relation to nursing because caring is so much a part of nursing and its image. However, key questions need to be asked: Does the caring come across to patients? Do nurses say and do things that really do not support caring?

3. *Paying quality attention:* With the variable nursing shortage today, it is very easy, and in some cases critical, to focus on quantity; healthcare facilities often do not have enough

staff. However, in doing this, quality becomes less visible. The skill of presence or mindfulness involves controlling attention. This allows the persons (patient, family, others) who are on the receiving end of the care to feel like the center at that moment. The nurse is not distracted, and the patient connects; caring occurs.

4. *Reducing patient anxiety:* This is where there is a clear deviation from what one typically thinks about when considering customers. Retail store sales staff want to make customers happy, but nurses and other healthcare staff want to reduce patient anxiety and support them. Making patients feel happy is not a bad result, but it may not reduce anxiety or provide support.

5. *Your personal calling:* Are you committed to improvement and caring, and how do you demonstrate this in your practice?

Critical in understanding patients is having knowledge about what they want and what they think their care outcomes should be. In the face of increasing out-of-pocket patient expenses, patients are compelled to know about their needs and care and to influence care decisions. If one compares this to shopping for a product such as an automobile, the buyer typically wants the best quality for the best price. Consumers are expressing concerns about the limits in their healthcare choices (e.g., employers offering fewer choices of health plans, offering plans with restricted or limited services, or placing restrictions on provider use). Although healthcare consumers may have changed over the years, quality of care and access to services remain important consumer issues. Managed care actually was a stimulus for consumers' greater engagement with the healthcare system; they became more active in their complaints about the changes made by managed care in healthcare reimbursement.

Patient Rights

The Patient Self-Determination Act of 1990 is a law that significantly impacts patient information and process. It applies to all healthcare organizations that receive Medicare or Medicaid reimbursement; thus, because few healthcare organizations do not receive this form of reimbursement, this law applies to most healthcare organizations. It requires that all these organizations or providers give their patients certain information that relates to confidentiality; consent; the right to make medical decisions, be informed about diagnosis and treatment, and refuse treatment; and use of advance directives. As yet, no federal legislation has been passed that specifically addresses patients' rights, although several attempts have been made. It is with the patient–healthcare provider (nurse) relationship that patient-centered care can best be actualized.

Information Resources and Consumers

Today, technology provides easy access to information not only for healthcare providers but also for consumers. The *Utilize Informatics* chapter discusses this trend in more detail, but healthcare informatics and technology also relate to patient-centered care. Through the use of new technologies, providers have multiple ways to communicate with current customers/consumers/patients, such as e-mail, the Internet, and cell phones, and extensive methods to collect, manage, and use healthcare information. Patients use such information to self-manage their health and care, expanding their knowledge of self-care and wellness. They seek medical advice, learn about their treatment options, and obtain information about reimbursement. Patients are also increasingly obtaining information to help them evaluate providers (physicians, hospitals, and so on), such as "report cards" about practice and outcomes, which are now more widely available to the public.

Customer or patient satisfaction is a critical topic in most healthcare organizations. Hospitals expend a great deal of energy and monies to assess how patients feel about their services. External companies, such as Press Ganey (listed in the "Linking to the Internet" section in this chapter), may assist in data collection and analysis. Customer/patient satisfaction data can be helpful, but this information must be viewed carefully. The following are some myths and related comments about satisfaction data that are important to consider (Zimmerman, 2001, pp. 255–256):

1. *Patient satisfaction is objective and straightforward.* This is not true. Surveys are difficult to develop, and they are often poorly designed.

2. *Patient satisfaction is easily measured.* Satisfaction is complex and not easily measured. Patient expectations influence the process, and many factors can affect patient responses that are not always easy to identify.

3. *Patient satisfaction is accurately and precisely measured.* This is not possible at this time. Attitudes are being measured.

4. *It is obvious who is the customer.* A healthcare organization actually has many different types of customers—more than just patients. For example, families, physicians, insurers, and internal customers (staff within the organization become customers to other staff; e.g., the laboratory provides services to the units and thus nursing staff on the units are the laboratory's customers) are also customers. A complete customer satisfaction analysis should include multiple types of customers in the healthcare organization.

Exhibit 9-2 identifies three key consumer or patient tips to better ensure safe health care and outcomes.

When it comes to quality of care, there is no clear universal definition of quality of care. A patient often sees quality of care and services differently than a nurse or physician would. An insurer may look at quality mostly from a cost perspective. This makes it difficult to analyze satisfaction data objectively. It is important to not assume that when a healthcare provider has a positive view of the quality of care and patient satisfaction, the patient agrees. For example, when patients receiving ambulatory care express different views of quality than do hospitalized patients, this is a concern. Root-cause analysis needs to be done in such a case. In examining the issues in this example, ambulatory care patients may be concerned with access to care, wait time for appointments, amount of time the provider spends with the patient, response from office or clinic staff, follow-up, access to information, or patient outcomes. Assumptions should not be made about what patients want or who they want to know about their health care.

Over time, a variety of methods to collect the data will undoubtedly emerge, but right now there are only a few reliable sources of data such as HCAHPS:

> The HCAHPS (Hospital Consumer Assessment of Healthcare Providers and Systems) survey is the first national, standardized, publicly reported survey of patients' perspectives of hospital care. HCAHPS

Exhibit 9-2   Consumer Tips for Safe Health Care

- Speak up if you have questions or concerns.
- Keep a list of all medications you take.
- Make sure you get the results of any test or procedure.

Source: Data from Agency for Health Resources and Quality. (2004). Five steps to safer health care. Publication No. OM 00-0004. Retrieved from http://www.ahrq.gov/consumer/5steps.htm

(pronounced "H-caps"), also known as the CAHPS Hospital Survey, is a survey instrument and data collection methodology for measuring patients' perceptions of their hospital experience. While many hospitals have collected information on patient satisfaction for their own internal use, until HCAHPS there was no national standard for collecting and publicly reporting information about patient experience of care that allowed valid comparisons to be made across hospitals locally, regionally and nationally. (U.S. Department of Health and Human Services [HHS], Centers for Medicare and Medicaid Services, 2013)

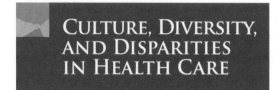

CULTURE, DIVERSITY, AND DISPARITIES IN HEALTH CARE

Healthy People 2020 identifies four major goals for the health of U.S. citizens, one of which emphasizes cultural diversity: "Achieve health equity, eliminate disparities, and improve the health of all groups" (HHS, 2010). This goal also indicates that providers throughout the healthcare system, including nurses, need to know more about culture, as indicated in the definition of patient-centered care.

Culture

Culture is "the accumulated store of shared values, ideas (attitudes, beliefs, values, and norms), understandings, symbols, material products, and practices of a group of people" (IOM, 2003b, p. 522). Nurses view patients through their personal experiences with culture and their personal histories. This may lead to problems, such as misinterpretation of communication and behavior that result in limitations in planning and implementing patient-centered care that meets the patient's needs. Culture and

language may influence the following aspects of care (HHS, 2008a):

- Health, healing, and wellness belief systems
- Patient/consumer perception of causes of illness and disease
- Patients/consumer behaviors and their attitudes toward healthcare providers
- Provider perceptions and values

In the United States, the diversity of racial and ethnic communities and linguistic groups is growing. Each of these subpopulations, with its own cultural traits and health profiles, presents a challenge to the healthcare delivery system and providers. The provider and the patient bring their individual learned patterns of language and culture to the healthcare experience, which in turn affects the care process and may further increase healthcare disparities. Demographic data indicate that more nurses are caring for patients from different cultural, racial, and ethnic backgrounds. In some areas, there are clusters of specific cultural populations, such as African Americans, Hispanics, Native Americans, and Asians. The United States' total minority population increased by 1.9% from 2011 to 2012 and accounted for 116 million people, or 37% of the total U.S. population, in July 2012 (U.S. Census Bureau, 2012). In 2011, Hispanics, Blacks, Asians, and other minorities accounted for 50.4% of U.S. births, 49.7% of all children younger than age 5, and slightly more than half of the 4 million children younger than age 1 (U.S. Census Bureau, 2011). Areas of the United States that have the highest diversity (in order of size) are the South, the West, the Northeast, and the Midwest. This presence of such diversity requires greater emphasis on providing care that is respectful of, and responsive to, the health beliefs, practices, and cultural and linguistic needs of the various patient populations.

Cultural Competence

Schools of nursing and healthcare organizations are working to improve cultural competence in students, faculty, and practicing nurses (Finkelman & Kenner, 2012). This trend has been driven by the IOM reports that indicate the presence of significant healthcare disparities in the healthcare delivery system. Competence "implies having the capacity to function effectively as an individual and as an organization within the context of the cultural beliefs, behaviors, and needs presented by consumers and their communities" (Anderson, Scrimshaw, Fullilove, Fielding, & Normand, 2003, pp. 68–69). The IOM describes three conceptual approaches to cross-cultural education: (1) focus on attitudes (cultural sensitivity/awareness approach); (2) knowledge (multicultural/categorical approach); and (3) skills (cross-cultural approach) (IOM, 2003b, p. 19). All three are necessary for improvement.

Disparities in Health Care

Disparities in health care are defined as "racial or ethnic differences in the quality of healthcare that are not due to access-related factors or clinical needs, preferences, and appropriateness of intervention" (IOM, 2003b, pp. 3–4). The IOM looked at two issues when determining the existence of disparities in health care. The first is how the U.S. healthcare system functions and which legal and regulatory issues may make it difficult for patients to get equal care. The second issue is discrimination at the patient provider level. Discrimination is defined as "differences in care that result from bias, prejudices, stereotyping and uncertainty in clinical communication and decision-making" (IOM, 2002, p. 4). What do some of these terms mean?

- **Bias**: Predisposed to a point of view.
- **Ethnicity**: Shared feeling of belonging to a group—peoplehood.
- **Ethnocentrism**: Belief that one's group or culture is superior to others.
- **Prejudice**: Making assumptions or judgments about the beliefs, behaviors, needs, and expectations of patients or other healthcare staff of a different cultural background

than one's own because of emotional beliefs about the population; involves negative attitudes toward the different group.
- **Race**: A biological designation of a group; belonging to the group based on biological factor(s).
- **Stereotyping**: A "process by which people use social groups (such as sex and race) to gather, process, and recall information about other people … these are labels" (IOM, 2002, p. 475). It is natural for people to organize information, and organizing information about people is part of this. However, this process can be negative if it involves unfairly classifying people or using incorrect information about an individual who may or may not meet the characteristics.

After the IOM report on disparities in health care indicated that there were problems in the United States, it was recognized that more effective monitoring of diversity in health care was necessary. In 2001, the National Healthcare Disparities Report was created. This annual report, which is accessible via the Internet, focuses on five critical areas (IOM, 2002, p. 2):

1. Measurement of socioeconomic status in disparities research
2. Measurement of disparities in healthcare services and quality
3. Measurement of disparities in healthcare access
4. Measurement of geographic units in disparities research
5. Subnational data sets

Critical issues of socioeconomic status, service and quality, and access, as well as geographic issues, are covered in this annual report. Healthcare disparities occur consistently across a variety of illnesses and delivery services and are associated not with specific types of illnesses but with a broad spectrum of characteristics. The annual disparities report was first completed in 2003, and this report and subsequent annual reports can be accessed through the

"Linking to the Internet" section at the end of the chapter.

In 2010, the Agency for Healthcare Research and Quality (AHRQ) asked the IOM to review past national quality and disparity reports and provide a vision so that the reports can contribute to advancing the quality of health care for all persons in the United States. The IOM formed the Committee on Future Directions for the National Healthcare Quality and Disparities Reports to address this task. Through research and deliberations, the Future Directions committee concluded that while the disparity reports alone will not improve the quality of health care, they assist in closing the gap between current performance levels and recommended standards of care. The committee recommended that the AHRQ take the following steps (HHS, AHRQ, 2010):

- Align the content of the reports with nationally recognized priority areas for quality improvement to help drive national action.
- Select measures that reflect healthcare attributes or processes that are deemed to have the greatest impact on population health.
- Affirm through the contents of the reports that achieving equity is an essential part of quality improvement.
- Increase the reach and usefulness of the AHRQ's family of report-related products.
- Revamp the presentation of the reports to tell a more complete quality improvement story.
- Analyze and present data in ways that inform policy and promote best-in-class achievement for all actors.
- Identify measure and data needs to set a research and data collection agenda.

This is a good example of how an initiative such as the IOM original recommendation that the United States use monitoring to provide a view of healthcare quality and healthcare disparities can be expanded and must be reviewed periodically to see if the process needs to be improved.

The Department of Health and Human Services (HHS, 2008b) has published information on its website about culture and health care. It describes health disparities as the persistent gaps between the health status of minorities and nonminorities in the United States. As defined by the IOM, equity in health services involves "providing care that does not vary in quality because of personal characteristics such as gender, ethnicity, geographic location and socioeconomic status" (2001, p. 6). Despite continued advances in health care and technology, racial and ethnic minorities continue to have more disease, disability, and premature death than nonminorities. African Americans, Hispanics/Latinos, American Indians and Alaska Natives, Asian Americans, Native Hawaiians, and Pacific Islanders have higher rates of infant mortality, cardiovascular disease, diabetes, human immunodeficiency virus infection/acquired immunodeficiency syndrome, and cancer, as well as lower rates of immunizations and cancer screening. Two major factors influence these results:

- *Inadequate access to care:* Barriers to care can result from economic, geographic, linguistic, cultural, and healthcare financing issues.
- *Substandard quality of care:* Even when minorities have similar levels of access to care, health insurance, and education, the quality and intensity of health care they receive are often poor. Lower-quality care has many causes, including patient–provider miscommunication, provider discrimination, stereotyping, and prejudice. Quality of care is now usually rated using the IOM-recommended four measures: effectiveness, patient safety, timeliness, and patient centeredness.

Disparities: Examples and Importance

Disparities in health status and health outcomes can be categorized by individual factors and healthcare system factors (Peters & Elster, 2002), including the following:

- *Individual factors:* Sociodemographic characteristics (e.g., age, race/ethnicity, gender), socioeconomic status (e.g., income, occupation, and education), or other personal characteristics such as disabilities, rural or urban residency, and sexual orientation. Although biological and genetic factors account for some of these group differences, other contributing factors include cultural norms and values, literacy levels, familial influences, environmental and occupational exposures, and patient preferences for care and treatment. Uneven distribution of societal resources, including social and political advantages such as knowledge and social connections, has a negative impact on health. Individual health behaviors also vary by race/ethnicity, income, and education; such factors may explain group differences in mortality and morbidity, but do not account for all of the disparities found in mortality and morbidity rates. Promoting healthy lifestyles and reducing health-risk behaviors are interventions that nurses and other healthcare providers can use to reduce healthcare disparities.

- *Healthcare system factors:* The rates of access to, and utilization of, health care vary among population groups. Explanations for these differences include insurance status and affordability, transportation and geographic barriers to needed services, health beliefs, attitudes, level of self-confidence in complying with treatment, racial concordance of patient and physician, cultural preferences for less invasive procedures, and provider bias, racism, and discrimination.

The Centers for Disease Control and Prevention's Health Disparities and Inequalities Report—United States 2012 (CDC, 2012) identifies some of the current major issues, which **Exhibit 9-3** further highlights. The summary of results from the most recent report (2012) indicate that overall quality is improving, access is getting worse, and disparities are not improving. This report was completed prior to implementation of the first major changes dictated by the Affordable Care Act, which were initiated in late 2013 and early 2014. These changes—particularly the expansion of insurance coverage among the U.S. population—should make a difference in the long term on these concerns. The disparities and quality national reports are always a few years behind the current year because it takes time to collect and analyze the data. The Health Disparities and Inequalities Report correlates with *Healthy People 2020* and with the National Partnership for Action to end health disparities and relates to the national disparity report published annually by the AHRQ.

It is probably not possible to totally eliminate disparities in health care; however, much can be done to improve care for all persons and to improve equity in health care. Ensuring access is critical. Can patients get the care they need from experts in a timely manner? Access involves multiple factors, such as appointments, transportation to appointments, availability of qualified staff, wait times, service hours, and so on. Disparity issues require that all healthcare professionals actively consider patient values and preferences (a critical component of patient-centered care). These values and preferences can vary between groups and within groups. It is easy to stereotype and assume that everyone in a specific ethnic group is the same, but this is not the case. Monitoring data on disparities is important to assist in identifying current status and to develop and improve effective interventions to reach desired outcomes. This monitoring is now being done annually in the National Disparities Report, but individual healthcare provider organizations such as hospitals can also monitor their own data and outcomes.

Diversity in the Healthcare Workforce

The Sullivan Commission report (Sullivan, 2004), which is separate from the IOM reports, examined disparities in health care from a different perspective. This commission concluded that a key contributor

---

Exhibit 9-3   Highlights from the Centers for Disease Control and Prevention Health Disparities and Inequalities Report—United States 2012

Disparities in quality of care are common:

▪ Blacks received worse care than Whites, and Hispanics received worse care than non-Hispanic Whites for approximately 40% of quality measures.
▪ American Indians and Alaska Natives (AI/ANs) received worse care than Whites for one-third of quality measures.
▪ Asians received worse care than Whites for one-fourth of quality measures but better care than Whites for a similar proportion of quality measures.
▪ Poor and low-income people received worse care than high-income people for approximately 60% of quality measures; middle-income people received worse care for more than half the measures.

Disparities in access are also common, especially among AI/ANs, Hispanics, and poor people:

▪ Blacks had worse access to care than Whites for one-third of measures, and AI/ANs had worse access to care than Whites for approximately 40% of access measures.
▪ Asians had worse access to care than Whites for approximately 20% of access measures but better access to care than Whites for a similar proportion of access measures.
▪ Hispanics had worse access to care than non-Hispanic Whites for approximately 70% of measures.
▪ Poor people had worse access to care than high-income people for all measures; low-income people had worse access to care for more than 80% of measures; and middle-income people had worse access to care for about 70% of measures.
▪ Review the report details at http://www.ahrq.gov/research/findings/nhqrdr/nhqr12/highlights.html or the details of the most current report that has been published.

Source: Modified from U.S. Department of Health and Human Services, Agency for Healthcare Research and Quality. (2012). 2012 National Healthcare Disparities Report. Retrieved from http://www.innovations.ahrq.gov/content.aspx?id=4008).

---

to the growing healthcare disparity problem is the disparities in the United States' health professional workforce. This limits minorities' access to health care and to healthcare providers who understand their needs. The commission suggested that there should be an increase in the number of minority health professionals. This suggestion came at a time when there was a shortage of nurses and other healthcare providers.

There must be greater efforts to increase minority admissions to nursing programs and retain students. The federal government is providing grants to encourage schools of nursing to increase minority enrollment, develop support services, and increase minority enrollment in graduate school to increase the number of minority nursing faculty. It will take time to improve the level of minority participation in nursing. The U.S. Census Bureau in 2012 reported that ethnic and racial minorities account for approximately 37% of the U.S. population. However, in 2013 the National Council of State Boards of Nursing (NCSBN) and the Forum of State Nursing Workforce Centers reported that only 19% of all U.S. registered nurses (RNs) were members of an ethnic or racial minority (American Association of Colleges of Nursing [AACN], 2014). Enrollment and graduation data in BSN and higher degree programs demonstrate that ethnic and racial minorities still lag behind, with minorities representing 28.3% of BSN students, 29.3% of students in master's-level programs, and 27.7% of students in PhD programs (AACN, 2014).

The AACN and the Robert Wood Johnson Foundation (RWJF) have partnered together to launch a new initiative entitled Doctoral Advancement in Nursing (DAN) project that aims to attract more minority students to PhD and DNP programs. These organizations also support another joint initiative called RWJF New Careers in Nursing Scholarship Program, which focuses on providing monies for minority students in accelerated programs. The AACN and Johnson & Johnson Campaign for the Minority Nurse Faculty Scholars Program focuses on preparing minority nurses for faculty roles (AACN, 2014). These are just a few of the initiatives that are attempting to address the ongoing shortage of minority nurses.

The American Organization of Nurse Executives (AONE) is an important organization for nurses in leadership and management positions. This organization's principles include diversity:

> The organizational mission, vision and strategic direction of AONE recognize that the success of nursing leadership is dependent on reflecting the diversity of the communities nurses serve. AONE moves forward with an active sensitivity toward promoting diversity in all forms. It is the position of AONE that diversity is one of the essential building blocks of a healthful practice/work environment. (AONE, 2007, p. 1)

organizations, and healthcare institutions, as well as those developed by accrediting organizations and other healthcare professional organizations, support advocacy and consumerism. Throughout the care delivery process, nurses participate in and support actions that emphasize patient advocacy. They support patient and family education, patient satisfaction and the complaint process, and efforts to improve care, and they support and ask for patient participation in healthcare decision making.

As each nurse provides care, he or she has numerous opportunities to serve as the patient's advocate. The nurse coordinates the care and in doing so represents the patient, but the nurse needs to recognize the patient's values and preferences in this process, thereby supporting patient-centered care. This means that the nurse must know about the patient's values and preferences—for example, cultural issues and how they might impact the patient. This should lead to an improved collaborative relationship with the patient. Collaboration is working with others to arrive at the best outcome. When the nurse acts as the patient advocate, the nurse remembers that the patient must be involved. Advocacy does not mean that the nurse makes the patient dependent on the nurse. The nurse must also be persuasive with other healthcare team members to ensure better care for the patient that meets the patient's needs (outcomes). Advocacy means that the nurse is active in respecting the patient and patient rights and in ensuring that the patient has the education to understand treatment and care needs. Support is given to the patient and family. When the patient makes a treatment decision, the nurse does not judge the patient's decision, even though the nurse may disagree with that decision.

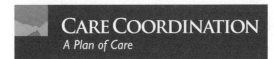

PATIENT ADVOCACY

Patient advocacy has always been a major aspect of the nursing role and requires leadership skills. Nursing standards developed by the American Nurses Association (ANA), nursing specialty

CARE COORDINATION
A Plan of Care

Care coordination is the first of the priority areas of care identified by the IOM. The purpose of care coordination is "to establish and support a continuous healing relationship, enabled by an integrated clinical environment and characterized by a proactive delivery of evidence-based care and follow-up" (IOM, 2003a, p. 49). To accomplish this, healthcare providers, including nurses, need to provide patient-centered care. The IOM also discusses the need for clinical integration and care coordination. The goal is care coordinated across people, functions, activities, and sites (including the community and home) so that the patient receives effective care. A critical issue today is the need to improve interprofessional teamwork in the care planning process for patients.

CRITICAL THINKING AND CLINICAL REASONING AND JUDGMENT

For a long time, nurse educators have included critical thinking in curricula; however, the content itself and the means by which it is taught need to be revised to include clinical reasoning and judgment. It is important to recognize that the processes of critical thinking and clinical reasoning and judgment relate to planning, implementing, and evaluating patient-centered care. Critical thinking and clinical reasoning and judgment should be used throughout the nursing process. They are important to effective nursing practice, but it takes time and experience to develop these skills and to use them effectively.

Critical thinking requires nurses to generate and examine questions and problems, use intuition, examine feelings, and clarify and evaluate evidence. It means being aware of change and willing to take some risks. Critical thinking allows the nurse to avoid using dichotomous thinking—seeing things either as good or bad, or black or white. This limits possibilities and clinical choices for patients (Finkelman, 2001).

Clinical reasoning and **clinical judgment** require more than recall and understanding of content or selection of the correct answer;

they also require the ability to apply, analyze, and synthesize knowledge (Del Bueno, 2005). Nursing clinical judgment is the process, or the "ways in which nurses come to understand the problems, issues or concerns of clients/patients, to attend to salient information, and to respond in concerned and involved ways" (Benner, Tanner, & Chesla, 1996, p. 2). This process includes both deliberate, conscious decision making and intuition. "In the real world, patients do not present the nurse with a written description of their clinical symptoms and a choice of written potential solutions" (Del Bueno, 2005, p. 282). Beginning nursing students, however, are looking for the clear picture of the patient that matches what the student has read about in the text. This patient really does not exist, so critical thinking and clinical reasoning and judgment become more important as the student learns to compare and contrast what might be expected with what is reality (Benner, Sutphen, Leonard, & Day, 2010).

Nursing Process

The **nursing process** is a systematic method for thinking about and communicating how nurses provide patient care. It is a step-by-step tool that guides nurses as they plan and provide care in a variety of clinical settings. The process requires that nurses use critical thinking and clinical reasoning and judgment. Students are asked to use this process often by developing extensive care plans for patients. As students become RNs and move into practice, this process is adapted for daily use with multiple patients.

The nursing process is similar to the problem-solving process in that there is a concern that requires more information to determine the best approach to solve it. In the nursing process, there are five steps, as described in **Figure 9-3**.

Assessment

Information or data about the patient is required to describe the patient's health status and needs. This

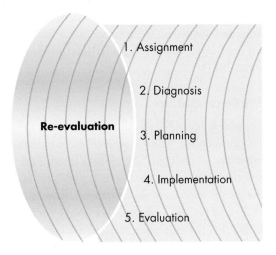

1. Assignment

2. Diagnosis

Re-evaluation

3. Planning

4. Implementation

5. Evaluation

Figure 9-3 Nursing Care Process

information is collected during assessment by multiple methods, such as a description of the patient's health history, interviews, observation, physical exam, and review of medical records.

The nursing process is not linear; it is ongoing, and one step leads to the next step and then begins again. Assessment begins the process; however, assessment is ongoing because a patient's health status and needs change, which may require a change in diagnosis, plan, and how a plan is implemented. This also impacts outcomes and evaluation. During assessment, the nurse must evaluate the quality of the information to determine if additional information is needed and which method would be best suited to obtaining the information. It is during this step that the nurse begins to establish the nurse–patient relationship.

Patient-centered care means that the patient's values, preferences, needs, culture, and history play a critical role in the planned care. The nurse needs to document the assessment in a manner that is clear and informs other staff. In today's healthcare settings, effective care is typically delivered by an interprofessional team. This means that the nursing plan of care should not be separate from other aspects of the patient's care needs. The team needs to

consider all aspects of care and collaborate. There needs to be greater movement toward a patient plan of care rather than a focus on a specific profession's plan of care, such as the nursing care plan or medical care plan.

Patients often complain that many staff from different healthcare disciplines ask them the same questions. Some healthcare organizations are trying to address this problem by eliminating repetition in assessment forms—for example, making sure that the assessment forms that physicians use and the nursing assessment forms are not repetitive unless a sufficient rationale exists for the repetition. Some healthcare organizations have been more successful than others in controlling unnecessary repetition.

Assessment time is a critical time to communicate to patients that they are the center of concern. Achieving this goal requires attention on the part of the nurse. Patient rights—for example, maintaining privacy during the assessment, ensuring confidentiality of information obtained, and explaining to the patient the process and patient rights—are also important.

Diagnosis

Diagnosis occurs as the nurse analyzes and interprets the information/data to determine the patient's nursing problems and needs—actual and potential. Nursing diagnoses have been identified and categorized through a system referred to as the North American Nursing Diagnosis Association (NANDA, 2011).

Planning

The care plan directs the care that will be given, promotes communication and sharing of information, and provides a record of the plan. The plan identifies the interventions or actions that the nurse may take to manage or resolve problems; to monitor the patient; to decrease risks of injury or illness; to promote health or prevent injury or illness; to support patient self-management; and to provide patient-centered care. Interventions may be direct or indirect care. Examples of direct care are administering medication, helping the patient get out of bed, changing a dressing, teaching the patient, and assessing or monitoring patient status—all interventions or actions that include the patient and the nurse. Examples of indirect care are documenting in the medical record, preparing medications, giving a report on a patient's status, talking to the physician about the patient, reviewing medical orders, and delegating care to **unlicensed assistive personnel**, such as explaining what needs to be done for the patient during daily care—all interventions or actions in which the patient is not directly involved in the process. Classification of nursing care and interventions includes the following categories: (1) dependent care, meaning that most nurses cannot legally prescribe medications or act without a physician order (after the physician orders the medical intervention, the nurse follows the orders unless the nurse assesses the situation and determines the physician needs to be consulted before implementing the orders); (2) independent care, meaning that the nurse may make decisions about interventions to prevent, reduce, or alleviate a problem; and (3) interdependent care, including care in which both the nurse and the physician collaborate. State nurse practice acts identify the types of care that are independent, dependent, and interdependent within each state. There is greater interest in practice to use interprofessional care plans; in such a case, nursing plans would be part of the treatment team's plan.

Planning takes time and must be connected to the assessment data and the diagnoses/problems identified for the patient. The patient needs to be part of the planning and the identification of care needs, with an explanation about the plan. This approach supports patient-centered care. The final decision about treatment is really up to the patient unless the patient is not physically able to make decisions.

The plan identifies interventions, responsibility for implementing interventions, a timeline, and expected outcomes. Outcomes are particularly important in evaluation. Some schools of nursing and

some hospitals use lists of typical nursing interventions and outcomes. The common list is the Nursing Intervention Classification (NIC) (University of Iowa, 2011).

Implementation

The plan is developed so that the patient can receive the care required, which is achieved through implementation of the plan. Change may be required at any time during this process. It is possible that as the plan is implemented, the patient's status might change, or perhaps an intervention might not be effective. Many factors affect implementation, such as the nurse's competency, the strategy used for delegation, staffing levels, acuity levels of all the patients whom the nurse is caring for at the time, availability of supplies and resources, the number of interruptions, the needs of the patient's family, patient cooperation and acceptance of the plan, time management and priorities, and much more.

Throughout the implementation step, it is critical that the nurse coordinate, collaborate, and communicate with the interprofessional team and other nursing staff. Delegation, therefore, is part of implementation.

Evaluation

Evaluation focuses on each of the nursing care process steps. The following questions are asked (the applicable nursing process step or steps follow each question in parentheses):

1. Was the assessment adequate? (assessment)
2. Are there changes in the patient's status that require attention? (assessment)
3. Are there new diagnoses/problems? (diagnosis)
4. What are the outcomes for the identified nursing diagnoses/problems? (diagnosis)
5. Were the interventions completed, and what were the outcomes? (planning, implementation)
6. Are new interventions required? (planning, implementation)

Reevaluation should take place throughout the process as the patient's health status changes. This may require that the nurse return to a previous step in the nursing process.

Getting patients involved in their own care can be challenging. Most patients want to be involved, but nurses must use strategies to support patient-centered care. It is important to be aware of your attitude and tone of voice when you speak with adult patients. Some nurses approach all patients as if they were children, which is not helpful in engaging patients in their care. For example, when patients are recovering from anesthesia, the nurse may speak to the patient in "baby tones"; this is not appropriate. Box 9-1 provides some examples of strategies to help encourage patient participation in the thinking process, which is an important part of care planning.

Care/Concept Mapping

The traditional format for the nursing care plan, which focuses on the five steps just outlined, has been used for a long time; however, it has been the subject of some criticism. Its length is one issue, but it might also limit critical thinking, clinical reasoning, and clinical judgment because of its rigid format. Another approach to care planning is the concept map or **care map**. "The concept map care plan is an innovative approach to planning and organizing nursing care. In essence, a concept map care plan is a diagram of patient problems and interventions. Your ideas (concepts) about patient problems and treatments are the 'concept' that will be diagrammed" (Schuster, 2007, p. 2). Using concept mapping for care plans develops your critical thinking and clinical reasoning.

Concept map plans are developed through the following steps:

1. *Develop the basic skeleton diagram.* Begin with the patient's reason for care (often the medical diagnosis), putting it in the center of the page or diagram. Around this central point, identify general problems (nursing problems). This is the first concept map.

Box 9-1	Strategies to Help Healthcare Providers Encourage Patient Participation in the Critical Thinking Process

- Stay in the room. Don't talk to patients from the doorway.
- Pay attention to your body language and to the patient's body language.
- Sit down so that you are at eye level with the patient.
- Use open questions and comments, such as "Tell me about …" instead of closed questions that imply you expect a short answer.
- Touch patients, but be respectful of their space and cultural norms.
- Use collaborative thinking language, such as "We should think this through," "Let's look at some possible conclusions," and "Can we analyze this together?"
- Use phrases that let the patient know that the patient's situation is not so unusual that the patient cannot discuss it. For example, "Some people feel anxious when …"
- Address patients respectfully. Find out if they prefer Mr. or Mrs., Doctor, Professor, Reverend, and so on. Do not use affectionate terms to address the patient, such as "sweetheart", "dear" and so on.
- Do not look at your watch, no matter how busy you are.
- Be direct and honest. For example, tell patients when the schedule is backed up and why.
- If you feel like avoiding a patient, reflect on why you feel that way.

Source: From Rubenfeld, M. G., & Scheffer, B. (2006). *Critical thinking tactics for nurses.* Sudbury, MA: Jones and Bartlett.

2. *Analyze and categorize data.* In this step, the focus is on the information (assessment data) that is known; categorization provides evidence for the medical and nursing diagnoses. The information is obtained from history, assessment, medical records, and interviews with the patient. This information is added to the care map—problems/diagnoses with related data.

3. *Analyze nursing diagnoses relationships.* Taking the data map that also includes the problems with related data identified per problem, begin to make connections by analyzing relationships among the diagnoses, drawing lines to identify the relationships, and numbering each problem/diagnosis. The goal is to achieve a holistic view of the patient.

4. *Identify goals, outcomes, and interventions.* On a separate page, identify the patient's goals and outcomes. Next, identify interventions to meet these goals and outcomes for each of the problems/diagnoses numbered on the care map. This step is similar to the planning process in the nursing care process.

5. *Evaluate the patient's responses.* On the page with the goals, outcomes, and interventions for each of the problems, add the patient's responses (outcomes) to each of the interventions after they have been implemented and evaluated. This information is then used in documentation.

With the concept map, you create a diagram describing the care and can add to it as needed. This document is similar to the traditional nursing care plan format in that all the components of care are included. However, the concept map allows for more creative thinking as you create a visual depiction of the patient's status, care needs, and the plan for care.

SELF-MANAGEMENT OF CARE

Regardless of whether healthcare providers accept it, patients are very active in managing their own care.

Even if they choose not to receive health care, they have made a decision about their health and what they want to do about it. In some cases, the patient is pushed into greater personal responsibility for care; the patient may have inadequate reimbursement or no reimbursement at all, or may not have support from family and others. It is recognized that critical strategies in preventing health problems and reducing healthcare costs are self-management, health promotion, and disease and illness prevention. When patients use **self-management of care** effectively and are supported by healthcare providers to use self-management, the outcomes are (1) greater collaboration with healthcare providers, (2) better understanding of treatment choices and patient and healthcare provider responsibilities, and (3) improved follow-up to treatment. Patients who are involved in their healthcare decisions are more satisfied with their health care and health status. The IOM (2003b) defines self-management of care support as "the systematic provision of education and supportive interventions to increase patients' skills and confidence in managing their health problems, including regular assessment of progress and problems, goal setting, and problem-solving approach" (p. 52). The Institute for Health Improvement (IHI) provides many self-management resources. (See "Linking to the Internet" at the end of the chapter.)

Based on this definition of self-management, it is critical to consider two important factors in nursing care: (1) health literacy and its impact and (2) patient education.

Health Literacy: A Barrier

Health literacy is important to effective self-management. Nearly 90 million Americans (almost half of all adults) have difficulty understanding and using health information. This serious problem has increased the rate of hospitalizations and the use of emergency services, and it increases healthcare costs. If a patient cannot understand directions or does not follow the directions, the patient may need more intensive care, including hospitalization. A patient who does not understand the diabetic diet or know how to use insulin correctly will have health problems; that person may then seek out help in the emergency room and consequently need to be hospitalized.

Healthcare literacy includes reading, writing, and arithmetic skills; listening and speaking abilities; and conceptual knowledge. Health literacy is defined as "the degree to which individuals have the capacity to obtain, process, and understand basic information and services needed to make appropriate decisions regarding their health" (IOM, 2004, p. 2). Even educated people can find themselves with a health literacy problem and not understand medical information. The Joint Commission (2008) notes that communication problems are the most common root cause of healthcare errors. Safety and errors are discussed in more detail in the *Apply Quality Improvement* chapter, but it is important in this discussion about patient-centered care to recognize the connection between healthcare literacy, self-management, and errors.

With the increase in the number of patients from diverse backgrounds, healthcare organizations are seeking more language interpreters, particularly those who speak Spanish, but also those who speak other languages. Families are not the best source for interpretation because they are not trained in medical terminology, and they may influence the communication and decision-making processes because of their personal connection to the patient. An interpreter interprets only the language or words and is not involved in how the patient should respond. Some healthcare organizations have bilingual staff who can be a useful source of interpreting services if they are easily accessible and still able to complete their usual work.

In 2006, the HHS Office of Minority Health issued a new guide to help healthcare organizations implement effective language access services and improve care for patients with limited

English skills. This report, *A Patient-Centered Guide to Implementing Language Access Services in Healthcare Organizations*, offers a practical and basic step-by-step approach to implementing language services.

In 2011, the AHRQ announced that low health literacy in older Americans is linked to poorer health status and a higher risk of death, more emergency room visits, and more hospitalizations. The agency noted that more than 75 million English-speaking adults in the United States have limited health literacy. In 2010, the HHS initiated an action plan to improve health literacy with the following goals (HHS, AHRQ, 2010):

- Providing everyone with access to accurate and actionable health information
- Delivering person-centered health information and services
- Supporting lifelong learning and skills to improve good health

Jargon needs to be reduced and information needs to be provided in easy-to-understand written information, clear forms, and understandable information on websites. Verbal communication with all patients needs to be improved.

Nurses are in direct contact with patients daily and encounter many patients who are experiencing health literacy problems. This has an impact on how effective nurses can be in providing care, in assisting patients with self-management of their care, and in teaching patients what they need to know to understand their health, illness, and care needs.

Patient/Family Education: Inclusion in the Plan of Care

Patient and family education has long been a part of nursing, but it is not easy to provide such education effectively. One can look at patient education from two perspectives: (1) helping the patient understand the illness experience and cope with it effectively and (2) providing information and direction for self-management of care.

One of the major nursing interventions is patient education. It is not an intervention that the nurse can delegate unless the learning need is best addressed by another healthcare professional. The RN cannot delegate patient education to non-RN nursing staff such as a licensed practical nurse or a nursing assistant because this is a professional nursing responsibility.

It is not easy to provide effective patient education. The barriers to meeting patient education needs may include the following:

- Inadequate assessment of the patient's education needs
- Inadequate patient education plan
- Lack of time to provide the education required
- Interruptions that limit concentration
- Medical status of the patient (inability of the patient to adequately participate)
- Unclear assessment of the role of the family/significant others (whether the family wants or needs to participate in the education)
- Patient education in settings such as ambulatory care typically not reimbursed; less emphasis placed on education as a result
- Confusion regarding who is responsible for patient education
- Lack of effective learning strategies and tools to meet individual patient education needs
- Lack of nursing staff (nurses seeing to other aspects of nursing that are more critical)
- Lack of follow-up and evaluation of patient outcomes related to the education provided

Given the realities of the healthcare workplace today, it is difficult to plan and implement education for patients and their families. This can be very frustrating for both the nurse and the patient. Patients are discharged early, but they are often still sick at that point. While in the hospital, they may not be able to concentrate on what they need to learn, and then they are sent home and feel at a loss. Home care is one solution, but most home care is not provided around the clock, and patients still need to know about their illness or injury and treatment. Home health nurses provide a lot of the education, but patient education needs to be provided in the hospital as well. Patients who do not have home health services are particularly vulnerable.

When nurses are rushed, the typical scenario is to hand the patient and/or family some written information. The nurse may ask if there are questions. This is not effective patient education. Effective education incorporates the following elements:

1. The nurse assesses the patient's education status and needs. What does the patient need to know? How much does the patient know?
2. The nurse identifies (diagnoses) learning needs. For example, the patient may need to know how to administer insulin and how to plan a diet.
3. The nurse develops a learning plan with specific interventions. These interventions are based on expected outcomes. The nurse identifies who is responsible for providing the learning intervention and creates the timeline. Here the nurse must consider the patient's values and preferences, age, family support, cultural background and issues, and health literacy. For example, the nurse will teach the diabetic patient about equipment and where to get it; how to draw up insulin, including checking dosage and so on; how to prepare the skin; and how to administer the medication. The nurse will talk about complications and aftercare needs. The patient is told how to track insulin administered and store insulin. The nurse plans several sessions with the patient and uses a variety of teaching–learning strategies, such as discussion, visual aids, equipment, demonstration, and return demonstration. The family is included as appropriate and with permission of the patient. The patient needs time to ask questions and express concerns.
4. The nurse implements the plan. Typically, this responsibility is not delegated unless assigned to another RN. Many of the barriers mentioned

earlier come into play when implementing the plan. It takes planned effort to make sure the patient gets the education that is needed at the proper time.

5. The nurse evaluates the plan/interventions. Were the expected outcomes met? This is commonly a weak link in the process, often because the patient goes on to another setting or home. It is important, whenever possible, to assess outcomes, such as through questions, return demonstrations, and so on, and to ask the patient how he or she feels about the process and outcomes. Often the patient is discharged, preventing complete evaluation of patient education.

For nursing care to be patient centered, with each patient developing effective self-management of health and care needs, each patient needs information and skills to meet his or her individual needs.

THERAPEUTIC USE OF SELF IN THE NURSE–PATIENT RELATIONSHIP

When you as a nurse begin to care for patients, eventually you realize that the relationship is different from other relationships that you have experienced. It is not a parent–child relationship, a teacher–student relationship, or a personal or friend relationship. As you progress in the nursing program and then become an RN, this difference becomes even more evident. In the beginning, students often try to make the nurse–patient relationship into something it is not (e.g., in many cases, the student tries to be friends with the patient). The key difference between the nurse–patient relationship and a friendship is that in a friendship, there is an expectation, on both sides, that friends will help each other, listen to each other, and be there for each other. This

is not the case in a nurse–patient relationship. There should not be any expectation that the patient will listen to the nurse's concerns, feelings, or problems, nor is the patient there to support the nurse. The nurse is expected to listen to the patient, work with the patient (even if the nurse does not really like the patient), and meet the patient's care needs. This is difficult to learn, but it does come with experience.

The nurse–patient relationship has been described as therapeutic. *Therapeutic* means treatment. Using this term to describe this special relationship emphasizes that this relationship is part of the care process. **Therapeutic use of self** requires the nurse

to use his/her personality consciously and in full awareness in an attempt to establish relatedness and to structure nursing intervention … . This requires self-insight, self-understanding, an understanding of the dynamics of human behavior, ability to interpret one's own behavior, as well as the behavior of others, and the ability to intervene effectively in nursing situations. (Travelbee, 1971, p. 19)

The importance of this relationship should not be minimized.

Professional successes, especially at the bedside, are most often measured objectively through such sources as patient outcome data, length of stay, response to treatment, patient satisfaction, and the like. But other measurements, which are often therapeutic but less tangible, cannot be discounted as measures of success. These patient outcomes may take the form of relief in a troubled countenance, tears of joy, or a peaceful, pain-free sleep. (Parker, 2006, p. 28)

In this relationship, the patient expects the nurse to be competent and to have expertise in nursing care. There is no such expectation of the patient. The nurse plans and initiates care for the patient, but patient-centered care must include the patient in the process. The center of the nurse–patient relationship is the patient. Even when a patient asks about the nurse's personal reactions, the patient is still more focused on self. Through the nurse–patient relationship, the patient is given support and guidance in coping with the illness experience. Patients with acute illness recover, but they still need help with coping during their illness, and they may need time to reflect on their illness after recovery. As has been discussed, more and more people have chronic illnesses that are not resolved through interventions. These patients need to receive support and to learn coping skills that can help them during the ups and downs of their illness process.

Communication is a critical component of the nurse–patient relationship. The nurse needs to be clear and consistent with the patient and provide explanations about the care. Both verbal and nonverbal communication are integrated throughout the communication process. Nurses need to be aware of their own communication patterns and nonverbal messages, as well as those of the patient and people around the patient (family, friends, and other members of the healthcare team). **Exhibit 9-4** identifies some examples of therapeutic communication responses.

Box 9-2 identifies examples of validation remarks to promote patient participation in decisions. These communication examples illustrate how communication, the nurse–patient relationship, and patient-centered care are interrelated.

The National Council of State Boards of Nursing (1996) identified key information about boundaries in the nurse–patient relationship. A professional boundary is an invisible line that provides limits to a nurse's behavior and focuses professional nurse–patient behavior that has the patient in the center. The patient expects that the nurse will act for the patient and respect his or her values and preferences. There should be no personal gain for the nurse. **Figure 9-4** lists critical descriptors of professional boundaries. The National Council of State

Exhibit 9-4	Therapeutic Communication Responses

- Using silence
- Accepting
- Giving recognition
- Offering self
- Giving broad openings
- Offering general leads
- Placing an event in time or sequence
- Making observations
- Encouraging description or perceptions
- Encouraging comparison
- Restating
- Reflecting
- Focusing
- Exploring more fully
- Seeking clarification
- Presenting reality
- Voicing doubt
- Verbalizing the implied, then asking for validation
- Attempting to translate words into feelings
- Formulating a verbal contract
- Assessing, evaluating with the patient

Boards of Nursing (1996) highlights the following guiding principles:

- The nurse's responsibility is to delineate and maintain boundaries (e.g., it is not the patient's responsibility to know the boundaries or enforce them).
- The nurse should work within the zone of helpfulness. (The zone of helpfulness falls between being underinvolved with the patient and being overinvolved with the patient. The most common boundary issue involves overinvolvement and, therefore, forgetting one's professional boundary.) **Figure 9-5** illustrates a continuum of professional behavior.
- The nurse should examine any boundary crossing, be aware of its potential implica-

Box 9-2   Validation Remarks to Promote Patient Participation in Decisions

- Here's what I think; do you agree?
- What would you say is going on here?
- How is all of this affecting you?
- Does it seem that way to you? It does to me.
- Let's think about this together for a minute.
- Only you know your daily living situation.
- Can we find a way through this together?
- Let me explain my thinking to you.
- What do you think?
- Does this feel okay?
- Do you agree with this?
- This is what I'm thinking; what do you think?
- I'm interested in your take on all of this.
- If you could change this, what would be different?
- If you had a magic wand, what would you have it do?

Source: From Rubenfeld, M. G., & Scheffer, B. (2006). *Critical thinking tactics for nurses*. Sudbury, MA: Jones and Bartlett.

tions, and avoid repeated crossings. (For example, if a patient offers the nurse a gift, the nurse does not accept the gift. The nurse should analyze the situation and may consider discussing this with a supervisor, mentor, or colleague to get feedback).

- Variables such as the care setting, community influences, patient needs, and nature of therapy affect the delineation of boundaries (e.g., patients in mental health settings are particularly vulnerable to boundary issues, and nurses have to be clear about the boundaries).
- Actions that overstep established boundaries to meet the needs of the nurse are boundary violations (e.g., the nurse does not describe his or her personal problems to patients; does not accept money or individual gifts from patients; and does not give money or gifts to patients).
- The nurse should avoid situations where the nurse has a personal or business relationship,

Professional boundaries are the spaces between the nurse's power and the client's vulnerability. The power of the nurse comes from the professional position and the access to private knowledge about the client. Establishing boundaries allows the nurse to control this power differential and allow a safe connection to meet the client's needs.	Boundary violations can result when there is confusion between the needs of the nurse and those of the client. Such violations are characterized by excessive personal disclosure by the nurse, secrecy or even a reversal of roles. Boundary violations can cause distress for the client, which may not be recognized or felt by the client until harmful consequences occur.
Boundary crossings are brief excursions across boundaries that may be inadvertent, thoughtless or even purposeful if done to meet a special therapeutic need. Boundary crossings can result in a return to established boundaries but should be evaluated by the nurse for potential client consequences and implications. Repeated boundary crossings should be avoided.	Professional sexual misconduct is an extreme form of boundary violation and includes any behavior that is seductive, sexually demeaning, harassing or reasonably interpreted as sexual by the client. Professional sexual misconduct is an extremely serious violation of the nurse's professional responsibility to the client. It is a breach of trust.

Figure 9-4 Professional Boundaries: Definitions

Source: From National Council of State Boards of Nursing. (1996). *Professional boundaries: A nurses's guide to the importance of appropriate professional boundaries*. Chicago, IL: Author. Reprinted with permission.

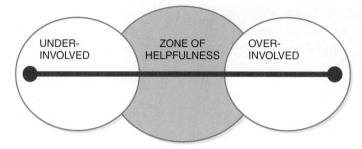

Figure 9-5 Continuum of Professional Behavior

as well as a professional one (e.g., the nurse should not date a patient; develop a friendship outside the nurse–patient relationship; or have a business transaction with a patient).

■ Post-termination relationships are complex because the patient may need additional services and it may be difficult to determine when the nurse–patient relationship is truly terminated (therefore, post-care personal relationships with patients are not recommended).

How does a nurse know that there may be a boundary violation with a patient? There are some red flags to watch for (Ohio Nursing Law, 2007):

■ Self-disclosure of one's own personal information to a patient

■ Secretive behavior between the nurse and a patient

■ "Super-nurse" behavior (the nurse thinks he or she is the only one who can care for the patient)

■ Special treatment by the nurse

■ Selective communication (not open communication)

■ "You and me against the world" thinking

■ Failure to protect the patient

All nurses need to watch for these red flags and respond to them by altering communication and behavior if boundary violation problems may be occurring.

Landscape © f9photos/Shutterstock, Inc.

CONCLUSION

This chapter discussed the first of the five IOM core competencies for healthcare providers: provide patient-centered care. Nurses work with patients with many different health problems and in many different settings. Through the nursing process, nurses need to consider how they can better provide patient-centered care. Such care puts the patient first and considers the patient's values, preferences, needs, culture, and background. The nurse–patient relationship can be an important element in supporting and recognizing the patient as the center of care. Nurses provide patient and family education to allow patients to more actively participate in their care and care decisions and to encourage effective self-management of health and illness.

CHAPTER HIGHLIGHTS

1. The IOM competency of "provide patient-centered care" refers to considering the patient's needs, cultural values, preferences, and unique situation instead of centering on the provider's prospective.

2. Four rules underpin patient-centered care: (1) care is based on continuous health relationships; (2) care customization is based on patient needs and preferences; (3) patients are the source of control; and (4) there is shared knowledge and free flow of information.

3. Patients who are involved in their care have better outcomes.

4. Examples of four nursing theories related to patient-centered care are Watson's theory on caring, Orem's self-care theory, Leininger's cultural diversity theory, and Peplau's interpersonal relations theory.

5. Macro consumers of health care are government and insurers.

6. Micro consumers of health care are the patient and family.

7. Patient satisfaction is a key factor that many healthcare institutions measure as a part of their delivery of care, although it is difficult to effectively quantify satisfaction.

8. The health disparities problem includes issues related access to care, level of care, and equality of care across races and ethnic groups.

9. Strategies to overcome disparities include addressing access-to-care issues, such as wait times,

appointment availability, and hours of service, to better meet the needs of the population served. Another strategy is to include patient values and preferences in the delivery of care.

10. Patient advocacy means the nurse is active in respecting patient rights and in ensuring that the patient has the education necessary to understand treatment and care needs.

11. Care coordination is a priority of the IOM's perspective on high-quality, patient-centered care, but it is an aspect of care that is not generally reimbursable. Interprofessional teamwork is an important part of coordination.

12. Clinical reasoning is different from critical thinking. It focuses on putting the care needs within the context that the patient presents—environment, values, and preferences—as gathered in the assessment.

13. The nursing process is a systematic method for thinking about and communicating how nurses provide patient care.

14. A concept map care plan is a diagram of patient problems and interventions that offers a more interactive plan than the traditional care plan.

15. Healthcare literacy includes reading, writing, and arithmetic skills; listening and speaking ability; and conceptual knowledge. Lack of healthcare literacy can present a barrier to care because patients may not understand aspects of their care.

16. A professional boundary is an invisible line that places limits on a nurse's behavior.

DISCUSSION QUESTIONS

1. What does *patient-centered care* mean, and why is it relevant to nursing?
2. Describe a nursing theory that relates to patient-centered care.
3. How is diversity related to patient-centered care?
4. Explain consumerism in health care and its relevance to nursing.

(continues)

DISCUSSION QUESTIONS (CONTINUED)

5. Describe healthcare disparity and its importance.
6. What is health literacy?
7. Why is patient advocacy important?
8. Compare and contrast the nursing process, nursing care plan, and concept mapping.

9. What is the relationship between care coordination and delegation?
10. What is self-management of care?
11. Discuss the importance of patient education.

CRITICAL THINKING ACTIVITIES

1. The Guidance for the National Healthcare Disparities Report (Institute of Medicine, 2002b) (http://www.nap.edu/openbook.php?record_id=10512) outlines the annual National Healthcare Disparities Report (http://www.innovations.ahrq.gov/content.aspx?id=4008). This report tracks four measurements: (1) socioeconomic status, (2) access to the healthcare system, (3) healthcare services and quality, and (4) geographic disparities in health care. Go to the site. What can you learn about disparities in health care? Summarize a key point related to each of the four measurements.

2. The Provider's Guide to Quality and Culture is an extensive compendium of information about diversity. Review one of the sections on this site that interests you (http://erc.msh.org/mainpage.cfm?file=1.0.htm&module=provider&language=English). (When you get to the end of the screen, note whether there is a "next" page noted; if so, click to continue the selected section.) In the content you reviewed, what is relevant to your view of nursing?

3. Watch an episode of a favorite TV show, including the commercials, if there are any. This program does not have to be a health-related TV show. As you watch the show, keep notes describing ethnic, racial, and culture issues that arise. Note who is playing which types of the roles. Also note the communication, clothing, attitudes, values, and any other factors related to diversity. Do the same for the commercials. Share your findings in an online course discussion forum.

4. Clearly and briefly respond to the following questions:
   a. How would you describe yourself ethnically/racially/culturally? Has your view of ethnicity/race/culture changed over time? If so, how?
   b. Describe the racial or ethnic group to which you belong.
   c. Do you think people are treated differently because of race or ethnicity? If so, describe an example.
   d. Have you been treated differently because of your own ethnicity or race? If so, how?
   e. When did you first become aware that people were different ethnically or racially?

5. If you were a member of a minority group, would you want to have a healthcare professional who is a member of that minority group care for you? Why?

6. Review the material on health literacy found at the following site: http://nnlm.gov/outreach/consumer/hlthlit.html. Discuss the identified vulnerable populations and their relevance to health literacy with a team.

7. Learn more about critical thinking by visiting these pages on the The Critical Thinking Community's website: Mission Statement (http://www.criticalthinking.org/pages/our-mission/599) and the Center for Critical Thinking (http://www.criticalthinking.org/pages/center-for-critical-thinking/401#3135). Describe how you might apply some of this information to your own critical thinking.

Landscape © f9photos/Shutterstock, Inc.

CRITICAL THINKING ACTIVITIES (CONTINUED)

8. Visit the Joint Commission website (http://www.jointcommission.org) and learn what this organization emphasizes regarding diversity in health care. What can you learn that might help you be more culturally competent? How does information like this improve health care?

9. Divide into teams. Have each team member review one of the following topics:

   a. What do healthcare consumers need to know about racial and ethnic disparities in health care? Search for information on the Internet and/or read commentary from the IOM's report, *What Health Care Consumers Need to Know About Racial and Ethnic Disparities in Healthcare* (http://www.iom.edu/Reports/2002/Unequal-Treatment-Confronting-Racial-and-Ethnic-Disparities-in-Health-Care/Report-Brief-What-Health-Care-Consumers-Need-to-Know-About-Racial-and-Ethnic-Disparities-in-Healthcare-PDF.aspx).

   b. What do healthcare system administrators need to know about racial and ethnic disparities in health care? Search for information on the Internet and/or read commentary from the IOM's report, *What Health Care Administrators Need to Know About Racial and Ethnic Disparities in Healthcare* (http://www.iom.edu/Reports/2002/Unequal-Treatment-Confronting-Racial-and-Ethnic-Disparities-in-Health-Care/Report-Brief--What-Health-Care-System-Administrators-Need-to-Know-About-Racial-and-Ethnic-Disparities-in-Healthcare-PDF.aspx).

   c. What do healthcare providers need to know about racial and ethnic disparities in healthcare? Find commentary in the report, *Unequal Treatment: Confronting Racial and Ethnic Disparities in Health Care* (http://www.nap.edu/openbook.php?record_id=10260&page=1).

   Discuss your findings together, noting similarities and differences with consumers, healthcare system administrators, and providers.

ELECTRONIC *Reflection Journal*

Circuit Board: ©Photos.com

In your journal, describe your personal views of patient-centered care and explain how your views might impact the care you provide. Design a concept map to provide a visual illustration of your views.

Landscape © f9photos/Shutterstock, Inc.

LINKING TO THE INTERNET

- Center for Nursing Classification: http://www.ncvhs.hhs.gov/970416w6.htm
- Commonwealth Fund: Health Care Disparities:
  http://www.commonwealthfund.org/Program-Areas/Archived-Programs/Health-Care-Disparities.aspx
- National Center for Complementary and Alternative Medicine: http://nccam.nih.gov/
- National Council State Boards of Nursing: https://www.ncsbn.org/index.htm
- National Disparities Report: http://www.innovations.ahrq.gov/content.aspx?id=4008

(continues)

Landscape © f9photos/Shutterstock, Inc.

LINKING TO THE INTERNET (CONTINUED)

- Department of Health and Human Services: Minority Health: http://minorityhealth.hhs.gov/
- NANDA International: http://www.nanda.org/
- Planetree Institute: http://www.planetree.org
- Press Ganey: Partners in Improvement: http://www.pressganey.com/
- Professional Patient Advocate Institute: http://www.patientadvocatetraining.com
- Six Sigma: http://www.sixsigmaonline.org/index.html
- Cultural Diversity Resources: http://www.aarc.org/resources/cultural_diversity/tools.cfm
- Patient Satisfaction: http://www.qualitymeasures.ahrq.gov/content.aspx?id=26774
- National Partnership for Action: http://minorityhealth.hhs.gov/npa/
- National Quality Forum: Cultural Competency Standards:
  http://www.qualityforum.org/projects/cultural_competency.aspx

CASE STUDIES

Case Study 1

A 45-year-old woman fell during an ice storm. She went to the emergency department because she thought she may have broken one or more ribs. When the X-ray results came back, the physician told the patient and her husband that they showed a carcinoid tumor in one lung. The patient had never smoked and was healthy. There was no history of lung cancer in her family. The couple left devastated, with a list of specialists for follow-up. They spent 3 weeks in testing. Both the patient and her husband assumed from the term *carcinoid* that the patient had malignant lung cancer. The patient and her husband had college degrees and held management positions. The physician in the emergency department did not discuss what "carcinoid" meant. The couple's anxiety rose with each passing day. At a later appointment, it became evident that the couple was not clear on what "carcinoid" meant and that the couple's interpretation included more life-threatening implications than necessary.

What does *carcinoid* mean? The National Cancer Institute (NCI) in the National Institutes of Health (NIH) defines "carcinoid" as a slow-growing type of tumor usually found in the gastrointestinal system (most often in the appendix) and sometimes in the lungs or other sites. Carcinoid tumors may spread to the liver or other sites in the body, and they may secrete substances such as serotonin or prostaglandins, causing carcinoid syndrome. This patient's tumor was localized, and it was removed.

Case Questions

1. What do you see in this case that could have been done differently?
2. Which role might a nurse have played, and what specifically might the nurse have done?
3. Is this an example of health literacy? If so, how is it an example?
4. How might patient-centered care be applied to this case? Be specific.

CASE STUDIES (CONTINUED)

Case Study 2

A nurse on a medical unit was caring for an elderly woman. The patient's family visited frequently. The nurse, patient, and family spent a lot of time together, and the nurse was very helpful to the family. The nurse had shared that her husband was out of work and her family was experiencing a difficult time. Her husband had applied for a job at many businesses, and it turned out that one of the businesses was owned by the patient's son-in-law. He was never called for an interview.

After the patient left the hospital, the family sent flowers to the nurse that were delivered to the unit where she worked. The nurse was surprised and happy to receive the flowers, which she took home. A week later, her husband received a call for an interview at the business owned by the patient's son-in-law; he received a job offer one week later. The couple was very happy.

Case Questions

1. How were professional boundaries crossed in this case?
2. Describe how this case relates to nurse–patient (and family) relationships as described in this chapter.
3. What should the nurse have done when she experienced issues related to boundaries?

Words of Wisdom

© Roobcio/Shutterstock, Inc.

Josepha Campinha-Bacote, PhD, MAR, APRN, BC, CNS, CTN, FAAN
President, Transcultural C.A.R.E. Associates

The literature clearly reveals a strong relationship between patient-centered care and culturally competent care, for both concepts center on the core essential of respecting and incorporating the patient's worldview into the delivery of care. The concept of culture and its relationship to health is critical to comprehend, for cultural values give an individual a sense of direction and meaning to life. One of the most influential factors for understanding an individual's health behaviors and practices is to understand his or her worldview. Compelling research and documentation support that a lack of cultural competence among healthcare professionals can result in poor health outcomes. Therefore, to have a positive impact on health outcomes, nurses must engage in the process of becoming culturally competent. Culturally competent nursing care can be viewed as the ongoing process in which the nurse continuously strives to achieve the ability and availability to work effectively within the cultural context of the patient (individual, family, community). Cultural competence, like patient-centered care, will render quality patient care that is individualized and equitable.

Landscape © f9photos/Shutterstock, Inc.

REFERENCES

Agency for Healthcare Research and Quality (AHRQ). (2011). Low health literacy linked to higher risk of death and more emergency room visits and hospitalizations. Retrieved from http://www.ahrq.gov

American Association of Colleges of Nursing (AACN). (2014). Enhancing diversity in the workplace. Retrieved from http://www.aacn.nche.edu/media-relations/fact-sheets/enhancing-diversity

American Organization of Nurse Executives (AONE). (2007). AONE guiding principle for diversity in health care organizations. Retrieved from http://www.aone.org

Anderson, L., Scrimshaw, S., Fullilove, M., Fielding, J., & Normand, J. (2003). Culturally competent healthcare systems: A systematic review. *American Journal of Preventive Medicine, 24*(3S), 68–79.

Balik, B., Conway, J., Zipperer, J., & Watson, J. (2011). *Achieving an exceptional patient and family experience of inpatient hospital care.* IHI Innovation Series white paper. Cambridge, MA: Institute for Healthcare Improvement. Retrieved from http://www.ihi.org/resources/Pages/IHIWhitePapers/AchievingExceptionalPatientFamilyExperienceInpatientHospitalCareWhitePaper.aspx

Benner, P., Sutphen, M., Leonard, V., & Day, L. (2010). *Educating nurses: A call for radical transformation.* San Francisco, CA: Jossey-Bass.

Benner, P., Tanner, C., & Chesla, C. (1996). *Expertise in nursing practice: Caring, clinical judgment and ethics.* New York, NY: Springer.

Boodman, S. (2007, February 20). A silent epidemic. *Washington Post.* Retrieved from http://www.washingtonpost.com/wp-dyn/content/article/2007/02/16/AR2007021602260.html

Centers for Disease Control and Prevention (CDC). (2012). Centers for Disease Control and Prevention health disparities and inequalities report—United States 2012. Retrieved from http://www.cdc.gov

Commonwealth Fund. (2008). Patient-centered care: An overview. Retrieved from http://www.commonwealthfund.org/Program-Areas/Archived-Programs/Delivery-System-Innovation-and-Improvement/Patient-Centered-Coordinated-Care.aspx

Davis, K., Schoenbaum, S., & Audet, A. (2005). A 2020 vision of patient-centered primary care. *Journal of General Internal Medicine, 15,* 953–957.

Del Bueno, D. (2005). A crisis in critical thinking. *Nursing Education Perspectives, 26,* 278–282.

Finkelman, A. (2001, December). Problem-solving, decision-making, and critical thinking: How do they mix and why bother? *Home Care Provider,* 194–199.

Finkelman, A., & Kenner, C. (2012). *Teaching IOM: Implications of the Institute of Medicine reports for nursing education* (3rd ed.). Silver Spring, MD: American Nurses Association.

Gerteis, M., Edgman-Levitan, S., Daley, J., & Delbanco, T. (Eds.). (1993). *Through the patient's eyes.* San Francisco, CA: Jossey-Bass.

Hagenow, N. (2003). Why not person-centered care? The challenges of implementation. *Nursing Administration Quarterly, 27,* 203–207.

Halpern, R., Lee, M., Boulter, P., & Phillips, R. (2001). A synthesis of nine major reports on physicians competencies for the emerging practice environment. *Academic Medicine, 76,* 606–615.

Hochbaum, G. (1958). *Public participation in medical screening programs: A sociological study.* Public Health Service Publication No. 572. Washington, DC: U.S. Government Printing Office.

Institute of Medicine (IOM). (1999). *To err is human.* Washington, DC: National Academies Press.

Institute of Medicine (IOM). (2001). *Crossing the quality chasm: A new health system for the 21st century.* Washington, DC: National Academies Press.

Institute of Medicine (IOM). (2002). *Guidance for the national healthcare disparities report.* Washington, DC: National Academies Press.

Institute of Medicine (IOM). (2003a). *Health professions education.* Washington, DC: National Academies Press.

Institute of Medicine (IOM). (2003b). *Unequal treatment.* Washington, DC: National Academies Press.

Institute of Medicine (IOM). (2004). *Health literacy: A prescription to end confusion.* Washington, DC: National Academies Press.

Joint Commission. (2008). Facts and figures. Retrieved from http://www.jointcommission.org/NewsRoom/PressKits/Health_Literacy/facts_figures.htm

Knowles, M. (1972). *The modern practice of adult education.* New York, NY: Associated Press.

Leebov, W. (2008). Beyond customer service. *American Nurse Today, 3*(1), 21–23.

Lewin, S., Skea, Z., Entwistle, V., Zwarenstein, M., & Dick, J. (2001). Interventions for providers to promote a patient-centered approach to clinical consultations. *Cochrane Database System Review, 4,* CD003267.

Masters, K. (2009). *Role development in professional nursing practice* (2nd ed.). Sudbury, MA: Jones and Bartlett.

National Council of State Boards of Nursing (NCSBN). (1996). *Professional boundaries: A nurse's guide to the importance of appropriate professional boundaries.* Chicago, IL: Author.

National Council of State Boards of Nursing (NCSBN). (2013). Supplement: The National Council of State Boards of Nursing and the Forum of State Nursing Workforce Centers 2013 national workforce survey of registered nurses. *Journal of Nursing Regulation, 4*(2), S1–S72.

North American Nursing Diagnosis Association (NANDA). (2011). Nursing diagnoses: Definitions and classification. Retrieved from http://nanda.org

Ohio Nursing Law. (2007, December 2). *2006 Ohio nursing law program-boundaries* (Vol. *4*). Columbus, OH: Ohio Board of Nursing.

Parker, D. (2006). Establishing a passion for nursing: The role of the nurse leader. *Nurse Leader, 4*(5), 28–32.

Peters, K. & Elster, A. (2002). *Roadmaps for clinical practice: A primer on population-based medicine*. Chicago, IL: American Medical Association.

Pew Health Professions Commission. (1995). *Critical challenges: Revitalizing the health professions for the twenty-first century.* San Francisco, CA: UCSF Center for the Health Professions.

Planetree Institute. (n.d.). About Planetree. Retrieved from http://planetree.org/about-planetree/

Rubenfeld, M., & Scheffer, B. (2006). *Critical thinking tactics for nurses*. Sudbury, MA: Jones and Bartlett.

Schuster, P. (2007). *Concept mapping: A critical thinking approach to care planning*. Philadelphia, PA: Davis.

Shaller, D. (2007). *Patient-centered care: What does it take?* New York, NY: Commonwealth Fund. Retrieved from http://www.-commonwealthfund.org/publications/publications_show.htm?doc_id=559715

Stewart, M. (2001). Towards a global definition of patient-centered care. *British Medical Journal, 322*(7284), 444–445.

Sullivan, L. (2004). *Missing persons: Minorities in the health professions: A report of the Sullivan Commission on diversity in the healthcare workforces*. Washington, DC: Sullivan Commission on Diversity in the Healthcare Workforce.

Travelbee, J. (1971). *Interpersonal aspects of nursing*. Philadelphia, PA: Davis.

University of Iowa, College of Nursing. (2011). Center for Nursing Classification and Clinical Effectiveness. Retrieved from http://www.nursing.uiowa.edu/excellence/nursing_knowledge/clinical_effectiveness/index.htm

U.S. Census Bureau. (2011). Minorities. Retrieved from http://www.census.gov/

U.S. Census Bureau. (2012). 2012 census. Retrieved from http://www.census.gov/newsroom/releases/archives/population/cb13-112.html

U.S. Department of Health and Human Services (HHS). (2008a). The Office of Minority Health. Retrieved from http://minorityhealth.hhs.gov/

U.S. Department of Health and Human Services (HHS). (2008b). National Partnership for Action to End Healthcare Disparities. Retrieved from http://minorityhealth.hhs.gov/npa/

U.S. Department of Health and Human Services (HHS). (2010). *Healthy people 2020*. Washington, DC: U.S. Government Printing Office.

U.S. Department of Health and Human Services (HHS), Agency for Health Research and Quality (AHRQ). (2010). National healthcare quality and disparities reports. Retrieved from http://www.ahrq.gov/qual/qrdr10.htm

U.S. Department of Health and Human Services (HHS), Centers for Medicare and Medicaid Services. (2013). HCAHPS: Patients' Perspectives of Care survey. Retrieved from http://www.cms.gov/Medicare/Quality-Initiatives-Patient-Assessment-Instruments/HospitalQualityInits/HospitalHCAHPS.html

Zimmerman, P. (2001). The problems with healthcare customer satisfaction surveys. In J. Dochterman & H. Grace (Eds.), *Current issues in nursing* (6th ed., pp. 255–260). St. Louis, MO: Mosby.

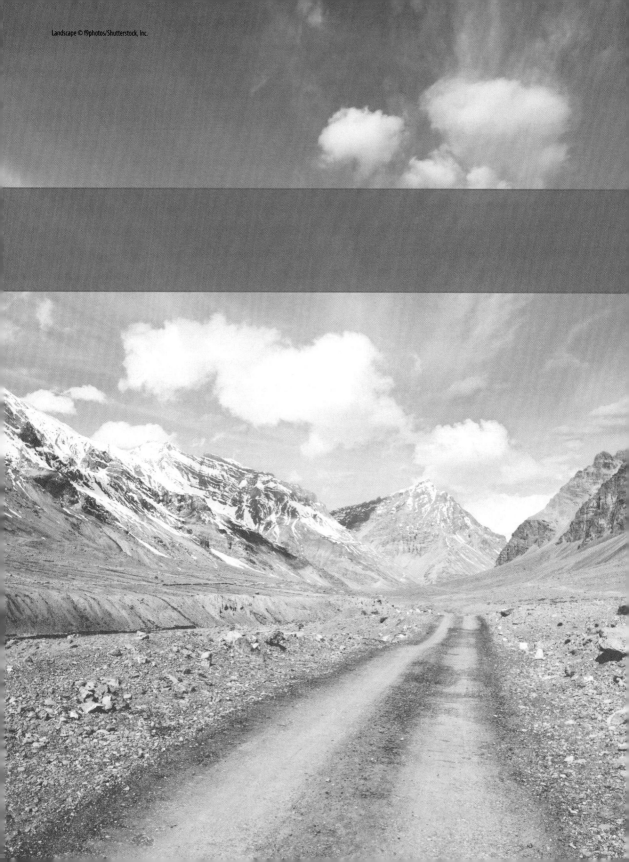

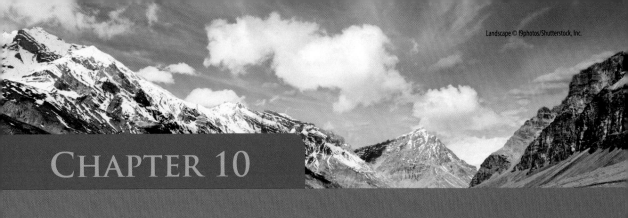

CHAPTER 10

Work in Interprofessional Teams

CHAPTER OBJECTIVES

At the conclusion of this chapter, the learner will be able to:

- Discuss the Institute of Medicine competency: work in interprofessional teams
- Define teamwork and types of teams
- Describe effective team functioning
- Discuss communication and its relationship to patient care and teams
- Examine collaboration and its relationship to patient care and teams

- Explain how coordination relates to patient care and teams
- Analyze the change process and implications for health care and teams
- Apply the delegation process
- Explain conflict and conflict resolution

CHAPTER OUTLINE

CHAPTER OUTLINE (CONTINUED)

KEY TERMS

Collaboration
Communication
Conflict
Conflict resolution
Coordination
Delegatee
Delegation
Delegator

Empowerment
Followers
Handoffs
Interprofessional team-based
  care
Interprofessional teamwork
Microsystem
Plan–do–study–act cycle (PDSA)

Power
Situation–background–
  assessment–recommendations
  (SBAR)
Team
Team leader
Teamwork
Types of power

INTRODUCTION

This chapter focuses on working in teams—both nursing teams and interprofessional teams. This is a critical competency for every nurse. The content includes an explanation of the Institute of Medicine (IOM) core competency, teams and teamwork, and critical components of effective teams: communication, collaboration, and coordination. Communication is a critical element of both collaboration and coordination. In addition, delegation is a part of the daily work for every nurse and is part of planning care and **teamwork**. Teams must cope with change and learn to make effective change decisions. The last topic in the chapter is conflict and conflict resolution—resolving issues to improve teamwork. Teams need to recognize the importance of patient-centered care and appreciate how the patient participates in the healthcare team. Through

its assessment of the U.S. healthcare system, the IOM (2001) has determined that the system

is in need of fundamental change. Many patients, doctors, nurses and healthcare leaders are concerned that the care delivered is not, essentially, the care we should receive. The frustration levels of both patients and clinicians have probably never been higher. Yet the problems remain. Healthcare today harms too frequently and routinely fails to deliver its potential benefits. (p. 1)

Technology and new drugs, among many other care advances, can improve health and health care, but something is wrong with the care delivery models. This set of problems is what the IOM is most concerned about, and what has resulted in the focus on core competencies. This chapter looks at the core competency that most directly addresses the need for

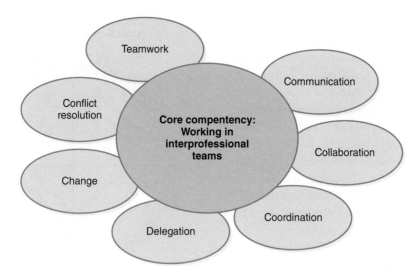

Figure 10-1 Working Interdisciplinary Teams: Key Elements

changes in the care delivery models. **Figure 10-1** highlights the key elements for this competency.

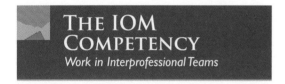

THE IOM COMPETENCY
Work in Interprofessional Teams

The first of the IOM healthcare professions core competencies is "provide patient-centered care." This chapter covers the second core competency, "work in interprofessional teams." The IOM (2003a) describes this competency as follows: "co-operate, collaborate, communicate, and integrate care in teams to ensure that care is continuous and reliable" (p. 4). As a reminder, these core competencies were developed for all healthcare professions, not just nursing; however, this chapter focuses on nurses who are members of interprofessional teams and also members of nursing teams. The IOM (2003b) further supports the need for effective interprofessional needs by identifying care coordination as one of the 20 priority areas of care.

One has to ask why there is such emphasis on this core competency. After all, it makes sense that teams are important—why would anyone question this? The critical issue is whether healthcare professionals are prepared to participate effectively in teams, particularly interprofessional teams. The IOM has concluded that they are not. Healthcare professional education takes place in isolation; each healthcare profession provides its own education, with limited reference to other healthcare professionals. The result is that nursing, medical, pharmacy, and allied health students (e.g., physical therapists, occupational therapists, and so on) have limited, if any, contact with one another in their educational programs (Finkelman & Kenner, 2012; Interprofessional Education Collaborative Expert Panel, 2011). As a consequence, they have limited knowledge of roles of the other professions and the ways in which they must collaborate and coordinate care to provide patient-centered care. This is a serious problem because when healthcare professionals graduate and meet licensure requirements, they are expected to work together—"deliberately working together with the common goal of building a safer and better patient-centered and community/population oriented U.S. healthcare system" (Interprofessional Education Collaborative Expert Panel, 2011, p. 3). The IOM states that at present there is limited effective interprofessional teamwork.

In addition, nurses need to know how to work with nursing teams whose focus is nursing care. In most cases, this, too, leads to isolation and limited recognition of the need for greater reaching out to other healthcare disciplines. Nurses tend to focus on the nursing care plan to the detriment of the total plan of care for the patient—a nursing care plan, as opposed to a patient-centered care plan. Nursing education reinforces this perspective by emphasizing just the nursing care plan. This is not to say that the same scenario does not exist in other healthcare professions, because it does. Nursing students need a broader view of health care along with the nursing perspective (Barnsteiner, Disch, Hall, Mayer, & Moore, 2007). Nurses also work together on teams related to service, such as committees and task forces. These teams require the same competencies as teams focused on patient care.

All healthcare providers should be focused on delivering patient-centered care—care that "alleviates vulnerability in all of its forms. That care should and must be delivered at the right time, at the right level, in the right place, and so on. If care were on a compass it would be true north and all other functions would stand in line to provide added value and service to that focus" (Hagenow, 2003, p. 204). Interprofessional teams are best suited to achieve this patient-centered care, because one individual healthcare profession cannot do it all alone.

Figure 10-2 describes the interprofessional collaborative practice core competency domains that support the World Health Organization (WHO) perspective on the need for and impact of interprofessional education that leads to effective interprofessional teams, which is also supported by the Interprofessional Education Collaborative Expert Panel (2011).

Interprofessional Collaborative Practice Core Competency Domains

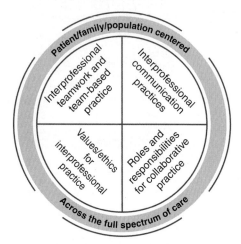

The learning continuum

Figure 10-2 Interprofessional Collaborative Practice Core Competency Domains

Source: © American Association of Colleges of Nursing, American Association of Colleges of Osteopathic Medicine, American Association of Colleges of Pharmacy, American Dental Education Association, Association of American Medical Colleges, and Association of Schools of Public Health. (2011).

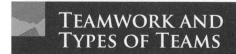

TEAMWORK AND TYPES OF TEAMS

According to the IOM (2003a):

An interdisciplinary/interprofessional team is composed of members from different professions and occupations with varied and specialized knowledge, skills, and methods. The team members integrate their observations, bodies of expertise, and spheres of decision making to coordinate, collaborate, and communicate with one another in order to optimize care for a patient or group of patients. (p. 54)

This definition is further supported in recent work that examined the need for greater interprofessional education and identified two key definitions:

Interprofessional teamwork: The levels of cooperation, coordination, and collaboration characterizing the relationship between professions in delivering patient-centered care.

Interprofessional team-based care: Care delivered by intentionally created, usually relatively small work groups in health care, who are recognized by others as well as by themselves as having a collective identity and shared responsibility for a patient or a group of patients, e.g., rapid response team, palliative care team, primary care team, operating room team. (Interprofessional Education Collaborative Expert Panel, 2011, p. 2)

With the increasing complexity of care and concerns about the fragmented healthcare system, interprofessional teams are becoming even more important. In addition to the complex needs of patients with chronic illness, providing critical acute care, geriatric care, and care at the end of life requires effective planning to ensure improved outcomes. The patients who require such care have multiple, complex needs. The types of settings, complexity of settings, and great need to share information and planning across settings require more teamwork. As noted by the IOM (2003a), use of interprofessional teams tends to result in improved quality and a decrease in healthcare costs.

Throughout this content, when the term **team** is used, it applies to both interprofessional teams and nursing staff teams. Nurses are members of interprofessional teams and also members of nursing teams (nursing teams include nursing staff such as registered nurses (RNs), licensed practical/vocational nurses, and unlicensed assistive personnel [UAP]). In this chapter, we will discuss the importance of teams in health care.

Clarification of Terms

The IOM used the term *interdisciplinary* in its report (IOM, 2003a), although recently the more widely accepted term has been *interprofessional*; however, in the literature and in practice, nurses encounter other terms that seem similar, such as *multidisciplinary*. Interdisciplinary/interprofessional "refers to people with distinct disciplinary training working together for a common purpose, as they make different, complementary contributions to patient-focused-care" (McCallin, 2001, p. 419). Multidisciplinary refers to "a team or collaborative process where members of different disciplines assess or treat patients independently and then share information with each other" (p. 420). The key difference between these two descriptors for teams is that multidisciplinary focuses on how individual team members do their work but encourages sharing of information with others who are providing care. For example, nurses share information about the nursing care plan with physicians and social workers, and vice versa. This typically is what has been done in health care, but it is not what the IOM recommends in this core competency. The descriptor interdisciplinary/interprofessional is much more involved, and emphasizes collective action and in-depth collaboration in planning and implementing care. Less emphasis is placed on what individual team members do, and more emphasis is placed on what individual members can do together to contribute to the joint team plan and initiatives. **Table 10-1** compares multidisciplinary, interdisciplinary, and interprofessional teams.

Use of interprofessional teams provides the following advantages:

- Decreased fragmentation in a complex care system
- Effective use of multiple types of expertise (e.g., medicine, nursing, pharmacy, allied health, social work, and so on)
- Decreased utilization of repetitive or duplicate services
- Increased creative or innovative solutions to complex problems
- Increased learning for team members about different roles and responsibilities, communication and coordination, and ways to better plan care

Table 10-1	Comparison of Multidisciplinary, Interdisciplinary, and Interprofessional Teams		
	Multidisciplinary Teams (adapted from Siegler, 1998)	**Interdisciplinary Teams (adapted from Siegler, 1998)**	**Interprofessional Teams (adapted from Simpson et al., 2001)**
Membership	Professionals from a variety of disciplines	All necessary disciplines	A partnership among professionals, individuals, families, and communities
Sources of information	Members contribute information from their own area of expertise within the roles of their specific discipline	Patients and/or significant others provide information along with members of the disciplines	Patients and/or significant others, along with members of the disciplines related to the patient's care, provide information
Leadership	Leadership and membership are fixed	Leadership and membership vary depending on the situation	Leadership is based on expertise that matches the situation
Decision making	One person makes the final treatment decisions	All members work together to come up with both alternative solutions and final decisions	Responsibility for decision making and problem solving is shared
Focus of care	Task orientation	Collaboration to see the bigger picture	A shared biopsychosocial paradigm

Source: From Rubenfeld, M. G., & Scheffer, B. (2006). *Critical thinking tactics for nurses.* Sudbury, MA: Jones and Bartlett.

- Provision of motivation and increased self-esteem in team and individual performance
- Greater sharing of responsibility
- Empowerment of members to speak up

Microsystem

Another way to describe the clinical team is to refer to it as a **microsystem** (Nelson et al., 2008). A microsystem in a healthcare system has been described as follows:

[A] small group of people who work together on a regular basis to provide care to discrete subpopulations including the patients. It has clinical and business aims, linked processes, [and a] shared information environment and produces performance

outcomes. [Microsystems] evolve over time and are (often) embedded in larger organizations. As a type of complex adaptive system, they must: (1) do the work, (2) meet staff needs, and (3) maintain themselves as a clinical unit. Clinical microsystems are the front-line units that provide most health care to most people. They are the places where patients, families, and care teams meet. Microsystems also include support staff, processes, technology, and recurring patterns of information, behavior, and results. Central to every clinical microsystem is the patient. Microsystems are the building blocks that form hospitals (Dartmouth College, 2010).

The microsystem is the place where:

- Care is provided.
- Quality, safety, reliability, efficiency, and innovation are critical elements.
- Staff morale and patient satisfaction are important aspects of the culture.

Team Leadership

Teams typically have designated **team leaders**. For a nursing team, the leader is an RN. Interprofessional teams may have different leaders, and in some cases, the leader may be a nurse. Regardless of who is the leader, all team members are critical to the success of a team. To be effective, a team leader must first recognize that it is the work of the team that is critical. The leader should not focus on personal success as a leader or on the success of any one team member. This is not always easy to do, but truly effective team leaders shine through the effectiveness of the entire team.

Leaders need to know when to guide, when to let the team function, and when to be directive. If the team is on task as planned, direction is not as critical. In contrast, if the team is floundering and not able to get work done, the leader needs to be more active in directing the team, engaging the team to assume more responsibility. Leaders need to encourage and accept members' ideas and actively seek information and ideas from team members. Some of the responsibilities of team leaders are as follows:

- Lead the team—at meetings and in the team's work.
- Determine or clarify the team's purpose and operating rules or guidelines. Some of this may be predetermined by the organization.
- Select team members. In many cases, selection of members is done by someone other than the team leader or by the structure; for example, team members may be assigned to a unit or a particular patient.
- Orient team members to the team, including coaching and training new members.

- Determine the plan of action with team members' participation. After the team reviews information, discusses issues, and arrives at team decisions, the team leader ensures that there is an effective plan of action. If it is a clinical team, keep the focus on the patient(s).
- Determine how to make the team more effective given the time constraints.
- Provide resources and information for the team as needed.
- Update the team as necessary.
- Ensure that the team's plan of action is implemented as designed.
- Recognize the team's work as well as the work of individuals.
- Resolve conflict when it occurs.
- Evaluate the team's outcomes and include input from all team members; strive for improvement.
- Encourage team learning to improve effectiveness.
- Ensure that required information about team functioning, decisions, and actions implemented is documented.
- Accept feedback from team members and others who may be involved.
- Provide feedback to team members and the team as a whole.
- Ensure that the team effectively uses collaboration, coordination, and delegation.

An important role for team leaders is to lead the team's activities, and much of this is done through team discussion. The process of leading discussion can be informal or formal. When the team leader seeks out individual team members to discuss team issues and the team's work, this is informal discussion. In this situation, the leader is seeking an open discussion of issues and sharing of ideas. Such an exchange can help the leader to better understand team members and to identify the issues. Informal discussion can be used for the team members to get to know the leader on a different level.

The term *team* does not include the letter *I*, and this is important to note. Teams are about groups of people who work collaboratively, not about individuals. However, it takes effort and time to move a team to a state where it is truly functioning as a team and not as a group of individuals (Weinstock, 2010). The most common scenario is that the team members work in "silos" most of the time and then come together periodically to collaborate and communicate. Unfortunately, this pattern leads to problems and errors. The development of a team is critical to the success of new and innovative interventions such as briefings before **handoffs**, checklists, and time-outs before surgery, such as the SBAR technique, TeamSTEPPS, and others. Organizations that just use these interventions without working on developing teams will not be as successful, but using them in combination with teamwork creates a more effective organization and improved care outcomes. Some of these methods are described next:

SBAR

The **situation–background–assessment–recommendations (SBAR)** method is used to improve team communication dealing with critical information about a patient that requires immediate attention and action. To ensure more effective communication, a consistent process is used that includes the following steps (Institute for Health Improvement, 2011b):

> **S**ituation: What is going on with the patient?
> **B**ackground: What is the clinical background or context?
> **A**ssessment: What do I think the problem is?
> **R**ecommendation: What would I do to correct it?

This process includes the call-out and the check-back. The call-out is used to communicate important or critical information that lets all team members hear the information at the same time and clarifies responsibilities. The check-back provides assurance that the team members heard and understood the information from the sender. **Exhibit 10-1** offers an example of SBAR in action.

Mindful Communication

Mindful communication is a process by which actively aware individuals engage in communication

---

Exhibit 10-1   SBAR Example

This is an example of how SBAR might be used to focus a telephone call between a nurse and a physician. The nurse would not wait for the physician to ask these questions, but rather would routinely provide the information in clear statements as indicated by SBAR.

Situation: *What is going on with the patient?*

A nurse finds a patient on the floor. She calls the doctor: "I am the charge nurse on the night shift on 5 West. I am calling about Mrs. Jones. She was found on the floor and is complaining of pain in her hip."

Background: *What is the clinical background or context?*

"The patient is a 75-year-old woman who was admitted for pneumonia yesterday. She did not complain of hip pain before being found on the floor."

Assessment: *What do I think the problem is?*

"I think the fall may have caused an injury. Her pain is level 9 out of 10."

Recommendation: *What would I do to correct it or respond to it?*

"I think we need to get an X-ray immediately and have her seen by the orthopedic resident."

that is meaningful, that is timely, and that responds continually as events unfold (Anthony & Vidal, 2010; O'Keefe & Saver, 2014, p. 9).

Describe–Express–Suggest–Consequences Scripts

Describe–express–suggest–consequences (DESC) is an approach for approaching a conflict (Agency for Healthcare Research and Quality [AHRQ], 2008; O'Keefe & Saver, 2014, p. 12). The goal is to arrive at consensus and keep the discussion on track. The DESC script includes the following elements:

- **D**escribe the specific conflict situation or behavior using concrete data.
- **E**xpress how the situation made you feel or identify your concerns.
- **S**uggest alternatives and seek agreement.
- State **c**onsequences in terms of effects on team goals; strive for **c**onsensus.

TeamSTEPPS

TeamSTEPPS is an evidence-based teamwork system aimed at optimizing patient outcomes by improving communication and teamwork skills among healthcare professionals. It includes a comprehensive set of ready-to-use materials and a training curriculum to successfully integrate teamwork principles into any healthcare system (AHRQ, 2011). (See "Linking to the Internet" at the end of the chapter for more information.). **Figure 10-3** describes the TeamSTEPPS model.

Checklists

Dr. Atul Gawande (2009) wrote *The Checklist Manifesto* to address safety in the surgical arena. His document mandates that all staff who work in the surgical arena must follow a checklist. This checklist itemizes a list of activities that must be examined by the team before surgery takes place to ensure clear communication and certainty about actions to be taken. Gawande based his work on the checklist approach used by pilots to ensure safety during takeoff, landing, and during other critical points in a flight.

Formal Team Meetings

Formal meetings are an important part of teamwork, and the team leader or someone designated by the leader usually leads these meetings. Formal meetings can be held in a variety of settings. The most common site is a conference room in the healthcare setting. The setting should be private and conducive to fostering communication. Space should be provided for team members to sit and take notes. In clinical settings, telephone access is important, although members should be encouraged to keep interruptions to a minimum.

Another method for conducting meetings today is virtual conferencing, including conference calls, video conferencing, and even Internet conferencing. These methods also require planning and equipment. Members must be informed about access requirements, and technological support may be needed to assist with possible connection problems.

The following guide recommends steps for conducting formal meetings:

1. *Planning the meeting:* Planning before the meeting is important. Avoid scheduling meetings just to have a meeting. Time is too limited. Staff will be reluctant to attend and may not be productive in meetings that they feel are not worthwhile. Prior to completing the final agenda, the leader can survey members via e-mail for additional agenda items.
2. *Steps prior to the meeting:* Arrange for meeting space. Send out the agenda, any necessary handouts, and minutes from the last meeting. Allow time for this material to be reviewed. Typically, these items are now sent electronically. If there is no designated minute taker or secretary, the leader may ask a member to assume this role.
3. *Meeting time:* Meetings should begin and end on time. All members should make an effort to be on time, come prepared, and follow the agenda. The leader should guide the meeting so

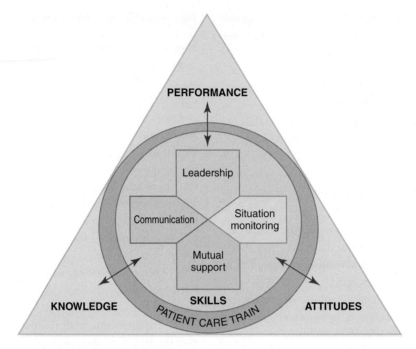

The TeamSTEPPS triangle logo is a visual model that represents some
basic but critical concepts related to teamwork training as explained below.
Individuals can learn four primary trainable teamwork skills. These are:
1. Leadership.
2. Communication.
3. Situation monitoring.
4. Mutual support.

If a team has tools and strategies it can leverage to build a fundamental level
of competency in each of those skills, research has shown that the team can
enhance three types of teamwork outcomes:
1. Performance.
2. Knowledge.
3. Attitudes.

Figure 10-3 TeamSTEPPS

Source: Reproduced from Agency for Healthcare Research and Quality, U.S. Department of Health & Human Services, http://teamstepps.ahrq.gov/teamsteppslogo.htm

that the agenda is followed. At the beginning of
the meeting, minutes should be reviewed and
approved—the minutes are the team's documentation. The leader is responsible for making sure all members have the opportunity to
participate. If the discussion digresses from the
agenda or becomes volatile, the leader needs to
guide the discussion back to the topic and away
from personal reactions. Decisions should be
clearly identified. The minutes should reflect

action items, persons responsible for those items,
and timelines for completion. Planning and conducting a meeting in an orderly fashion indicates
that a team member's time is valued and that accountability for actions is an expectation.

4. *Post meeting:* Minutes are finalized. The leader
and members take up actions that require follow-up or as designated by the decision plan. A
report of these actions should be addressed at
the next meeting.

5. *Evaluation of meetings:* Consider these questions: (1) Was there a clearly defined purpose (agenda) for the meeting? (2) Were there measurable outcomes (do the minutes provide data, and were they met?) (3) What was the attendance level? (4) Did members participate in the meeting(s), or was the leader doing all of the talking?

Another type of meeting that is common among clinical teams is the patient planning meeting. Such meetings may take place daily, each shift, or several times a week. The purpose of these meetings is to assess patient care and determine the patient plan of care. This type of meeting is typically less structured than the formal meeting (e.g., no structured agenda or minutes). However, the team leader does need to plan the topics for discussion. The team may develop a common order in which patient issues are discussed. Notes should be kept, although they need not be formal minutes. The team may add changes to the patient's plan of care or other standard clinical document. The responsibilities noted earlier for team leaders remain the same for the clinical planning team as for other types of teams.

In many hospitals, patient rounds are also used for planning. Staff go to the patient's bedside to talk with the patient and assess needs. The patient should be an active participant in the rounds, although this is not always the case. Rounds may be interprofessional (the ideal method) or focused on a specific profession (such as nursing rounds or physician rounds).

Healthcare Team Members: Which Knowledge and Skills Do They Need?

Team members can be viewed as **followers**. This is not a negative term. If there were no members or followers, there would be no need for a leader. There may be times when a follower, leader of a subgroup, or another member must take over the leadership role, such as in the absence of the team leader; however, in most cases, team members are followers. The follower role should not be a passive one, but rather a very active one. Each member needs to feel a responsibility to participate actively in the work of the team and feel that the members have the right to help the team determine its rules, structure, and activities.

Effective teams require members (healthcare professionals) who engage in the work of the team in the following ways (IOM, 2003a):

- Learn about other team members' expertise, background, knowledge, and values.
- Understand individual roles and processes required to work collaboratively.
- Demonstrate basic group/team skills, including communication, negotiation, delegation, time management, and assessment of group/team dynamics.
- Ensure that accurate and timely information reaches those who need it at the appropriate time.
- Customize care and manage smooth transitions across settings and over time, even when the team members are in entirely different physical locations.
- Coordinate and integrate care processes to ensure excellence, continuity, and reliability of the care provided.
- Resolve conflicts with other members of the team.
- Communicate with other members of the team in a shared language, even when the members are in entirely different physical locations.

Development of Effective Teams

The word *team* implies there is a group of people, but how do they develop into a team? To just say, "Today this group of staff is a team," does not mean that the group is actually functioning as a team. It takes time to develop a team. Within a team, members have informal and formal roles, and some members may assume multiple roles at different times as the team members interact. Heller (1999, p. 42) defines some of these roles:

- *Coordinator:* Pulls together the work of the team
- *Critic:* Keeps an eye on the team's effectiveness
- *Idea person:* Encourages the team to be innovative
- *Implementer:* Ensures that the team's functioning is effective
- *External contact:* Looks after the team's external contacts and relationships
- *Inspector:* Ensures that standards are met
- *Team builder:* Develops the team spirit

The IOM noted four areas of particular concern that need to be considered when evaluating team effectiveness (Fried, Topping, & Rundall, 2000, as cited in IOM, 2001, p. 132):

1. Team makeup, such as having the appropriate team size and composition of members, and the ability to reduce status differences (for example, between the nurse manager and staff nurses or between nurses and physicians).
2. Team processes, such as communication structure, conflict management, leadership that emphasizes excellence, and clear goals and expectations.
3. Nature of team tasks, such as matching roles with knowledge and experience, and promoting cohesiveness when work is highly interdependent.
4. Environment context, such as obtaining needed resources and establishing appropriate rewards.

"Effective teams have a culture that fosters openness, collaboration, teamwork, and learning from mistakes" (IOM, 2001, p. 132). Health care has a problem with development of effective teams because it overemphasizes personal accountability of healthcare professionals such as nurses and physicians. Teams often resort to uncoordinated or sequential action rather than collaborative work, which is required for effective teams (IOM, 2001).

Interprofessional Team Competencies

Recent work that has sought to clarify ways to ensure interprofessional team education has identified key competencies for all healthcare professions related to teamwork (Interprofessional Education Collaborative Expert Panel, 2011, pp. 19, 21, 23, 25). The following competencies might look like they form a to-do list. In a way they do, because these are the expected actions/competencies of the healthcare team:

- Work with individuals of other professions to maintain a climate of mutual respect and shared values.
- Use the knowledge of one's own role and the roles of other professions to appropriately assess and address the healthcare needs of patients and populations served.
- Communicate with patients, families, communities, and other health professionals in a responsive and responsible manner that supports a team approach to the maintenance of health and treatment of disease.
- Apply relationship-building values and the principles of team dynamics to perform effectively in different team roles to plan and deliver patient/population-centered care that is safe, timely, efficient, effective, and equitable.

Accomplishing these competencies requires greater emphasis on interprofessional education for all healthcare profession students.

Teams and Decision Making

Teams make decisions about the work that they need to do. The amount and quality of information that is required and the number of possible solutions for a problem affect decisions. The schedule is very important; for example, is an immediate decision required, or can time be taken to consider options carefully? Many clinical teams must act quickly in response to clinical problems. These teams need to develop quick thinking and analytic skills (depending on the expertise of team members), trust one another, weigh benefits and risks, and move to a decision. At other times, teams may have more time to fully analyze an issue or problem, brainstorm possible solutions, and develop a consensus regarding the best decision. Teams must recognize that there may not be a perfect solution (there rarely is) and that there is risk, but decisions need to be made. Not making a decision is really making a decision—to do nothing is a decision.

Several decision-making styles may be used (Milgram, Spector, & Treger, 1999):

- Decisive decision making depends on minimal data to arrive at a single solution or decision.
- The integrative style uses as much data as possible to arrive at several reasonable solutions or decisions.
- The hierarchic style uses a large amount of data and organizes the data to arrive at one optimal decision.

- The flexible style relies on minimal data but generates several different options or will shift focus as the data are interpreted.

A team leader and the team typically use more than one decision-making style, depending on the issue or problem.

Key questions that are asked during decision making are: (1) What is the issue, problem, or task to be done and the desired outcome? (2) Which kind of data is needed? (3) How complicated and substantial is the issue, problem, or task? (4) How many possible solutions or approaches are there, and what are they? (5) Can the desired outcome(s) be met with acceptable cost-benefit standards? (Note that cost is more than financial; it could refer to the patient's health status if an outcome is not achieved or an error occurs due to a decision-making problem, for example.)

Figure 10-4 illustrates team thinking. **Box 10-1** provides an example of a team thinking inventory that teams can use to assess their thinking.

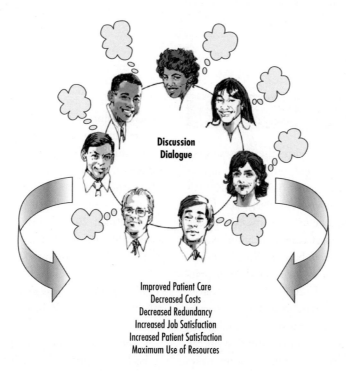

Discussion
Dialogue

Improved Patient Care
Decreased Costs
Decreased Redundancy
Increased Job Satisfaction
Increased Patient Satisfaction
Maximum Use of Resources

Figure 10-4 Interprofessional Team Thinking
Source: Rubenfeld, M., & Scheffer, B. (2006). *Critical thinking tactics for nurses.* Sudbury, MA: Jones and Bartlett.

- Which strategies are used to help team members think about the big picture as well as the parts?
- Which strategies are used to help team members see the situation from different perspectives?
- Which strategies are used to help team members see their biases and assumptions?
- Which strategies help team members think about patterns and interrelationships of issues and parts of problems?
- Which strategies are used to help team members think beyond cause-and-effect consequences?
- Does the thinking that occurs in the team resemble simple sharing of information or discussion/dialogue? Why? How can you move in the direction of discussion/dialogue?
- What is done to encourage team members to share their thinking or feel comfortable enough to talk about it?
- How is conflict managed in the team to promote thinking instead of discouraging it?
- Which other sources of gratification, besides interdisciplinary teamwork, are available for team members to socialize, obtain recognition, and interact?
- How were the interdisciplinary team members prepared for their thinking roles?
- How does the team deal with ambiguity? How long can team members tolerate not having a solution?
- How does the team examine its own thinking processes (e.g., how it works, not what it is doing), and who is doing it?

Sources: From Rubenfeld, M. G., & Scheffer, B. (2006). *Critical thinking tactics for nurses.* Sudbury, MA: Jones and Bartlett. Data adapted from Senge, P. (1998). *The fifth discipline: The art and practice of the learning organization.* New York, NY: Doubleday; Bensimon, E., & Neumann, A. (1993). *Redesigning collegiate leadership: Teams and teamwork in higher education.* Baltimore, MD: Johns Hopkins University Press; and Brookfield, S., & Peskill, S. (1999). *Discussion as a way of teaching: Tools and techniques for democratic classrooms.* San Francisco, CA: Jossey-Bass.

 # COMMUNICATION

All nurses communicate—with other nurses, other staff, patients, families, and others who impact patient care. The assumption is that individuals know how to communicate effectively, and this is not always true. Effective **communication** takes practice and awareness of communication. Nurses have an ethical mandate to become skilled communicators; doing so is an essential standard of practice (Kupperschmidt et al., 2010; O'Keefe & Saver, 2014, p. 7). What is important is the effectiveness of this communication. Teams must communicate, too. The effectiveness of team communication can also vary, but it is clear that communication makes a difference in results and decreases errors.

Individuals have communication styles, and understanding one's style is important. Some people are more passive; others use a lot of nonverbal communication; others prefer to see important information in writing; and so on. Using professional jargon often creates a barrier, limiting clear communication (Interprofessional Education Collaborative Expert Panel, 2011). This is why using practices such as SBAR, call-out, and check-back is important in reducing communication barriers. Within these methods, all healthcare providers use the same terminology and process so that they do not have to take time to figure out the process or what someone else means.

The Joint Commission analyzed data related to healthcare quality from 2004 to 2012 and concluded that communication issues were the major reasons for deaths related to a delay in treatment. Data from 2010 to 2012 indicated that communication was the third highest root cause of sentinel events (Joint Commission, 2013; O'Keeffe & Saver, 2014). Not communicating is the major issue in communication breakdown. Situations that are most at risk for communication breakdown include those involving broken rules or taking shortcuts, mistakes or use of poor clinical judgment, lack of support, incompetence, poor teamwork, disrespect, and micromanagement when someone abuses authority (Maxfield, Grenny, McMillan, Patterson, & Switzler, 2005). Clearly, effective communication is critical for delivery of quality health care and something that must be improved and frequently monitored.

The relationships and communication between nurses and physicians have long been important healthcare issues because they have an impact on the quality of care and work satisfaction. One small study that included 20 medical and surgical residents examined their attitudes toward nurses (Weinberg, Miner, & Rivlin, 2009). In this study, 19 of the 20 residents shared examples of poor communication or problematic relationships with nurses, but the important result was the residents did not feel such issues presented a problem for patient care because the nurses' role was to follow orders and nothing more. The residents did say that when nurses were knowledgeable and collaborative, such qualities had positive effects on the residents and on patient care—which, of course, contradicts their view of the importance of nurses' roles. Such knowledgeable and collaborative nurses were able to anticipate and respond to needs and then work with residents to identify patient needs and interventions, and this working relationship was part of the residents' positive comments. However, this was not the common experience. This type of result indicates that residents view nurses with more education and experience in a more positive light, suggesting there might be a more collaborative relationship formed in this circumstance. Because this study focused on residents, transferring these results to experienced

physicians is not possible, because they represent a different sample. This study also did not examine nurses' views of the medical residents.

In reality, this is not a one-sided perspective, and blame for poor communication with nurses cannot just be placed on the medical residents. Nurses have responsibilities in the communication process, and their role in this partnership is complicated, too. More of a power struggle is also apparent today because of the increased number of female physicians, increased number of nurse practitioners, increased nursing autonomy, and decreased perception of physician esteem due to accessibility of information online (Nair, Fitzpatrick, McNulty, Click, & Glembocki, 2012). Researchers tend to focus on physician–nurse communication, but there is much more to communication in healthcare settings—for example, communication from nurse to nurse, nurse to unlicensed personnel, nurse to other healthcare professionals, and nurse to administrators/managers. All of these staff are critical to effective functioning of the healthcare delivery systems, yet problems occur in all of these combinations of interactions.

Another recent study that focused on quality care reached an interesting conclusion that relates to the issue of interprofessional teamwork (Curry et al., 2011). This study examined the factors that may be related to better performance in care of patients with an acute myocardial infarction diagnosis, which the study measured by assessing risk-standardized mortality rates. The sample included 11 hospitals and 158 staff members. The high-performing hospitals demonstrated organizational cultures that supported improved care for this patient population. The conclusion was that evidence-based protocols and processes are important but not sufficient to reach high hospital performance. These hospitals had clear organizational values and goals; senior management was involved; communication and coordination were evident in broad staff presence and expertise; and problem solving and learning were important. These are all elements of effective teamwork. Teamwork does make a difference in patient outcomes, and depending on the effectiveness of the team, it can be negative or positive.

Relational coordination is a theory about work: Successful work is accomplished when high-quality relationships and communication are present (Gittel, 2002; Gittel, Weinberg, Pfefferle, & Bishop, 2008; Weinberg et al., 2009). The theory suggests that successful work flows from two sources:

- Frequent, high-quality communication that is timely, is accurate, and uses problem solving
- High-quality relationships that include shared goals, shared knowledge, and mutual respect

These characteristics are in line with the IOM core competency of interprofessional teamwork and descriptions of quality. Based on Gittel's theory, the key dimensions of relational coordination are frequent communication, timely communication, accurate communication, problem-solving communication, mutual respect, shared knowledge, and shared goals.

Assertiveness

Assertiveness is a communication style that is often confused with aggression and, therefore, may be viewed negatively. Assertiveness, however, is important, though many nurses have to learn how to use this style. Using assertiveness, a person stands up for what he or she believes in but does not push or control others. The assertive nurse uses *I* statements when communicating thoughts and feelings and *you* statements when persuading others (Fabre, 2005). Other suggestions for improving assertiveness include the following (Fabre, 2005, p. 78):

- Intervene in situations calmly and confidently.
- Respond to problems in a timely way to avoid accumulation of negative feelings. Those who are passive for a long time run the risk of overreacting to small incidents.
- Clearly articulate the importance of using nursing perspectives.

- Use language that others (the audience; for example, the team or management) understand.

Communication is the sharing of a message between one person or group and another. It is important to know if the message was received as sent. Interpretation has a major impact on effective communication, and sometimes interpretation confuses or changes the original message. Nonverbal communication also has an impact on the message sent. If a team member verbally affirms commitment to an action but the team member's facial expression shows a lack of interest (such as no eye contact or a hurried manner), the message of commitment may be viewed as noncommitment. As team members get to know one another, they learn each other's communication styles, including nonverbal methods. This knowledge confers an advantage in that it can improve and speed up communication. Nevertheless, in some cases, team members may jump to conclusions, and communication may not be clear.

Nurses need to break the code of silence (Fabre, 2005). Nurses are often silent, keeping their opinions to themselves rather than being open with the treatment team. This pattern most likely reflects the low self-esteem of the profession as a whole, which has a very negative impact—namely, loss of valuable nursing input. Speaking up brings a risk, but the results can be worthwhile. It may take time for team members to value one another's opinions and expertise. If done in a professional manner with the goal of collaboration and coordination, however, over time most team members begin to respect and trust one another and see value in the team's diversity of multiple healthcare professionals and variety in experience.

Listening

Listening is an important skill to develop. It is important when delivering care—listening to the patient and family—and when listening in work teams and to colleagues. Most people probably would say that they listen, but listening takes practice. There are also a number of barriers to effective listening:

- Anxiety and stress
- Interruptions
- Too many tasks to do
- Fatigue and hunger
- Lack of self-esteem
- Anger
- Reaction from the past
- Confusing message

In addition, the team member may not think that individual team members' opinions are valued, leading the member to tune out or exhibit a lack of concern or respect for the communicator. The opposite can also occur with the team member thinking he or she knows enough and thus does not need to listen.

When you recognize that you are not listening, you should think about what is interfering with listening. What is the barrier(s) at the moment? Through this self-examination, you can learn more about the listening process and improve your listening skills—and, in turn, your communication skills. Fabre (2005) identifies why listening is important beyond generally improving communication:

- Listening helps us identify problems.
- Listening exposes feelings—those invaluable, but sometimes inconvenient, traits that make us truly human. We need to manage our feelings and give them a positive focus instead of denying them.
- Listening jump-starts the solution process because answers may pop up during candid conversations.
- Listening relieves stress. Bottling up thoughts and feelings simply depletes our energy.
- Active listening is more than hearing; it requires communicating to the other person that you are listening.
- Saying "yes" and "no" is not active listening.
- Paraphrasing communicates that you have listened; you repeat what you have heard to make sure the message is clear.

Nurse–physician communication has long been an important topic, probably more so in nursing than in medicine. In addition to the studies mentioned earlier, other studies have examined this issue and the impact of collaboration on care (Baggs et al., 1999; Fairchild, Hogan, Smith, Portnow, & Bates, 2002; Higgins, 1999; Thomas, Sexton, & Helmreich, 2003). These studies indicate the ongoing existence of communication problems, which in turn can impact collaboration and, consequently, patient outcomes.

For example, two nurses and one physician conducted a study using focus groups of nurses and physicians. They identified methods to improve nurse–physician communication (Burke, Boal, & Mitchell, 2004). The researchers noted that some communication problems require major organizational changes—system changes. The suggested methods that are not as system focused but rather are more individual focused include these steps:

1. Develop a personal connection, which helps to increase colleagueship.
2. Use humor.
3. Make the assumption that you are on the same team.
4. Recognize that team members are equal in their expertise that can be important to patient care.
5. If you speak frequently to a physician over the phone, arrange to meet in person.
6. Report good news about patients—improvements, not just problems.
7. Recognize that conflict will occur, but this does not mean that communication and collaboration cannot be maintained.
8. Discuss preferred methods of communication (telephone, e-mail, pager, in person, voice message) and under which circumstances they should be used.
9. Ask for parameters regarding when the physician wants to be called.
10. Plan ahead for meetings or times of contact so that you are prepared with information and

know what you want to communicate. Provide clinically pertinent information.

11. Work with the physician to determine the best methods for communicating with the family and determine who should contact whom and for what purposes.

COLLABORATION

Collaboration is an integral part of patient-centered care and safe, quality care. When staff or team members work in a collaborative environment, it is a satisfying work experience with limited conflict. Collaboration means that all the people involved are listened to and that decisions are developed together. Views are respected; however, at some point, decisions must be made, and not all views or opinions will be part of the final decision. Compromise is part of effective collaboration. The goal is to arrive at the best possible decision. Working with others increases the possibility of having the best decision because there is greater availability of ideas and dialogue about ideas and solutions. This diversity improves decision making.

The American Nurses Association (ANA) standard on collaboration states, "The registered nurse collaborates with healthcare consumer, family, and others in the conduct of nursing practice" (2010, p. 57). The focus of the standard supports patient-centered care. It requires nurses to communicate, collaborate with the plan of care, promote conflict management, build consensus, engage in teamwork, cooperate, and partner with others to effect change and produce positive outcomes while adhering to professional standards and codes of conduct.

Collaboration requires that open communication take place and that team members feel comfortable expressing their opinions even when they disagree. Team members of different healthcare professions must work across professional boundaries to develop a team culture of working together. The goal is not to make an individual's profession look

good, but rather to focus on the team as a whole. Even when the team is composed of members from the same healthcare profession, such as a nursing team, the focus is on the team, not individuals. This does not mean that conflicts will not occur, but some can be prevented. When conflict does occur, the team uses effective methods for coping to reach a common goal.

Nurses work closely with physicians, and this relationship has a long history of conflict. Often it is stereotyped as "us versus them," which is an unhealthy approach. With the greater emphasis on teamwork, nurses and physicians are slowly being forced into improving their work relationships. As has been discussed, this change in attitude really needs to begin at the student level. Organizations need to stand behind efforts to improve team collaboration, coordination, and communication.

One area that has received special attention is abuse—usually verbal—from physician to nurse. Unfortunately, this is also a problem from nurse to nurse—incivility or bullying among nurses is now found in healthcare organizations as well as in schools of nursing.

In schools of nursing, incivility is found among students and faculty, in both the student–faculty and faculty–student directions. Students also experience such bullying with nurses during their clinical experiences. In 2008, the National Student Nurses Association published an article about incivility in its journal (Luparell, 2008). Involvement in this type of behavior can lead to physical and emotional responses, even causing the victim to feel traumatized, powerless, or stressed; lose sleep; and develop depression. People may try to avoid one another for fear of another negative encounter leading to distrust. When students and faculty are in situations where evaluation occurs, distrust on both sides can prevent objective faculty evaluation of students and student evaluation of faculty. This behavior can be disruptive in the classroom and in clinical experiences, and it interferes with student learning both for the students directly involved and for the students on the sidelines. The community of learning then becomes a place where no one wants to be.

Incivility demonstrates disrespect. When this type of behavior occurs, decreasing the escalation is critical. Many times incivility occurs from misunderstanding, so trying to talk about the issue—albeit in a calm manner—is important. Students may feel that they have no power. If the issue cannot be worked out directly with those involved, all schools have a process for discussing difficult issues, and these guidelines should be followed.

Before you go to talk to the person (another student or faculty member) about the situation that you found unacceptable, think about what you will say and even practice. Doing so will help you cope with your emotions, as you do not want to have a repeat of the uncivil behavior.

Another method for dealing with verbal abuse is to try to remove the emotion from the situation—step back for a breather, and then discuss the issue or problem on a factual basis. This strategy may require a third party to act as neutral mediator in the discussion. This is not easy to do when parties are emotional and often tired and stressed, but it does make a difference. Such an approach provides time to gain more objective perspective.

Organizations associated with health care have made statements about the problem of incivility. In 2008, The Joint Commission issued a sentinel alert on incivility and, as the problem has increased in healthcare organizations (HCOs), in 2010 required HCOs to have standards in place to address this type of behavior. The American Association of Critical Care Nurses (2005) also issued a statement about healthy work environments.

When students observe or are involved in uncivil encounters in clinical experiences, this has a negative impact on their professional socialization. Such behaviors are all connected to communication, ability to compromise and listen, and respect and trust, which in turn affect the ability to work collaboratively as a team member.

Concern has also emerged about the impact of verbal abuse and disruptive behaviors among team members on patient care. Examples of disruptive behaviors include verbal abuse, negative behavior, and physical abuse (e.g., profanity, innuendo, demeaning comments), reprimanding or insulting another person in public and inappropriately, threatening, telling racial or ethnic jokes, undermining team cohesion, scapegoating, silence (not speaking to a team member), assaulting another person, throwing objects, and outbursts of rage (Lower, 2007).

One study sought to explore the impact of work relationships on clinical outcomes (Rosenstein & O'Daniel, 2005). This research was published in a nursing journal, conducted by a physician and a healthcare administrator, and was a follow-up to an earlier study that looked at the impact of disruptive behavior on job satisfaction and retention (Rosenstein, 2002). In the 2005 study, 1500 surveys from nurses and physicians were evaluated. Nurses were reported to exhibit disruptive behavior as frequently as physicians. Both groups felt that disruptive behavior (which included verbal abuse) negatively impacted relationships and created stress, leading to frustration, lack of concentration, poor communication, and inability to effectively collaborate and provide effective information transfer in the workplace. Given that this chapter discusses the need for greater use of effective interprofessional teams to provide quality, safe, patient-centered care, it is easy to see how these results may be perceived as disturbing. The participants also felt that disruptive behavior was adversely affecting patient safety, patient mortality, the quality of care, and patient satisfaction. This point further emphasizes the need to improve teamwork and professional relationships.

The researchers recommended that the following steps be taken in organizations to improve workplace relationships (Rosenstein & O'Daniel, 2005):

- The organization should conduct a self-assessment to determine the prevalence of disruptive behavior and better understand its nature.

- The organization should share the results of this self-assessment with staff to increase awareness of the problem.
- The organization should open up lines of communication between nurses and physicians (and any other staff who are experiencing disruptive behavior) in a non-antagonistic environment to discuss issues.
- The organization should provide education about mutual respect among coworkers and the benefits of team collaboration; communication; team building; and conflict management. (This is a good way to emphasize the IOM interprofessional team core competency.)
- The organization should develop and implement policies and procedures that reinforce acceptable codes of behavior.

All these strategies should promote better patient care and clinical outcomes.

Many organizations now have zero-tolerance policies related to this type of abuse as well as code-of-conduct policies. However, the existence of a written policy does not guarantee on its own that attitudes and behaviors will automatically improve. Staff need to know both the policy content and the consequences of violating the policy, and these consequences must be meted out when necessary.

It is very easy to say that poor attitudes and abusive behaviors are all the physicians' fault when, in fact, they are not. Many nurses enter the profession with a negative attitude toward physicians and feel that they do not want to be controlled by physicians. The better approach is for new nurses to enter the profession with a positive attitude toward nursing as a profession, to be knowledgeable about what nursing is, to be competent, and to possess a reasonable level of self-esteem. Nurse–nurse incivility is all too prevalent and a serious problem; thus the problem involves more than just nurse–physician incivility. What is needed to prevent incivility is someone who wants to work with others, not against others, and someone who approaches

issues and problems with an open mind and who is not tied to an "I know better" mind-set. If all healthcare professionals could approach practice in this manner, then collaboration, coordination, and communication would improve. There would be limited incidence of verbal abuse, and the work environment would be positive and healthy for all team members.

COORDINATION

Nurses coordinate patient care through planning and implementing care, and they have been involved in the development of care **coordination** throughout its evolution (Lamb, 2013). "Care coordination involves deliberately organizing patient care activities and sharing information among all of the participants concerned with a patient's care to achieve safer and more effective care. This means that the patient's needs and preferences are known ahead of time and communicated at the right time to the right people, and that this information is used to provide safe, appropriate, and effective care to the patient" (AHRQ, 2014). Effective coordination needs to be interprofessional. Indeed, coordination and collaboration should be interconnected. Dessler (2002) described coordination as "the process of achieving unity of action among interdependent activities" (pp. 143–144). Care is complex, and patients require healthcare providers with different expertise to meet these needs. With this type of situation, the different providers need to collaborate to reach a plan and then implement care in a manner that makes sense—meeting the timeline required, with minimal conflict and confusion.

Although the need for care coordination is clear, there are obstacles within the American health care system that must be overcome to provide this type of care. Redesigning a health care system in order to better coordinate patients' care is important for the following reasons:

- Current healthcare systems are often disjointed, and processes vary among and between primary care sites and specialty sites.
- Patients are often unclear about why they are being referred from primary care to a specialist, how to make appointments, and what to do after seeing a specialist.
- Specialists do not consistently receive clear reasons for the referral or adequate information on tests that have already been done. Primary care physicians do not often receive information about what happened in a referral visit.
- Referral staff deal with many different processes and lost information, which means that care is less efficient. (AHRQ, 2014)

Coordination—working to see that the pieces and activities fit together and flow as they should—can help to meet desired patient outcomes. "Conscious patient-centered coordination of care not only improves the patient experience, it also leads to better long-term health outcomes, as demonstrated by fewer unnecessary trips to the hospital, fewer repeated tests, fewer conflicting prescriptions, and clearer advice about the best course of treatment" (U.S. Department of Health and Human Services [HHS], 2013). Patients often complain about the number of care providers. They may not know who is responsible for which aspects of their care, and they receive confusing and often conflicting communication and information. The patient needs to have an anchor—a healthcare provider to whom the patient can turn for support and knowledge of the plan. Basically, patients are saying that they are not the center of care and that their care is fragmented. This leads to an increased risk of errors and decreases the quality of care. Consequently, the ANA (2010) standards of practice include coordination of care. Care is coordinated through the implementation of the care plan, documentation of care, and teamwork.

Barriers and Competencies Related to Coordination

Coordination is not easy to achieve even when team members want to achieve it. Some of the barriers to effective coordination are listed here:

- Failure of team members to understand the roles and responsibilities of other team members, particularly members from different healthcare professions
- Lack of a clear interprofessional plan of care
- Limited leadership
- Overwork and excessive burden of team member responsibilities
- Ineffective communication, both oral and written
- Lack of inclusion of the patient and family/significant others in the care process
- Competition among team members to control decisions

Despite these barriers, coordination can be achieved. First, the team must recognize that coordination is critical and strive to ensure that it is implemented. The team needs to understand the purpose and goals of coordination and work to achieve them. To do so, the team must evaluate its work and be willing to identify weaknesses and figure out methods to improve coordination. Team members need to communicate openly and in a timely manner. Teams that effectively solve problems together will improve their coordination. Delegation, discussed elsewhere in this chapter, is an important part of coordination. One person cannot do everything (and that one person may not even be the best person for the task or activity). Coordination requires team members who understand the different roles and expertise of the members, determine the best member to make or deliver care and in which timeline, and evaluate the outcomes.

Tools to Improve Coordination

Health care has developed a variety of tools and methods to increase coordination. From a chronic illness perspective, disease management is a tool to improve coordination and collaboration. Two other methods are practice guidelines and clinical protocols or pathways.

A clinical protocol or pathway is a written guide to provide direction for specific clinical problems. The protocol content includes interventions, timeline, and resources needed; it identifies expected outcomes and provides a sequencing of interventions to reach the outcomes. Typically, a pathway is laid out in a chart, as illustrated in **Figure 10-5**, which provides examples of information categories that might be found in a clinical pathway.

Pathways are developed in a number of ways. In some situations, healthcare organizations may create them by identifying focus areas based on needs—for example, pathways that focus on the care of a diabetic patient who has been hospitalized, a patient who needs a hip replacement, or a patient who is severely depressed and suicidal. An interprofessional team of experts then develops the pathway. This team should use current literature and evidence from research while constructing the pathway, and team members may even seek out examples from other hospitals or examples found in professional literature. In other situations, the healthcare organization may decide to use a published clinical pathway. After the clinical pathway is developed or selected, staff need training about the pathway and its use. Pathways can be used to evaluate care and outcomes by collecting data about their use and the

patients' outcomes. The question to be addressed during such an evaluation is simple: Does the pathway, or specific interventions within a pathway, make a difference?

There are a number of advantages to using clinical protocols or pathways. First, this type of tool improves coordination and increases the likelihood of meeting outcomes. Because clinical protocols or pathways are written and based on evidence, there is a standard for care and greater consistency, which in turn enhances quality of care and facilitates evidence-based practice. However, whenever a pathway is used, it must be reviewed to ensure that it meets the individual needs of the patient and then adapted accordingly. Other advantages of using clinical protocols or pathways include more effective use of expertise and resources, better management of healthcare costs, improved collaboration and communication, decreased errors, improved patient satisfaction (because patients feel that their care is organized and they are more informed), improved care documentation (because it follows a consistent plan), improved identification of responsibilities, and a clear statement of interventions.

DELEGATION

Delegation is part of the daily work of nurses. Care is planned and coordinated to meet patient needs, but at some point the RN may need to delegate work to others. Much of the work is done in a team model, in which it is not cost-effective for all care to be provided by the RN. Delegation involves giving another staff member the responsibility and authority to complete a task or activity. Before an RN can delegate, the RN needs to have responsibility and authority, or the power over the activity or task. An RN cannot delegate something that is outside approved nursing practice as determined by the nurse practice act in the state where the nurse practices. An extreme example is that an RN cannot delegate prescriptive authority (prescribing of

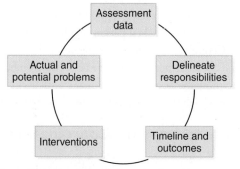

Figure 10-5 Categories of Information Found in Clinical Pathways

medications) because an RN typically cannot do this activity. An advanced practice nurse may have prescriptive authority because this nurse has met special requirements and the state allows it, but even this nurse cannot delegate prescriptive authority to someone who does not meet the legal requirements for having such authority.

When an RN delegates to another staff member, such as unlicensed assistive personnel (UAP) or a licensed practical nurse/licensed vocational nurse (LPN/LVN), the RN is not avoiding work and is still held accountable for the outcomes, but the care is provided in a more efficient manner. Accountability is "being responsible and answerable for actions or inactions of self or others in the context of delegation" (National Council of State Boards of Nursing [NCSBN], 2006). The UAP is an unlicensed staff member who is trained to function in an assistive role to the licensed nurse in the provision of patient activities as delegated by the nurse. The UAP may have several different titles, such as nursing assistant or nurse's aide. There is no national standard that is accepted and enforced in every state as to employment requirements, training, or position descriptions for the UAP. The RN (the delegator) is still responsible for supervising the work (activity, task) that the other staff member (the delegatee) is to do.

Supervision, *assignment*, and *delegation* are key terms that are easy to confuse. They are related to one another. When a nurse is monitoring care and work done, this is supervision. The nurse may be in a formal management position, such as a nurse manager, a team leader, or an RN staff nurse who has delegated work to another and then ensures that it is done effectively. Assignment is the process that moves an activity from one person to another, including the responsibility and accountability. For example, the nurse manager might assign an RN to lead a team or to administer medications to the patients. An assignment can be given only to staff who have the required qualifications to complete the tasks and can assume the responsibility and

accountability; however, the accountability is still shared. The person doing the activity has the accountability for the actual action or activity, whereas the person who made the assignment is responsible for the assignment decision.

Importance of Delegation

Why is delegation important, and why is it part of care coordination and teamwork? One RN or one team member cannot always do everything that is required for a patient. There must be effective use of resources—expertise and time. Through delegation, work can be allocated to those who can most effectively accomplish it. Delegation is a critical part of providing cost-effective care. In some situations, it is more cost-effective if care can safely be provided by a UAP or a licensed practical nurse, whose salary is lower than that of an RN, with the RN providing overall supervision.

Delegation is also critical to quality care (Anthony & Vidal, 2010). Quality care requires that patient outcomes are achieved with no harm to the patient. Through delegation, the RN determines which tasks should be done, by whom, when, and how. The Centers for Medicare and Medicaid (CMS) conditions identify unfavorable outcomes such as falls and lack of turning resulting in pressure ulcers as being related to quality care, and delegation has a major impact on these conditions.

Communication and information are critical elements of delegation. If communication is not effective or there is inadequate information, delegation can be ineffective, which can in turn lead to problems for the patient and interfere with the team's ability to achieve the desired patient outcomes. It is often difficult to provide clear communication in rushed healthcare environments, but doing so has never been more important if care is to be improved. Mindfulness—staying alert to key information, and evaluating and updating that information as necessary—is an active process that can improve communication during delegation. The goal is not to share as much information as possible, but rather to share the critical information—that is, information that has meaning in the situation.

> When mindful communication is integrated as a principle of delegation, it involves more than knowing the facts regarding the care plan. Mindful communication practice is recognizing the significance of the facts and how they pertain to the patient situation. When nurses engage in mindful communication, information processing is redirected, resulting in a unique set of decisions and actions. Historically, RNs have relied on job descriptions and delegated skills lists to guide delegation practices.... hospitals value standardization as a means to improve safety through consistent practices. Paradoxically, however, overreliance on standards that results in routine interpretations and behaviors may jeopardize patient safety when nurses do not engage in mindful communication about the task at hand. (Anthony & Vidal, 2010)

The National Council of State Boards of Nursing, through the state boards of nursing, has identified delegation standards and described the delegation process. The NCSBN (2006) defines delegation as "transferring to a competent individual authority to perform a selected nursing task in a selected situation. The nurse retains the accountability for the delegation." This definition really says the following:

1. *Transferring* means that the RN can do something that will be passed on to someone else to do. The RN has the right to do this. The RN cannot delegate something that the RN has no right to do. (For example, suppose a patient needs a bed bath. The RN can do the bed bath, but it is more efficient to have the UAP complete the bed bath while the RN assesses the patient's overall status at the beginning of a shift.)

2. The RN transfers this activity to a *competent* person—someone who can complete the task because that person has the skills and experience to do so. (For example, the UAP has been trained to give bed baths and report to the nurse any problems encountered.)

3. In the delegation process, the delegator or RN is giving the delegatee the authority or power to do the act or task. (For example, RNs have overall responsibility and authority for all nursing care—from basic care, such as a bed bath, to complex care needs. The RN determines who is the best staff member to complete a task. In some cases, the RN may decide that because of the critical status of the patient and the need for intensive interaction and assessment, the RN should complete the bed bath; alternatively, the RN may decide that the UAP is best suited to handling this task.)

4. The delegatee must then do something—this action is specific and is attached to a specific situation. (For example, the UAP completes the bed bath, documents the care, and informs the RN that there was nothing unusual to report.)

Five Rights

It is natural to wonder who is responsible for the care. The **delegatee** is responsible for the care that the delegatee provides or the delegatee performance. The **delegator** is responsible for the delegation process. This process is not a simple one and requires experience. The RN must consider the five rights of delegation (NCSBN, 2006).

1. *Right task:* The task must be delegatable for a specific patient or situation. If the RN or delegator is not clear about what the task is, the RN will not be able to clearly identify what needs to be done and by whom.

2. *Right circumstances:* The appropriate setting, available resources, and other relevant factors need to be considered. Perhaps the RN needs to tell the delegatee where to complete the task

and to identify which supplies, equipment, and other resources are needed to complete the task effectively.

3. *Right person:* The right person delegates the right task to the right person, to be performed by the right person. The RN must consider the best staff member to complete the task (type of staff, experience and skills, availability of time to complete task without negatively impacting other work, and so on).

4. *Right direction/communication:* Providing a clear, concise description of the task, including its objective, limits, and expectations, is part of effective delegation. The delegator must explain to the delegatee what is to be done, how to do it (if that is not already clear), the time frame, outcomes, and so on. The delegatee needs to feel comfortable asking questions for clarification or expressing concern about the delegatee's inability to complete the task. The delegator must be an effective communicator and must be sensitive to concerns and issues to establish a communication environment that allows for open discussion. This is critical to ensure patient-centered care that is focused on quality. If the delegatee is afraid of speaking up and saying, "I do not know how to do something" or "Would you explain more about what you want done?", then this is an ineffective delegation process that may harm the patient. The delegatee may need help in organizing work and setting priorities, or the delegatee may need to be told what to report to the RN and when. The delegator needs to ask directly if there are questions or concerns and be open to the response. All of this is part of providing clear directions and guidance.

5. *Right supervision:* Appropriate monitoring, evaluation, intervention (as needed), and feedback are part of delegation. The RN as a delegator does not just delegate a task and then forget about it. Instead, the RN needs to supervise as required. Monitoring methods include observation, verbal

feedback, written feedback, and review of records in which the delegatee documented what was done. In some situations, supervision is minimal; in other situations, there may be a greater need for monitoring. Factors such as the expertise of the delegatee, the patient's status, the complexity of the task, and timing may all affect the monitoring process.

Another factor that cannot be ignored is how comfortable the delegator feels in delegating, and how well the delegator knows the delegatee. New RNs may be very nervous about delegating; trusting another person to complete a task can be risky. Some new RNs may be overly concerned because they feel that they could perform the task better. In both situations, the result could be excessive hovering or over-monitoring; the delegatee may interpret the delegator's behavior or attitude as indicating a lack of confidence in the delegatee. This message can have a negative impact on staff team relationships. Finding the right balance takes experience. New RNs need time to learn how to delegate effectively, and they need to seek guidance from their own supervisors or mentors to assess their delegation competencies.

Figure 10-6 highlights the five delegation rights.

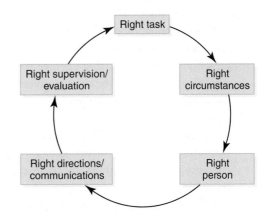

Figure 10-6 Five Rights for Effective Delegation

Delegation Principles

The American Nurses Association (ANA) and the National Council of State Boards of Nursing (NCSBN) collaborated to identify the key delegation principles that should be applied by every RN (ANA & NCSBN, 2006, pp. 2–3):

- The RN takes responsibility and accountability for the provision of nursing practice.
- The RN directs care and determines the appropriate utilization of any assistant involved in providing direct patient care.
- The RN may delegate components of care but does not delegate the nursing process itself. Nursing judgment cannot be delegated.
- The decision of whether to delegate or assign is based on the RN's judgment concerning the condition of the patient, the competence of all members of the nursing team, and the degree of supervision that will be required of the RN if a task is delegated.
- The RN delegates only those tasks that the RN believes the other healthcare worker has the knowledge and skill to perform, taking into consideration training, cultural competence, experience, and facility/agency policies and procedures.
- The RN individualizes communication regarding the delegation to the nursing assistive personnel and patient situation, and the communication is clear, concise, correct, and complete. The RN verifies comprehension with the nursing assistive personnel and ensures that the assistant accepts the delegation and the responsibility that accompanies it.
- Communication must be a two-way process. Nursing assistive personnel should have the opportunity to ask questions and clarify expectations.
- The RN uses critical thinking and professional judgment when following the five rights of delegation.

- Chief nursing officers are accountable for establishing systems to assess, monitor, verify, and communicate ongoing competence requirements in areas related to delegation.
- There are both individual accountability and organizational accountability for delegation. Organizational accountability for delegation relates to providing sufficient resources.

It is important that the RN, as the delegator, thanks the delegatee and recognizes the work that the delegatee has done. The RN should provide positive feedback when work is done well and constructive feedback as needed, which means that the RN does not criticize work negatively but rather discusses the work and outcomes and makes recommendations for improvement. It is easy to take things for granted and not recognize the work of team members. It really takes little time to give positive feedback and a "thank you," yet this step can go a long way toward building teams.

Will there be times when the RN as delegator must change a decision about delegation? If so, why would this occur? In the monitoring process, the delegatee could ask for help. The RN needs to listen to this request and intervene. There may be times when the patient's condition changes, and someone else, including the RN, may be better suited to completing the task. The RN may recognize that the delegatee is not as qualified to complete the task as originally thought. The RN must be aware of the need to avoid being negative, hurting the delegatee's self-confidence, or embarrassing the delegatee in front of others. How the RN communicates and intervenes can make the situation a positive learning experience for the delegatee. In addition, the RN must recognize the impact on the patient—how the patient views the change of assignment and if the patient wonders what is going on.

Supervision is a critical part of delegation. The ANA and the NCSBN have similar definitions of supervision. The ANA defines supervision as the "active process of directing, guiding, and influencing the outcome of an individual's performance of a task" (ANA & NCSBN, 2006), whereas the NCSBN defines it as "the provision of guidance or direction, oversight, evaluation and follow-up by the licensed nurse for the accomplishment of a delegated nursing task by assistive personnel" (ANA & NCSBN, 2006). It is important to note that supervision does not necessarily mean that the RN is in a management position. RNs who are not in management positions must also supervise when they delegate. **Figure 10-7** describes the decision tree for delegation.

Evaluation

How does the RN evaluate the delegation? The first focus is the role of the delegator. Were the right tasks delegated, and why? The second concern is the directions. Were the directions clear? The RN should consider to whom the task was delegated and the delegatee's strengths and limitations. Did the delegatee have the resources to complete the task? Did the delegatee have the time to complete the task? What impact did performing the specific task have on other responsibilities that the delegatee may have had? Did the delegatee have the authority to complete the task? Was the delegator available to the delegatee if questions arose or problems occurred? This availability is more than just physical; it concerns not only whether the delegatee is able to reach the delegator, but also whether the delegator is able to listen and hear the delegatee and then respond effectively.

Effective Delegation

RNs want to be effective delegators, and all new RNs struggle with how to delegate. The following are some characteristics of effective delegation (Milgram et al., 1999, p. 245):

- Do not give employees just menial tasks; include tasks that offer opportunities for learning and growth.
- Distribute tasks with an understanding of each employee's position description and job status, abilities, and total workload.

- Delegate when there is someone skilled available or when the task can be completed by a subordinate whose time is less expensive.
- Use benchmarks to monitor progress along the way; having only a final deadline can be overwhelming. (This applies to activities or tasks that take a longer time to complete.)
- Do not micromanage subordinates. Experienced employees usually have the skills necessary for managing complex tasks on their own (particularly if the tasks are typically done by them).
- Establish what needs to be done, and then provide support to the employee so that the employee can decide how to effectively accomplish the activity or task.

The focus of this discussion thus far has been on RNs delegating to other nursing staff—staff who are not RNs. It is important to recognize that RNs may assign work or tasks to other RNs. A team may include several RNs, and one may be the team leader. The nurse manager or nurse coordinator of a unit assigns work to RN staff routinely.

Effective delegation takes practice; it does not "just happen." There are barriers to delegation. Staff may be uncomfortable with delegating and with criticism, depending on whether they are the delegator or the delegatee. This can interfere with effective delegation and positive outcomes. RNs typically delegate to UAPs. Consequently, RNs need to know about UAP roles and job responsibilities. UAPs cannot do the following or be delegated these activities: health counseling; teaching; and activities that require independent, specialized nursing knowledge, skills, or judgment. The ANA (1997) has identified the UAP direct and indirect patient care activities as follows:

- *Direct patient care activities* assist the patient in meeting basic human needs (settings may be hospitals, home, long-term care, and other). Activities include assisting with feeding, drinking, ambulation, grooming, toileting, dressing, and socializing. Collection,

Step One — Assessment and Planning

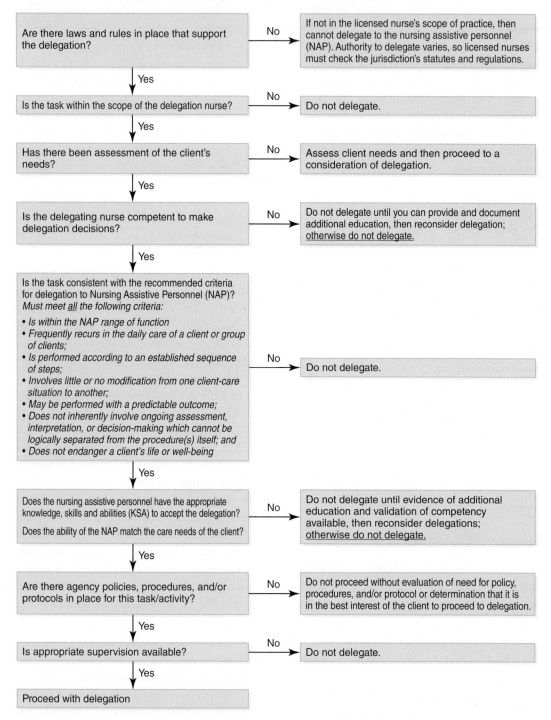

Figure 10-7 National Council of State Boards of Nursing Decision Tree for Delegation to Nursing Assistive Personnel

Source: From American Nurses Association and National Council of State Boards of Nursing. (2006). Joint statement on delegation. Retrieved from https://www.ncsbn.org/Delegation_joint_statement_NCSBN-ANA.pdf

reporting, and documentation of data related to these activities are important. UAPs need to report data to RNs; data then are used to make clinical judgments about patient care.

- *Indirect patient care activities* support the patient and the patient's environment, such as providing a clean, efficient, and safe patient care milieu. Activities might include companion care; simple meal preparation; housekeeping; providing transportation; and clerical, stocking, and maintenance tasks. Many of these activities would take place in the patient's home, where UAPs may be working one-on-one with patients through a home health agency or some type of community agency.

Generally, tasks that can be delegated are those that have the following characteristics (NCSBN, 2006):

- Frequently occur
- Are considered technical by nature
- Are considered standard and unchanging
- Have predictable results
- Have minimal potential for risks

Figure 10-8 illustrates the key to delegation and highlights the key aspects of delegation.

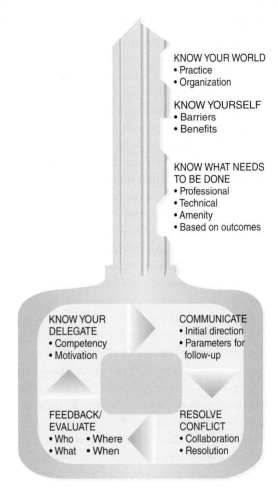

Figure 10-8 The Key to Delegation

Source: From Hansten, R. I., & Jackson, M. (2004). *Clinical delegation skills: A handbook for professional practice.* Sudbury, MA: Jones and Bartlett.

CHANGE

Change can be discussed in relation to changes in the healthcare delivery system. Change is also a part of collaboration and coordination, which are difficult to accomplish without some change; change may be required from an individual team member, the entire team, a unit, or the organization. Patients are asked to change all the time. Why do team members often not like change? They may be fearful of the results, particularly of the unknown; they may fear losing something of value, such as control, job responsibility, and so on; or they may have a belief that change will not make things better. The other view of change is its potential as an opportunity for improvement. Sometimes, however, change does not lead to positive outcomes. This situation has to be dealt with, but not changing means stagnation and lack of improvement.

The **plan–do–study–act cycle (PDSA)** is used more today by healthcare professionals and teams to assist in decision making, make changes, and ensure better coordinated care (Institute for

Health Improvement, 2011a). This cycle is used to test changes. During the first step (*plan*), the team identifies the objective(s) and discusses predictions as to what might happen and why; the team then develops a plan to implement the change. In the next step (*do*), the team institutes the change and collects and analyzes outcome data. In the third step (*study*), there is more in-depth analysis of the data and problem. In the last step (*act*), the change may be modified and then fully initiated.

Which methods can be used to decrease barriers to change and increase team involvement in change? Explanation and education about the issue or problem and the need for change is the first step. Including team members in the discussion about the need for change and possible solutions allows members to buy into the change process. They will participate more fully and be more invested in the results. Change is stressful; this stress needs to be recognized and, when possible, interventions to reduce stress implemented. Experiencing too many changes at one time or too quickly can make effective change difficult. Sometimes there are situations in which change is dictated. When this occurs, team members still need an explanation, and attempts to include them in some aspects of the change process should be encouraged. Asking for feedback and listening are important.

Change is risky—and sometimes it will fail. Teams need to learn from their errors and ineffective decisions and then move on. Effective collaborative teams do not place blame on individuals; rather, they look at results in an objective manner and realize that the team works together and sometimes can make mistakes.

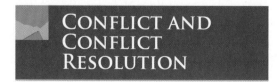

CONFLICT AND CONFLICT RESOLUTION

Conflict is inevitable; however, what is important is how it is handled. In many cases, conflict can

be prevented. It is natural for misunderstandings to occur among people who work together, such as in teams. Often, causes of conflict relate to whether resources are shared equitably; insufficient explanation of expectations, leading to performance being questioned; unexplained changes that disturb routines and process and for which team members are not prepared; and stress resulting from changes that team members do not understand and may see as threatening. Each of these causes can be prevented from developing into conflict, or at least conflict can be lessened, by engaging in clear, timely communication and including team members in the process.

There is another cause of conflict that is more difficult to manage: an individual's personal responses and behavior that may increase team conflict. Examples include the team member who does not do expected work; the team member who is late to meetings; the team member who does not listen to others; the team member who complains; the team member who is overly critical of others, the team member who does not know how to communicate effectively; and the team member who wants to be the star and take all the credit. **Figure 10-9** shows a conflict flowchart.

Conflict resolution requires leadership and participation from team members. When difficult issues or problems arise, it is best to deal with them rather than postpone decisions (which usually means that the problem has time to get worse). Using threats and negativity with little positive feedback can lead to conflict, so these approaches need to be avoided. Listening can go a long way toward preventing conflict and, if conflict does occur, resolving it. When team members treat one another with respect and communicate clearly, conflict can be decreased. Respect means to recognize another's right to have opinions and to listen and discuss these opinions. Nonverbal communication can give important clues as to when conflict is increasing. When teams or individual members experience stress, the risk of conflict increases. Open communication is

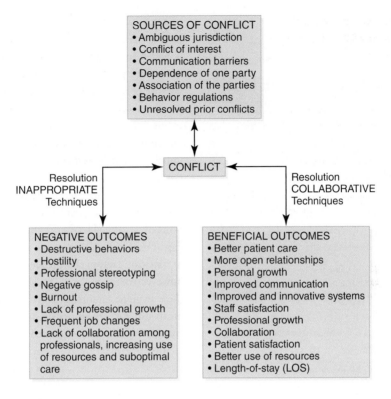

Figure 10-9 Conflict Flowchart

Source: From Hansten, R. I., & Jackson, M. (2004). *Clinical delegation skills: A handbook for professional practice.* Sudbury, MA: Jones and Bartlett.

key to resolution of conflict, and it is key to preventing conflict when possible.

When conflict occurs, it is important to provide opportunities to identify the facts, determine the purpose of the actions or activities at the time, and review team member perspectives. When members are emotional, this factor can interfere with effective resolution, so sometimes the best first approach is to step back and allow some time for all parties involved to temper their emotional reactions. However, the issue needs to be resolved, so this time period needs to be monitored—it should not go on too long. Sometimes one or two members need to be persuaded to reexamine the issue. This effort may or may not be successful. Teams need to learn that individual team members will not always get their viewpoint accepted

by all. Compromise is required; however, when this occurs, it must be done in a manner that respects divergent opinions and that does not use negativity or reduce self-esteem. All of these facets of conflict resolution require leadership—on the part of the designated team leader and from the members who commit to the team and its effectiveness. **Figure 10-10** describes a collaborative resolution method.

Power and Empowerment

As people work together, the issue of power arises. Simply put, **power** can be described as when healthcare provider A wants something that healthcare provider B has and may or may not need or want as much; healthcare provider B then has more

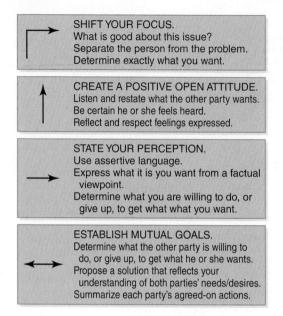

SHIFT YOUR FOCUS.
What is good about this issue?
Separate the person from the problem.
Determine exactly what you want.

CREATE A POSITIVE OPEN ATTITUDE.
Listen and restate what the other party wants.
Be certain he or she feels heard.
Reflect and respect feelings expressed.

STATE YOUR PERCEPTION.
Use assertive language.
Express what it is you want from a factual
  viewpoint.
Determine what you are willing to do, or
  give up, to get what what you want.

ESTABLISH MUTUAL GOALS.
Determine what the other party is willing to
  do, or give up, to get what he or she wants.
Propose a solution that reflects your
  understanding of both parties' needs/desires.
Summarize each party's agreed-on actions.

Figure 10-10 Hansten & Washburn's Collaborative
Resolution Method
Source: From Hansten, R. I., & Jackson, M. (2004). *Clinical delegation skills: A handbook
for professional practice.* Sudbury, MA: Jones and Bartlett.

power in the relationship. Typically, there is not a balance of power in a team, particularly when it is first formed. This is most commonly seen with nurses and physicians; physicians have more power because of their profession, experience, and history. This balance, however, can shift and should change as the team develops, with members recognizing one another's value and experience. Nevertheless, an imbalance can be difficult to overcome and makes the work situation stressful.

How a person feels about his or her work and job has an impact on how that person functions on a team. Herzberg's theory, as described in **Figure 10-11**, identifies job maintenance factors or extrinsic factors that influence job satisfaction; however, there is more to job satisfaction than these hygiene factors, as Herzberg calls them. The motivator factors (intrinsic factors) must also be considered. Herzberg suggested that because of these factors, organizations that increase accountability,

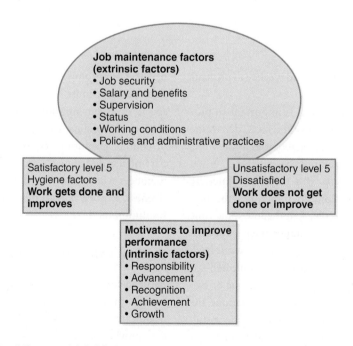

**Job maintenance factors
(extrinsic factors)**
• Job security
• Salary and benefits
• Supervision
• Status
• Working conditions
• Policies and administrative practices

Satisfactory level 5
Hygiene factors
**Work gets done and
improves**

Unsatisfactory level 5
Dissatisfied
**Work does not get
done or improve**

**Motivators to improve
performance
(intrinsic factors)**
• Responsibility
• Advancement
• Recognition
• Achievement
• Growth

Figure 10-11 Herzberg's Theory on Job Satisfaction

Exhibit 10-2	Types of Power

Type of Power	Description
Legitimate/formal power	Power that originates from serving in a formal position (e.g., a team leader, nurse manager, or chief nursing officer).
Referent/informal power	Power that originates from others recognizing that an individual has leadership qualities and choosing to follow that person.
Informational power	Power that originates from information a person has and others need.
Expert power	Power that originates from a person's expertise, which can be useful to others and enable the person to provide guidance (e.g., a nurse clinical specialist).
Reward power	Power that originates from a person's ability to reward others (e.g., the ability to grant a salary increase, promotion, or assign an interesting project) if they agree to do something.
Coercive power	Power that originates from a person's ability to punish others (e.g., the ability to assign an unpleasant task or project, or deny a promotion) if they do not do what is asked.

create teams, remove controls, provide feedback, introduce new tasks, allocate special assignments, and grant additional authority may increase staff motivation (Michalopoulos & Michalopoulos, 2006). Staff will then feel increased personal achievement and more **empowerment**. The same authors noted that the factors to increase staff motivation are part of the need for nurses to "increase responsibility, control over their work, and the opportunity to use their own initiative, all of which are offered in team nursing and the nursing process" (pp. 54–55). **Exhibit 10-2** describes the **types of power**.

Empowering teams means that the leader of the team needs to be less assertive over time and allow the team to lead itself. The team needs to find the best solutions by using the expertise of all the members and then assuming more leadership. This actually strengthens the team leader's leadership— with the result of better team outcomes.

CONCLUSION

This chapter includes content that is important to the healthcare profession's core competency, work in interprofessional teams. The content explored the meaning of this competency, its relationship to nursing, and what is involved in teams and teamwork. Collaboration, coordination, communication, delegation, and conflict and conflict resolution are major team activities.

CHAPTER HIGHLIGHTS

1. The essential features of the interprofessional team include examination of self as it relates to the team effort, interprofessional communication and conflict resolution, and the impact of the team's efforts on quality, safety, patient-centered care, and overall delivery of care.

2. Care coordination is a key factor in healthcare delivery and requires an interprofessional team effort.

3. Healthcare professional education takes place in isolation, with each healthcare profession providing its own education with limited regard to other healthcare professionals. This has limited the development of effective interprofessional teams.

4. A team leader must first recognize that it is the work of the team that is critical and avoid focusing on personal success as a leader.

5. Formal meetings are an important part of teamwork.

6. Planning before any team meeting is very important to the overall success of the meeting itself.

7. Effective teams value openness and collaboration.

8. Communication is the sharing of a message between one person or team/group and another. It is important to know if the message was received as sent. Interpretation plays a major role in effective communication, and sometimes interpretation confuses or changes the original message sent. Practices such as SBAR and checklists help to reduce communication problems.

9. Listening is critical to good communication.

10. Collaboration means that all people involved are listened to and that decisions are developed together.

11. Coordination—working to see that the pieces/activities fit together and flow as they should—can help to meet desired patient outcomes.

12. A clinical protocol or pathway is a written guide that provides direction for specific clinical problems; considers the interventions, timeline, and resources needed; and identifies expected outcomes.

13. Delegation refers to the process of transferring responsibility for a task to another person. The person delegating must have the authority to transfer this task; the task must then be handed off to someone whose scope of responsibilities includes this work.

14. There are five rights of delegation: right task, right circumstances, right person, right direction, and right supervision.

15. Change is part of collaboration and coordination, which are difficult to accomplish without some change; change may be required from an individual team member, the entire team, a unit, or the organization. The plan–do–study–act (PDSA) cycle is one method for planning and implementing change that a team might use.

16. Causes of conflicts may relate to inequitable sharing of resources; insufficient explanation of expectations leading to performance being questioned; unexplained changes that disturb routines and process and for which team members are not prepared; and stress resulting from changes that team members do not understand and may see as threatening.

17. Resolving conflict requires leadership and participation from team members.

18. Empowering teams means that the leader of the team must be less assertive over time and allow the team to lead.

Landscape © f9photos/Shutterstock, Inc.

DISCUSSION QUESTIONS

1. Explain the healthcare core competency "work in interprofessional teams." Why is this issue important to address in healthcare education, and what is its impact on practice?
2. What is a team, and how does it function?
3. How does collaboration influence team effectiveness?

4. Why is coordination a key activity of a clinical interprofessional team? Of a nursing team?
5. Explain the communication process.
6. Discuss the five delegation rights.
7. What is conflict resolution? How can conflict be prevented?

Landscape © f9photos/Shutterstock, Inc.

CRITICAL THINKING ACTIVITIES

1. For a week, keep a log of your critical communications. Note who was involved in the communication; the context or situation in which it occurred; the time of day and day of the week; the message; the effectiveness of the communication; and what could have been done to improve communication. Compare four communication examples from your log.
2. Make a list of how you would like to improve your communication. Why are those items on the list important to you?

3. Why do you think delegation might be easy or difficult for you as an individual?
4. Have you been a member of a team/group or in a work situation in which there was conflict? Describe the situation, the events that occurred, your role in the situation, and the resolution. How did you feel about the experience? Could something have been done to prevent the conflict? Were you satisfied with the resolution? If not, what could have improved it?

ELECTRONIC Reflection Journal

Circuit Board: ©Photos.com

Describe a team/group experience that you have had. Consider the structure, process, and communication of the team/group. For example, you might use a committee that you have been on, a group that you were in for a course project, a community service group, and so on. Consider how your experience relates to content in this chapter. Be sure and include your role(s) in the team/group.

Landscape © f9photos/Shutterstock, Inc.

LINKING TO THE INTERNET

- National Council of State Boards of Nursing: https://www.ncsbn.org/index.htm
- District of Columbia Area Health Education Center: http://dcahec.gwumc.edu/education/session3/members.html
- TeamSTEPPS: http://teamstepps.ahrq.gov/
- Institute of Health Improvement: http://www.ihi.org/
- Video on incivility in the workplace: http://www.youtube.com/watch?v=NujWmw8z7sg

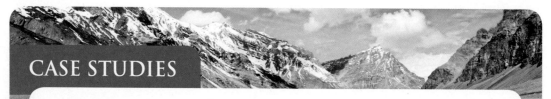

CASE STUDIES

Landscape © f9photos/Shutterstock, Inc.

Case Study 1

A 96-year-old man in very good health experiences a syncopal episode after standing unsupported for 20 minutes. His pulse was 46 and color ashen with circumoral cyanosis. Paramedics were called, and he was taken to the nearest emergency department. After extensive tests and 3 weeks of home monitoring, it was determined that the patient needed a pacemaker. Following the pacemaker insertion, it was determined that his cholesterol was elevated, and he was started on medication. The patient stated that he had been put on statins once before by his primary care physician and was not able to tolerate them. This time, the medication was to be closely monitored.

One month following his pacemaker insertion and the start of this medication, the patient saw his primary care physician. The physician went over his lab tests, for which samples were drawn prior to the visit. When the patient asked about his cholesterol, he was told that no lipid levels had been measured. When the patient further asked about the report on his pacemaker surgery, the physician replied that he had no report.

This case presents a lack of care coordination, a lack of effective communication among team members, and potential for error, resulting in patient safety and quality-of-care issues.

Case Questions

1. What could have been done to prevent the confusion that this patient experienced?
2. Where and when might errors have occurred?
3. How does this case reflect the need for interprofessional teamwork?
4. Have you or a family member experienced similar situations when receiving health care? What happened? Now that you know more about teamwork, safety, and quality, what is your perspective of the experience?

CASE STUDIES (CONTINUED)

Case Study 2

Examine the important topic of care coordination at the AHRQ website: http://www.ahrq.gov/professionals/prevention-chronic-care/improve/index.html. Content and presentations on the topic are provided on the site. Based on this information consider how care coordination will impact you as a nurse.

Case Questions

1. What are some examples of effective care coordination that you have seen in your clinical experiences?
2. What are some examples from your clinical experiences when you thought care coordination should have been used?

Words of Wisdom

Gayla D. Freeman, RN, MS
Acting Associate Chief Nurse, Specialty Services, Department of Veterans Affairs Medical Center, Oklahoma City, Oklahoma

I have been the operating room nurse manager for the past 5 years; I was the nurse manager for the surgical intensive care unit from 1988 to 1999, and nurse manager of the surgical clinics from 1999 to 2003.

Teamwork is one of the most important tasks of our time. Teamwork is like the invasive kudzu vine that covers everything in its path and is found growing everywhere in the southern part of the United States. Teamwork allows the healthcare team to bond together in a manner that promotes timely completion of patient care and support of each other's life struggles. Without teamwork, we are ineffective in our efforts; we struggle to pull all of the factors together; and we are obligated to duplicate the efforts of others. Without teamwork, health care is like a single stalk growing in the desert without anyone to nurture us. With teamwork, we are the kudzu vine, grasping, connecting, and supporting one another. I learned a long time ago that I was nothing without my staff, my patients, my doctors, and ancillary staff. In fact, I couldn't exist without all of the team members.

References

Agency for Healthcare Research and Quality (AHRQ). (2008, November). Pocket guide: TeamSTEPPS: Strategies and tools to enhance performance and patient safety. Retrieved from http://www.ahrq.gov/provessionals/education/curriculum-tools/teamstepps/instructor/essentials/pocketguide.html

Agency for Healthcare Research and Quality (AHRQ). (2011). TeamSTEPPS. Retrieved form http://teamstepps.ahrq.gov/

Agency for Healthcare Research and Quality (AHRQ). (2014). Care coordination. Retrieved from http://www.ahrq.gov/professionals/prevention-chronic-care/improve/coordination/index.html

American Association of Critical Care Nurses (AACN). (2005). AACN standards for establishing and sustaining healthy work environments: A journey to excellence. Retrieved from http://www.aacn.org/wd/hwe/content/hwehome.pcms?menu=hwe

American Nurses Association (ANA). (1997). *Position statement: Registered nurse utilization of unlicensed assistive personnel.* Washington, DC: Author.

American Nurses Association (ANA). (2010). *Scope and standards of practice.* Silver Spring, MD: Author.

American Nurses Association (ANA) & National Council of State Boards of Nursing (NCSBN). (2006). Joint statement on delegation. Retrieved from https://www.ncsbn.org/Delegation_joint_statement_NCSBN-ANA.pdf

Anthony, M. & Vidal, K. (2010). Mindful communication: A novel approach to improving delegation and increasing patient safety. *OJIN, 15* (2). Retrieved from http://nursingworld.org/MainMenuCategories/ANAMarketplace/ANAPeriodicals/OJIN/TableofContents/Vol152010/No-2May2010/Mindful-Communication-and-Delegation.html

Baggs, J. G., Schmitt, M. H., Mushlin, A. I., Mitchell, P. H., Eldredge, D., Oakes, D., & Hutson, A.D. (1999). Association between nurse–physician collaboration and patient outcomes in three intensive care units. *Critical Care Medicine, 27*, 1991–1998.

Barnsteiner, J., Disch, J., Hall, L., Mayer, D., & Moore, S. (2007). Promoting interprofessional education. *Nursing Outlook, 55*, 144–150.

Burke, M., Boal, J., & Mitchell, R. (2004). Communicating for better care: Improving nurse–physician communication. *American Journal of Nursing, 104*(12), 40–47.

Curry, L., Spatz, E., Charlin, E., Thompson, J. W., Decker, C., Krumholtz, H. M., & Bradley, E. H. (2011). What distinguishes top-performing hospitals in acute myocardial infarction mortality rates? *Annals of Internal Medicine, 154*, 384–390.

Dartmouth College. (2010). Clinical microsystems. Retrieved from http://dms.dartmouth.edu/cms/

Dessler, G. (2002). *Management: Leading people and organizations in the 21st century.* Upper Saddle River, NJ: Prentice Hall.

Fabre, J. (2005). *Smart nursing.* New York, NY: Springer.

Fairchild, D., Hogan, J., Smith, R., Portnow, M., & Bates, D. (2002). Survey of primary care physicians and home care clinicians. *Journal of General Internal Medicine, 17*, 243–261.

Finkelman, A., & Kenner, C. (2012). *Teaching IOM: Implications of the Institute of Medicine reports for nursing education* (3rd ed.). Silver Spring, MD: American Nurses Association Publishing.

Fried, B., Topping, S., & Rundall, T. (2000). Groups and teams in health services organizations. In S. Shortell & A. Kaluzny (Eds.), *Healthcare management: Organization and design behavior* (4th ed., pp. 233–250). Albany, NY: Delmar.

Gawande, A. (2009). *The checklist manifesto: How to get things right.* New York, NY: Metropolitan Books.

Gittell, J. (2002). Coordinating mechanisms in care provider groups: Relational coordination as a mediator and input uncertainty as a moderator of performance. *Management Science, 48*(11), 1408–1426.

Gittell, J., Weinberg, D., Pfefferle, S., & Bishop, C. (2008). Impact of relational coordination on job satisfaction and quality outcomes: A study of nursing homes. *Human Resource Management, 18*(2), 154–170.

Hagenow, N. (2003). Why not person-centered care? The challenges of implementation. *Nursing Administration Quarterly, 27*(3), 203–207.

Heller, R. (1999). *Learning to lead.* New York, NY: DK Publishing.

Higgins, L. (1999). Nurses' perceptions of collaborative nurse–physician transfer decision making as a predictor of patient outcomes in a medical intensive care unit. *Journal of Advanced Nursing, 29*, 1434–1443.

Institute for Health Improvement. (2011a). PDSA cycle. Retrieved from http://www.ihi.org/resources/Pages/Tools/PlanDoStudyActWorksheet.aspx

Institute for Health Improvement. (2011b). SBAR. Retrieved from http://www.ihi.org

Institute of Medicine (IOM). (2001). *Crossing the quality chasm.* Washington, DC: National Academies Press.

Institute of Medicine (IOM). (2003a). *Health professions education: A bridge to quality.* Washington, DC: National Academies Press.

Institute of Medicine (IOM). (2003b). *Priority areas for national action: Transforming healthcare quality.* Washington, DC: National Academies Press.

Interprofessional Education Collaborative Expert Panel. (2011). *Core competencies for interprofessional collaborative practice: Report of an expert panel.* Washington, DC: Interprofessional Education Collaborative.

Joint Commission. (2008). Sentinel event alert: Behaviors that undermine a culture of safety. Retrieved from http://www.jointcommission.org/sentinel_event_alert_issue_40_behaviors_that_undermine_a_culture_of_safety

Joint Commission. (2013). Sentinel event data: Root causes by event type 2004–2012. Retrieved from http://www.joint-commission.org/sentinel_event.aspx

Kupperschmidt, B., Kientz, E., Ward, J., & Reinholz, B. (2010, January). A healthy work environment: It begins with you. *OJIN: The Online Journal of Nursing, 15*(1). Retrieved from http://www.nursingworld.org/MainMenuCategories/AN-AMarketplace/ANAPeriodicals/OJIN/TableofContents/Vol152010/No1Jan2010/A-Healthy-Work-Environment-and-You.html

Lamb, G. (2013). Care coordination, quality, and nursing. In G. Lamb (Ed.), *Care coordination: The game changer. How nursing is revolutionizing quality care* (pp. 1–10). Silver Spring, MD: American Nurses Association.

Lower, J. (2007, September). Creating a culture of civility in the workplace. *American Nurse Today*, pp. 49–51.

Luparell, S. (2008, April–May). Incivility in nursing education: Let's put an end to it. *NSNA Imprint*, 42–46.

Maxfield, D., Grenny, J., McMillan, R., Patterson, K., & Switzler, A. (2005). Silence kills: The seven crucial conversations in healthcare. Retrieved from http://www.silenttreatmentstudy.com/silencekills/SilenceKills.pdf

McCallin, A. (2001). Interdisciplinary practice—a matter of teamwork: An integrated review. *Journal of Clinical Nursing, 10*, 419–428.

Michalopoulos, A., & Michalopoulos, H. (2006). Management's possible benefits from teamwork and the nursing process. *Nurse Leader, 4*(3), 52–55.

Milgram, L., Spector, A., & Treger, M. (1999). *Managing smart.* Houston, TX: Gulf Publishing.

Nair, D. M., Fitzpatrick, J. J., McNulty, R., Click, E. R., & Glembocki, M. M. (2012). Frequency of nurse–physician collaborative behaviors in an acute care hospital. *Journal of Interprofessional Care, 26*(2), 115–120.

Nelson, C., Godfrey, M., Batalden, P., Berry, S., Bothe, A., McKinley, K., & Nolan, T. (2008). Clinical microsystems, Part 1: The building blocks of health systems. *The Joint Commission Journal on Quality and Patient Safety, 34*(7), 367–378.

O'Keeffe, M., & Saver, C. (2014). *Communication, collaboration, and you.* Silver Spring, MD: American Nurses Association.

Rosenstein, A. (2002). Original research: Nurse–physician relationships: Impact on nurse satisfaction and retention. *American Journal of Nursing, 102*(6), 26–34.

Rosenstein, A., & O'Daniel, M. (2005). Disruptive and clinical behavior outcomes. *American Journal of Nursing, 105*(1), 54–63.

Rubenfeld, M. G., & Scheffer, B. (2006). *Critical thinking tactics for nurses.* Sudbury, MA: Jones and Bartlett.

Siegler, E. (1998). *Geriatric interdisciplinary team training.* NY: Springer.

Simpson, E., Rabin, D., Schmitt, M., Taylor, P., Urban, S., & Ball, J. (2001). Interprofessional healthcare practice: Recommendations of the National Academies of Practice expert panel on health care in the 21st century. *Issues in Interdisciplinary Care, 3*(1), 5–19.

Thomas, E., Sexton, J., & Helmreich, R. (2003). Discrepant attitudes about teamwork among critical care nurses and physicians. *Critical Care Medicine, 31*, 956–959.

U.S. Department of Health and Human Services (HHS). (2013). 2013 annual progress report to Congress: National strategy for quality improvement in health care. Retrieved from http://www.ahrq.gov/workingforquality/nqs/nqs2013annlrpt.htm

Weinberg, D., Miner, D., & Rivlin, L. (2009). "It depends": Medical residents' perspectives on working with nurses. *AJN, 109*(7), 34–43.

Weinstock, M. (2010). Team-based care. *Hospital Health Network, 84*(3), 6, 28.

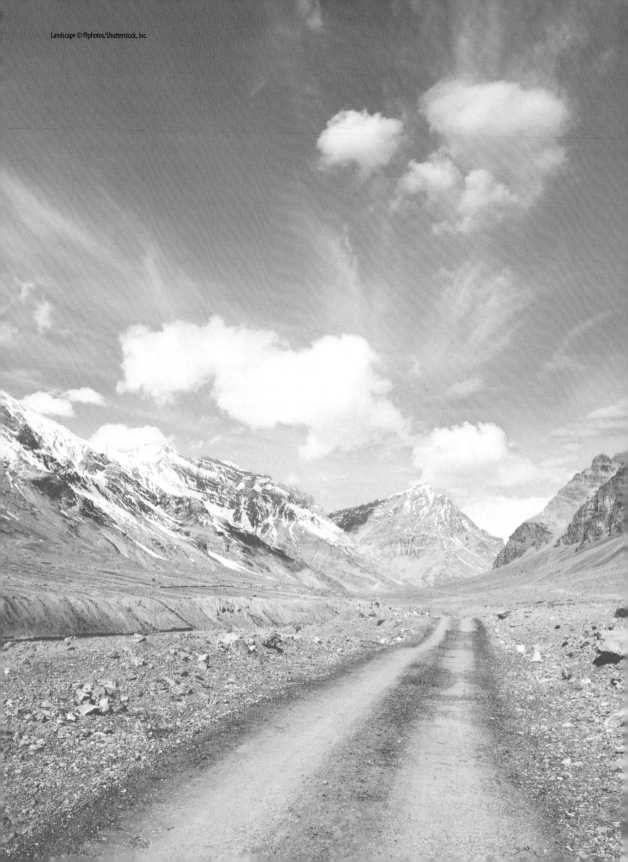

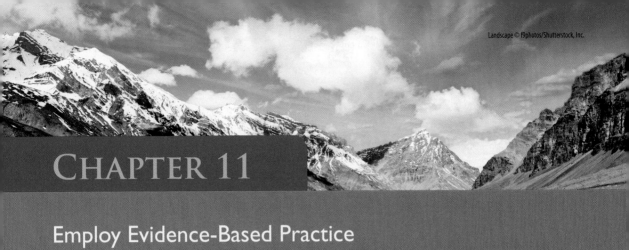

Landscape © f9photos/Shutterstock, Inc.

CHAPTER 11

Employ Evidence-Based Practice

CHAPTER OBJECTIVES

At the conclusion of this chapter, the learner will be able to:

- Discuss the core competency, "employ evidence-based practice"
- Define research
- Describe the research steps
- Discuss the relevance of nursing research
- Define evidence-based practice
- Describe the evidence-based practice process
- Analyze two key evidence-based practice tools
- Compare and contrast evidence-based practice and evidence-based management

- Discuss the barriers to implementing evidence-based practice and evidence-based management in nursing practice
- Compare and contrast evidence-based practice with research and quality improvement
- Examine the impact that evidence-based practice has had over the last decade on nursing practice, nursing models and frameworks, nursing education, and research

CHAPTER OUTLINE

KEY TERMS

Applied research
Basic research
Evidence-based management (EBM)
Evidence-based practice (EBP)
Experimental study
Hypothesis
Outcomes research

Patient–intervention–comparison–outcome–time (PICOT)
Procedures
Qualitative study
Quality improvement (QI)
Quantitative study
Randomized controlled trial (RCT)

Research
Research analysis
Research design
Research problem statement
Research proposal
Research purpose
Research question
Systematic review

INTRODUCTION

This chapter focuses on the third Institute of Medicine (IOM) core competency, "the need to use **evidence-based practice (EBP)** by all healthcare professionals, including nurses." **Evidence-based management (EBM)** is also critical for effective healthcare delivery in all settings. The content provided in this chapter explores this core competency. Because research is an important component in understanding and using EBP and is a part of nursing content, a brief introduction to nursing research is offered as well. EBP and its impact on nursing care and the nursing profession are described.

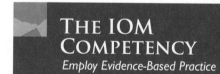

THE IOM COMPETENCY
Employ Evidence-Based Practice

The third healthcare profession core competency is to employ EBP. The IOM (2003) definition of EBP is to "integrate best research with clinical expertise and patient values for optimum care, and participate in learning and research activities to the extent feasible" (p. 4). EBP as a core competency is connected to providing patient-centered care and to interprofessional teams. Teams need to use EBP and EBM to provide the most effective patient-centered care. Nurse managers and other nursing leaders also need to actively apply EBM. "The lag between the discovery of more effective forms of treatment and their incorporation into routine patient care is, on average, 17 years" (Balas, 2001, as cited in IOM, 2003, p. 33). Clearly, there is a great need to get research results to the patient sooner. Increasing use of evidence can improve the quality of care and avoid underuse, misuse, and overuse of care (Chassin, 1998). To the nurse, this means the ability to get to the evidence, know what the evidence is;, and apply it, as appropriate, at the point of care. Using evidence might impact interventions such as prevention, diagnostic tests, or therapy; affect the ability to compare alternatives; and, in some cases, lead to the decision that no intervention is the best choice. **Figure 11-1** illustrates the key elements related to this core competency.

In 2011, the IOM published additional information about the relevance of EBP to health care:

> We seek the development of a learning health system that is designed to generate and apply the best evidence for the collaborative healthcare choices of each patient and provider; to drive the process of discovery as a natural outgrowth of patient care, and to ensure innovation, quality, safety, and value in health care. Our vision is for a healthcare system that draws on the best evidence to provide the care most appropriate to each patient, emphasizes prevention and health promotion, delivers the most value, adds to learning throughout the delivery of care, and leads to improvements in the nation's health. By the year 2020, 90 percent of clinical decisions will be supported by accurate, timely, and up-to-date clinical information, and will reflect the best available evidence. We feel that this presents a tangible focus for progress toward our vision, that Americans ought to expect at least this level of performance, that it should be feasible with existing resources and emerging tools, and that measures can be developed to track and stimulate progress. (IOM, 2011a, p. xi)

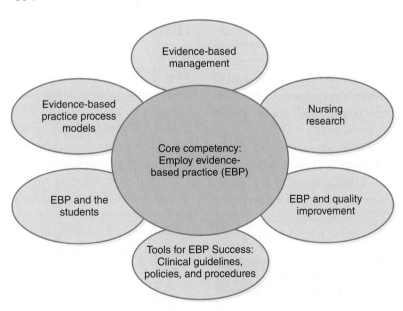

Figure 11-1 Employ Evidence-Based Practice: Key Elements

Research results that can make a difference in health care in general, and in nursing in particular, need to be implemented in practice. Currently, it takes too long for this to happen. EBP is the major initiative to increase the use of best practice or evidence in making clinical decisions. EBP requires that nurses "integrate best research with clinical expertise and patient values for optimum care" (IOM, 2003, p. 4). It is important to note that this definition of EBP includes more than just research results. Best practice clinical decisions also require healthcare provider expertise and patient assessment, as well as inclusion of the patient's perspective (patient preferences and values).

A critical question is: How much EBP is actually being used? Research done for research's sake, without ever influencing clinical research or making it into practice, has limited value. There are growing efforts to change this by increasing EBP content—not just research content—in all levels of nursing education, undergraduate through graduate. Efforts are also being made to improve staff education about EBP so that nurses in practice can gain and maintain essential competencies to increase EBP in clinical settings. In this chapter, it is important to recognize that research cannot be discussed without considering EBP; research and EBP should be interconnected. As part of this relationship, science must be accessible. EBP provides methods for making science more accessible to the practitioner who does not have a lot of time to pore over research study reports to determine what works and what does not work and to compare one study with another in detail.

It is easy to confuse research utilization and EBP. Research utilization usually involves using knowledge gained from one study, with limited regard to provider expertise, patient assessment, and patient preferences and values. EBP, by comparison, is a much more organized approach to getting research into practice.

NURSING RESEARCH

The first step in using EBP effectively is to understand research. **Research** is a systematic investigation that includes research development, testing, and evaluation. It is designed to develop or contribute to generalizable knowledge. Knowledge about research and the research process is important to understanding EBP. One of the major sources of best evidence for practice comes from research results. Nursing is considered a science discipline in that much of the knowledge base for nursing practice includes theoretical and evidence-based knowledge (American Nurses Association [ANA], 2010a).

Two major types of research approaches exist: basic and applied. **Basic research** is designed to broaden the base of knowledge, rather than solve an immediate problem, and is typically done in a laboratory setting. Results from basic research may be used to develop applied research. **Applied research** is designed to find a solution to a practical problem. It is often referred to as clinical research and is usually carried out in a nonlaboratory setting. Nurses typically are also involved in applied research, although some nurses are involved in basic research. **Outcomes research** is a newer approach. This type of research focuses on determining the effectiveness of healthcare services and patient outcomes.

Historical Background

How has the nursing profession developed nursing research (ANA, 2010b)? Florence Nightingale was interested in clinical research, but no such activity occurred in nursing in her era. Although Nightingale used the data she collected to measure patient outcomes and improve care, the nursing community really did not pay much attention to research early in its history.

When nurses began to earn advanced degrees, this trend resulted in some studies about nurses and nursing education, but research was still not an important part of nursing. In the 1920s and 1930s, a few very early studies focused more on nursing care. Some of these studies were published in the *American Journal of Nursing*, making them the first studies to be published in a nursing journal, although the conduct of nursing studies remained very rare. It took time for more studies to be done.

In the 1950s, greater interest in nursing research emerged, and the journal *Nursing Research* was launched. In the 1970s and 1980s, more nurses conducted studies and more nurses obtained graduate degrees (including doctoral degrees); thus nursing researchers were more qualified. Nursing theorists were very active in the 1960s and 1970s, adding to the scholarly work.

Nursing organizations in the United States and internationally support nursing research and have described their views of research. The International Council of Nurses (ICN, 2010) describes it in the following way:

> The International Council of Nurses is committed to supporting nursing research as a powerful tool for generating new knowledge and evidence to underpin nursing practice. Nursing has an obligation to society to provide care that is continually researched and evaluated. Nurses working singly or in multidisciplinary research teams can offer new insights and unique perspectives to the research process. Nursing research provides opportunities for linkages between those involved in the research process, practicing nurses, other health professionals, policy makers, and the public. With the rapid advances in knowledge and technology, nursing research serves as a framework for organizing facts and evidence into a coherent and usable format. A research network provides a vehicle for continual exchange of knowledge and experience. The ICN Research Network will serve as a forum for exchange of ideas, experience and expertise and as a vital resource bank for global nursing and health research.

The American Association of Colleges of Nursing (AACN, 2006) statement on research includes the following principles:

> Nursing researchers bring a holistic perspective to studying individuals, families, and communities; their research takes a biobehavioral, interdisciplinary (interprofessional), and translational approach to science. The priorities for nursing research reflect nursing's commitment to the promotion of health and healthy lifestyles, the advancement of quality and excellence in health care, and the critical importance of basing professional nursing practice on research.

The AACN position statement also identifies major research focus areas. The first area, clinical research, includes interventions that might be used, from acute to chronic care experiences across the entire life span; health promotion and preventive care to end-of-life care; and care for individuals, families, and communities in diverse settings. The second area is health systems and outcomes research, which focuses on identifying ways that the organization and delivery of health care influence quality, cost, and the experience of patients and their families. The third focus is on nursing education—research that explores more effective and efficient educational processes and new teaching–learning practices to incorporate technology in the learning process; intergenerational learning differences and their impact on education; and the development of methods to improve lifelong learning and commitment to leadership.

National Institute of Nursing Research

The National Institute of Nursing Research (NINR), established in 1985, is part of the National Institutes of Health (NIH). It is important that nursing have a presence in the most prestigious national research system in the United States. NINR conducts research that has an impact within the discipline of nursing and allocates funding for nursing studies conducted in other institutions such as universities and clinical organizations; interprofessional research is also encouraged and funded by this organization. NINR (2014) describes how nursing research develops knowledge for the following purposes:

- Build the scientific foundation for clinical practice
- Prevent disease and disability
- Manage and eliminate symptoms caused by illness
- Enhance end-of-life and palliative care

NINR is physically located at the NIH campus in Rockville, Maryland. When funded research is conducted at the NINR campus, it is referred to as an intramural or internal study. Grants are also awarded for outside, or extramural, studies that are conducted at the researcher's home institution or in collaboration with several institutions. The

NINR's current (2011, updated 2013) strategic plan identifies its goals to invest in research focused on the following areas:

- Enhance health promotion and disease prevention
- Improve quality of life by managing symptoms of acute and chronic illness
- Improve palliative and end-of-life care
- Enhance innovation in science and practice
- Develop the next generation of nurse scientists

The Research Process

The research process is similar to the nursing process; it is a problem-solving method. **Exhibit 11-1** describes the steps of the quantitative research process.

Exhibit 11-1   Steps in the Quantitative Research Process

I. Describe problem statement, including background and significance

II. Identify research question(s) and hypothesis

III. Identify the purpose(s) of the study

Explain how the findings might be used.

IV. Review of literature

Provide a summary of critical literature (theoretical and research literature) that applies to the study.

V. Theoretical framework

Use theories and conceptual models to organize research findings into a broader conceptual context. Include conceptual and operational definitions of the variables (independent and dependent) in the framework. Identify assumptions. (This step is not done for all studies.)

VI. Ethical considerations

Follows the consent and institution review board process.

VII. Research design and methods

A. Research design

1. Identify the research design. Is the study a quantitative study or a qualitative study? Which specific subdesign (e.g., experimental, quasi-experimental, descriptive) is used?
2. Provide an adequate rationale for choosing the research design.
3. Identify independent and dependent variables (if required).

Or

B. Sample and sample selection

1. Describe the sample population.
2. Provide sample criteria (inclusion and exclusion criteria).
3. Describe sample size using power analysis.
4. Describe how those participants/subjects who met the criteria were selected as study subjects, sampling method. (How were eligible participants/subjects selected and located?)
5. If applicable, describe how groups or treatments/interventions were assigned.

Exhibit 11-1 *(continued)*

C. Setting

   1. Briefly describe the setting for the study.

D. Measurement and instrumentation

   1. Discuss the origin and type of measurement instruments.

   2. Describe why the instrument(s) is (are) appropriate to study the problem (i.e., why the instrument can produce data that can answer the study question).

   3. Ensure that the instrument is compatible with the conceptual/theoretical framework.

   4. If an instrument was developed for the study, describe how it was developed and how it was tested for reliability/validity; pilot-test it before using it in the study.

   5. Describe the reliability and validity of the instrument. Evaluate and report relevant reliability and validity data from previous research.

E. Data collection

   1. Describe how access to the study setting will be obtained.

   2. Describe the data collection process and procedures chronologically and clearly enough to allow for replication

(describe them in sufficient detail so that a stranger could use this procedure and collect the data as intended).

   3. Identify who will collect the data and the training required. Provide data collection forms as required.

   4. Discuss control features of study procedures.

F. Data analysis (This step is completed after the previous steps are completed, but the proposal plan needs to describe the data analysis plan.)

   1. Answer each hypothesis or study question according to a specific plan for each.

   2. Identify appropriate statistical tests and the rationale for their use in analyzing each study question or hypothesis and participant demographic data. Include the level of measurement of each variable and selected level of significance.

   3. Specify and justify the level of significance (i.e., 0.05, 0.01) for statistical results and findings.

G. Limitations

   1. Ensure that limitations are clearly identified and appropriate.

VIII. Results and conclusions

First, the researcher develops a plan or proposal. This written document describes recent relevant literature on the problem area, describes the research topic or problem, and defines the processes or steps that will be followed to answer the research question(s). The **research proposal** is used to plan the research and also may be used to apply for research funding. The proposal is written in the future tense because the research has not yet been done.

There must be an assessment to identify and describe the problem, formulating the **research problem statement**. The researcher does this

assessment using the researcher's individual expertise and by reviewing the literature. The review of literature is included in the research proposal and in the subsequent research report of results. The researcher (or researchers) primarily examines previous studies by reading their published reports of results.

The researcher then identifies the study question(s) and hypothesis(ses). The **research question** is concise; it is developed before the research is conducted. It is stated in the research proposal.

The **hypothesis** is the formal statement of the expected relationship or relationships between two or more variables in a specified population, which is the sample. The hypothesis is stated before the research is conducted, and it is included in the proposal. Some studies do not have hypotheses, such as qualitative studies in which the emphasis is on describing a situation or perception rather than on measuring the variable of interest. The question and hypothesis flow from the description of the research problem statement and the research question. The researcher also needs to consider the **research purpose**—describing the potential uses the results.

In nursing research, particularly qualitative studies, the researcher may identify a theory or a conceptual model to organize the findings. The theory or model is described and related to the research question. For example, if a study was developed to investigate patient education about diabetes, Orem's theory on self-care might be used as the framework for the study. Not all nursing research that uses a conceptual framework relies on nursing theory. It is important that the framework represents the phenomenon of interest and guides the question and the way in which the variable is to be measured. For example, if the nurse is studying blood pressure in a premature infant, the study would most likely use a scientific, physiologically based framework to support factors that influence blood pressure.

This all sets the stage for the actual research, which requires that the assessment and problem identification are clear. These steps are similar to the assessment and nursing diagnosis phases. The specific plan for conducting the study is the research design and methods. In the proposal, the researcher describes what will be done, and in the research report or published article, poster, or presentation after the study, the researcher describes what was done.

The **research design** and methods are complex. They include the details related to type of study (research approach and design); the sample and the means by which the sample is selected; the setting for the study; measurement and instrumentation to collect data; the data collection process

(What exactly will be done to collect the data?) and data analysis (How will the data be analyzed?); and a description of potential limitations. The plan should be clear and detailed. The research proposal can be compared to the nursing care plan. This information, or the plan, is called a proposal until the research is conducted. The study is conducted after funding is received. This step could be compared to implementing a care plan.

The last part of the research process is the **research analysis** and description of the results and conclusions. The proposal describes how the data will be analyzed, but the actual analysis of data cannot occur until the study has been conducted and data collected. What did the analysis of data demonstrate, and what are the implications of the data? The researcher has to consider the proposal—what was planned, how the study was implemented, and how the data were to be analyzed—so that the outcomes are identified, just as would be done in the nursing process. This can be compared to the evaluation that determines whether patient outcome goals were met based on the nursing process or care plan.

Types of Research Design

The research design describes the plan for the study in detail. It can be compared to a nursing care plan in that the design provides information about the study and explains how the study will be conducted, as well as planned assessment or analysis of the results. Research study designs are categorized as either quantitative or qualitative. In **quantitative studies**, the research question focuses on how many or how much; in **qualitative studies**, the research question focuses on feelings or experiences.

All quantitative research is not **experimental**; to be experimental, a study must meet three criteria:

1. *Manipulation of intervention:* The researcher administers an intervention to the participants/subjects (sample). This intervention represents

the independent variable or variables. The researcher wants to identify the effect of the independent variable on the dependent variable or determine if the independent variable causes the dependent variable.

2. *Control:* The researcher controls some of the experimental situation and uses a control group. Total control is not usually possible, but efforts must be made to have as much control of the situation as possible. This is more difficult in applied or clinical research as compared with a laboratory setting.

3. *Randomization:* The researcher assigns participants in the sample to the experimental or control groups using systematic methods, randomization. The control group does not experience the intervention identified as the independent variable.

Data collection in a quantitative study is highly structured. Examples of data collection methods include structured interviews; collection of biophysiological data, such as blood pressure, blood, urine, and other physiological parameters; questionnaires; rating scales; structured observation; and many other methods. In quantitative studies, data analysis involves the use of statistics.

Data collection in qualitative studies is less structured than in a quantitative study. A qualitative study might use focus groups, diaries, logs, observation, and open-ended interviews; analysis of data does not rely on statistics or mathematical equations. The researcher is less detached and may interact actively with the participants/subjects to obtain the best data possible. In fact, the researcher is often considered the instrument of the qualitative research. Data are analyzed as the study progresses and may lead the researcher in a different direction or to collect additional data. However, data that are not covered in the informed consent cannot be collected without institutional review board (IRB) approval for the change. The goal is to understand the issue deeply, not to intervene, and also to see results or compare groups.

Research Funding

Funding is a critical part of any research because it provides the resources to conduct the research. Funding sources vary widely: universities, private donations, foundations and organizations, local and state governments, and the federal government. The federal government is the largest source of grant monies.

There are three approaches that a researcher can take to obtain funding:

1. Identify a problem and develop a proposal. This proposal is sent to funding sources that would have an interest in the particular problem.

2. Develop a research proposal that specifically addresses a problem area that a funding source has identified as a critical need area. This is called a request for proposals or request for applications.

3. Sometimes funding sources require that the researcher conduct a pilot study or have data that indicate greater need for research about a particular problem. Indeed, in many cases, having data is critical to getting funding for a study.

Once the written proposal is completed and submitted, it is scrutinized to see whether it meets a set of very specific requirements. These requirements can vary from one funding source to another, and deadlines differ. The proposal then goes through the grant review process, which can take months. Typically, peer groups identified by the funding source review grant proposals.

It is extremely difficult to get funding. The federal government grants are highly competitive, and the major source of such funds is the NIH. Congress sets the NIH's budget. Nursing research is funded by similar sources, as is other healthcare research. Funds are also available to support training programs and service programs—for example, to develop a new graduate program for nurse practitioners or doctors of nursing practice, offer a nurse residency program, implement programs to increase student retention, and establish a nurse managed clinic. Funding for these types of projects and programs typically comes from the Health Resources and Services Administration (HRSA), which is part of the U.S. Department of Health and Human Services (HHS). These funds are not research grants, but rather program grants.

Ethics and Legal Issues

When ethics and legal issues are considered in relation to research, the first concern is to protect the rights of human participants/subjects. A second area that the researcher considers is how best to balance benefits and risks in the studies. There are many studies in which participants might potentially be harmed. Research ethics emphasizes the need to be clear about participant/subject risks whenever possible. The third ethical and legal issue is informed consent, which is also important in healthcare service delivery. The last concern is institutional review—that is, review of the proposal to ensure that participant/subject rights are protected and that the study is planned in an effective manner that meets the sponsoring organization's standards.

Several major historical research projects have been influential in increasing attention to the ethical conduct of research, particularly studies that involve human subjects. The most familiar may be the Nazi medical experiments conducted during World War II. These "research" studies violated many aspects of basic human rights and led to few gains in scientific knowledge. In 1947, after World War II had ended, 27 Nazi physicians were tried in Nuremberg, Germany, for research atrocities that they performed during the war. The U.S. Holocaust Memorial Museum maintains a website where the official trial record can be accessed. The transcripts of testimony by persons who were forced to serve as subjects in these experiments reveal incredible violations of human rights. An important outcome of this experience and the trial was the publication of the first internationally recognized code of research ethics, the Nuremberg Code, which has served as a prototype

for the development of many later codes of research ethics. The core of the research code comprises the following rights that must be protected:

- Right to self-determination
- Right to privacy
- Right to anonymity and confidentiality
- Right to fair treatment
- Right to protection from discomfort and harm

Other important examples of human rights violations have occurred in the United States. The two best known are the Tuskegee syphilis study (1932–1972) and the Willowbrook study (mid-1950s–1970s). The Tuskegee study used African Americans in the sample to examine the natural course of syphilis. Many of the participants did not give informed consent, and some did not even know that they were participants in a study. Even though it was clear within a few years of the study's progress that participants with syphilis had severe complications and high death rates, nothing was done to institute treatment. The Willowbrook study examined hepatitis at an institution for mentally retarded individuals. The children at this facility were deliberately infected with hepatitis.

In all three of these examples, researchers abused vulnerable subjects and there were few, if any, controls. Today, because of standards and ethics, there is greater control to prevent these types of experiences from happening again. An example is the extensive required informed consent process and documentation requirements. The ANA's *Code of Ethics with Interpretive Statements* focuses on five rights:

1. Right to anonymity and/or confidentiality
2. Right to self-determination
3. Right to privacy
4. Right to fair treatment
5. Right to protection from discomfort and harm (ANA, 2001)

After these experiences of abuse in research, efforts were instituted to prevent further problems. One of the strategies was the creation of the institutional research board (IRB). This committee reviews research before it is conducted to ensure that the study is conducted ethically. Researchers conducting any study that involves human subjects have to obtain approval from their institution's IRB. IRBs are mandated to review all research that involves human subjects in institutions that receive federal funds. The purpose is to protect subjects from unnecessary risk or from risks that outweigh potential benefits. Particularly vulnerable populations include the following groups:

- Neonates (newborns)
- Children
- Pregnant women and fetuses
- Persons with mental illness
- Persons with cognitive impairment
- Terminally ill persons
- Persons confined to institutions (e.g., prisons, long-term care hospitals)

Examples of questions that might be considered by an IRB include the following:

1. Is the subject being deceived, and if so, is it necessary for the integrity of the research?
2. Does the subject understand the purpose of the project and completely understand his or her role in the project?
3. Are there obvious costs or hidden costs to people if they participate? Can they withdraw at any time?
4. What are the benefits, if any, to the subject?
5. What are the risks, immediate and long term (if known), to the subject?
6. How will the researcher protect the subject's right to confidentiality?
7. Whom should the subjects contact with questions?
8. What will be done with the results of the study?

Barriers to and Facilitators of Research

Research is not easy to accomplish. Barriers need to be turned into facilitators for research to be successful. Barriers could include any of these issues:

1. *Lack of funding:* Researchers need to obtain adequate funding; most research is costly to implement.
2. *Lack of sufficient time:* Good research takes planning and time to accomplish. The researcher needs blocks of time to work on a study. Some investigators do research on a full-time basis.
3. *Lack of research competencies:* Research expertise is developed over a period of years. Finding a mentor or mentors is important; working with researchers who have been successful can assist a novice researcher.
4. *Lack of participants/subjects for the sample:* If the study requires participants/subjects, it is not always easy to find them in the number required or for the circumstances required. This takes time and creativity, and ethical principles must be considered. Participants/subjects may leave a study at any time.
5. *Inability to find the right setting:* Finding and securing a setting that agrees to participate in the study can be problematic because it requires contacts and communication, and on the setting side does have an impact on their functioning.
6. *Lack of statistical expertise:* Researchers should find a statistical expert to consult; researchers work in teams and need to work with different experts.

Other Influential Organizations: Impact on Research

The ANA identifies research as an important issue for professional nursing.

The mission statement of the American Nurses Association (ANA) is *nurses advancing our profession to improve health for all.* Central to this mission is that ANA serves as the profession's advocate for nursing quality outcomes. Quality outcomes require the use of research for evidence-based practice. ANA's goal in developing this research agenda is to identify gaps in evidence for practice. The following agenda provides direction for research activities to ANA's members, its constituent and state nurses associations and organizational affiliates, health care organizations and clinical and academic researchers; priority areas for consideration when submitting a proposal for the National Database for Nursing Quality Indicators (NDNQI) data use, consideration and potential funding opportunities. (ANA, 2011).

Key research agenda items identified by the ANA include the following topics:

- The value of nursing contributions to safety, reliability, quality, and efficiency
- Factors that increase the impact of nurses on quality and efficiency
- Use of NDNQI to enhance patient safety, quality care, and efficiency
- Nurse workforce issues
- Population health issues

The Improvement Science Research Network (ISRN) is a new organization. Its purpose is to "… to accelerate interprofessional improvement science in a systems context across multiple sites." (ISRN, 2014). This organization is based at the University of Texas–San Antonio and offers programs each summer focusing on quality improvement. The ISRN is the only NIH-supported improvement research network to accelerate interprofessional improvement science in a systems context across multiple sites.

The IOM provides in-depth analysis of research issues. Some of these reports are briefly described here:

- *Knowing What Works in Health Care: A Roadmap for the Nation* (IOM, 2008): This report emphasizes the need to use EBP and to identify diagnostic, treatment, and prevention services based on what works effectively. Cost must also be considered in clinical decisions, and it impacts quality care. Critical factors that need to be considered are constraining healthcare

costs, reducing geographic variation in the use of healthcare services, improving quality, empowering healthcare consumers, and making healthcare coverage decisions.

- *Clinical Practice Guidelines We Can Trust* (IOM, 2011b): This report discusses the importance of developing effective clinical guidelines based on best evidence and then applying those guidelines when appropriate. The guidelines should be based on systematic reviews; developed by knowledgeable multidisciplinary experts; consider important patient subgroups and patient preferences; provide clear explanations of the logical relationships between alternative care options and health outcomes; and be revised as needed.

- *Finding What Works in Health Care: Standards for Systematic Reviews* (IOM, 2011c): This report focuses on research and EBP and emphasizes the importance of systematic reviews. Standards to ensure quality care should be based on systematic reviews that include assessment of individual studies and synthesis of the evidence, with this information then being shared through publication so that it can be applied.

EVIDENCE-BASED PRACTICE

What is the purpose of EBP? The use of EBP in nursing leads to more effective decision making to guide the use of limited resources, control costs, and improve quality (Jennings & Loan, 2001). An EBP nursing review is not nursing research; an EBP review involves looking for evidence, including (1) evidence of research results, (2) evidence from a patient's assessment and other sources, (3) evidence from clinical expertise, and (4) evidence from information about patient preferences and values.

How do you get from EBP to research? You might not. At the conclusion of an EBP review,

Exhibit 11-2	Five-Step Approach for Evidence-Based Nursing Practice
Ask	Identify the research question. Determine if the question is well constructed to elicit a response or solution.
Acquire	Search the literature for preappraised evidence or research. Secure the best evidence that is available.
Appraise	Conduct a critical appraisal of the literature and studies. Evaluate for validity and determine the applicability in practice.
Apply	Institute recommendations and findings and apply them to nursing practice.
Assess	Evaluate the application of the findings, outcomes, and relevance to nursing practice.

Source: Schmidt, N. A., & Brown, J. M. (2015). *Evidence-based practice for nurses: Appraisal and applications of research.* Burlington, MA: Jones & Bartlett Learning. Adapted from Straus, S. (2005). *Introduction to teaching evidence-based health care.* University of Toronto knowledge translation program (PowerPoint Presentation). Retrieved from http://www.cebm.net/?o=1021

you might find that there is sufficient evidence to answer the clinical question. If this is the case, no more research is needed. Thus an EBP review does not mean that research is conducted or that it must be conducted. If an EBP review indicates that evidence is already available, there is no need to perform additional research. In most cases, however, sufficient nursing research is not available to settle most nursing questions. This means that research may be needed to fill the gap in the knowledge base. **Exhibit 11-2** shows a five-step approach for EBP.

Definitions

According to the 2008 IOM report on EBP,

> Decisions about the care of individual patients should be based on the conscientious, explicit, and judicious use of current best evidence. This means that individual clinical expertise should be integrated with the best information from scientifically based, systematic research and applied in light of the patient's values and circumstances. (p. 2)

This does not mean that all patient care decisions are based on research evidence or only research

evidence characterized by factors such as clinical expertise and patient values and circumstances. Multiple sources of knowledge or evidence exist (Melnyk & Fineout-Overholt, 2010), including the following resources:

- *Best research evidence:* This evidence is ranked and described in **Figure 11-2**.
- *Clinical expertise:* The knowledge and experience of the clinician (nurse, physician, and others on the healthcare team).

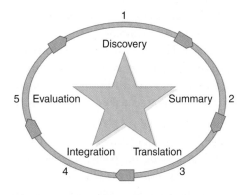

ACE Star Model of Knowledge Transformation

Figure 11-2 Rating EBP
Source: UT San Antonio Health Science Center. (n.d.). ACE Star Model. Retrieved from http://www.acestar.uthscsa.edu/acestar-model.asp

- *Patient values and preferences/circumstances:* These are the individual patient's own concerns, preferences, expectations, and social and financial resources that impact health and health care. These factors can change over time and with each unique healthcare need and encounter.
- *Clinical data (assessment) and history:* A patient's assessment includes important evidence that should be considered in treatment decisions.

As nursing students soon discover when they search for nursing EBP literature, there is a problem in this field: The nursing and allied health professions are not as far along in implementing EBP as medicine is. The amount of nursing research must increase—not just in quantity, but also in quality and relevance to nursing practice. Also, nursing health interventions are not captured effectively in medical records, which impacts whether nursing data are included in research studies (IOM, 2003). Examples of nursing data include those related to patient pain, dehydration, skin breakdown, lifestyle change, patient knowledge deficiencies, and non-adherence with treatment. Furthermore, nursing interventions often are evaluated in descriptive or qualitative studies rather than in quantitative studies. Quantitative studies are ranked higher than qualitative studies when evaluating or ranking evidence from research studies.

The **PICOT** question should be part of every search for evidence to improve practice. The goal is to ask a searchable and answerable question to identify the best evidence to answer the question. The acronym stands for the patient/population, intervention, comparison, outcome, and time (Melnyk & Stillwater, 2010, pp. 29–30):

1. The *P* (patient/population) needs to be specific—describing the population such as age, gender, diagnosis, ethnicity, or other.
2. The *I* (intervention) can be related to prognostic factors, risk behaviors, exposure to disease, or clinical intervention or treatment.

3. The *C* (comparison) can be with another treatment or no treatment.
4. The *O* is the outcome—what will it be, such as risk of disease, complication, side effect, or adverse outcome.
5. The *T* is time—meaning the time involved to demonstrate the outcome.

The PICOT process includes five steps (Melnyk & Stillwater, 2010):

1. Identify a burning clinical issue or question.
2. Collect the best evidence relevant to the question.
3. Critically appraise that evidence before it is used.
4. Integrate the evidence with the other parts of EBP: patient preferences and values, your clinical expertise, assessment information about the patient and the patient's history.
5. Evaluate the practice decision or change.

Exhibit 11-3 provides examples of templates that can be used to develop PICOT questions.

Types of EBP Literature

EBP literature is different from typical clinical literature and research literature (i.e., published articles about studies). The key component of EBP literature is a systematic review. A **systematic review** is a "summary of evidence typically conducted by an expert or a panel of experts on a particular topic, that uses a rigorous process (to minimize bias) for identifying, appraising, and synthesizing studies to answer a specific clinical question [PICOT question] and draw conclusions about the data gathered" (Melnyk & Fineout-Overholt, 2010, p. 582). Another definition of systematic review is that it is "the consolidation of research evidence that incorporates a critical assessment and evaluation of the research (not simply a summary) and addresses a focused clinical question using methods designed to reduce the likelihood of bias" (DiCenso, Guyatt, & Ciliska, 2005, p. 570). The key characteristic of systematic reviews that identifies their value is their critique of multiple studies related to the same research question to determine best evidence available.

Exhibit 11-3	Templates for PICOT Questions

Intervention: In _____, what is the effect of _____ on _____ compared with _____ within _____?

Etiology: Are _____ who have at risk for/of _____ compared with _____ with/without _____ over _____?

Diagnosis or diagnostic test: Are (is) _____ more accurate in diagnosing _____ compared with _____?

Prevention: For _____, does the use of _____ reduce the future risk of _____ compared with _____ within _____?

Prognosis/Prediction: Does _____ influence _____ in patients who have _____ over_____?

Meaning: How do _____ diagnosed with _____ perceive _____ during _____?

Source: From Melnyk, B., & Fineout-Overholt, E. (2010). *Evidence-based practice in nursing and healthcare* (p. 31). Philadelphia, PA: Lippincott Williams & Wilkins. Reprinted with permission.

There are several types of systematic reviews, but all types (1) have prescribed criteria for conducting the review process, (2) review not only research reports but also some data from large databases and may include published articles that are opinion or essay, and (3) try to find as much available evidence as possible (Brown, 2009). During the assessment process, when evidence is reviewed, a standard hierarchy or rating system is used (shown in Figure 11-2).

Searching for EBP Literature: Evidence

The first step in finding evidence is to look for a systematic review that addresses the identified PICOT question. If these reviews cannot be found, randomized controlled trials/studies should be sought. **Randomized controlled trials (RCT)** are often referred to as the gold standard in research design. They involve a true experiment; there is control over variables, randomization of the sample with a control group and an experimental group, and manipulation of an intervention or interventions (independent variable). The results of a randomized controlled trial provide the strongest support for a cause-and-effect relationship. Not all studies meet these criteria.

Two important EBP literature databases are the Cochrane database and the Joanna Briggs Institute EBP database. A third source is the Agency for Healthcare Research and Quality (AHRQ) and its collection of evidence-based national clinical guidelines. A description of each of these databases follows:

- *The Cochrane collaboration:* This center develops, maintains, and updates systematic reviews of healthcare interventions to allow practitioners to make informed decisions.
- *Joanna Briggs Institute:* This organization represents an international collaboration among nursing and allied health centers. The main purpose is to train professionals to conduct systematic reviews.
- *AHRQ national clinical guidelines:* This source is government based, although the guidelines come from many different sources. Guidelines are discussed further elsewhere in this chapter. The guidelines are available at http://www.guideline.gov/.

Sigma Theta Tau International (STTI), the nursing honor society, is also active in the area of EBP through its online publication, *Online Journal of Knowledge Synthesis for Nursing.* This journal provides full-text systematic reviews to guide nursing practice. It is available by subscription. University libraries may have access via a university subscription, so students may be able to access the journal through their university library.

The Roles of Staff Nurses as Related to Systematic Reviews

Nurses may be involved in developing systematic reviews by reviewing studies based on specific criteria, but this is not common for most nurses (Jennings & Loan, 2001). Reviewing studies using systematic review procedures takes special expertise and in-depth knowledge of statistics, so this would not be something every nurse could do. It should not be an expectation that staff nurses will do these reviews. The staff nurse's most important role is that of consumer of the systematic reviews. Using the PICOT method to guide them, nurses search for the systematic reviews through databases (e.g., Cochrane and Joanna Briggs). After evidence is found, nurses look

at the validity of the evidence, its relevance, and its applicability to the focus question and then apply the evidence in their practice.

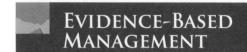

EVIDENCE-BASED MANAGEMENT

Most nurse managers or even non-nurse managers do not actively use evidence from research to assist in making management decisions. Many do use the professional literature, which does not usually describe research but rather provides more content and descriptions of experiences. One of the American Organization of Nurse Executives' (AONE) strategic objectives is to "utilize evidence-based management practice and sound research in the development of future patient care delivery systems and practice environments[; explore] and support the interrelations of technology, facility design and patient care delivery models" (AONE, 2010, p. 2). The definition of EBM is not much different from the definition for EBP. EBM is the "systematic application of the best available evidence to the evaluation of managerial strategies for improving the performance of health services organizations" (Kovner & Rundall, 2009, p. 56). There needs to be more research that focuses on nursing management and leadership; the results of these studies may then be considered evidence and incorporated into leadership and management decisions.

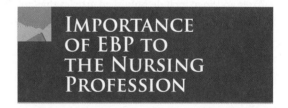

IMPORTANCE OF EBP TO THE NURSING PROFESSION

As noted by the IOM, EBP can improve care (Gawlinksi, 2008). Nursing care should be supported by evidence, but it is not uncommon for nursing care to be provided in a manner that is best described as "we have always done it this way." This type of approach may not always lead to quality care that best meets patient outcomes, and it may not be the most cost-effective approach. "Evidence-based practice is a problem-solving approach to making clinical, educational, and administrative decisions that combines the best available scientific evidence with the best practical evidence" (Newhouse, 2006, p. 337). In this process, EBP increases nurses' clinical knowledge; this in turn leads to greater freedom to act, increasing nurses' autonomy (Kramer & Schmalenberg, 2005). EBP can empower nurses. The following are the critical questions for each nurse to ask:

1. Will the evidence help me provide quality care?

2. Were all clinically relevant outcomes considered?

3. Are the benefits worth the potential harm and costs?

Changing how care is delivered is a major undertaking because there are always barriers to change. It takes an organized approach to implement EBP into a healthcare delivery system. Reimbursement for services—medical and nursing—is increasingly based on whether the guidelines for care are evidence based. As the financial incentive to implement EBP grows, so will integration of EBP. **Exhibit 11-4** describes nursing role criteria for the staff nurse, nurse manager, advanced practice nurse, and nurse executive related to EBP functions.

Exhibit 11-4   Sample EBP Performance Criteria for Nursing Roles

Staff Nurse

- Questions current practices
- Participates in implementing changes in practice based on evidence
- Participates as a member of an EBP project team
- Reads evidence related to the nurse's practice
- Participates in quality improvement initiatives
- Suggests resolutions for clinical issues based on evidence

Nurse Manager

- Creates a microsystem that fosters critical thinking
- Challenges staff to seek out evidence to resolve clinical issues and improve care
- Role-models EBP
- Uses evidence to guide operations and management decisions
- Uses performance criteria about EBP in evaluation of staff

Advanced Practice Nurse

- Serves as a coach and mentor in EBP
- Facilitates locating evidence
- Synthesizes evidence for practice
- Uses evidence to write/modify practice standards
- Role models use of evidence in practice
- Facilitates system changes to support use of EBPs

Nurse Executive

- Ensures the governance reflects EBP if initiated in councils and committees
- Assigns accountability for EBP
- Ensures explicit articulation of organizational and department commitment to EBP
- Modifies the mission and vision to include EBP language
- Provides resources to support EBP by direct care providers
- Articulates the value of EBP to the chief executive officer and governing board
- Role-models EBP in administrative decision making
- Hires and retains nurse managers and advanced practice nurses with knowledge and skills in EBP
- Provides a learning environment for EBP
- Uses evidence in leadership decisions

Source: Schmidt, N. A., & Brown, J. M. (2015). *Evidence-based practice for nurses: Appraisal and applications of research.* Burlington, MA: Jones & Bartlett Learning. Adapted from Titler, M. G. (2014). Developing an evidence-based practice. In G. LoBiondo-Wood & J. Haber (Eds.), *Nursing research: Methods and critical appraisal for evidence-based practice* (8th ed, pp. 418-440). St Louis, MO: Mosby Elsevier.

Barriers to EBP Implementation

It has not been easy to incorporate EBP into practice. Some healthcare organizations have been more successful than others. Over time, greater use of EBP will occur, but some barriers still need to be overcome by most organizations:

- *Lack of knowledge about EBP and its value:* EBP has been added to nursing curricula in only the last 5 to 10 years, so many practicing nurses have limited knowledge of EBP. This gap in the knowledge base requires healthcare organizations to play catch-up to improve staff knowledge of EBP.
- *Limited time in practice settings:* Staff are rushed and often just able to keep up with required care, so adding more responsibilities is difficult.
- *Nursing shortage:* There are insufficient staff to allow nurses time to consider EBP effectively.
- *Greater need to emphasize both knowledge and practical approaches:* This barrier applies to both nursing education and practice settings.
- *Concern that EBP represents a cookbook approach to care:* EBP can be considered a cookbook approach if it is used without assessment and clinical reasoning and judgment. Every patient must be viewed as an individual (patient-centered care).
- *Lack of knowledge about EBP resources:* To make evidence available and usable, more information is needed regarding searching for resources, accessing resources, and analyzing resources.
- *Lack of resources to find information:* For example, staff may not have easy access to the Internet, access to appropriate databases, and library support.
- *Limited recognition by employers regarding the value of EBP:* Nurses are not given time to find EBP evidence and then apply it.

Improving EBP Implementation

The IOM recommends that for EBP to be used more effectively, healthcare professionals should have these abilities (IOM, 2003, pp. 57–58):

- Know where and how to find the best possible sources of evidence
- Formulate clear clinical questions
- Search for the relevant answers to the questions from the best possible sources of evidence, including those that evaluate or appraise the evidence for its validity and usefulness with respect to a particular patient or population
- Determine when and how to integrate these new findings into practice

Nursing services within a healthcare organization (or any type of healthcare organization) need to plan carefully how to prepare staff to effectively apply EBP and evaluate the outcomes. The first step is staff preparation. Most of today's staff are not ready to engage in EBP. Given that most staff did not graduate from nursing education programs within the last few years (the average age of nurses is older than 45 years) and, therefore, few staff had any EBP content in their nursing programs, this is a major hurdle. In an effort to remedy this staff knowledge deficit, many healthcare organizations have integrated EBP content into their staff education programs.

In a study published in 2005 (Pravikoff, Tanner, & Pierce, 2005), 760 registered nurses responded to a 93-item questionnaire about readiness of nurses for EBP. The results indicated:

[A]lthough these nurses acknowledge that they frequently need information for practice, they feel much more confident asking colleagues or peers and searching the Internet and World Wide Web than they do using bibliographic databases such as PubMed or CINAHL to find specific information. They don't understand or value research and have received little or no training in the use of tools that would help them find evidence on which to base their practice. (Pravikoff et al., 2005, p. 40)

Table 11-1 describes strategies to overcome barriers to EBP.

Tools to Ensure a Higher Level of Use of EBP

EBP evidence should be incorporated into standards of care that guide nursing practice and education. This can reduce practice variation and provide greater consistency based on evidence to improve

Table 11-1	Strategies to Overcome Barriers to Adopting EBP

Barrier	Strategy
Lack of Time	Devote 15 minutes a day to reading evidence related to a clinical problem
	Sign up for e-mails that offer summaries of research studies in your area of interest
	Use a team approach when considering policy changes to distribute the workload among members
	Bookmark websites having clinical guidelines to promote faster retrieval of information
	Evaluate available technologies (i.e., personal digital assistant) to create time-saving systems that allow quick and convenient retrieval of information at the bedside
	Negotiate release time from patient care duties to collect, read, and share information about relevant clinical problems
	Search for established clinical guidelines because they provide synthesis of existing research
Lack of value placed on research in practice	Make a list of reasons why healthcare providers should value research and use this list as a springboard for discussions with colleagues
	Invite nurse researchers to share why they are passionate about their work
	When disagreements arise about a policy or protocol, find an article that supports your position and share it with others
	When selecting a work environment, ask about the organizational commitment to EBP
	Link measurement of quality indicators to EBP
	Participate in EBP activities to demonstrate professionalism that can be rewarded through promotions or merit raises
	Provide recognition during National Nurses Week for individuals involved in EBP projects
Lack of knowledge about EBP and research	Take a course or attend a continuing education offering on EBP
	Invite a faculty member to a unit meeting to discuss EBP
	Consult with advanced practice nurses
	Attend conferences where clinical research is presented and talk with presenters about their studies

(continues)

Table 11-1	Strategies to Overcome Barriers to Adopting EBP (continued)

Barrier	Strategy
	Volunteer to serve on committees that set policies and protocols
	Create a mentoring program to bring novice and experienced nurses together
Lack of technological skills to find evidence	Consult with a librarian about how to access databases and retrieve articles
	Learn to bookmark important websites that are sources of clinical guidelines
	Commit to acquiring computer skills
Lack of resources to access evidence	Write a proposal for funds to support access to online databases and journals
	Collaborate with a nursing program for access to resources
	Investigate funding possibilities from others (i.e., pharmaceutical companies, grants)
Lack of ability to read research	Organize a journal club where nurses meet regularly to discuss the evidence about a specific clinical problem
	Write down questions about an article and ask an advanced practice nurse to read the article and assist in answering the questions
	Clarify unfamiliar terms by looking them up in a dictionary or research textbook
	Use one familiar critique format when reading research
	Identify clinical problems and share them with nurse researchers
	Participate in ongoing unit-based studies
	Subscribe to journals that provide uncomplicated explanations of research studies
Resistance to change	Listen to people's concerns about change
	When considering an EBP project, select one that interests the staff, has a high priority, is likely to be successful, and has baseline data
	Mobilize talented individuals to act as change agents
	Create a means to reward individuals who provide leadership during change
Lack of organizational support for EBP	Link organizational priorities with EBP to reduce cost and increase efficiency
	Recruit administrators who value EBP
	Form coalitions with other healthcare providers to increase the base of support for EBP
	Use EBP to meet accreditation standards or gain recognition (i.e., Magnet recognition)

Source: Schmidt, N. A., & Brown, J. M. (2015). *Evidence-based practice for nurses: Appraisal and applications of research.* Burlington, MA: Jones & Bartlett Learning.

quality and safety (Newhouse, 2006, 2007). In practice, two major tools are commonly used to ensure a higher level of EBP: (1) healthcare organization policies and procedures and (2) clinical guidelines.

Policies and Procedures Based on EBP

Much of the care in healthcare organizations is defined by policies and **procedures**. Policies and procedures are important guides for care within healthcare settings. Organizations develop these written guides to inform staff about expectations related to specific policies and procedures. Policies and procedures are not new to health care, and many policies and procedures have been developed by reviewing resources such as research results. However, in many cases, they have been developed without an EBP approach.

What is the evidence to support a policy or procedure? The difficulty in nursing is that there may not yet be evidence such as research, but policies and procedures should state the research evidence used (if it exists) to support the content. Many healthcare organizations are now trying to improve their policies and procedures by reviewing them from an EBP perspective. Unfortunately, this is a time-consuming process.

Clinical Guidelines Based on EBP

Clinical practice guidelines are developed by expert panels or professional organizations and are EBP based. An important source for guidelines is the National Guideline Clearinghouse, which is sponsored by the AHRQ. The Guideline Clearinghouse is a searchable database of guidelines that are used to improve patient outcomes.

> Variation in practice patterns and a continued gap between evidence and practice has resulted in recognition for the need to assess the value of interventions and to use evidence-based decision-making. Practice guidelines and other forms of standardized protocols such as clinical pathways have been defined as both the engines and the vehicles for improving an organization. (Goode, Tanaka, Krugman, & O'Connor, 2000, p. 202)

An EBP guideline is one of the strongest sources for EBP, along with systematic reviews (Melnyk & Fineout-Overholt, 2010). Clinical guidelines are described as follows:

> [S]ystematically developed statements to assist clinicians and patients in making

decisions about care; ideally the guidelines consist of a systematic review of the literature, in conjunction with consensus of a group of expert decision-makers, including administrators, policy-makers, clinicians, and consumers who consider the evidence and make recommendations. (Melnyk & Fineout-Overholt, 2010, p. 572)

CONFUSION
Difference in Research, EBP, and Quality Improvement

Research, EBP, and **quality improvement (QI)** are not the same. Although QI is not discussed in detail in this chapter, it is important to clarify the differences in these three terms and processes for the purposes of this discussion. Research is systematic investigation of a problem, question, issue, or topic that uses a specific scientific process to gain new knowledge. Results from studies can be used as evidence to support clinical decisions, although not all research deals with clinical decisions or has an impact on quality care. An example of research that is clinically focused and would have an impact on quality is a nurse who questions the best method for preventing patient falls in a long-term care facility and wants to consider new interventions. This nurse might develop a study to gather data to examine how two different groups of patients respond to a new intervention to prevent falls. In doing so, the nurse would follow the research process described elsewhere in this chapter.

By comparison, EBP focuses on systematic review and appraisal of evidence, including research results but also the patient's assessment and history data, the clinician's expertise, and the patient's preferences and values. In this case, the same nurse who wondered about factors related to falls might take a different approach, the EBP approach. The nurse would pose a PICOT question, such as "Which factors influence patient falls in a long-term care facility?" The nurse would look for systematic reviews to answer this question and would use systematic reviews, if found, to guide practice; doing so would impact quality care.

Quality improvement is "a process by which individuals work together to improve systems and processes with the intention to improve outcomes" (Committee on Assessing the System for Protecting Human Research Participants, 2002, as cited in Newhouse, 2007, p. 433). Healthcare organizations are involved in QI on a daily basis as the healthcare organization staff try to understand outcomes and improve them. In the same example noted with falls, a QI project might include a monthly collection of data related to the number of falls and specific information about the falls (i.e., factors related to the falls). The healthcare organization would examine the seriousness of the problem by using root-cause analysis. The healthcare organization might then institute a change, such as requiring that patients at risk for falls be identified in medical records and on labels in the patient areas. The healthcare organization would then track data to see if there is any change in the number of falls for at-risk patients.

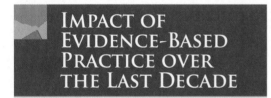

IMPACT OF EVIDENCE-BASED PRACTICE OVER THE LAST DECADE

Since the publication of the IOM reports on quality, covering the last decade, and the publication of *The Future of Nursing* report (IOM, 2011d), there have been many changes in the delivery of care by nurses. Notably, EBP has influenced these changes in nursing practice, nursing models and frameworks, education, and nursing research. The following are examples as described by Stevens (2013).

Nursing Practice

It was recognized early on that to integrate EBP into the healthcare delivery system, nurses as individual care providers, microsystem and system leaders, and policy makers at all levels of government would have to implement EBP. The Magnet Recognition Program includes EBP as one of its recognition elements—a factor that has encouraged an increasing number of healthcare organizations to adopt nursing EBP and actively pursue staff knowledge of EBP so that EBB can be effectively implemented. Evidence has also been used more extensively to support new practice initiatives such as TeamSTEPPS. However, even when a program is based on evidence and is well developed, it is not easy to implement and sustain an EBP program. Much more is needed to improve practice and to use evidence to do so.

Nursing Models and Frameworks

In addition to practice models and frameworks, many models and frameworks have been developed for EBP. In fact, as of 2013, the literature described 47 EBP models. These models can be categorized as (1) EBP, research utilization, and knowledge transformation processes; (2) strategic/organizational change theory to promote update and adoption of new knowledge; and (3) knowledge exchange and synthesis for application and inquiry (Mitchell, Fisher, Hastings, Silverman, & Wallen, 2010).

Nursing Education

EBP was included in the five healthcare professions core competencies, which in turn provided more support for the call to include EBP in nursing education (IOM, 2003). To prepare their students in these core competencies, schools of nursing began to include EBP in courses and to develop courses that focused on EBP at both the undergraduate and graduate levels.

Nursing Research

The IOM work led to recognition of the dire need for evidence to support strategies employed to improve care. Examples of two initiatives that were developed to meet this need are the Clinical and Translational Science Awards (CTSA) and the Patient-Centered Outcomes Research Institute (PCORI). The CTSA's goal is to decrease the time taken to move research into practice; as a consequence, this initiative has driven translational research. Translational research had been described in two ways: (1) the application of discoveries generated in the laboratory and in preclinical studies to the development of trials and studies in humans, and (2) research aimed at enhancing the adoption of best practices in the community. The comparative effectiveness of prevention and treatment strategies, for example, is part of translational science (NIH, 2010). PCORI focuses on research that addresses patient-centered outcomes (PCORI, 2014).

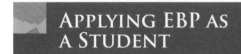

Applying EBP as a Student

Nursing curricula are including more content on EBP for both undergraduate and graduate students. The location of this content in the curriculum can vary from school to school, but typically it is associated with nursing research content and then emphasized throughout the curriculum.

This content is not something that should be presented in isolation from other nursing content and clinical experiences. Instead, students need to actively pursue understanding of EBP and use of evidence in their practice. When you are assigned or select patients for clinical experiences, part of the preparation for clinical experience or practicum should be to search for current research evidence found in professional literature and incorporate this evidence into the care plan and practice. This search should extend beyond the patient diagnosis to nursing problems. Students typically use certain types of EBP data— for example, patient values and preferences, patient history, and assessment data— but they rarely include research evidence and often do not know how to consider their own clinical expertise level.

The more you examine and use EBP, the more it will become an integral part of your practice as a student, as well as your practice after graduation. Merely completing a few assignments on EBP or taking an exam on EBP will not cause you to develop the IOM core competency to use EBP practice. Instead, you need to make a commitment to practice at the best possible level; to get there takes practice, and that practice should include EBP.

Landscape © f9photos/Shutterstock, Inc.

Conclusion

This chapter examined the important core competency of using EBP. Research was discussed as a major source of evidence to support effective patient care interventions, as well as management decisions. The research process and some elements used to describe studies are necessary information for understanding how research is reviewed and used in EBP. Every nurse needs to use EBP, and doing so requires understanding the topic and implications for nursing practice and the profession.

CHAPTER HIGHLIGHTS

1. Evidence-based practice as a core competency is connected to providing patient-centered care, quality improvement, and interprofessional teams.

2. EBP's use has increased because of the recognition of the large translation gap between bench (scientific) research and its impact (i.e., its use in practice).

3. Research is a systematic investigation of a specific problem.

4. The relationship between research and EBP centers on the fact that the best evidence comes from research findings.

5. Basic research is designed to broaden the base of knowledge rather than to solve an immediate problem.

6. Applied research is designed to find a solution to a practical problem.

7. Nursing research is inextricably linked to the profession's mandate to protect the public and promote the best possible patient outcomes.

8. The NINR was established in 1985, providing nursing with representation at the National Institutes of Health.

9. The research process, like the nursing process, is based on problem solving.

10. Research can be either quantitative or qualitative. In quantitative studies, the research question(s) focus(es) on how many or how much; in the qualitative design, the research question(s) focus(es) on feelings or experiences.

11. Institutional review boards (IRBs) focus on participant/subject rights. The IRB is charged with the responsibility of ensuring that a research participant/subject's rights are protected and that the study is planned in an effective manner that meets scientific standards, particularly theory and informed consent.

12. The Nuremberg Code established the need to protect human research subjects.

13. EBP uses evidence from research results, patient assessment and other sources, clinical expertise, and information about patient preferences and values.

14. The key component of EBP literature is systematic reviews.

15. The involvement of staff nurses in the EBP process is critical to its eventual integration into the organization's culture of care delivery.

16. EBM is critical for effective management of care in all types of settings.

17. Research, EBP, and quality improvement are not the same. Research focuses on the scientific method to deduce answers to questions; EBP focuses on the use of supporting data to ground interventions; and QI focuses on a system or process to measure and systematically examine quality of care at a macro (or system) level or a micro (or patient) level.

18. Nursing education has begun to shift from pure research content with additive information on EBP to a focus on EBP while teaching how research underlies much of EBP.

DISCUSSION QUESTIONS

1. What does the core competency "employ evidence-based practice" mean?

2. What is the research process?

3. How does research relate to EBP?

DISCUSSION QUESTIONS (CONTINUED)

4. What is a systematic review? How do systematic reviews relate to EBP? What is their value to practice?

5. Why is EBP important to nursing practice?

6. What are the barriers to implementing EBP, and how might some of them be overcome?

7. Why is EBM important to healthcare delivery?

8. Which factors would you consider when implementing EBP in a nursing unit?

CRITICAL THINKING ACTIVITIES

1. Visit the website for the Academic Center for Evidence-Based Practice, University of Texas School of Nursing, San Antonio, to learn more about the school's EBP center (http://www.ace-star.uthscsa.edu/). What is the ACE Star Model? What do you think about this model? Can you connect this model to what you know about nursing practice?

2. In an EBP review, you begin by describing the clinical problem or scenario. At the University of Washington's website (http://libguides.hsl.washington.edu/content.php?pid=231619&sid=1931590), you will find examples of clinical problems and scenarios. The PICOT method is used to clearly define a specific clinical problem. This site shows you how to move from the clinical problem/scenario to a clinical question using a PICOT question. How would you summarize this process?

3. Write a PICOT question using one of the templates described in this chapter. After you have written your PICOT question, compare it with questions developed by other students (this can be done in a small group). Ask members of the group to identify the *P, I, C, O,* and *T* in your question, and do the same with the other questions. Select one PICOT question and see if the

group can find a systematic review dealing with it. If you cannot find a systematic review, then discuss what this means. Identify PICOT questions for your clinical patients.

4. Visit the National Institute of Nursing Research website and review the current strategic plan (http://www.ninr.nih.gov/AboutNINR/NINRMissionandStrategicPlan/). Which examples are given on the site to demonstrate how nursing research is making a difference? Do any of these examples surprise you (nursing involvement, type of study, results)? What is your own school doing in the area of nursing research?

5. Visit the NIH's ethics program website (http://ethics.od.nih.gov/default.htm). Review one of the posted topics. Why did you select this topic? Summarize what you have learned from this site.

6. If you are interested in learning more about the Tuskegee study, visit The National Academics online ethics center (http://www.onlineethics.org/CMS/edu/precol/scienceclass/sectone/cs3.aspx). What happened in this study? What were the ethical issues that should have been considered? Does your school have an IRB office? If so, visit its website and review the informed consent forms and Health Insurance Portability and Accountability Act forms.

ELECTRONIC *Reflective Journal Log*

Circuit Board: ©Photos.com

Consider how you can improve your practice first as a student and then as a nurse. Develop the steps you will take to work to improve and then track your results annually.

Landscape © f9photos/Shutterstock, Inc.

LINKING TO THE INTERNET

- Academic Center for Evidence-Based Practice, University of Texas, San Antonio (ACE Star Model): http://www.acestar.uthscsa.edu/
- Agency for Healthcare Research and Quality: http://www.ahrq.gov/
- Arizona State University College of Nursing Center for Advancement of Evidence-Based Practice: http://nursingandhealth.asu.edu/evidence-based-practice/index.htm
- Health Resources and Services Administration: http://www.hrsa.gov/
- Joanna Briggs Institute: http://www.joannabriggs.org
- National Guideline Clearinghouse (reviews EBP guidelines on many topics): http://www.guideline.gov/
- National Institute of Nursing Research: http://www.ninr.nih.gov/
- National Institutes of Health: http://www.nih.gov/ and http://www.ahrq.gov/clinic/epcix.htm
- Patient-Centered Outcomes Research Institute: http://www.pcori.org/

CASE STUDIES

Landscape © f9photos/Shutterstock, Inc.

Case Study 1

Health professionals noticed that ventilator-dependent adults often developed pneumonia. They started questioning what might be going on. They reviewed the literature and found that there was little evidence to support this phenomenon, although a few studies had addressed the topic. Subsequently, more and more institutions examined ventilator-associated pneumonia (VAP). Based on these reviews, guidelines or best practices were developed to decrease the incidence of VAP in adults. Now, research and EBP studies examine VAP as a measure of quality of care; consider costs associated with VAP versus preventive costs; and use VAP as a benchmarking tool for quality care and patient safety (Ruffell & Adamcova, 2008; Uckay, Ahmed, Sax, & Pittet, 2008).

Case Questions

1. Can you find a systematic review focusing on VAP and related care issues? If so, which evidence does it provide?
2. Can you find a clinical guideline on VAP? Which evidence is provided?
3. Which care approach is used in a clinical setting in which you have practicum? How does it relate to what you have learned from the systematic review and/or clinical guideline?

Case Study 2

You have just taken a new position in a cardiac care unit. A month after you start the job, you have a question about a procedure and the rationale for its use. You go to your staff mentor, and she tells you to just follow the procedure as written, as it makes work easier. This is not what you expected.

Case Questions

1. What might be your response to your mentor?
2. How might this interaction affect your view of your mentor?
3. At your next monthly meeting with the nurse manager, what might you say about this issue?
4. What does this tell you about EBP on the unit?
5. What might be improved in this unit's practice?

Words of Wisdom

Lisa English Long, PhD(c), RN, CNS
Expert Evidence-Based Practice Mentor, Clinical Instructor, Center for Transdisciplinary Evidence-Based Practice, College of Nursing, The Ohio State University
Former Evidence-Based Practice Mentor, Director, Evidence-Based Practice, Cincinnati Children's Hospital Medical Center, Cincinnati, Ohio

EBP is an approach that promotes scholarly inquiry, a sense of autonomy, and control over practice. The growth that nurses have experienced through the use of EBP has been instrumental in leading practice changes that improve patient, family, and staff outcomes. My experiences in working with staff whose goal is to establish a practice based on evidence is exciting and one that instills a sense of pride. I have found point-of-care staff eager to learn, work collaboratively, and support each other in

(continues)

Words of Wisdom (*continued*)

establishing and sustaining that questioning attitude. Engaging in the EBP process motivates staff to learn about change theory, use of EBP models in guiding work, and the barriers to implementation of EBP. The challenges that permeate the evidence relate, many times, to system issues over which staff have less control. Even so, these barriers have not limited staff in their efforts to change practice from "the way we have always done it" to "the way that is the best based on critically appraised research, clinical expertise, and patient/family preferences." My experiences with those involved in evidence work have allowed me to witness change in policy, policy and procedure development, dissemination of findings, and presentations at regional, local, national, and international forums. The growth in colleagues both personally and professionally is truly impressive, as they not only grow but also improve outcomes in patients, families, and colleagues through engagement in EBP.

REFERENCES

American Association of Colleges of Nursing (AACN). (2006). *AACN position statement on nursing research*. Washington, DC: Author.

American Nurses Association (ANA). (2001). *Code of ethics with interpretive statements*. Silver Spring, MD: Author.

American Nurses Association (ANA). (2010a). *Nursing's social policy statement* (2nd ed.). Silver Spring, MD: Author.

American Nurses Association (ANA). (2010b). *Scope and standards of practice*. Silver Spring, MD: Author.

American Nurses Association (ANA). (2011). Research agenda. Retrieved from http://www.nursingworld.org/MainMenu Categories/ThePracticeofProfessionalNursing/Improving-Your-Practice/Research-Toolkit/ANA-Research-Agenda/Research-Agenda-.pdf

American Organization of Nurse Executives (AONE). (2010). 2013–2015 strategic plan. Retrieved from http://www .aone.org/membership/about/docs/2013.2015.AONE .StratPlan.Graphic.pdf

Balas, E. (2001). Information systems can prevent errors and improve quality. *Journal of the American Medical Informatics Association*, 8, 398–399.

Brown, S. (2009). *Evidence-based nursing*. Sudbury, MA: Jones and Bartlett.

Chassin, M. (1998). Is healthcare ready for Six Sigma quality? *Milbank Quarterly*, 76, 565–591.

Committee on Assessing the System for Protecting Human Research Participants. (2002). *Responsible research: A systems approach to protecting research participants*. Washington, DC: National Academies Press.

DiCenso, A., Guyatt, G., & Ciliska, D. (2005). *Evidence-based nursing: A guide to clinical practice*. St. Louis, MO: Elsevier Mosby.

Gawlinksi, A. (2008). The power of clinical nursing research: Engage clinicians, improve patients' lives, and forge a professional legacy. *American Journal of Critical Care*, 17(4), 315–326.

Goode, C., Tanaka, D., Krugman, M., & O'Connor, P. (2000). Outcomes from use of an evidence-based practice guideline. *Nursing Economics*, 18, 202–207.

Improvement Science Research Network (ISRN). (2014). What is the Improvement Science Research Network? Retrieved from http://isrn.net/about/what_is_isrn.asp

Institute of Medicine (IOM). (2003). *Health professions education: A bridge to quality*. Washington, DC: National Academies Press.

Institute of Medicine (IOM). (2008). *Knowing what works in health care: A roadmap for the nation*. Washington, DC: National Academies Press.

Institute of Medicine (IOM). (2011a). *Clinical data as the basic staple for health learning: Workshop summary*. Washington, DC: National Academies Press.

Institute of Medicine (IOM). (2011b). *Clinical guidelines we can trust*. Washington, DC: National Academies Press.

Institute of Medicine (IOM). (2011c). *Finding what works: Standards for systematic reviews*. Washington, DC: National Academies Press.

Institute of Medicine (IOM). (2011d). *The future of nursing: Leading change, advancing health*. Washington, DC: National Academies Press.

International Council of Nurses (ICN). (2010). Nursing research network. Retrieved from http://www.icn.ch/networks/icn-networks/

Jennings, B., & Loan, L. (2001). Misconceptions among nurses about EBP. *Journal of Nursing Scholarship, 33*, 121–127.

Kovner, A. & Rundall, T. (2009). Evidence-based management reconsidered. In A. Kovner, D. Fine, & R. D'Aquila (Eds.), *Evidence-based management in health care* (pp. 53–78). Chicago, IL: Health Administration Press.

Kramer, M., & Schmalenberg, C. (2005). Best quality patient care: A historical perspective on Magnet hospitals. *Nursing Administration Quarterly, 29*, 275–287.

Melnyk, B., & Fineout-Overholt, E. (2010). *Evidence-based practice in nursing and healthcare*. Philadelphia, PA: Lippincott Williams & Wilkins.

Melnyk, B., & Stillwater, S. (2010). Asking compelling, clinical questions. In B. Melynik & E. Fineout-Overholt (Eds.), *Evidence-based practice in nursing and healthcare* (pp. 25–39). Philadelphia, PA: Lippincott Williams & Wilkins.

Mitchell, S. A., Fisher, C. A., Hastings, C. E., Silverman, L. B., & Wallen, G. R. (2010). A thematic analysis of theoretical models for translational science in nursing: Mapping the field. *Nursing Outlook, 58*(6), 287–300.

National Institute of Nursing Research (NINR). (2011; update 2013). Bringing science to life: NINR strategic plan. Retrieved from https://www.ninr.nih.gov/sites/www.ninr.nih.gov/files/ninr-strategic-plan-2011.pdf

National Institute of Nursing Research (NINR). (2014). What is nursing research? Retrieved from http://www.ninr.nih.gov/

National Institutes of Health (NIH). (2010). Institutional clinical and translational science award (US4). Retrieved from http://grants.nih.gov/grants/guide/rfa-files/RFA-RM-10-001.html#SectionI

Newhouse, R. (2006). Examining the support for evidence-based nursing practice. *Journal of Nursing Administration, 36*, 337–340.

Newhouse, R. (2007). Diffusing confusion among evidence-based practice, quality improvement, and research. *Journal of Nursing Administration, 37*(10), 432–435.

Patient-Centered Outcomes Research Institute (PCORI). (2014) About us. Retrieved from http://www.pcori.org/about-us/landing/

Pravikoff, D., Tanner, A., & Pierce, S. (2005). Readiness for U.S. nurses for evidence-based practice. *American Journal of Nursing, 105*(9), 40–50.

Ruffell, A., & Adamcova, L. (2008). Ventilator-associated pneumonia: Prevention is better than care. *Nursing Critical Care, 13*(1), 44–53.

Stevens, K. (2013). The impact of evidence-based practice in nursing and the next big ideas. *OJIN, 18*(2). Retrieved from http://www.nursingworld.org/MainMenuCategories/ANAMarketplace/ANAPeriodicals/OJIN/TableofContents/Vol-18-2013/No2-May-2013/Impact-of-Evidence-Based-Practice.html

Uckay, I., Ahmed, Q., Sax, H., & Pittet, D. (2008). Ventilator-associated pneumonia as a quality indicator for patient safety? *Clinical Infectious Diseases, 46*(4), 557–563.

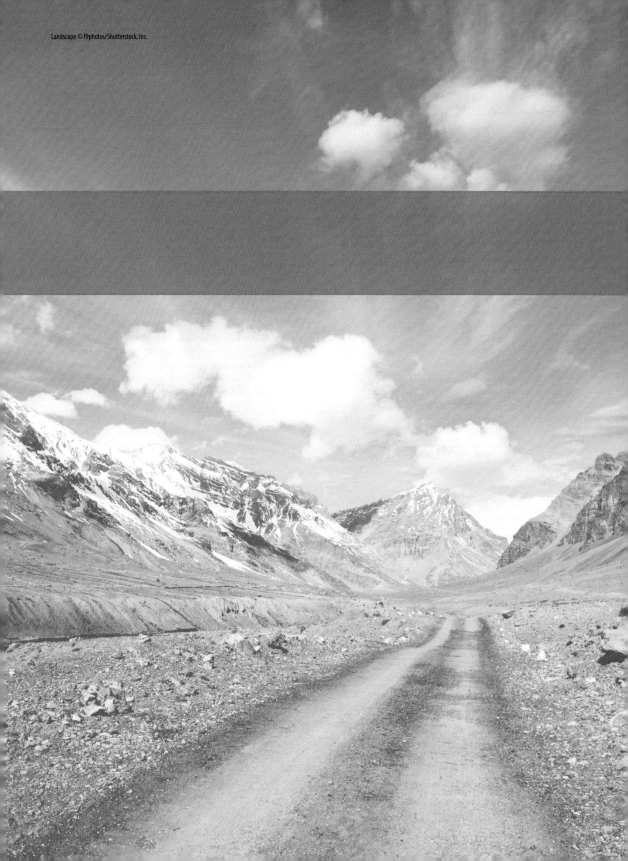

CHAPTER 12

Apply Quality Improvement

CHAPTER OBJECTIVES

At the conclusion of this chapter, the learner will be able to:

- Discuss the relevance of the core competency: Apply quality improvement
- Describe the status of safety in health care today
- Explain the need for a blame-free culture of safety
- Identify staff safety issues in the healthcare workplace environment
- Discuss the need for quality improvement and strategies to improve care

- Examine how the Institute of Medicine reports on quality care have affected nursing and healthcare delivery
- Describe healthcare organization accreditation and the role of The Joint Commission
- Define the tools and methods used to monitor and improve health care
- Discuss the roles of nurses and nursing as a profession in improving health care

CHAPTER OUTLINE

CHAPTER OUTLINE (CONTINUED)

- Benchmarking
- Assessment of Access to Healthcare Services
- Evidence-Based Practice
- Clinical Pathways/Protocols
- Medication Reconciliation
- Institutional Review Board
- Healthcare Policy and Legislation
- Patient Outcomes and Nursing Care: Do We Make a Difference in Quality Improvement?

- Conclusion
- Chapter Highlights
- Discussion Questions
- Critical Thinking Activities
- Electronic Reflection Journal
- Linking to the Internet
- Case Studies
- Words of Wisdom
- References

KEY TERMS

Accreditation	The Joint Commission	Root-cause analysis
Adverse event	Misuse	Safety/safe care
Benchmarking	Near miss	Sentinel event
Blame-free environment	Outcomes	Structure
Clinical pathways	Overuse	Surveillance
Effective care	Patient-centered care	System
Efficient care	Process	Timely care
Equitable care	Protocols	Underuse
Error	Quality	Utilization review
Failure to rescue	Quality improvement (QI)	
Healthcare report card	Risk management (RM)	

INTRODUCTION

This chapter's content discusses the fourth Institute of Medicine (IOM) healthcare core competency: apply quality improvement. The content includes information about the key IOM quality and associated safety reports and their recommendations. Through further exploration of safety issues and quality care, the role of accreditation of healthcare organizations (HCOs) is also related to the need to improve care. Nurses and nursing as a profession assume major roles in ensuring that care is safe and outcomes are reached, resulting in quality care.

THE IOM COMPETENCY

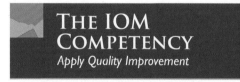

Apply Quality Improvement

The fourth healthcare profession core competency is to apply quality improvement (QI). The IOM's (2003) description of this core competency follows:

> [I]dentify errors and hazards in care; understand and implement basic safety design principles, such as standardization and simplification; continually understand and measure quality of care in terms of structure, process, and outcomes in relation

to patient and community needs; and design and test interventions to change processes and systems of care, with the objective of improving quality. (p. 4)

Current data indicate that there are serious problems with health care in the United States—its safety, its quality, and waste and inefficiency. In 2014 the U.S. Congressional Subcommittee on Primary Health and Aging held a meeting to examine healthcare errors, as noted in a press release dated July 17, 2014:

> Preventable medical errors in hospitals are the third leading cause of death in the United States, a Senate panel was told today. Only heart disease and cancer kill more Americans… "Medical harm is a major cause of suffering, disability, and death – as well as a huge financial cost to our nation," Sen. Bernie Sanders (I-Vt.)"

The press release went on to state that each year as many as 440,000 people die due to a preventable medical error in hospitals. Compared with other nations, the United States is about average.

In addition to deaths and injuries, medical errors also cost billions of dollars. One study conducted in 2011 put the figure at $17 billion a year. Counting indirect costs like lost productivity due to missed work days, medical errors may cost nearly $1 trillion each year…

There has been improvement since the IOM's 1999 report, *To Err Is Human*, but there has not been enough. This information indicates major problems still exist.

The healthcare system is the focus of QI. The system is fragmented and in need of improvement. A **system**

> can be defined by the coming together of parts, interconnections, and purpose. While systems can be broken down into parts, which are interesting in and of themselves, the real power lies in the way the parts come together and are interconnected to fulfill some purpose. The healthcare system in the United States consists of various parts (e.g., clinics, hospitals, pharmacies, laboratories) that are interconnected (via flows of patients and information) to fulfill a purpose (e.g., maintaining and improving health). (Plsek, 2001, p. 309)

This does not mean that individual patient needs and improvement of individual patient care are not important. Each patient's care is part of this overall emphasis on healthcare improvement and is integrated in the system. Ultimately, the goal is that each patient's outcomes will be met. **Figure 12-1**

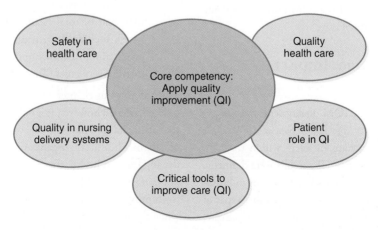

Figure 12-1 Apply Quality Improvements: Key Elements

illustrates the key elements related to this core competency as discussed in this chapter.

The Institute for Healthcare Improvement (IHI, 2007) suggests that new designs can and must be developed to simultaneously accomplish three critical objectives—that is, the IHI triple aim:

1. Improve the health of the population
2. Enhance the patient experience of care (including quality, access, and reliability)
3. Reduce, or at least control, the per capita cost of care

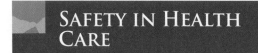

SAFETY IN HEALTH CARE

Safety is a critical component of quality care. There is no question that healthcare providers, including nurses, have long been concerned about providing safe care for their patients. If one interviewed healthcare providers, there is no doubt that they would say that they want to keep their patients safe and that care is safe. This belief was somewhat shattered when the IOM was directed by the U.S. Congress to begin an exploration of healthcare safety and quality and make recommendations based on its findings. Here we explore the topic of safety in health care: what it is and what can be done to better ensure safe care for all. Safety as a component of quality care is part of the IOM core competency "improve the quality of care."

To Err Is Human: Impact on Safety

The first report in the IOM quality series was *To Err Is Human: Building a Safer Health System* (1999). This report explored the status of safety within the U.S. healthcare delivery system. The results were dramatic, with data indicating serious safety problems in hospitals. This investigation did not include other types of healthcare settings, such as ambulatory care, home care,

long-term care, and many other types of sites. More research is needed to provide data about the quality of care and safety in these settings. A recent example of such research is the report published by the Agency for Health Research and Quality (AHRQ, 2013) describing studies in this area, but noting that more information is needed to support strong conclusions.

The media took note of *To Err Is Human* and its recommendations, and soon worrisome stories appeared on the evening news and in newspapers; special in-depth news reports asked, "How safe are you when you go in for health care?" The consumer began to ask questions. Some of the data that disturbed the public and healthcare providers included the following findings (IOM, 1999, pp. 1–2):

- When data from one study were extrapolated, the result suggested that at least 44,000 Americans die each year as a result of a medication error. Another study indicated the number of deaths from this cause could be as high as 98,000 (American Hospital Association [AHA], 1999).
- More people die in a given year as a result of medical errors than from motor vehicle accidents (43,458), breast cancer (42,297), or acquired immunodeficiency syndrome (AIDS) (16,516) (Centers for Disease Control and Prevention [CDC], National Center for Health Statistics, 1998).
- Healthcare delivery costs represent over more than half of total healthcare national costs, which includes lost income, lost household production, disability and the actual healthcare delivery costs (Thomas et al., 1999).

Later in this chapter, HCO accreditation is discussed in detail; however, it is important to note here that accreditation, focusing on evaluating the quality of care in a healthcare organization, has long been a driving force in health care. It is clear from *To Err Is Human* (IOM, 1999) that this has not been enough to improve care at the level needed. What happens when there are errors? Why is it so important?

- *Complications may occur and increase costs.* In 2007, the Centers for Medicare and Medicaid Services (CMS) introduced a major change in its reimbursement policy. It will no longer pay for complications that occur in the hospital that could have been prevented—so-called hospital-acquired complications (HACs). Specific types of complications that are no longer covered include falls, hospital-acquired decubiti, performing the wrong procedure, and administering the wrong blood type. In early 2008, some of the major insurers came out in support of this approach, announcing zero tolerance for hospital-acquired complications. This policy has major implications: Who will pay for these episodes? Ultimately, the HCO may hold the bill and have to pay for it. HCOs are limited in what they can charge a Medicare patient personally. This issue is complex and serious, but the major message from CMS and other insurers is that when errors are made, there are costs involved and performance is associated with cost. For many reasons, HCOs have problems maintaining a stable budget. This change in reimbursement practices has had a major impact on the financial status of hospitals, and it is uncertain how hospitals will respond to this change.

- In addition, in 2011, Medicaid issued its list of about two dozen HACs that might occur in hospitals. In July 2012, Medicaid implemented a policy of not paying for these HACs if they occurred in hospitalized patients covered by Medicaid. Examples of some of these events, similar to Medicare's list, are blood incompatibility, falls and trauma, hypoglycemic coma, and surgery on the wrong patient or wrong body part (Galewitz, 2011). The list of HACs may change over time based on data related to common complications

and errors. In addition, nongovernmental insurers now have similar lists of nonreimbursable events.

- *Opportunity costs increase.* Opportunity costs relate to situations in which diagnostic tests must be repeated or in which a change in the plan of care is needed because of adverse reactions to treatment. This may put the patient at greater risk for harm depending on the test and may increase costs of care.

- *Decrease in patient trust.* As mentioned, the report *To Err Is Human* had a major impact on consumers, and its content was shared via the media across the United States. The result is that patients and families now question their care more. Some patients do not want to be in the hospital without having a family member or friend with them at all times. When a patient experiences an error, the patient's trust level drops, and this has an impact on how the patient approaches future care. There is a positive side to this situation: More patients are demanding that they be informed about their care and, therefore, are becoming more involved in the care process.

The first important issue when trying to do something to prevent errors is that there is not a specific answer to this problem; the IOM report (1999) makes this clear. Changing the status of quality care requires multiple planned strategies in practice and an increase in safety education in professional healthcare programs and staff training.

Critical Safety Terms

Through the IOM's emphasis on healthcare quality, this organization has expanded knowledge about safety and errors, in part by undertaking identification and definition of key terms. This development of a common language is an important step in addressing the issue. To effectively collect and analyze data nationally, there must be a shared language. The following terms are part of this effort, and they have relevance to nurses who need to be directly involved in initiatives to improve care, including decreasing errors and improving safety. Definitions are identified by the IOM (Chassin & Galvin, 1998; IOM, 1999).

- **Safety**: Freedom from accidental injury. Example: The patient leaves the hospital after surgery and a 3-day stay with no complications and expected outcomes reached.
- **Error**: The failure of a planned action to be completed as intended or the use of the wrong plan to achieve an aim. Errors are directly related to outcomes. There are two types of errors: error of planning and error of execution. Errors harm the patient, and some that injure the patient may have been preventable adverse events. Example: The patient is given the wrong medication.
- **Adverse event**: An injury resulting from a medical intervention; in other words, an injury that is not a result of the patient's underlying condition. Not all adverse events are caused by errors, and not all are preventable. It requires greater investigation and analysis to determine the possible relationship between an error and an adverse event. When an adverse event is the result of an error, it is considered a preventable adverse event. Example: A patient is given the wrong medication and experiences a seizure. If the patient does not have a seizure disorder, this is more likely to be an adverse event, but much more needs to be known about the causes. How did the error that led to the adverse event happen? The following factors are expected to increase the risk of adverse events in the future: development of new medications, discovery of new uses for older medications, aging of the U.S. population, and greater use of medications for disease prevention (CDC, 2012).

- **Misuse**: Avoidable complications that prevent patients from receiving the full potential benefit of a service. Example: The patient receives a medication that is not prescribed and conflicts with the patient's allergies; the patient experiences anaphylaxis.
- **Overuse**: The potential for harm from the provision of a service that exceeds the possible benefit. Example: An elderly patient is on multiple medications, and the patient's multiple healthcare providers do not know the medications that have been prescribed by different specialists.
- **Underuse**: Failure to provide a service that would have produced a favorable outcome for the patient. Example: The patient is not able to get a specialty service needed for cancer because of distance from resources, or the patient's insurer will not cover a medication for arthritis that could make the patient more mobile.
- **Near miss**: Recognition that an event occurred that might have led to an adverse event. This does not mean that the error happened, but that it almost happened. It is important to understand these errors because they provide valuable information for preventing future actual errors. Example: The surgical team is preparing for surgery to repair the patient's knee. The right knee is prepped, but soon after, the team checks the records and goes through a safety check prior to beginning surgery, the call-out and check-back, to ensure that the correct knee is exposed—only to find out that it is the left knee that requires surgery. The team stops and replans the surgery. If there is no consideration of why this error almost happened, then the team cannot learn from it and hopefully prevent an error in the future.

One model for understanding near misses and prevention of an error is the Endhoven model (van der Schaaf, 1992), which has been adapted by Henneman and Gawlinski (2004) to nursing (**Figure 12-2**). According to this model, there are three sources of errors:

1. *Technical failure (system error):* Physical items such as software, equipment, or other materials are not designed correctly, are working incorrectly, or are not available when needed.

2. *Organizational failure (system error):* Such errors relate to complex factors that affect how work is carried out in the healthcare setting, such as new staff orientation, protocols, procedures, clinical pathways, management priorities, and organizational culture.

3. *Human failure:* This failure results from behaviors related to skills, rules, and knowledge. Safety mechanisms are reliable system defenses and the availability of adequate human recovery. Human intervention such as nursing can prevent adverse outcomes even when high-risk incidents develop into error incidents.

- **Sentinel event**: An event that had a serious negative patient outcome (unexpected death, serious physical or psychological injury, or serious risk). A root-cause analysis or a systematic review of the event is conducted to assess the process, not the individual staff who were involved; blame is not the goal, but rather prevention of further events. Example: A patient commits suicide while in the hospital for treatment of diabetes.

- **Root-cause analysis**: An in-depth analysis of an error to assess the event and identify causes and possible solutions. The Joint Commission's (2009) root-cause analysis matrix includes the following dimensions that need to be assessed:

1. What happened?

2. Why did it happen? (The process or activity in which the event occurred)

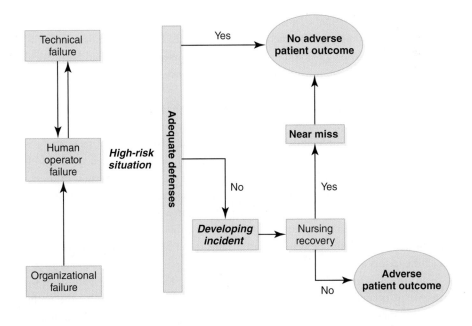

Figure 12-2 Near-Miss Model

Source: Reprinted from Henneman, E., & Gawlinski, A. (2004). A "near-miss" model for describing the nurse's role in the recovery of medical errors. *Journal of Professional Nursing, 20*(3), 196–201. Copyright 2004, with permission from Elsevier.

3. What were the most proximate factors? (Human, equipment, controllable environmental factors, uncontrollable external factors, other)

4. Which systems and processes underlie those proximate factors? (Human resources issues, information management issues, environmental management issues, leadership issues [corporate culture, encouragement of communication, clear communication of priorities], uncontrollable factors)

After an interprofessional team analyzes the event or conducts a root-cause analysis, an action plan is developed.

Root-cause analysis is now used by many HCOs to better understand errors. This approach is based not on a blame culture approach, but rather on a just culture approach, and recognizes the importance of system issues. Reporting of errors should be done anonymously; otherwise, staff will be reluctant to report them. The best reporting systems also let staff know about results from reporting—what is improved from doing this routinely. In addition, the best systems provide a method for reporting near misses. Near misses can teach staff a lot about potential errors and need for improvement.

The root-cause analysis process should be conducted by an interprofessional healthcare team—including representatives from critical clinical areas, administration, medical records, QI, pharmacy, laboratory, and any other department that might be involved in the type of situation. The focus is on the system, not on individuals. This process requires that the team be willing to be open and honest and to dig deep into the issues to analyze the process. When one describes all the factors and steps in the process that resulted in an error, it is usually quite complex.

Some safety experts identify errors as honest mistakes or mistakes that are not discussed. "Each category has a different cause, produces a different range of outcomes, and requires different solutions.

Honest mistakes include accidental or unintentional slips and errors—for example: poor handwriting, confusing labels, difficult accents, competing tasks, language barriers, distractions, etc." (Maxwell, Grenny, Lavandero, & Groah, 2011, p. 1). James Reason (2000) describes these honest mistakes as the human equivalent of gravity—they are inevitable. Awareness of the existence of honest errors means staff must be alert to the possibility of them occurring and prevent them.

The American Association of Critical-Care Nurses conducted a study to examine calculated decisions of nurses to not speak up when nurses have knowledge of errors (Maxwell et al., 2011). One aspect of the study looked at the use of four common survey safety tools (universal protocol checklist; World Health Organization [WHO] checklist; SBAR [situation, background, assessment, recommendations] as used with a handoff protocol; and drug-interaction warning systems). In the study, the nurses were asked how often they had been in situations where one of these tools worked, warning them of a problem that might have been missed and harmed a patient if it had not been used. The results indicated that 85% (2020) of the nurses said they had been in this situation at least once, and 29% (693) said they were in this situation at least a few times a month. This would indicate that these tools do make a difference and lead to improved care.

Other data from the same study were not so positive, however. Maxwell et al. (2011) also documented that the effectiveness of these safety tools may be undercut by "undiscussables": 58% (1403) of the nurses said they had been in situations where it was either unsafe to speak up or they were unable to get others to listen. Seventeen percent (409) said they were in this situation at least a few times a month. This type of data attests to the complexity of quality improvement—the problems themselves; the challenges in identifying, monitoring, and measuring the problems; and the impact of human factors. Findings reported in this "Silent

Treatment" study show that only a small minority of nonsupervisory nurses spoke up when they had a concern related to dangerous shortcuts, incompetence, or disrespect. Only 9% spoke up in all three of these situations, and only 14% spoke up in two of the three.

> The goal is to connect to people's existing values to stimulate their passion for keeping patients safe. The most effective way to make this connection is through sharing personal experiences. The least effective way is to resort to verbal persuasion: data dumps, lectures, sermons, and rants. (Maxwell et al., 2011, p. 10)

Thus it is important to get staff to share stories of near misses, patient injuries, or examples of when speaking out prevented errors and harm to a patient. Staff can relate more to stories, and they will remember them.

If the IOM had stopped its investigation of healthcare quality with the *To Err Is Human* report, the major impact of the report and its recommendations would most likely have been diluted. This, however, did not happen. In 2004, due to recognition that much more needed to be known about the quality of health care, the IOM published a follow-up report. The approach of the IOM has been to describe a problem area, identify recommendations to respond to the problem, and then identify monitoring methods. *Patient Safety: Achieving a New Standard for Care* (IOM, 2004a) focuses on the need to establish a national information infrastructure and the need for data standards. These elements will help healthcare providers and payers better monitor outcomes. Having a common language with which to discuss safety and errors is critical in meeting this goal of having a national information infrastructure. It also addresses the fifth IOM healthcare professions core competency, which focuses on informatics. This is another example that illustrates how the IOM reports, data, recommendations, and methods to monitor change are all interconnected; they are clearly interwoven with the need to develop core competencies so that healthcare providers can meet the need to improve care.

A Culture of Safety and a Blame-Free Work Environment

The typical approach to errors in health care has been to identify the staff member who made the error or to ask staff to report their errors by completing an incident report that describes the error. This type of approach has been punitive in nature and has not been effective in reducing errors, as noted in the IOM's 1999 report. It has not been effective because most errors are not made by an individual, but rather are complex and are described as system errors. When an error occurs, the question should not be, "Who is at fault?" but rather "Why did our defenses fail?" (Reason, 2000). Communication, collaboration, and coordination (interprofessional teamwork); lack of staff; patient acuity level; equipment; delivery processes; the role of the patient in care; and many other factors affect any action taken or not taken in health care. In *To Err Is Human*, the IOM (1999) reported that the healthcare system was focusing on the blame game and not really finding out more about all the factors related to an error. Staff members need to feel comfortable—not fearful—in reporting errors. The goal should be a **blame-free environment** in which staff can practice and openly discuss potential errors or near misses as well as actual errors. If staff worry about implications such as impact on their position or performance, they may not report an error, and this can have serious consequences for patients and prevent the system from improving. This type of fear may also prevent staff from communicating near misses, from which much can be learned about potential errors.

In the past, if a nurse made a medication error, the nurse might have been required to take a medication review course and an exam with no consideration of analyzing the causes of the error.

The following questions are important to consider in this situation.

- Does this intervention really get to an understanding of the error?
- Does it consider factors such as the question, Was the correct medication sent by pharmacy?
- Did the error involve placing a patient medication in the wrong patient medication box?
- Was the prescription transcribed correctly?
- Was there a computer error?
- What were the distractions and interruptions when the medication was prepared and administered?
- Did the nurse check the patient's identification correctly?
- Was an error made in what the physician intended to order or what the team agreed would be the best approach?

The five rights of medication administration have been part of safe medication administration for some time: right patient, right medication, right dose, right time, and right route. The right time consideration has been a problem, particularly as more HCOs use electronic medical records and bar codes. A common accepted policy that is supported by CMS is that medications should be administered within 30 minutes of the ordered time. The Institute for Safe Medication Practice (2011) has expressed concern about what happens when nurses cannot meet this standard. The typical response is to use workarounds or shortcuts. The Institute for Safe Medication Practice conducted a survey that included 17,500 nurses, and the majority believed that trying to meet the 30-minute deadline leads to problems and errors. With electronic methods, more data are now available regarding the times at which medications are administered, and this has led to negative views, with late administration being considered an error. This viewpoint does not consider that most nurses are capable of making common-sense clinical decisions and are aware of medications for which administration time is a critical element.

There is a strong recommendation to move to a culture of safety within a blame-free environment. To accomplish this goal, there must be (1) greater understanding of its essential elements, (2) a decrease in barriers to creating the culture, (3) development and implementation of strategies to create the safety culture, and (4) evaluation of outcomes (IOM, 2004a). Trust is important in this type of culture. Moving away from blame means that staff must trust that they will not be automatically individually blamed or punished for errors that are out of their individual control. Another aspect of this issue is related to individual staff expectations; nurses feel that they should not make mistakes, that the care they provide should be perfect. This is not a reality-based perspective. Errors will inevitably be made that are caused by many factors. Improvement is, of course, critical, but to think that errors will never be made is not realistic. There is no doubt that the number of errors needs to decrease. Moreover, there is no doubt that what has been done to address errors has not yet been fully effective.

Hospitals and other HCOs are moving toward cultures of safety, but it will take time and effort to change attitudes and behaviors. Particularly important is how the HCO leadership guides and supports the development of a culture of safety (Anderson, 2006). A topic that comes up often from all types of healthcare professionals is concern about revealing errors and near misses. This is based on past experiences. To be truly effective, disclosure must be present with maximum transparency. Ensuring transparency and involving patients are the most difficult aspects of ensuring a culture of safety (Anderson, 2006). "A fundamental principle of the systems approach to error reduction is the recognition that all humans make mistakes and that errors are to be expected, even in the best organizations" (Reason, 2000, p. 768).

It is important to note that a no-blame culture of patient safety does not mean a lack of individual accountability (Wachter & Pronovost, 2009). Yes, there is greater emphasis on and recognition of the impact of the system on errors, but nurses and other healthcare providers must still have accountability for their own practice. When an individual fails to adhere to a safety standard that one would be expected to know and there are no system issues for this failure, then that individual is accountable for the error.

Despite all of these reports, data, and initiatives to improve care and respond to errors—for example, with checklists to ensure that the correct side or body part is operated on in surgery—major problems persist. Data in 2011 indicated that wrong-site surgery continues to be a major problem, with The Joint Commission estimating that this error occurs 40 times per week in U.S. hospitals (Boodman, 2011). Such errors are increasing, not decreasing. For example, consider what might happen in a hospital with a patient who is scheduled to have cardiac bypass surgery. When a nurse asks the patient to sign the consent form, it lists a different procedure. The patient, who is a physician, points out the error and refuses to sign. An hour later, another nurse brings the patient a second consent form to sign, but it is also incorrect. The third consent form is correct and signed by the patient. This should never happen. What if the patient had not noticed or did not have the background to understand that the surgical procedure described was not what was agreed upon between the physician and the patient? This experience also took staff time and increased stress for the patient. It highlights the fact that much more needs to be done to improve care and that changing the culture is much more complicated than thought. In addition, the issue of a blame culture continues, and there needs to be more attention given to the personal reaction of staff who are involved in errors, particularly errors that lead to the death of a patient. How much debriefing occurs, and are they blamed and how?

In 2011, a neonatal nurse with 24 years' experience was involved in fatal medication error that led to the death of an 8-month-old child, though at the time it was not clear the error was the actual cause of the death. Immediately after the incident, the nurse was escorted from the hospital, put on administrative leave, and then fired several weeks later. Seven months later, the nurse committed suicide. The hospital in which this event occurred had been following a "just culture" approach for more than 3 years (Aleccia, 2011). Does this incident send a message not to mention mistakes? How effective was the organization's "just culture"? How can employers help staff who may become secondary victims if they cannot cope with the result of an error? It is important for students who are involved in a near miss or error to discuss this experience openly with faculty and to ask for support, and faculty need to provide the support to students when these situations occur.

Staff Safety

The IOM's 1999 report, *To Err Is Human*, focused on patient safety, not staff safety, but the report did state the committee believes that "creating a safe environment for patients will go a long way in addressing issues of worker safety as well" (p. 20). This does not mean that staff safety is not important—it is very important. Another IOM report, *Keeping Patients Safe: Transforming the Work Environment of Nurses* (2004b), includes content related to staff safety, particularly nurses. Nursing staff are not immune to injury at work. The Occupational Safety and Health Administration (OSHA) is the federal agency that is responsible for monitoring safe workplaces.

The American Nurses Association (ANA) is a strong advocate for safety for nurses in all types of healthcare settings. Its position statements on staff safety provide guidelines for work environments for staff. Examples of some of the position statements are available at the ANA website (http://www.nursingworld.org), such as *Personnel Policies and HIV in the Workplace*, *HIV Infection and Nursing Students*, *HIV Testing*, and others. Some of the key safety issues for nursing staff other than those mentioned are highlighted here.

Needlesticks

Healthcare workers suffer between 600,000 and 1 million injuries from conventional needles and sharps annually. These exposures can lead to hepatitis B, hepatitis C, and human immunodeficiency virus (HIV), the virus that causes AIDS. At least 1000 healthcare workers are estimated to contract serious infections annually from needlestick and sharps injuries. Registered nurses (RNs) working at the bedside experience the majority of these exposures. More than 80% of needlestick injuries could be prevented with the use of safer needle devices. More disturbing is the fact that fewer than 15% of U.S. hospitals use safer needle devices and systems.

Infections

As noted, healthcare workers are often exposed to communicable diseases via needlesticks, including HIV and hepatitis B and C. Other examples of infections transmitted via this route are tuberculosis (whose incidence is increasing in the United States), *Staphylococcus*, cytomegalovirus, influenza, and bacteria. Influenza spread has been linked to suboptimal vaccination levels of healthcare workers (Polygreen et al., 2008). Bacterial infections have sometimes been linked to glove contamination (Diaz, Silkaitis, Malczynski, Noskin, Warren, & Zembower, 2008).

Ergonomic Safety

Nurses experience a significant number of work-related back injuries and other musculoskeletal disorders. ANA's Handle with Care campaign addressed work-related musculoskeletal disorders (Castro, 2004). Because of these injuries, nurses may transfer to other units or other healthcare settings, and sometimes they may leave nursing. Typical injuries are to the neck, shoulder, and back. Nursing practice requires a lot of patient handling, and factors such as the patient's weight, height, body shape, age, dependency, and medical status are important to consider as ergonomic issues. There has been an increase in weight in the U.S. adult population in general, and this has increased the risk of injury. The physical setting also is a factor in increasing risk. There should be enough room to move around in a room when moving the patient, and nurses should consider the types of equipment available to assist with moving patients.

The national campaign known as Handle with Care was established in September 2003 by the ANA. Its goal is to develop and implement a proactive, multifaceted plan to promote the issue of safe patient handling and the prevention of musculoskeletal disorders among nurses in the United States. Through a variety of activities, the campaign seeks to educate and to advocate and facilitate change from traditional practices of manual patient handling to emerging technology-oriented methods. Nursing education needs to include content and experiences to facilitate the use of the most effective handling methods. In addition, more emphasis should be placed on assistive patient handling equipment and devices. Students need to learn how to use this equipment, too.

In 2013, the ANA expanded its initiative on safe patient handling by publishing *Patient Handling and Mobility: Interprofessional National Standards*. These standards were developed in collaboration with an interprofessional group to establish safe environments for nurses and patients (ANA, 2013). The standards focus on the following topics:

Standard 1. Establish a culture of safety.

Standard 2. Implement and sustain a safe patient handling and mobility (SPHM) program.

Standard 3. Incorporate ergonomic design principles to provide a safe environment of care.

Standard 4. Select, install and maintain SPHM technology.

Standard 5. Establish a system for education, training and maintaining competence.

Standard 6. Integrate patient-centered SPHM assessment, plan of care, and use of SPHM technology.

Standard 7. Include SPHM in reasonable accommodation and post-injury return to work.

Standard 8. Establish a comprehensive evaluation system.

Violence

Violence may not be a typical staff safety concern that a student would first think of when asked about safety in the healthcare workplace, but it is a concern. There is greater risk for violence in emergency departments, psychiatric/substance abuse departments, and long-term care facilities; however, such incidents could occur anywhere. Patients and families may not be able to control their anger appropriately. The nurse may also be in a situation in which violence that is not directly related to the nurse or health care occurs, such as providing home care in a community in which there is violence. The four types of workplace violence are (1) violence committed during a robbery or similar crime (which accounts for 85% of all workplace homicides); (2) violence that involves customers who become violent during the course of a transaction; (3) violence related to worker-on-worker assault; and (4) violence as a spillover of domestic violence (Gates & Kroeger, 2007).

Staff need training so that they can prevent violence when possible—particularly training on how to identify signs of escalation and how to deescalate a situation when possible—and they need to know how to protect themselves when violence cannot be prevented. In areas such as psychiatry, this training is more common. Signs of escalation include a sudden change in behavior, clenched jaws or fists, threats, pacing, increased movement, shouting, use of profanity, increased respirations, and staring or pointing. These signs do not mean that the person will become violent, but rather that the nurse should be more aware of the person's behavior and communication to determine if the person is escalating. Protecting oneself is very important; the nurse may leave the room, stay near the door or keep the door open, ask other staff to be present, or call for security assistance.

Chemical Exposure

OSHA (2004) has developed guidelines for preventing workplace injuries caused by exposure to chemicals, which is something nurses may encounter during the course of their work. An online survey of workplace exposures and disease conditions among 1500 nurses was conducted by the Environmental Working Group and Healthcare Without Harm, in collaboration with the ANA and the Environmental Health Education Center of the University of Maryland's School of Nursing, and supported by numerous state and specialty nursing organizations. This comprehensive survey indicated that participating nurses who were exposed frequently to sterilizing chemicals, housekeeping cleaners, residues from drug preparation, radiation, and other hazardous substances reported increased rates of asthma, miscarriage, and certain cancers, as well as increased rates of cancers and birth defects (in particular, musculoskeletal defects) in their children. There are workplace safety standards for only six of the hundreds of hazardous substances to which nurses are exposed on the job (Environmental Working Group, 2007). Specific risks identified for nurses include anesthetic gases, hand and skin disinfection, housekeeping chemicals, latex, medications such as antiretroviral medications and chemotherapeutic agents, mercury-containing devices, personal care products, radiation, and sterilization and disinfectant agents such as ethylene oxide and glutaraldehyde.

Examples of Safety Initiatives

A number of important safety initiatives have been stimulated by the IOM's work on safety. The Institute for Healthcare Improvement (IHI), for example, was established in 1991. It describes itself as "a reliable source of energy, knowledge, and support for a never-ending campaign to improve healthcare worldwide. The Institute helps accelerate change in healthcare by cultivating promising concepts for improving patient care and turning those ideas into action" (IHI, 2014). It focuses on safety, effectiveness, patient-centeredness, timeliness, efficiency, and equity, all of which are emphasized in the IOM quality series. The 5 Million Lives campaign is one example; this voluntary initiative sought to protect patients from 5 million incidents of medical harm over 2 years (December 2006–December 2008). This initiative led the IHI to further develop its resources to improve healthcare quality, such as an improvement map designed to help hospitals deal with the multiple requirements they face and to focus on high-leverage changes to transform health care (IHI, 2011a).

Another initiative, a collaborative effort between the IHI and the Robert Wood Johnson Foundation, is called Transforming Care at the Bedside (TCAB). TCAB is a "unique innovation initiative that aims to create, test, and implement changes that will dramatically improve care on medical/surgical units, and improve staff satisfaction as well" (IHI, 2011b).

Another example of a safety initiative is The Joint Commission's annual safety goals, which were first introduced in 2003. Each year, The Joint Commission identifies safety goals that should be the focus of every Joint Commission–accredited HCO. These goals are based on the critical, current safety concerns. Surveyors also emphasize the goals during accreditation visits. HCOs typically provide staff education related to the goals and monitor related progress. The current goals are available on The Joint Commission website (http://www.jointcommission.org).

QUALITY HEALTH CARE

There is no universal definition of healthcare quality—a fact that has made it difficult to assess quality in this setting. For this discussion, the IOM definition of quality care will be used; this is the definition used throughout the IOM quality series of reports. The IOM defines **quality** as the "degree to which

health services for individuals and populations increase the likelihood of desired health outcomes and are consistent with current professional knowledge" (1990, p. 4). Quality is a complex concept, and who is defining it can make a difference; for example, a nurse, a physician, and a patient may all have different definitions of quality.

The IOM definition of quality includes three elements, which usually are included in the discussion of quality care and monitoring care (**Figure 12-3**) (Donabedian, 1980):

1. **Structure**: The environment in which services are provided; inputs into the system, such as patients, staff, and environments.
2. **Process**: The manner in which services are provided; the interactions between clinicians and patients.
3. **Outcomes**: The results of services; evidence about changes in patients' health status in relation to patient and community needs.

Crossing the Quality Chasm: Impact on Quality Care

Crossing the Quality Chasm (IOM, 2001a) is the report that followed *To Err Is Human* (IOM, 1999) within the IOM quality series. This report's major message is that the U.S. healthcare system is in need of fundamental improvement. Although this system has undergone many changes—such as the development of new drugs, medical technology, and informatics that have improved care and care options—more needs to be done. The 2001 report provides valuable information to help nurses better

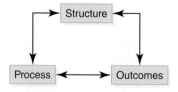

Figure 12-3 Three Elements of Quality

understand quality issues in the healthcare system; however, if this information is not applied to improve care, it serves little purpose.

The *Crossing the Quality Chasm* report identifies six aims or goals for improvement. These aims state that care should have the following characteristics (IOM, 2001a, pp. 5–6):

1. **Safe care**: Avoiding injuries to patients from the care that is intended to help them.
2. **Effective care**: Providing services based on scientific knowledge (evidence-based practice [EBP]) to all who could benefit and refraining from providing services to those not likely to benefit (avoiding underuse and overuse).
3. **Patient-centered care**: Providing care that is respectful of and responsive to individual patient preferences, needs, and values and ensuring that patient values guide all clinical decisions.
4. **Timely care**: Reducing waits and harmful delays for both those who receive and those who give care.
5. **Efficient care**: Avoiding waste, including waste of equipment, supplies, ideas, and energy.
6. **Equitable care**: Providing care that does not vary in quality because of personal characteristics such as gender, ethnicity, geographic location, and socioeconomic status (disparity concern).

All of the IOM healthcare professions' core competencies relate to these aims.

The IOM quality series is unique in that each report does not stand alone, but rather expands on previous reports in the series. This interconnectedness makes it important that readers understand the general information in each report, the ways in which the reports relate to one another, and the recommendations and joint implications for nursing and health care.

To ensure an improved healthcare system meets the six aims identified in the *Crossing the Quality Chasm* report, the IOM developed new rules for the 21st century to guide care delivery. These rules are directly related to the six aims and to the healthcare professions' core competencies. The information provided here describes this vision of the HCO system and indicates how the elements relate to nursing (IOM, 2001a, p. 67):

1. Care based on continuous healing relationships. Patients should receive care whenever they need it—access is critical. *Consider these related factors and examples: nurse–patient relationship, continuum of care, HCO services and systems, diversity, interprofessional teams.*
2. Customization based on patient needs and values. This rule relates directly to patient-centered care. Patient needs and values also constitute one of the sources of evidence for EBP. *Consider these factors and examples: nursing care and planning, interprofessional teams, patient-centered care, diversity, and patient education.*
3. The patient as the source of control. Patients need information to make decisions about their own care—this is essential to patient-centered care. Healthcare systems and professionals need to share information with patients and bring patients into the decision-making process. *Consider these factors and examples: plan of care, interprofessional care, and informed consent provides patient information to be the decision maker, patient education, informatics.*
4. Shared knowledge and the free flow of information. Patients need access to their medical information, and clinicians also need access. This rule relates to all the core competencies, and particularly to the fifth competency—applying informatics. *Consider these factors and examples: informatics, interprofessional teams, sharing information in the nursing care process, patient-centered care, patient education, computerized documentation.*
5. Evidence-based decision making. Patients need care that is based on the best possible evidence available. Care should not vary illogically from clinician to clinician or from place to place. *Consider these factors and examples: patient-centered care, nursing research and other areas of research, and plan of care.*

6. Safety as a system property. Patients need to be safe from harm that may occur within the healthcare system. There needs to be more attention placed on system errors rather than individual errors. *Consider these factors and examples: patient-centered care, nursing care provided in a safe manner, inclusion of safety in the plan of care, patient safety and errors, staff safety, and reimbursement (e.g., Medicare rules limit reimbursement if a patient experiences a fall—government, insurers).*

7. The need for transparency. The healthcare system should make information available to patients and their families that allows them to make informed decisions when selecting a health plan, hospital, or clinical practice, or when choosing among alternative treatments. This should include information that describes the system's performance on safety, EBP, and patient satisfaction. *Consider these factors and examples: interprofessional teams, informatics, informed consent, research, patient education, report cards, and national reports on quality and disparity.*

8. Anticipation of needs. Healthcare providers and the health system should not just react to events that may occur with patients, but should anticipate patient needs and provide care needed. *Consider these factors and examples because anticipation of needs is part of each: assessment, interprofessional teams, nursing care process, plan of care, HCO services, patient satisfaction, diversity, outcomes.*

9. Continuous decrease in waste. Resources should not be wasted—including patient time. *Consider these factors and examples of how the nurse must consider how resources are used: care delivery, costs of care, access to care and services, and issues of misuse, overuse, and underuse.*

10. Cooperation among clinicians. Collaboration and communication are critical among healthcare professionals and systems (interprofessional teamwork). *Consider these factors and examples: interprofessional team, plan of care requires team collaboration.*

Exhibit 12-1 compares the current approach, or "old rules," to the new rules recommended by the IOM.

Exhibit 12-1   Simple Rules for the 21st-Century Healthcare System

Current Approach (Old Rule)	New Rule
Care is based primarily on visits.	Care is based on continuous healing relationships.
Professional autonomy drives variability.	Care is customized according to patient needs and values.
Professionals control care.	The patient is the source of control.
Information is a record.	Knowledge is shared and information flows freely.
Decision making is an individual responsibility.	Decision making is evidence based.
Do no harm is an individual responsibility.	Safety is a system property.
Secrecy is necessary.	Transparency is necessary.
The system reacts to needs.	Needs are anticipated.
Cost reduction is sought.	Waste is continuously decreased.
Preference is given to professional roles over the system.	Cooperation among clinicians is a priority.

Source: Reprinted with permission from Crossing the Quality Chasm: A New Health System for the 21st Century, 2001 by the National Academy of Sciences, Courtesy of the National Academies Press, Washington, D.C.

Envisioning the National Healthcare Quality Report

Envisioning the National Healthcare Quality Report (IOM, 2001b) is the follow-up to the *Crossing the Quality Chasm* (IOM, 2001a) report. It describes a framework for collecting annual national data about healthcare quality and focuses on how the U.S. healthcare delivery system performs in providing personal health care. The Agency for Healthcare Research and Quality, which is part of the U.S. Department of Health and Human Services (HHS), is mandated to collect data using this framework and to publish an annual report, which is made available on the Internet. This report should "serve as a yardstick or the barometer by which to gauge progress in improving the performance of the healthcare delivery system in consistently providing high-quality care" (IOM, 2001b, p. 2). Elsewhere in this chapter, healthcare report cards are discussed. An annual national report card does not replace the need for individual HCOs to monitor their own quality. The information from the national annual report can be used by HCOs in developing services, by insurers and health policy makers, and by nurse educators in planning curricula and teaching–learning strategies.

The framework for the annual report uses a matrix. "The matrix is a tool to visualize possible combinations of the two dimensions (consumer perspectives and components of healthcare quality) of the framework and better understand how various aspects of the framework relate to one another" (IOM, 2001b, p. 8). This matrix was changed in 2010, and the current version is shown in **Figure 12-4**. The annual national report is designed to meet the following needs (p. 31):

- Supply a common understanding of quality and how to measure it that reflects the best current approaches and practices
- Identify aspects of the healthcare system that improve or impede quality
- Generate data associated with major quality initiatives
- Educate the public, the media, and other audiences about the importance of healthcare quality and the current level of quality
- Identify for policy makers the problem areas in healthcare quality that most need their attention and action, with the understanding that these priorities may change over time and differ by geographic location

Crosscutting dimensions	Components of quality care	Types of care		
		Preventive care	Acute treatment	Chronic condition management
E Q U I T Y / V A L U E	Effectiveness			
	Safety			
	Timeliness			
	Patient/family-centeredness			
	Access			
	Efficiency			
	Care coordination			
	Health systems infrastructure capabilities			

Figure 12-4 Updated Conceptual Framework for Categorizing Healthcare Quality and Disparities Measurement

Source: Reprinted with permission from Future Directions for the National Healthcare Quality and Disparities Reports, 2010 by the National Academy of Sciences, Courtesy of the National Academies Press, Washington, D.C..

- Provide policy makers, purchasers, healthcare providers, and others with realistic benchmarks for quality of care in the form of national, regional, and population comparisons
- Make it easier to compare the quality of the U.S. healthcare system with the systems of other nations
- Stimulate the refinement of existing measures and the development of new ones
- Stimulate data collection efforts at the state and local levels (mirroring the national effort) to facilitate targeted QI
- Incorporate improved measures as they become available and practicable
- Clarify the many aspects of healthcare quality and how they affect one another and quality as a whole
- Encourage data collection efforts needed to refine and develop quality measures, and ultimately stimulate the development of a health information infrastructure to support quality measurement and reporting

The annual report tracks outcomes for the priority areas of care identified by IOM and the adjusted priorities based on annual results.

The Current National Healthcare Quality report and the National Healthcare Disparities report of 2012 can be accessed at the AHRQ's website (HHS, AHRQ, 2010; see the "Linking to the Internet" section). This is the 10th year these reports have been completed; all have been based on recommendations from the IOM's *Crossing the Quality Chasm* report. The report is typically 2 years behind the current year. The monitoring approach is reviewed periodically to ensure the usefulness and quality of the data.

QUALITY IMPROVEMENT

Implementing the IOM's **quality improvement (QI)** approaches "requires that health professionals be clear about what they are trying to accomplish,

what changes they can make that will result in an improvement, and how they will know that the improvement occurred" (IOM, 2003, p. 59). Healthcare complexity is mentioned many times as a barrier to understanding safety and quality and to improving healthcare delivery.

Health care is complex. Its consumers are very diverse in their needs, diagnoses, ethnic and cultural backgrounds, and overall health status, including genetic background, socioeconomic factors, patient preferences for health care, community differences, and healthcare coverage/reimbursement. Health care cannot be viewed in the same manner as other businesses (such as the automobile industry) that might manufacture or sell one product or a series of highly related products. Healthcare products vary based on the medical problem and the patient, the setting, the expertise of clinical staff, the desires of the patient, treatment options, patient prognosis, the expertise of the healthcare providers and HCOs, and health policy and legislation. In specialty areas such as obstetrics, psychiatry, emergency care, intensive care, home care, and long-term care, there is great variation within services—in their interventions, roles of the patient and family, patient education needs, prognosis and outcomes, and so on. It is expensive to develop and maintain effective QI programs, but The Joint Commission requires such programs for all its accredited organizations. QI programs can lead to improved safety and quality, making them critical regardless of any pressure from The Joint Commission.

Because of the complex nature of quality, developing a QI program that addresses monitoring and improving healthcare quality is in and of itself a complex process. Effective appraisal of the scientific facts suggests that health care can be improved by closing the wide gaps between prevailing practices and the best-known approaches to care, and by inventing new forms of care. This requires planning and careful evaluation of results. One model for improvement focuses on three key questions (Berwick & Nolan, 1998):

1. What is the HCO trying to accomplish?
2. How will the HCO know whether a change is an improvement?
3. Which change can the HCO try that it believes will result in improvement?

For an HCO to have an effective QI program, nurses and other health professionals need to be knowledgeable and competent in the following areas (IOM, 2003, p. 59):

- Continually understand and measure quality of care in terms of structure, or the inputs into the system, such as patients, staff, and environments; process, or the interactions between clinicians and patients; and outcomes, or evidence about changes in patients' health status in relation to patient and community needs.

- Assess current practices and compare these practices with relevant better practices elsewhere as a means of identifying opportunities for improvement.
- Design and test interventions to change the process of care, with the objective of improving quality.
- Identify errors and hazards in care; understand and implement basic safety design principles, such as standardization and simplification and human factors training.
- Both act as an effective member of an interdisciplinary/interprofessional team and improve the quality of one's own performance through self-assessment and personal change.

Figure 12-5 illustrates the importance of quality in the healthcare system.

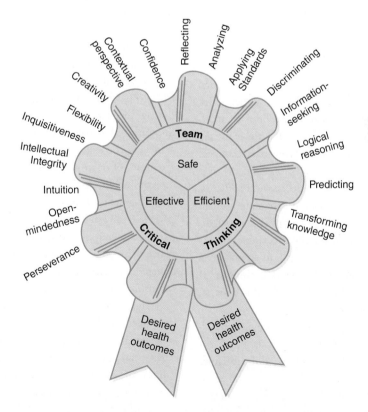

Figure 12-5 Medallion of Quality Health Care Through Critical Thinking

Source: From Rubenfeld, M. & Scheffer, B. (2006). *Critical thinking tactics for nurses.* Sudbury, MA: Jones and Bartlett.

Other changes in QI have focused on sharing information with patients and rewards for QI. Public reporting is more common. This sharing of predetermined quality and efficiency measures with performance data informs patients and stakeholders about provider performance (Dunton, Gonnerman, Montalvo, & Shumann, 2011). Value-based purchasing is also used today. Value-based purchasing is a payment system that provides financial rewards for performance. Such a system, in addition to the public reporting and opportunity to get referrals, incentivizes providers to improve outcomes.

The Joint Commission

Accreditation is the process by which organizations are evaluated on their quality, based on established minimum standards. The major organization that accredits HCOs is **The Joint Commission**, a nonprofit organization that accredits more than 20,500 HCOs, including hospitals, long-term care organizations, home care agencies, clinical laboratories, ambulatory care organizations, behavioral health organizations, and healthcare networks or managed care organizations. It has been accrediting HCOs since 1951, and over that time, the accreditation requirements and process have changed. Participating in a Joint Commission survey is time consuming and costly, but is necessary for HCOs. For example, nursing education programs need to use HCOs with current Joint Commission accreditation for student practicum/clinical experiences. As The Joint Commission has changed, its emphasis on quality and safety has also changed. Continuous QI is now the major focus of the accreditation process, which includes safety.

Nurses serve on the Joint Commission Nursing Advisory Council, which advises its parent organization about nursing concerns and care issues related to safety and quality. All nurses who work in HCOs eventually experience a Joint Commission survey. The Joint Commission makes a visit to the HCO every 3 years to complete its intensive survey and may even make unscheduled visits. For the scheduled visits, the HCO is given a date and has 9–12 months to prepare for the visit. Preparing for the visit involves gathering information and data for The Joint Commission, educating staff about the standards, conducting mock surveys to prepare staff, and so on. The HCO should meet standards at all times, not just at the time of a survey. In the past, great emphasis was placed on getting ready for the Joint Commission visit and surviving it; afterward, the HCO was less vigilant until it came time to prepare for the next visit. This approach of just focusing on the survey eventually changed, and now accredited HCOs must submit reports on certain data to The Joint Commission annually, with a plan of action for areas noted in the self-assessment requiring improvement (periodic performance review); in addition, HCOs must be prepared for possible unscheduled visits.

Nurses are very active in preparing for the survey and during the survey visit. The Joint Commission now involves more direct care staff in its survey visits by including them in meetings to discuss care in the HCO and asking individual staff questions during the survey. Students may even be asked questions. The goal is to find out if the patients are achieving the expected outcomes, and if not, why. Examples of outcomes that The Joint Commission assesses include mortality rates, length of stay, adverse incidents, complications, readmission rates, patient/family satisfaction, referrals to specialists, patient adherence to discharge plans or treatment plans, achievement of safety goals, and prevention adherence services (e.g., mammograms, Pap smears, immunizations).

The Joint Commission standards have been developed, evaluated, and changed over the years to meet the changing needs of healthcare delivery. These standards form the framework for accreditation. The accreditation of hospitals, for example, focuses on the following areas:

- Environment of care
- Emergency medicine

- Human resources
- Infection prevention and control
- Information management
- Leadership
- Life safety
- Medication management
- Medical staff
- National patient safety goals
- Nursing
- Provision of care, treatment, and services
- Performance improvement
- Record of care, treatment, and services
- Rights and responsibilities of the individual
- Transplant safety

Because The Joint Commission accredits a broad range of HCOs, there are differences in which minimum standards apply and in how the various healthcare settings might monitor their safety and quality. Consider home care agencies: These agencies use other national evaluation approaches that are not related to or led by The Joint Commission. The home care outcome-based approach to QI, known as the Outcome and Assessment Information Set (OASIS), was developed in the 1990s by the Department of Health and Human Services to provide a "systematic process that would yield consistent data to improve care outcomes" (Mosocco, 2001, p. 205). This database focuses on a group of data elements that represent core items of a comprehensive assessment of home care patients. The key question is this: Did the patient benefit from the home care services? In this type of system, home care agencies from all over the country input their QI data. OASIS is managed through the CMS.

Other organizations that focus on quality and safety in health care include those listed in **Table 12-1**.

Table 12-1	Selected Quality and Safety Organizations and Sample of Initiatives Affecting RNs in Hospitals
Organization	**Major National Initiatives Since 2000 Related to Nurses**
Institute of Medicine	Published high-profile reports on quality and safety of patient care: *To Err Is Human: Building a Safer Health System* (1999); *Crossing the Quality Chasm: A New Health System for the 21st Century* (2001); *Keeping Patients Safe: Transforming the Work Environment of Nurses* (2004) Advocated six aims to improve the quality of healthcare systems (patient centered, safe, effective, equitable, timely, and efficient) (2001)
National Quality Forum	Endorsed 15 national voluntary consensus standards for nursing-sensitive care in hospitals (2004)
Institute for Healthcare Improvement	Implemented the national hospital 100,000 Lives campaign (2005) Implemented the national hospital 5 Million Lives campaign (2006–2008)
The Joint Commission	Established a national Nursing Advisory Committee (2003) Endorsed the National Quality Forum's 15 national voluntary consensus standards for nursing-sensitive care in hospitals (2005) Included nursing-sensitive measures in the hospital accreditation process (2005)
Robert Wood Johnson Foundation	Developed the Transforming Care at the Bedside initiative (2005) Developed the Interdisciplinary Nursing Quality Research initiative (2006) Partnered with the Institute for Healthcare Improvement and American Organization of Nurse Executives (2007)

Source: From Buerhaus, P. I., Staiger, D. O., & Auerbach, D. I. (2009). *The future of the nursing workforce in the United States: Data, trends and implications.* Sudbury, MA: Jones and Bartlett.

Healthcare Report Cards

Healthcare report cards provide specific performance data about an organization at specific intervals, with a focus on quality and safety. Such a report can be used by the HCO to compare its outcomes with report cards published by other HCOs or with a large state or national database (benchmarking). This information can be helpful in improving care in the HCO by identifying what the HCO is doing well and what needs improvement as compared with other similar HCOs. Some of these report cards are now accessible on the Internet and can be used by consumers (patients, families). Nurses can also use them when searching for new jobs to obtain evaluation data about a specific HCO. In some cases, insurers use healthcare report cards to assess an HCO and compare it with similar HCOs. The goal is to examine performance based on clearly defined criteria.

In 1994, the ANA began an investigation of the impact of workforce restructuring and redesign on the safety and quality of patient care in acute care settings. This was around the time that the IOM was also beginning to work on this issue. The ANA wanted to "explore the nature and strength of the linkages between nursing care and patient outcomes by identifying nursing quality indicators" (Pollard, Mitra, & Mendelson, 1996, p. 1). "The National Database of Nursing Quality Indicators® (NDNQI) was established by the ANA in 1998 and has been in operation for 10 years. NDNQI is a program of ANA's National Center for Nursing Quality (NCNQ). ANA's NCNQ encompasses various nursing quality activities that identify and promote nurses' roles in quality. NDNQI is managed by the University of Kansas School of Nursing, under contract to ANA" (Dunton & Montalvo, 2009, p. VII). This initiative provided a framework for educating nurses, consumers, and policy makers to evaluate the contributions of nursing within the acute care setting by tracking the quality of nursing care provided in such settings. Databases and report cards

that focus on measuring quality and include nursing-specific quality indicators are needed, however. Patients come into the acute care setting primarily because they need around-the-clock care, which is the focus of nursing care. This early study made it clear that data on nursing and outcomes were lacking—that is, the methods of collecting data used at that time were not nursing specific.

The ANA initiative identified 10 nursing-sensitive indicators that reflect characteristics of the nursing workforce, nursing processes, and patient outcomes. The ANA also identified examples for each of these indicators (Montalvo & Dunton, 2007, p. 1):

- *Nursing workforce:* Measures of the supply of nursing (e.g., total nursing hours per patient day); nursing skill (percentage of nursing hours provided by RNs).
- *Nursing processes:* Risk assessment; **protocol** implementation.
- *Patient outcomes:* Fall rates that are related to nursing hours; hospital-acquired pressure ulcer rates that are related to skill mix.

After the 1994 survey, the ANA collaborated with seven state nurses associations to test whether it was possible to collect data on these indicators from a large number of sites. As a result, in 1998, the ANA established the NDNQI. As of 2007, more than 1000 hospitals were participating in the effort to collect data via this database, and even more had joined this program by 2014. This initiative "provides each nurse the opportunity to review the evidence, evaluate their practice, and determine what improvements can be made" (Montalvo & Dunton, 2007, p. 3). The participating institutions submit their nursing-sensitive indicator data to the database, which allows for the collection of a large amount of data for evaluation and for research. The following are the nursing indicators that are the most current focus of this database (ANA, NDNQI, 2014):

- Nursing hours per patient day (also a National Quality Forum [NQF] consensus measure)
  - Registered nurses (RN) hours per patient day

- Licensed practical/vocational nurses (LPN/LVN) hours per patient day
  - Unlicensed assistive personnel (UAP) hours per patient day
- Nursing turnover
- Nosocomial infections (also an NQF consensus measure)
- Patient falls (also an NQF consensus measure)
- Patient falls with injury (also an NQF consensus measure)
  - Injury level
- Pressure ulcer rate
  - Community acquired
  - Hospital acquired
  - Unit acquired
- Pediatric pain assessment, intervention, and reassessment (AIR) cycle
- Pediatric peripheral intravenous infiltration
- Psychiatric physical/sexual assault
- RN education/certification
- RN survey
  - Job Satisfaction Scales
  - Practice Environment Scale (PES) (also an NQF consensus measure)
- Restraints (also an NQF consensus measure)
- Staff mix (also an NQF consensus measure)
  - RNs
  - LPN/LVNs
  - UAPs
  - Percent agency staff

Additional data elements collected include the following items:

- Patient population—adult or pediatric
- Hospital category (e.g., teaching, non-teaching)
- Type of unit (critical care, step-down, medical, surgical, combined medical–surgical, rehabilitation, psychiatric)
- Number of staffed beds designated by the hospital

Some of these nursing-sensitive indicators are now included in public reporting such as data collected by the National Quality Forum (noted as NQF consensus measures in the list of indicators), but there needs to be more representation of nursing-sensitive indicators in public reporting on the status of healthcare quality (Dunton et al., 2011). Data are collected by the hospitals using the NDNQI electronic database. To assist with more effective comparisons, reports are provided to hospitals with information about patient population, unit type, and hospital bed size. The result is the nursing profession's quality report card. Participation in the process is voluntary.

The list of NDNQI indicators identifies some of the critical quality issues in health care that relate to nursing care, and others are added by the NDNQI as needed. Other common issues addressed by hospitals today are hand washing; medication errors; methicillin-resistant *Staphylococcus aureus* infection; wrong patient identification and consequences; wrong procedure; operating on the wrong area or limb; administration of the wrong blood type; and use of contaminated supplies, devices, and drugs. In nursing programs, students learn how to provide safe care through didactic content, simulation, laboratory experiences, and practicum/clinical experiences. It is very important that as this learning occurs, students understand the need to protect the patient and provide quality care in all aspects of nursing care. This major nursing initiative has had an impact on the presence of nursing in some of the healthcare monitoring programs. For example, the 12 NQF consensus standards related to nursing care include some of the NDNQI indicators; however, more needs to be done to recognize the impact that nursing care has on patient outcomes (Dunton et al., 2011).

The NDNQI provides useful data that can help all parties to better understand nursing processes, outcomes, and costs. Examples of data and NDNQI results follow (ANA, 2014a):

- Average cost per ventilator-associated pneumonia (VAP) incident: $40,144
- Average cost per fall: $13,316
- Average cost per central line–associated bloodstream infection (CLABSI): $5814
- Average cost per hospital-acquired pressure ulcer (HAPU): $10,700

Other examples of data are found in an ND-NQI study that examined patient outcomes related to falls and HAPU rates (Dunton, Gajewski, Klaus, & Pierson, 2007). The conclusions support the importance of three workforce characteristics on these patient outcomes: (1) total nursing hours per patient day, (2) percentage of hours supplied by RNs, and (3) years of experience in nursing. The last factor is especially important because with nursing turnover and increasing retirement, there may be fewer experienced nurses on units to provide critical expertise to staff who have less experience and expertise.

The National Quality Forum is an important national quality initiative, and one with which the NDNQI collaborates. The NQF (2010) focuses on three purposes:

1. Setting national priorities and goals for performance improvement
2. Endorsing national consensus standards for measuring and publicly reporting on performance
3. Promoting the attainment of national goals through education and outreach programs

The NQF has examined some of the critical care issues that need to be considered to meet these purposes. Specifically, it defined 28 healthcare "never events"—patient safety events that pose serious harm to patients, but should be considered entirely preventable. Specific categories of never events include surgical events (e.g., wrong-site surgery), device events (e.g., air embolism), care management events (e.g., death or disability due to medication errors), patient protection events (e.g., patient suicide), environmental events, and criminal events. Since the development and dissemination of this list of 28 never events, many states have mandated that healthcare facilities report all instances of these events. When such an event occurs, many institutions require that the organization undertake a root-cause analysis (NQF, 2010).

Root-cause analysis is now used by many HCOs to better understand errors. This approach is based not on a blame culture approach, but rather on a just culture approach and the need to recognize the importance of system issues. Reporting of errors should be done anonymously; otherwise, staff will be reluctant to report them. The best reporting systems also let staff know about results from reporting—what is improved from doing this routinely. In addition, the best systems provide a method for reporting near misses—those times when an error almost happens, but staff catch it before the error actually occurs. Near misses can teach staff a lot about potential errors and areas in need of improvement. When errors and near misses are reported, the reporting should include responses to the following questions:

- What happened?
- Who was involved?
- When did it happen?
- Where did it happen?
- What is the severity of the actual or potential harm?
- What is the chance this could happen again?
- What are the consequences?

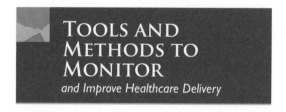

TOOLS AND METHODS TO MONITOR
and Improve Healthcare Delivery

HCOs use a variety of tools and methods to monitor safety and quality and to ensure improvement of quality. Nurses are involved in the use of all these tools and methods. Some examples follow.

Standards of Care

A standard is an authoritative statement that provides a minimum description of accepted actions that are expected from an HCO or an individual healthcare provider, such as a nurse who has specific skill and knowledge levels. Standards are expectations about what should be done. Standards are typically developed by professional organizations and may be derived from legal sources such as nurse practice acts and federal and state laws. Standards are also developed by regulatory agencies such as accreditation bodies and federal and state agencies as well as by individual HCOs. These standards should be evidence based. There are standards of practice and standards for professional performance. The ANA publishes many nursing standards, and some specialty-area standards have been developed by specialty-focused nursing organizations. As discussed, The Joint Commission also uses standards that it develops for its accreditation process, as do nursing education accreditation organizations.

Policies and Procedures

Policies and procedures set standards within an HCO that guide which decisions are made and how care is provided. Use of policies and procedures supports greater consistency in how care is delivered and can help to improve care. Policies and procedures should be evidence based, although only limited research evidence is available for some care issues in nursing at this time. Policies and procedures for nurses and nursing care should not conflict with regulatory issues in the state (such as the state's nurse practice act), and they should be in agreement with nursing standards.

A nurse uses policies and procedures daily in practice—for example, in following the accepted procedure in the hospital for administering blood products and medication administration and for ensuring safety for patients at risk of falling. Consequently, policies and procedures need to be readily available to staff. Many HCOs have put their policies and procedures into their computer systems, reducing the need for hard-copy policy and procedure manuals and making it easier for staff to access the information when needed. Nurses are expected to follow the HCO policies and procedures, which means that they need to know about them and how to seek out the information. Policies and procedures related to nursing care should be developed by nurses

in the HCO and updated annually or as needed. Many HCOs that are emphasizing evidence-based practice are reviewing and updating their policies and procedures based on EBP, and employing EBP is one of the IOM's five healthcare professions core competencies.

Licensure and Credentialing

Professional licensure verification is an important activity in all HCOs to better ensure quality care. This includes licensure for RNs, LPNs/LVNs, doctors of medicine, and others. A license means that the person has met expected minimal standards set by the state practice act. State laws require that certain healthcare providers have licenses. If an HCO allows someone to practice without a license, both the HCO and the individual are breaking the law.

Credentialing is different from checking licensure, although it is part of the latter process. Credentialing is a more in-depth review process that includes evaluation of licenses, certification if required in a specialty area, evidence of malpractice insurance as required, history of involvement in malpractice suits, and education. Credentialing is not done for all healthcare staff; it is primarily used for physicians, nurse–midwives, and nurse practitioners who want to practice or admit patients to an HCO. Credentialing would not typically be required for RNs who are not in an advanced practice position. Licensure and credentialing information is kept on file and may be reviewed by The Joint Commission during a survey.

Utilization Review/Management

Utilization review/management (UR/UM) is the process of evaluating the necessity, appropriateness, and efficiency of healthcare services for specific patients or in patient populations. Utilization review data are used by the HCO in a number of ways—for example, to assess access and usage of services; to determine that a service is no longer needed; to determine that a new service is needed; and to review the relationship of data to patient outcomes. Utilization review data are connected to financial concerns for the HCO and its budget (e.g., whether the HCO is serving enough patients to meet its budget, types of procedures and their reimbursement, and so on). **Utilization review** is administered by the HCO administration, although nurses may participate as data collectors and in the analysis process. Data are primarily obtained from medical records to determine necessity, appropriateness, and timeliness of healthcare services.

Risk Management

The goal of **risk management (RM)** is "to maintain a safe and effective healthcare environment and prevent or reduce loss to the healthcare organization" (Pike, Jansen, & Brooks, 2002, p. 3). RM is concerned with decreasing HCO financial loss that is the result of legal and malpractice issues. This function monitors errors and incidents and works with QI to decrease errors. If an error occurs, RM would evaluate the risk for a lawsuit and take actions as required. HCO attorneys are very involved in RM, and in some HCOs, RNs with a legal background are hired to work in the RM department or to consult with the department. RNs have considerable knowledge about healthcare delivery and can be excellent resources.

Benchmarking

Many hospitals and other types of HCOs use benchmarking. **Benchmarking** is

> the concept of discovering what is the best performance being achieved, whether in your company, by a competitor, or by an entirely different industry. Benchmarking is an improvement tool whereby a company measures its performance or process against other companies' best practices,

determines how those companies achieved their performance levels, and uses the information to improve its own performance. Benchmarking is a continuous process whereby an enterprise measures and compares all its functions, systems and practices against strong competitors, identifying quality gaps in the organization, and striving to achieve competitive advantage locally and globally. (Six Sigma, 2008)

One popular benchmarking approach is Six Sigma. This rigorous and systematic methodology utilizes information (management by facts) and statistical analysis to measure and improve an HCO's operational performance, practices, and systems by identifying and preventing defects in manufacturing and service-related processes, with the goal of anticipating and exceeding expectations of all stakeholders to accomplish effectiveness (Six Sigma, 2008).

Assessment of Access to Healthcare Services

Access to healthcare services is important to monitor and improve as part of the QI process. Communities are concerned about whether their citizens have access to care. *Healthy People 2020* (HHS, 2010) considers access to be a critical issue across the United States for all types of healthcare needs. When a patient does not have access, the patient's health status is at risk, and further complications may occur.

Evidence-Based Practice

EBP is relevant here because it is a method of improving the quality of care. Basing care decisions on evidence can better ensure that care needs are met in an effective manner. For example, clinical guidelines are a source of evidence to improve care and implement EBP. The IOM (1990) defines clinical guidelines as "systematically developed statements to assist practitioner and patient decisions about appropriate healthcare for specific clinical circumstances" (p. 38).

The AHRQ is a government agency that develops such guidelines and serves as a repository of those guidelines (see http://www.guidelines.gov). The AHRQ's goals are to (1) support improvements in health outcomes, (2) promote patient safety and reduce medication errors, (3) advance the use of information technology for coordinating patient care and conducting quality and outcomes research, and (4) establish an office of priority populations (this office should ensure that low-income groups, minorities, women, children, the elderly, and individuals with special needs receive care).

Clinical Pathways/Protocols

Clinical pathways describe how care is best provided for a specific patient population with specific problem(s); however, a pathway needs to be assessed for applicability to an individual patient's needs. The pathway helps the healthcare provider focus on outcomes and the assessment of achievement; in doing this, outcomes serve as a benchmarking method for individual patients. If outcomes are not met, the provider can consider the variances for the individual patient, and collecting and reviewing data from multiple patients can help to improve care for a certain patient population with certain problems. Thus it is important to recognize clinical pathways' use in the assessment of quality and cost of health care and how they increase consistency of care.

Medication Reconciliation

Patients often take many medications, and a key concern is how these medications mix together. Medication reconciliation is "creating the most accurate list possible of all medications a patient is taking, including drug name, dosage, frequency, and route, and comparing that list against the physician's admission, transfer, and/or discharge orders with the goal of providing correct medications to the patient at all transition points within the hospital (could be throughout continuum of care)" (Ketchum, Grass, & Padwojski, 2005, pp. 78–79). Responsibility for completing the medication reconciliation needs to be clarified in a policy and procedure. The tracking that is done routinely is important. HCOs should have a standardized form on which to record the information. Medication reconciliation can take time if the patient takes a lot of medications and in some cases cannot remember all the information. The Joint Commission, however, now requires this process in accredited HCOs. If problems arise in reconciling medications, then errors can result in omitted medications, incorrect dosage, incorrect route, incorrect timing, use of the same medications that are different formulations, and failure to discontinue contraindicated medications (Rozich, Howard, Justeson, Macken, Lindsay, & Resar, 2004).

Institutional Review Board

Use of an institutional review board (IRB) is the key method for ensuring informed consent and protection of human participants in research. This method also ensures, through its process, that patients who are participants in studies are not harmed unnecessarily.

Healthcare Policy and Legislation

Healthcare policy and legislation may mandate how care should be delivered to ensure safe, quality care. A current example is legislation related to whether hospitals may require mandatory overtime. This issue is important because there are questions about how many hours a nurse can work without increasing the risk for errors.

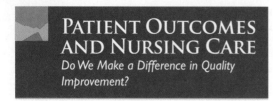

PATIENT OUTCOMES AND NURSING CARE
Do We Make a Difference in Quality Improvement?

Keeping Patients Safe: Transforming the Work Environment of Nurses (IOM, 2004b) focuses on acute care or care that is provided in the hospital setting; however, it is relevant here because much of the content can be applied to nursing in other types of settings. As the report states, "When we are hospitalized, in a nursing home, or managing a chronic condition in our own homes—at some of our most vulnerable moments—nurses are the healthcare providers we are most likely to encounter, spend the greatest amount of time with, and be dependent upon for our recovery" (IOM, 2004b, p. ix). The report emphasizes designs for a work environment in which nurses can provide safer, higher-quality patient care. The content discusses the nursing shortage, healthcare errors, patient safety risk factors, the central role of the nurse in patient safety, and work environment threats to patient safety. In discussing errors, the IOM emphasizes moving away from a punitive, blaming environment and states that errors need to be viewed more from a system perspective. Some of the factors that influence errors from a system perspective are highlighted in this report, including equipment failures, inadequate staff training, lack of clear supervision and direction, and inadequate staffing levels. The central message in the report is that we need to transform the healthcare work environment.

This critical report identifies six major concerns for direct care in nursing (IOM, 2004b):

1. Monitoring patient status or surveillance, which, according to the report, is different from assessment. **Surveillance** is defined as "purposeful and ongoing acquisition, interpretation, and synthesis of patient data for clinical decision-making" (McCloskey & Bulechek, 2000, p. 629). If surveillance is not successful, the result may be termed **failure to rescue**—missing an opportunity to prevent complications.

2. Physiologic therapy, the most common visible interventions that nurses perform.

3. Helping patients compensate for loss of function; many related activities are performed by unlicensed assistive personnel under the direction of RNs, but RNs may choose to do this work themselves rather than delegate it.

4. Providing emotional support, which is critical for patients and their families.

5. Education for patients and families, which has become more difficult for practicing nurses to provide because of work conditions, staffing shortages, patient acuity, and shorter lengths of stay.

6. Integration and coordination of care. Patients' needs are complex, and care is complex, often resulting in multiple forms of care provided by multiple providers. There is a high risk of failures in communication and inadequate collaboration, both of which increase the risk of errors. There is a critical need for interprofessional teams.

This IOM report (2004b) recommends (1) adopting transformational leadership and evidence-based management, (2) maximizing the capability of the workforce, (3) understanding work processes so that they can be improved, and (4) creating and sustaining cultures of safety. Nursing leadership must be very active throughout the HCO. Nurse leaders must represent staff, support the need for effective change, facilitate input from direct care nursing staff, and expand communication and collaboration. Leadership has been a reoccurring theme throughout this text. The HCO needs to support ongoing learning—for example, through effective orientation for appropriate length of time; ongoing training; nursing residency programs; funding support for nurses to return to school; establishing partnerships with schools of nursing; providing opportunities for interprofessional educational experiences; and so on. All this requires resources that administrators must ensure are available—for example, adequate staffing is critical. All HCOs struggle with the challenges of how best to fill positions and retain staff. Excessive documentation can lead to less time for patients, which can impact safety and quality. There is a need for computerized documentation with decision-making support. Work design is discussed in depth in the *Keeping Patients Safe* report; physical space and design—for example, lighting, size of the unit, and the ability to get to equipment easily and quickly—and how these may impact safety are addressed.

Staffing issues also include scheduling, nurse–patient ratios, and workloads. The IOM report on nursing comments on 12-hour shifts and the potential for greater risk of errors when staff members are tired and stressed.

Registered nurses have long acknowledged and continue to emphasize that staffing issues are an ongoing concern, one that influences the safety of both the patient and the nurse. There is a strong relationship between adequate nurse-to-patient ratios and safe patient outcomes. Rising patient acuity and shortened hospital stays have contributed to staffing challenges. Finding an optimal nurse-to-patient ratio has been a national challenge. Ensuring adequate staffing levels has been shown to:

- Reduce medical and medication errors
- Decrease patient complications
- Decrease mortality
- Improve patient satisfaction
- Reduce nurse fatigue
- Decrease nurse burnout
- Improve nurse retention and job satisfaction (ANA, 2014b)

Staffing approaches should consider patient acuity; strategies for using unlicensed assistive personnel; staff skills and competencies, education, and training required for specific settings; and effective use of delegation. Staffing is related to quality care and to meeting patient outcomes, as well as staff satisfaction and

a healthy work environment. For example, a recent study reported that staffing in 71 acute care hospitals in two states indicated that work schedules are related significantly to mortality when staffing levels and characteristics were controlled (Trinkoff et al., 2011). This study relates to earlier work done by Dr. Aiken about the impact of nurse staffing on patient mortality and quality care (Aiken et al., 2002).

"The safety of nurses from workplace-induced injuries and illnesses is important to nurses themselves as well as to the patients they serve. The presence of healthy and well-rested nurses is critical to providing vigilant monitoring, empathic patient care, and vigorous advocacy" (Trinkoff et al., 2008, p. 2473). The HCO needs to commit to developing and maintaining a culture of safety, and this must include staff safety issues.

Woven throughout all of the IOM's recommendations is the need for EBP and the need to base decisions on evidence. "As nurses are the largest component of the healthcare workforce and are also strongly involved in the commission, detection, and prevention of errors and adverse events, they and their work environment are critical elements of stronger patient safety defenses" (IOM, 2004b, p. 31).

Based on what is known about quality improvement and its importance, it is natural to assume that nurses are very active in QI and have assumed leadership in improving care, but this is not necessarily the case, particularly with new nurses. When a 2008 survey on this topic was sent to nurses who graduated between 2004 and 2005, 436 responded (a rate of 69.4%). According to the researchers, "Overall, 159 (38.6%) of new nurses thought that they were 'poorly' or 'very poorly' prepared about or had 'never heard of' QI. Their perceptions of preparation varied widely by the specific topic. Baccalaureate (BSN) graduates reported significantly higher levels of preparation than associate degree (ADN) graduates in evidence-based practice; assessing gaps in practice, teamwork, and collaboration; and many of the research-type skills such as data collection, analysis, measurement and measuring resulting changes" (Kovner, Brewer, Yingrengreung, & Fairchild, 2009). The authors of this study indicate that more needs to be done in nursing education on this critical content to help students see the connection between QI concepts and practice.

Subsequently, a second study was done that compared the 2004–2005 graduates with graduates from 2007–2008 (539 RNs who worked in 15 states). Not much difference was apparent in their responses, indicating little had changed in nursing education to better prepare new nurses for QI (Djukic, Kovner, Brewer, & Bernstein, 2013). Although more hospitals are providing staff education for new graduates, hospitals in general need to collaborate more with schools of nursing so that the graduates are better prepared and require less staff education, which is costly for the hospitals.

Although the Patient Protection and Affordable Care Act of 2010 primarily focuses on reimbursement, it does include an initiative to address quality improvement, known as the National Quality Strategy (NQS). Nurses need to participate actively in this initiative, although historically nurses have provided weak QI leadership. The *Future of Nursing* report (IOM, 2011) also emphasizes the need for more effective nursing leadership in quality improvement. Means by which nurses can participate include the National Priorities Partnership (NPP), Measures Application Partnership (MAP), and the NDNQI (Kennedy, Murphy, & Roberts, 2013). Nurses need to engage in the national quality agenda.

To achieve improved health care, health information technology is critical for effective performance measurement.

Health IT is a foundational tool to change the healthcare industry; however, it is not an instant fix. Rather, it is one tool in the arsenal of health reform. Health IT impacts quality by providing users the unique ability and opportunity to truly capture and derive the benefits from data. This allows users to translate seemingly independent pieces of data into meaningful conclusions that, if applied and implemented correctly, can improve the health of individuals and populations; lower costs; and help tailor healthcare to individual patient needs. Health IT can be implemented and employed in such a way as to support the National Quality Strategy and help achieve the 3-part aim of better care, better health, and lower cost. (Kennedy et al., 2013)

Some nurses may have active roles in health informatics, but all nurses should be aware of the connection of informatics with QI measurement.

Another example of the increasing relevance of nursing QI initiatives is the purchase of NDNQI in 2014. Press Ganey purchased the system from the ANA to integrate it into its performance evaluation options, providing greater visibility for nursing-sensitive data measurement (ANA, 2014).

Other ways that more nurses can participate in the quality agenda is through development and implementation of standards; involvement in shared governance and decision making about QI; serving on QI committees in healthcare organizations and for professional organizations; engaging in health policy development at the local, state, and national levels; undertaking research and using evidence to improve practice; and engaging in active discussions with colleagues and other healthcare professions about QI.

Nurses cannot provide quality care without the right information to make the right decisions when caring for patients. Nursing has become an information-based profession that provides healthcare. Technology gives nurses access to information at the point of care for decision-making. It can also remind or inform them of best practices. Nurses who are aware of the multiple changes in access and portability of information can help to inform development and adoption of new technologies facilitate quality healthcare. (Kennedy et al., 2013)

Landscape © f9photos/Shutterstock, Inc.

CONCLUSION

The IOM notes that with the need for change in the healthcare system, the following is critical:

> The 21st century healthcare system envisioned by the committee—providing care that is evidence based, patient centered, and systems oriented—also implies new roles and responsibilities for patients and their families, who must become more aware, more participative, and more demanding in a care system that should be meeting their needs. And all involved must be united by the overarching purpose of reducing the burden of illness, injury, and disability in our nation. (IOM, 2001a, p. 20)

Landscape © f9photos/Shutterstock, Inc.

CHAPTER HIGHLIGHTS

1. The IOM has published a number of critical reports related to quality health care in the United States.

2. Quality improvement is aimed at processes that critically examine the level of care, any problems with care, and how to make patient outcomes better.

3. Safety is a critical component of quality care and improved patient outcomes.

4. In 2007, the Centers for Medicare and Medicaid Services introduced a major change in its reimbursement policy, stating that the CMS will not pay Medicare benefits for certain patient complications that occur in the hospital that could have been prevented. In 2011, new regulations added Medicaid patients to this requirement.

5. Opportunity costs relate to situations in which diagnostic tests must be repeated or a change in the plan of care is necessary because of adverse reactions to treatment.

6. Because of a lack of trust of healthcare delivery, more patients are demanding that they be informed about their care and involved in the care process.

7. Critical terms that require consistent definitions related to safety and are important to understand and use in the practice setting in-clude the following: safety, error, adverse event, misuse, overuse, underuse, near miss, sentinel event, and root-cause analysis.

8. Errors are generally systems errors, not individual problems.

9. There is a strong recommendation to move to a culture of safety. To accomplish this, there must be (1) greater understanding of the essential elements of safety, (2) a decrease in barriers to creating the culture, (3) development and implementation of strategies to create a safety culture, and (4) evaluation of outcomes (IOM, 2004a).

10. Some of the key safety issues for nursing staff are needlesticks, infections, ergonomic safety, violence, and chemical exposures.

11. Examples of safety initiatives include the IHI's 5 Million Lives campaign; the IHI and Robert Wood Johnson Foundation's Transforming Care at the Bedside initiative; and The Joint Commission's annual safety goals.

12. Quality of care is usually measured by structure, process, and outcomes.

13. The IOM's six aims or goals for improvement state that care should be safe, effective, patient-centered, timely, efficient, and equitable (IOM, 2001a).

(continues)

CHAPTER HIGHLIGHTS (CONTINUED)

14. The IOM developed new rules for the 21st century to guide care delivery. These rules, which are directly related to the six aims and to the healthcare professions core competencies, are (1) care based on continuous healing relationships, (2) customization based on patient needs and values, (3) the patient as control source, (4) shared knowledge and free flow of information, (5) evidence-based decision making, (6) safety as a system property, (7) the need for transparency, (8) anticipation of needs, (9) continuous decrease in waste, and (10) cooperation among clinicians.

15. The IOM has recommended collecting national healthcare quality data annually. The data collected focus on delivery of care within the context of personal health care and are published in report form to make health care transparent. The report uses a matrix to visually depict consumer perspectives and components of quality of care.

16. The Joint Commission's standards for QI focus on patient-focused functions, organizational functions, and structural functions.

17. Healthcare report cards provide specific performance data about an organization at specific intervals, with a focus on quality and safety.

18. Nursing's report card (NDNQI) resulted in the provision of a framework for educating nurses, consumers, and policy makers about nursing's contributions within the acute care setting by tracking the quality of nursing care provided in acute care settings. Data are collected for nursing-sensitive indicators that reflect the nursing workforce, nursing process, and patient outcomes.

19. Examples of methods used to measure and monitor safety and quality include standards of care, policies and procedures, licensure and credentialing, utilization review/management, risk management, benchmarking, access to care, EBP, clinical pathways, institutional review boards, and healthcare policy and legislation.

20. Nursing care contributes to health care because nurses are the interface between the patient and the system.

21. *Keeping Patients Safe* (IOM, 2004b) recommended the following: (1) adopting transformational leadership and evidence-based management, (2) maximizing the capability of the workforce, (3) understanding work processes so that they can be improved, and (4) creating and sustaining cultures of safety.

22. Much more needs to be done to prepare nurses for QI and to assume leadership in QI.

DISCUSSION QUESTIONS

1. How do the IOM aims to improve quality relate to the IOM rules for the 21st century and the healthcare core competencies?
2. Describe the culture of safety. How does this compare to the blame culture?
3. What is accreditation? Also describe the major source of accreditation for HCOs.
4. Discuss the definition of quality.
5. If you had to explain the importance of the quality reports to someone outside health care, how would you do this?
6. Describe four tools and methods used to improve care.

Landscape © f9photos/Shutterstock, Inc.

CRITICAL THINKING ACTIVITIES

1. Divide up into teams, with each team taking one of the rules for the 21st century. Develop a defense for this rule and share with the other teams.

2. Visit the National Healthcare Quality and Disparities Reports website to review the current reports on healthcare quality and disparities (http://www.ahrq.gov/research/findings/nhqrdr/index.html). After reviewing data on the dimensions of quality, what have you learned? Select one of the areas monitored and summarize key issues. Share this with others who have reviewed different clinical conditions.

3. Learn more about NDNQI by going to http://www.nursingquality.org/FAQ. Review some of the frequently asked questions that interest you. Discuss your findings in a small group.

4. Visit the OSHA Workplace Violence website (http://www.osha.gov/SLTC/workplaceviolence/) to learn about this important staff safety problem and possible solutions. Review the guidelines for healthcare workplace violence. Which solutions are recommended, and what is your opinion of the solutions?

5. Select one of the common quality care issues, such as hand washing, decubiti, and so on, and search for information about the topic and how care can be improved.

6. Select two of the online patient safety resources found at National Patient Safety Foundation website (http://www.npsf.org/for-patients-consumers/tools-and-resources-for-patients-and-consumers/). How might nurses use this resource?

ELECTRONIC *Reflective Journal*

Circuit Board: ©Photos.com

In your journal, describe an example of QI problem that you observed or were directly involved in while in clinical practice. Remember to follow the Health Insurance Portability and Accountability Act (HIPAA) rules when recording your information.

Landscape © f9photos/Shutterstock, Inc.

LINKING TO THE INTERNET

- Agency for Healthcare Research and Quality, National Health Care Quality and Disparities Reports: http://www.ahrq.gov/qual/qrdr10.htm
- American Nurses Association: http://www.nursingworld.org
- Consumer Assessment of Healthcare Providers and Systems (CAHPS): https://cahps.ahrq.gov Centers for Medicare and Medicaid Services, OASIS Program: http://www.cms.gov/OASIS
- Institute for Healthcare Improvement: http://www.ihi.org (Open-source courses such as those found on the IHI website can assist nurses is obtaining more knowledge about QI in general, and then applying that knowledge to the nurse's role.)
- The Joint Commission: http://www.jointcommission.org

(continues)

Landscape © f9photos/Shutterstock, Inc.

LINKING TO THE INTERNET (CONTINUED)

- National Nursing Database:
  https://www.ncsbn.org/3873.htm, http://www.nursingworld.org/MainMenuCategories/
  ThePracticeofProfessionalNursing/PatientSafetyQuality/Research-Measurement/The-National-
  Database/NDNQIBrochure.aspx
- National Quality Measures Clearinghouse: http://www.qualitymeasures.ahrq.gov
- Nursing Alliance for Quality Care: http://www.naqc.org
- Nursing Quality Initiatives:
  http://nursingworld.org/MainMenuCategories/ThePracticeofProfessionalNursing/
  PatientSafetyQuality/Advocacy
- List of Quality Improvement Organizations, brief description and links:
  http://nursingworld.org/MainMenuCategories/ThePracticeofProfessionalNursing/
  PatientSafetyQuality/Quality-Organizations
- U.S. Department of Labor, Occupational Safety and Health Administration: http://www.osha.gov
- U.S. Department of Labor, Occupational Safety and Health Administration, Workplace Violence:
  http://www.osha.gov/SLTC/workplaceviolence

CASE STUDIES

Landscape © f9photos/Shutterstock, Inc.

Case Study 1

A 21-year-old woman presented to the emergency department of an urban hospital with a history of systemic lupus. Her complaint was dehydration, dizziness, and feeling faint. The woman also had a recent history of being dehydrated, complicated by renal involvement from lupus and having to receive bolus fluids. She was on multiple medications, including steroids and methotrexate. An intravenous (IV) line was started, and blood was drawn for labs. The emergency department physician returned to report that the lab values were within normal limits, yet the young woman felt no better. She stated that she still felt dehydrated, that her blood pressure felt low, and that she normally received more IV fluids and a steroid injection when she felt this way. The physician indicated that he felt no need for this treatment, but when the patient insisted on more fluids, he agreed to continue them for a while and to give her an injection of steroids. The patient asked, "Do you want to give me antinausea medication first?" The physician stated that there was no indication. The patient told him that she was always nauseated following steroids and had sometimes vomited if no antiemetic were administered first. The physician argued but finally grew tired and walked away. The steroid injection was given, and nausea ensued. When the patient got home a few hours later, the patient called her rheumatologist and urologist (neither had been available when the illness

CASE STUDIES (CONTINUED)

occurred because of the late hour). They repeated her labs the next day, only to find that she was severely dehydrated, and many values, including renal panel, were outside normal limits.

Case Questions

1. What are the critical issues in this case description?
2. Consider the six aims that the IOM recommends to better ensure quality care. How might they apply to this patient?
3. Is this patient-centered care? Why or why not?
4. If you were the nurse assigned to this patient in emergency department, what could you have done?

Case Study 2

A patient has been admitted to an ambulatory surgical unit for a hernia repair. He is a physician, and his wife is a nurse. After his surgery, his wife is taken to the post-anesthesia care unit (PACU; also known as recovery) to see her husband. The unit is configured with cubicles with curtains. In the patient area, there is the stretcher with the patient, monitors, and a computer with a stool in front of it. The patient is recovering from anesthesia and can communicate. The nurse is glued to the computer, rarely looking at the patient when speaking to him. The patient has a history of atrial fibrillation and takes a number of cardiac medications. The nurse says he is going to put a medication into the IV; he indicates the medication name, and begins to do so. At the same time, the patient becomes alert and says, "No." Just at that time the curtain opens and the anesthesiology resident says loudly, "Stop that order." Both physicians knew (the patient and the resident, although the resident should not have made the order) that there was a contraindication for mixing certain drugs.

A few hours later, the patient is getting ready for discharge in the ambulatory surgical unit, and his wife is present. During the admission process, the nurse was also glued to computer when assessing the patient, rarely looking at the patient and being more concerned with typing in information rather than assessment. At the time of discharge, the nurse comes in and reads through a list of discharge directions, strongly emphasizing that the patient should take all of his routine medications when he gets home. The patient says, "All of them?" (He is testing the nurse, as he knows the answer to this question.) The nurse says, "Yes." The patient says, "I don't think so. Aspirin should not be taken right after surgery, and I take it daily as routine medication." The nurse did not seem to understand what he said and did not respond.

In this situation, the doctor should not have written an order for all medications after discharge; however, in both incidents the nurse had responsibilities and provided ineffective, unsafe care that was stopped by the patient before a serious problem occurred. The patient and his wife left the hospital fed up with the quality of care. Both incidents were described in the patient satisfaction survey the patient received, and the patient never heard from the hospital. This was a university hospital with a medical school and nursing school attached to the university. The patient will not return to this hospital for surgery.

(continues)

CASE STUDIES (CONTINUED)

Case Questions

It is clear that physician errors led to near misses in this clear, but it is also clear that nursing actions led to near misses.

1. What is a "near miss"?
2. Describe each of the near misses and the roles of the physicians and the nurses in each incident.
3. Which system issues might have been involved?
4. What could have been done to prevent these near misses?
5. What do you think hospitals should do when patients describe incidents like these in patient satisfaction surveys?
6. What was the impact of technology in this case?

Landscape © f9photos/Shutterstock, Inc.

Words of Wisdom

© Roobcio/Shutterstock, Inc.

Carole Kenner, PhD, RNC-NIC, FAAN

Carol Kuser Loser Dean, School of Nursing, Health and Exercise Science, The College of New Jersey

I have been in nursing for more than three decades. Never has there been a time when there is more emphasis on quality in health care. With the passage of the Affordable Health Care Act, there has been more recognition that nurses are at the forefront of providing "quality" to care. We are the ones who are at the point of care. We often recognize potential and real patient safety risks. When I have worked with students, I have been amazed that in their zealous effort to be prepared for a clinical day, they will oftentimes identify a potential drug interaction or a wrong dose of a medication that has been given more than once. When students raise issues and question treatments: Listen. They may be right, and their contribution may increase quality and decrease patient errors.

Landscape © f9photos/Shutterstock, Inc.

REFERENCES

Agency for Health Research and Quality (AHRQ). (2013). AHRQ information technology: Ambulatory safety and quality. Retrieved from http://healthit.ahrq.gov/sites/default/files/docs/page/alternate-findings-and-lessons-from-the-ahrq-ambulatory-safety-and-quality-program.pdf

Aiken, L. H., Clarke, S. P., Sloane, D. M., Sochalski, J., & Silber, J. H. (2002). Hospital nurse staffing and patient mortality, nurse burnout, and job dissatisfaction. *JAMA, 288*(16), 1987–1993.

Aleccia, J. (2011). Nurse's suicide highlights twin tragedies of medical errors. Retrieved from http://www.msnbc.msn.com/id/43529641/ns/health-health_care/#.Tm0By09A8j8

American Hospital Association (AHA). (1999). *Hospital statistics*. Chicago, IL: Author.

American Nurses Association (ANA). (2013). *Safe patient handling and mobility: Interprofessional national standards across the care continuum*. Retrieved from http://www.nursingworld.org/handlewithcare

American Nurses Association (ANA). (2014a) NDNQI. Retrieved from http://www.nursingquality.org/#intro

American Nurses Association (ANA). (2014b). Workforce advocacy. Retrieved from http://nursingworld.org/workforceadvocacy

American Nurses Association (ANA), National Database for Nursing Quality Indicators. (2014). NDNQI indicators. Retrieved from ww.nursingworld.org/MainMenuCategories/ThePracticeofProfessionalNursing/PatientSafetyQuality/ResearchMeasurement/The-National-Database/Nursing-Sensitive-Indicators_1

Anderson, D. (2006). Creating a culture of safety: Leadership, teams, and tools. *Nurse Leader, 4*(5), 28–41.

Berwick, D., & Nolan, T. (1998). Physicians as leaders improving healthcare. *Annals of Internal Medicine, 128*, 289–292.

Boodman, S. (2011, June 20). Effort to end surgeries on wrong patient or body part falters. Retrieved from http://www.kaiserhealthnews.org/stories/2011/june/21/wrong-site-surgery-errors.aspx

Castro, A. (2004). Handle with Care: The American Nurses Association's campaign to address work-related musculoskeletal disorders. *Online Journal of Issues in Nursing, 9*(3). Retrieved from http://www.nursingworld.org/MainMenuCategories/ANAMarketplace/ANAPeriodicals/OJIN/TableofContents/Volume92004/No3Sept04/HandleWithCare.aspx

Centers for Disease Control and Prevention (CDC). (2012). Adverse drug events. Retrieved from http://www.cdc.gov/medicationsafety/basics.html

Centers for Disease Control and Prevention (CDC), National Center for Health Statistics. (1998). Births and deaths: Preliminary data for 1998. *National Vital Statistics Report, 47*(25), 6.

Chassin, M., & Galvin, R. (1998). The urgent need to improve healthcare quality. *Journal of the American Medical Association, 280*, 1000–1005.

Diaz, M. H., Silkaitis, C., Malczynski, M., Noskin, G. A., Warren, J. R., & Zembower, T. (2008). Contamination of examination gloves in patient rooms and implications for transmission of antimicrobial-resistant microorganisms. *Infection Control and Hospital Epidemiology, 29*(1), 63–65.

Djukic, M., Kovner, C., Brewer, C., & Bernstein, I. (2013). Early career registered nurses' participation in hospital quality improvement *Journal of Nursing Care Quality, 39*(1), 198–207.

Donabedian, A. (1980). *Explorations in quality assessment and monitoring, Vol. I: The definition of quality and approaches to its assessment*. Ann Arbor, MI: Health Administration Press.

Dunton, N., Gajewski, B., Klaus, S., & Pierson, B. (2007). The relationship of nursing workforce characteristics to patient outcomes. *On-line Journal of Issues in Nursing, 12*(3). Retrieved from http://www.nursingworld.org/MainMenuCategories/ANAMarketplace/ANAPeriodicals/OJIN/TableofContents/Volume122007/No3Sept07/NursingWorkforceCharacteristics.aspx

Dunton, N., Gonnerman, D., Montalvo, I., & Schumann, M. (2011). Incorporating nursing quality indicators in public reporting and value-based purchasing initiatives. *American Nurse Today, 6*(1), 14–17.

Dunton, N., & Montalvo, I. (Eds.). (2009). *Sustained improvement in nursing quality: Hospital performance on NDNQI indicators, 2007–2008*. Silver Spring, MD: American Nurses Association.

Environmental Working Group. (2007). Nurses' health and workplace exposures to hazardous substance. Retrieved from http://www.ewg.org/research/nurses-health

Galewitz, P. (2011). Medicaid to stop paying for hospital mistakes. Retrieved from http://www.kaiserhealthnews.org

Gates, D., & Kroeger, D. (2007, December). Violence against nurses: The silent epidemic. *Ohio Nurse*, pp. 8–10.

Henneman, E., & Gawlinski, A. (2004). A "near-miss" model for describing the nurse's role in the recovery of medical errors. *Journal of Professional Nursing, 20*(3), 196–201.

Institute for Healthcare Improvement (IHI). (2007). Triple aim. Retrieved from http://www.ihi.org/offerings/initiatives/tripleaim/Pages/default.aspx

Institute for Healthcare Improvement (IHI). (2011a). Five Million Lives campaign. Retrieved from http://www.ihi.org/IHI/Programs/Campaign

Institute for Healthcare Improvement (IHI). (2011b). Transforming Care at the Bedside. Retrieved from http://www.ihi.org/offerings/initiatives/paststrategicinitiatives/tcab/Pages/default.aspx

Institute for Healthcare Improvement (IHI). (2014). Institute for Healthcare Improvement. Retrieved from http://www.ihi.org

Institute for Safe Medication Practice. (2011). Medication errors. Retrieved from http://www.ismp.org/pressroom/PR20100909.pdf

Institute of Medicine (IOM). (1990). *Clinical practice guidelines: Directions for a new program*. Washington, DC: National Academies Press.

Institute of Medicine (IOM). (1999). *To err is human: Building a safer health system*. Washington, DC: National Academies Press.

Institute of Medicine (IOM). (2001a). *Crossing the quality chasm: A new health system for the 21st century*. Washington, DC: National Academies Press.

Institute of Medicine (IOM). (2001b). *Envisioning the national healthcare quality report*. Washington, DC: National Academies Press.

Institute of Medicine (IOM). (2003). *Health professions education: A bridge to quality*. Washington, DC: National Academies Press.

Institute of Medicine (IOM). (2004a). *Patient safety: Achieving a new standard for care*. Washington, DC: National Academies Press.

Institute of Medicine (IOM). (2004b). *Keeping patients safe: Transforming the work environment of nurses*. Washington, DC: National Academies Press.

Institute of Medicine (IOM). (2011). *The future of nursing: Leading change, advancing health*. Washington, DC: National Academies Press.

The Joint Commission. (2009). A framework for a root cause analysis and action plan in response to a sentinel event. Retrieved from http://www.jointcommission.org/Framework_for_Conducting_a_Root_Cause_Analysis_and_Action_Plan/

Kennedy, R., Murphy, J., & Roberts, D. (2013, September 30). An overview of the national quality strategy: Where do nurses fit? *Online Journal of Issues in Nursing, 18*(3). doi Retrieved from http://www.nursingworld.org/MainMenuCategories/ANAMarketplace/ANAPeriodicals/OJIN/TableofContents/Vol-18-2013/No3-Sept-2013/National-Quality-Strategy.html

Ketchum, K., Grass, C., & Padwojski, A. (2005). Medication reconciliation. *AJN, 105*(11), 78–85.

Kovner, C., Brewer, C., Yingrengreung, S., & Fairchild, S. (2009). New nurses' views of quality improvement education. Retrieved from http://www.rwjf.org/en/research-publications/find-rwjf-research/2009/09/the-rn-work-project/new-nurses--views-of-quality-improvement-education.html

Maxwell, D., Grenny, J., Lavandero, R., & Groah, L. (2011). *The silent treatment: Why safety tools and checklists aren't enough to save lives*. VitalSmarts, AORN, & AACN. Retrieved from http://www.aacn.org

McCloskey, J., & Bulechek, G. (2000). *Nursing interventions classification (NIC)*. St. Louis, MO: Mosby.

Montalvo, I., & Dunton, N. (2007). *Transforming nursing data into quality care: Profiles of quality improvement in U.S. healthcare facilities*. Silver Spring, MD: American Nurses Association.

Mosocco, D. (2001). Data management using outcomes-based quality improvement. *Home Care Provider, 12*, 205–211.

National Quality Forum (NQF). (2010). Mission and vision. Retrieved from http://www.qualityforum.org/About_NQF/Mission_and_Vision.aspx

Occupational Safety and Health Administration (OSHA). (2004). Guidelines for preventing workplace violence for health care & social service workers. Retrieved from http://www.osha.gov/Publications/OSHA3148/osha3148.html

Pike, J., Jansen, R., & Brooks, P. (2002). Role and function of a hospital risk manager. *Journal of Legal Nurse Consultants, 13*(2), 3–13.

Press Ganey. (2014). Press Ganey acquires national database of nursing quality indicators. Retrieved from http://pressganey.com/pressRoom/2014/06/10/press-ganey-acquires-national-database-of-nursing-quality-indicators-%28ndnqi-%29

Plsek, P. (2001). Redesigning healthcare with insights from the science of complex adaptive systems. In Institute of Medicine, *Crossing the quality chasm* (pp. 309–322). Washington, DC: National Academies Press.

Pollard, P., Mitra, K., & Mendelson, D. (1996). *Nursing report card for acute care*. Washington, DC: American Nurses Publishing.

Polygreen, P. M., Chen, Y., Beekmann, S., Srinivasan, A., Neill, M. A., Gay, T., & Cavanaugh, J. (2008). Elements of influenza vaccination programs that predict higher vaccination rates: results of an emerging infections network survey. *Clinical Infectious Diseases*, *46*(1), 14–19.

Reason, J. (2000). Human error: Models and management. *British Medical Journal*, *320*(7237), 768–770.

Rozich, J., Howard, R., Justeson, J., Macken, P., Lindsay, M., & Resar, R. (2004). Standardization as a mechanism to improve safety in healthcare. *Joint Commission Journal Quality and Safety*, *30*(1), 5–14.

Six Sigma. (2008). Retrieved from http://www.isixsigma.com/new-to-six-sigma/getting-started/what-six-sigma/

Thomas, E., Studdert, D., Newhouse, J., Zbar, B., Howard, K., Williams, E., & Brennan, T. (1999). Costs of medical injuries in Utah and Colorado. *Inquiry*, *36*, 255–264.

Trinkoff, A., Geiger-Brown, J., Caruso, C., Lipscomb, J., Johantgen, M., Nelson, A., & Selby, V. (2008). Personal safety for nurses. In R. Hughes (Ed.), *Patient safety and quality: An evidence-based handbook for nurses* (pp. 473–502). Washington, DC: Agency for Healthcare Research and Quality.

Trinkoff, A., Johantgen, M., Storr, C., Gureses, A., Liang, Y., & Han, K. (2011). Nurses' work schedule characteristics, nurse staffing and patient mortality. *Nursing Research*, *60*(1), 1–8.

U.S. Congress, Subcommittee on Primary Health and Aging. (2014, July 17). Medical mistakes are 3rd leading cause of Death in U.S. Retrieved from http://www.sanders.senate.gov/newsroom/press-releases/medical-mistakes-are-3rd-leading-cause-of-death-in-us

U.S. Department of Health and Human Services (HHS). (2010). *Healthy people 2020*. Washington, DC: U.S. Government Printing Office.

U.S. Department of Health and Human Services (HHS), Agency for Healthcare Research and Quality (AHRQ). (2010). National healthcare quality and disparities reports. Retrieved from http://www.ahrq.gov/qual/qrdr10.htm

van der Schaaf, T. W. (1992). *Near miss reporting in the chemical process industry*. (Unpublished doctoral dissertation). Eindhoven University of Technology, Eindhoven, Netherlands.

Wachter, R., & Pronovost, P. (2009). Balancing "no blame" with accountability in patient safety. *New England Journal of Medicine*, *361*(14), 1401–1406.

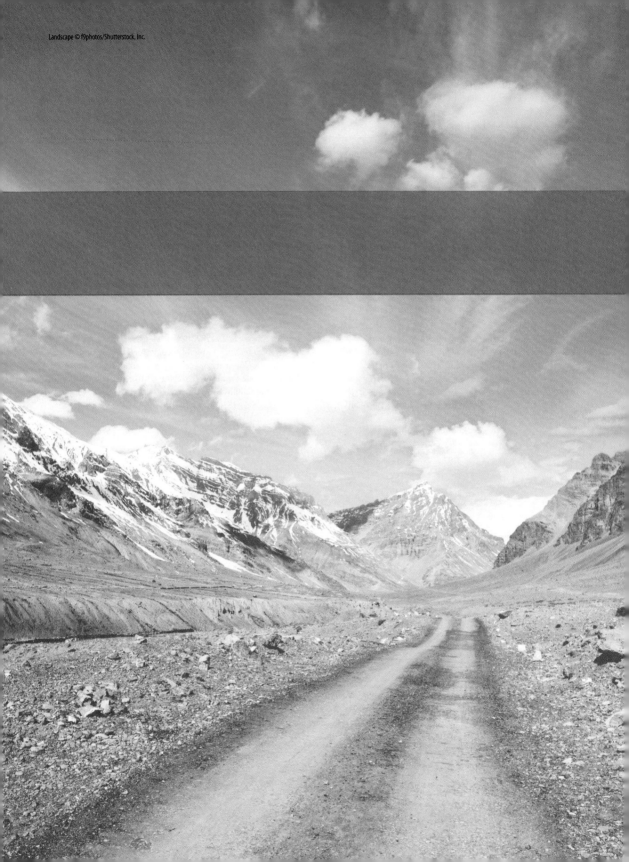

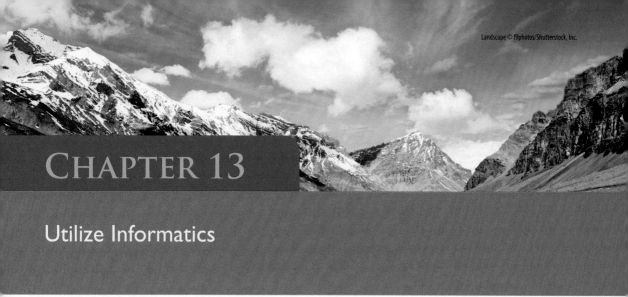

CHAPTER 13

Utilize Informatics

CHAPTER OBJECTIVES

At the conclusion of this chapter, the learner will be able to:

- Discuss the Institute of Medicine competency: Utilize informatics
- Describe informatics and its relationship to nursing
- Explain the purpose of documentation and key issues related to informatics and documentation
- Identify informatics tools used in healthcare delivery
- Describe telehealth and its relationship to healthcare delivery and nursing
- Examine the impact of the use of biomedical equipment on nursing care
- Compare and contrast high-touch care with high-tech care

CHAPTER OUTLINE

KEY TERMS

Clinical data repository
Clinical decision support systems
Clinical information system
Coding system
Computer literacy
Data
Data analysis software
Data bank
Data mining
Database
Electronic medical record (EMR)
E-mail list

E-measurement
Encryption
Health Insurance Portability and Accountability Act of 1996 (HIPAA)
Informatics
Information
Information literacy
Knowledge
Minimum data set
National Database of Nursing Quality Indicators

Nomenclature
Nursing informatics
Personal health record (PHR)
Provider order entry system
Security protections
Software
Standardized language
Telehealth
Telenursing
Wisdom

INTRODUCTION

This chapter concludes the section that focuses on the Institute of Medicine (IOM) healthcare profession core competencies with a discussion of the fifth core competency: utilize informatics. Informatics/information technology (IT) is an important topic in all areas of life today; with the explosion of technology, there are many opportunities for communication and sharing of knowledge. The impact of informatics on nursing care is explored here. Other issues that need to be addressed are documentation,

confidentiality and privacy of information, and telehealth. This chapter also includes content about biomedical equipment, an expanding area in healthcare technology that impacts nurses and nursing care. Some of this equipment also uses IT. Nurses today cannot avoid technology, whether it is used for communication, for care provision, or for monitoring the quality of care. The chapter concludes with a discussion about the potential conflict between high-touch care versus high-tech care and the need for nursing leadership in health informatics—important issues for nurses to consider. **Figure 13-1** identifies key elements in this chapter.

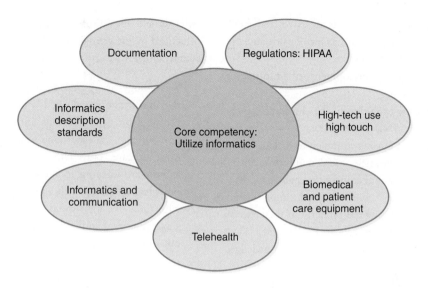

Figure 13-1 Utilize Informatics: Key Elements

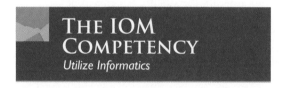

THE IOM COMPETENCY
Utilize Informatics

The IOM's description of the fifth healthcare profession core competency is "communicate, manage knowledge, mitigate error, and support decision making using information technology" (IOM, 2003, p. 4). **Informatics** entails more than just understanding what health informatics technology (HIT) is; it also includes how that technology is used to prevent errors and improve care. From the initial use of computers to management of financial records to the current use of informatics, there has been a major move toward HIT application in care. Some examples are greater use of informatics to find evidence to implement evidence-based practice; use of informatics in research; greater consumer access to information via the Internet; and more specific clinical applications, such as reminder and decision systems, telehealth, teleradiology, online prescribing, and use of e-mail for provider–provider communication and patient–provider communication.

The IOM (2003, p. 63) concludes that every healthcare professional should meet the following informatics competencies:

- Employ word processing, presentation, and data analysis software.
- Search, retrieve, manage, and make decisions using electronic data from internal information databases and external online databases and the Internet.
- Communicate using e-mail, instant messaging, e-mail lists, and file transfers.
- Understand security protections such as access control, data security, and data encryption, and directly address ethical and legal issues related to the use of IT in practice.
- Enhance education and access to reliable health information for patients.

A position statement from the Healthcare Information and Management Systems Society (HIMSS, 2011) addressed the IOM report *The Future of Nursing* from the perspective of informatics. The following recommendations were made and align with the IOM report on the key points of leadership, education, and practice:

- Partner with nurse executives to lead technology changes that advance health and the delivery of health care.
- Support the development of informatics departments.
- Foster the evolution of the chief nursing informatics (NI) officer role.
- Transform nursing education to include informatics competencies and demonstrable behaviors at all levels of academic preparation.
- Promote the continuing education of all levels of nursing, particularly in the areas of electronic health records (EHRs) and HIT.
- Ensure that data, information, knowledge, and wisdom form the basis of 21st-century nursing practice by incorporating informatics competencies into practice standards in all healthcare settings.
- Facilitate the collection and analysis of interprofessional healthcare workforce data by ensuring data can be collected from existing IT systems.

The statement also indicates that nurses play a critical role in healthcare informatics and need to continue to do so.

Nurses are key leaders in developing the infrastructure for effective and efficient health information technology that transforms the delivery of care. Nurse informaticists play a crucial role in advocating both for patients and fellow nurses who are often the key stakeholders and recipients of these evolving solutions. Nursing informatics professionals are the liaisons to successful interactions with technology in healthcare. (HIMSS, 2011)

INFORMATICS

Informatics is complex, and the fact that it is changing daily makes it even more difficult to keep current

with this field. Healthcare delivery has been strongly influenced by the changes in informatics, but what is informatics?

Technology is revolutionizing the way that healthcare is delivered with a steady infusion of new solutions into clinical environments. At the same time, outside of healthcare, both clinicians and consumers are learning to incorporate technological solutions into their daily lives with tools like high-speed data networks, smart phones, handheld devices, and various forms of patient engagement in social media exchanges. Bringing these types of technologies into the healthcare marketplace will transform the time and place for how care is provided. Having individuals who understand the unique complexities of healthcare practices along with how to best develop technological tools that positively affect safe patient care is essential. Nurses integrating informatics solutions into clinical encounters are critical for the transition to an automated healthcare environment that promotes the continuum of care across time and place, in addition to wellness and health maintenance activities. (HIMSS, 2011)

Just as mobile forms of informatics are increasing, mobile applications are used more by nurses, for example for discharge teaching and follow-up care. Nurses are also designing some of the applications for use in a variety of ways to promote patient safety and health.

Definitions and Description

Informatics has opened doors to many innovative methods of communication with patients and among providers, individuals, and healthcare organizations (HCOs) of all types. It often saves time, but can also lead to information overload. Today, physicians are using e-mail to communicate with patients (e.g., sending appointment reminders, sharing lab results, and answering questions). The Web has provided opportunities to build communities of people with common chronic diseases to help them with disease management. HCOs have developed websites to share information about their organizations with the public (a marketing tool for services). In addition, these websites provide HCOs with an effective method for internal communication; staff can access some parts of the sites with special passwords. With these changes comes greater risk of inappropriate access to information through hacking and other means. Informatics is also used to evaluate the performance of the HCO and individual healthcare providers. IT has a major impact on quality improvement; today, it is much easier to collect, store, and analyze large amounts of data that in the past were collected by hand. Insurers rely heavily on informatics to provide insurance coverage, manage data, and analyze performance, which has a direct impact on whether care is covered for reimbursement. Informatics allows governments at all levels—local, state, national, and international— to collect and use data for policy decision making and evaluation.

Informatics has its own language and is a highly specialized area. Nurses do not have to be informatics experts, but they do need to understand the basics. Some terms have become so common that the majority of people know what they are (such as *Internet* and *e-mail*). Other terms that are useful to know are highlighted here:

- **Clinical data repository**: A physical or logical compendium of patient data pertaining to health; an "information warehouse" that stores data longitudinally and in multiple forms, such as text, voice, and images (American Nurses Association [ANA], 2008).
- **Clinical decision support systems**: Computer applications designed to facilitate human decision making. Decision support systems are typically rule based. These systems

use a knowledge base and a set of rules to analyze data and information and provide recommendations (ANA, 2008).
- **Clinical information system**: An information system that supports the acquisition, storage, manipulation, and distribution of clinical information throughout an HCO, with a focus on electronic communication. This system uses IT that is applied at the point of clinical care. Typical clinical information system components include electronic medical records (EMRs), clinical data repositories, decision support programs (such as application of clinical guidelines and drug interaction checking), handheld devices for collecting data and viewing reference material, imaging modalities, and communication tools such as electronic messaging systems.
- **Coding system**: A set of agreed-on symbols (frequently numeric or alphanumeric) that are attached to concept representation or terms to allow exchange of concept representations or terms with regard to their form or meaning. Examples are the Perioperative Nursing Data Set and the Clinical Care Classification System (ANA, 2008).
- **Computer literacy**: The knowledge and skills required to use basic computer applications and computer technology.
- **Data**: Discrete entities described objectively without interpretation.
- **Data analysis software**: Computer software that is used to analyze data.
- **Data bank**: A large store of information; may include several databases.
- **Database**: A collection of interrelated data that are organized according to a scheme to serve one or more applications. The data are stored so that several programs can use the data without concern for data structures or organization. An example is the **National Database of Nursing Quality Indicators** (NDNQI) (ANA, 2008).

- **Data mining**: Locating and identifying unknown patterns and relationships within data.
- **E-mail list**: A list of e-mail addresses that can be used to send an e-mail to many addresses simultaneously.
- **Encryption**: To change information into a code, usually for security reasons, so as to limit access to that information.
- **Information**: Data that have been interpreted, organized, or structured.
- **Information literacy**: The ability to recognize when information is needed and to locate, evaluate, and effectively use that information (ANA, 2008).
- **Knowledge**: Information that has been synthesized so that relationships are identified and formalized (ANA, 2008).
- **Minimum data set**: The minimum categories of data with uniform definitions and categories; they concern a specific aspect or dimension of the healthcare system that meets the basic needs of multiple data users. An example is the Nursing Minimum Data Set (ANA, 2008).
- **Nomenclature**: A system of designations (terms) that is elaborated according to pre-established rules. Examples include Systematized Nomenclature of Medicine—Clinical Terms International and International Classification for Nursing Practice (ANA, 2008).
- **Security protections** (access control, data security, and data encryption): Methods used to ensure that information is not read or taken by unauthorized persons.
- **Software**: Computer programs and applications.
- **Standardized language**: A collection of terms with definitions for use in informational systems databases. A standardized language enables comparisons to be made because the same term is used to denote the same condition. Standardized language

is necessary for documentation in EHRs (ANA, 2008).
- **Wisdom**: The appropriate use of knowledge to solve human problems; understanding when and how to apply knowledge (ANA, 2008).

The role of health IT in e-measurement and quality care has become increasingly more important in recent years (Dykes & Collins, 2013). **E-measurement** is the secondary use of electronic data to populate standardized performance measures (National Quality Forum [NQF], 2013). The NQF is developing e-measures to make sure that data used for clinical documentation can be reused to measure patient outcomes. This endeavor, which is very complex, remains far from complete at this time. Getting the data in a consistent form into systems that can reuse the data and relate them to patient outcomes in languages that are clear and consistent will require much more work to be done.

Nursing Standards: Scope and Standards of Nursing Informatics

Nursing informatics (NI) is a specialty that integrates nursing science, computer science, and information science to manage and communicate data, information, knowledge, and wisdom in nursing practice. NI supports consumers, patients, nurses, and other providers in their decision making in all roles and settings. This support is accomplished through the use of information structures, information processes, and IT. The goal of NI is to improve the health of populations, communities, families, and individuals by optimizing information management and communication (ANA, 2008, p. 1).

This specialty area has expanded, and all nurses need to understand basic IT concepts and their application to nursing practice. Undergraduate nursing programs may include IT in the curriculum, sometimes as a course on informatics, but not all programs include this content. This omission from nursing educational programs is now a problem because of the emphasis on informatics as a healthcare professions core competency. Some schools of nursing offer master's degrees in NI.

Three major concepts related to information are important to understand (Englebardt & Nelson, 2002):

1. *Data* are discrete entities that are described objectively without interpretation.
2. *Information* is defined as data that are interpreted, organized, or structured.
3. *Knowledge* is information that is synthesized so that relationships are identified and formalized.

The flow from data to wisdom can be described as data naming, collecting, and organizing, following this pattern: (1) information—organizing and interpreting; (2) knowledge—interpreting, integrating, and understanding; and (3) wisdom—understanding, applying, and applying with compassion. **Figure 13-2** illustrates this flow.

"Wisdom is defined as the appropriate use of knowledge to manage and solve human problems. It is knowing when and how to apply knowledge to deal with complex problems or specific human needs" (Nelson & Joos, 1989, p. 6). "While knowledge focuses on what is known, wisdom focuses on the appropriate application of that knowledge. For example, a knowledge base may include several options for managing an anxious family, while wisdom would help decide which option is most appropriate

for a specific family" (ANA, 2008, p. 5). Nurses first need to understand the importance of data collection and data analysis, and then need to understand how to apply data and knowledge—leading to wisdom. Data are important to the delivery of nursing care. In hospitals, data can be used to evaluate outcomes, identify problems for a specific group of patients, and assist in making plans for change to improve care. In the community, aggregated data are often collected to better understand the health issues in a population or community and to formulate a plan of action.

Certification in Informatics Nursing

Nurses who practice in the area of informatics can be certified if they meet the eligibility criteria and complete the certification examination satisfactorily. The following list provides examples of application eligibility criteria required for the informatics certification exam sponsored by the American Nurses Credentialing Center (ANCC, 2014). The nurse must:

- Hold a current, active registered nurse license within a state or territory of the United States or the professional, legally recognized equivalent in another country
- Have practiced the equivalent of 2 years full time as a registered nurse
- Hold a baccalaureate or higher degree in nursing or a baccalaureate degree in a relevant field
- Have completed 30 hours of continuing education in informatics within the last 3 years
- Meet one of the following practice hour requirements:
    a. The nurse must have practiced a minimum of 2000 hours in informatics nursing within the last 3 years.
    b. The nurse must have practiced a minimum of 1000 hours in informatics nursing in the last 3 years and must have completed a minimum of 12 semester hours of academic

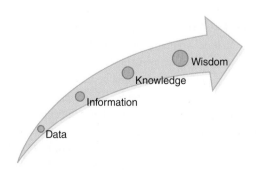

Figure 13-2 From Data to Wisdom

credit in informatics courses that are a part of a graduate-level NI program.

c. The nurse must have completed a graduate program in NI containing a minimum of 200 hours of faculty-supervised practicum in informatics.

These are not simple criteria; they take time to meet, and they provide a good overview of the need for expertise in this area. All criteria must be met before a nurse can apply for the ANCC certification examination.

The informatics nurse is involved in activities that focus on the methods and technologies of information handling in nursing. Informatics nursing practice includes the development, support, and evaluation of applications, tools, processes, and structures that help nurses to manage data in direct care of patients as well as in nursing education and research. The work of an informatics nurse can involve any and all aspects of information systems, including theory formulation, design, development, marketing, selection, testing, implementation, training, maintenance, evaluation, and enhancement. "Informatics nurses are engaged in clinical practice, education, consultation, research, administration, and pure informatics" (ANCC, 2014). It is clear that a nurse who wants to function in this specialty area must have excellent computer skills, understand practice needs for information, and know how best to apply IT to nursing practice. The nurse must also be able to work collaboratively in interprofessional teams and demonstrate leadership. By speaking for the needs of the practicing nurse, the informatics nurse represents all nurses in practice—clinical, education, and research—as applies to the specific situation.

Informatics: Impact on Care

The IOM recommendations indicate that informatics can lead to safe, quality care—and it truly can. Application of informatics, however, does not guarantee perfection.

There is a perception that technology will lead to fewer errors than strategies that focus on staff performance; however, technology may in some circumstances lead to more errors. This is particularly true when the technology fails to take into account end users, increases in staff time, replicates an already bad process or is implemented with insufficient training. The best approach is not always clear, and most approaches have advantages and disadvantages. (Finkelman & Kenner, 2012, p. 192)

Nurses need to assume an active role in the development of HIT for patient care and not wait to be asked to participate. When an HCO is choosing a system for an EMR, nurses need to be involved to ensure that the system meets nursing care documentation requirements and that relevant data can be collected to assist nurses in providing and improving care. Nurses may serve in key IT roles to guide development and implementation, and they may have special training or education in informatics. Nurses may also serve as resources in identifying needs and testing systems to ensure that the systems are nurse user friendly. Many nurses who provide feedback about systems do not have special IT training; they review the system to determine if it is user friendly for nurses who have limited informatics knowledge and help to determine if the system meets documentation needs and standards. All nurses need be skilled in managing and communicating information, and they are primarily concerned with the content of that information.

In today's dynamic healthcare environment, coordination of care is very important. One of the barriers to seamless coordination is the lack of interoperable computerized records (Bodenheimer, 2008). In 2007, only 34.8% of physician offices used computerized records, though this was a major increase from 2005, when that proportion was only 23.9%; also in 2007, 49.8% of U.S. hospitals had adopted the EMR, with more embracing this technology each year. Data for 2009 (U.S. Department of Health and Human Services [HHS], 2013) indicate that 41% of office-based physicians and 81% of hospitals planned on taking advantage of the federal incentive payments for adoption and meaningful use of certified EHR technology. To improve information sharing and coordination of care, ideally this percentage should be 100%, but implementing the EMR is a costly, complex process of change (National Center for Health Statistics, 2010). Nevertheless, the federal government's incentive program may make a significant difference in adoption of this critical healthcare informatics technology. From 2012 to 2013, the number of hospitals using EHRs tripled, with 4 out of every 10 hospitals now employing such records (Thompson, 2013). "HHS has met and exceeded its goal for 50 percent of doctor offices and 80 percent of eligible hospitals to have EHRs by the end of 2013" (HHS, 2013). A continuing problem is that information can rarely be shared from one system to another, which is a limitation that needs to be resolved for better coordination of care. For example, it should be possible to share current information among healthcare providers in private practice and clinics and the hospitals when it is needed.

Innovative methods to improve coordination that focus on informatics have been developed. One method is to use electronic referral (e-referral.) This approach allows a healthcare provider to send an e-mail to another provider, such as a specialist, with information about the patient and to ask for consultation. In many situations, such communication eliminates the need to see the patient. The specialist reviews information such as lab reports, surgical reports, and so on, and can share his or her opinion with the other healthcare provider. It is critical that reimbursement be provided for this type of service, or it will not be used. Health Insurance Portability and Accountability Act (HIPAA) requirements must also be considered, with all parties working together to ensure patient privacy. Timely information flow from the hospital to posthospital care should improve patient coordination. Not having this is a major drawback; even though the technology to improve it is available, it is not freely used.

Implications for Nursing Education and Nursing Research

Informatics is important not only for practice, but also for nursing education and nursing research. Today, there is greater use of IT in nursing education than was the case in the past. The increased use of online courses throughout the nursing curriculum, at both the undergraduate and graduate levels, has revolutionized nursing education. It has required that faculty consider more interactive learning methods. Informatics also impacts simulation, allowing faculty to create complex learning scenarios that use the computer and computerized equipment. Moreover, as students use more technology in their personal lives, they expect correspondingly greater use of IT in education. Such tools as iPods, tablets, and smartphones, and Internet tools and apps such as Facebook, Instagram, and Twitter provide instant information and can be very interactive. These methods can also be used to increase student–faculty communication and have the potential to provide different means of student–faculty supervision in the clinical area. This is particularly true in areas such as community health, when students visit multiple sites and faculty move from site to site to see students.

Nursing research uses informatics in data collection and analysis; it saves time and improves the quality of data collection and analysis.

> The capacity for a mega-repository of clinical and research findings will allow for a richer science derived from multiple perspectives. Nurses have the responsibility to initiate practice-based inquiry, participate in clinical nursing research, and use nursing research to enhance patients' well-being and contribute to the body of nursing knowledge. (Appleton, 1998, as cited in Richards, 2001, p. 10)

This quote is not current, but the message is the same today, though we have yet to really reach this status.

DOCUMENTATION

Over time, nursing documentation has increased in terms of its relevance to nurses and to other healthcare professionals, thus increasing its impact on patient care and patient outcomes.

> Clear, accurate, and accessible documentation is an essential element of safe, quality, evidence-based nursing practice. Nurses practice across settings at position levels from the bedside to the administrative office; the registered nurse (RN) and the advanced practice registered nurse (APRN) are responsible and accountable for the nursing documentation that is used throughout an organization. This may include either documentation on nursing care that is provided by nurses—whether RN, APRN, or nursing assistive personnel—that can be used by other non-nurse members of the health care team or the administrative records that are created by the nurse and used across organization settings. (ANA, 2010, p. 3)

According to the ANA (2010), nursing documentation is used for the following purposes:

- Communicate within the healthcare team
- Communicate with other professionals
- Verify credentialing—to monitor performance
- Provide legal support
- Learn about regulation and legislation—to provide data for audits and monitoring
- Receive reimbursement—determine services for reimbursement
- Support research—data for studies
- Conduct quality process and performance improvement

The ANA principles for nursing documentation are found in **Exhibit 13-1**.

The format and content of nursing documentation have also changed. It is a professional responsibility to document planning, actual care provided, and outcomes. Care coordination and continuity are supported by documentation. With many different staff caring for patients around the clock, it is critical that a clear communication mechanism exists, and this mechanism is documentation. Verbal communication is important, but a written document must be available. Staff can refer to such documentation when other care providers are not available. Documentation serves as a record of the patient's care; it provides data for reimbursement and quality improvement and staff performance; and it supports interprofessional teamwork. Through documentation, outcomes and evaluation of patient care are made clear.

The medical record is a legal document, and as such, rules must be followed when creating and amending it. Once documentation has been created, changes to it must be accompanied by a note indicating who made the change(s) and when (date and time). Only certain staff can document; they must note the date and time on the documentation and include their name and credentials. If there are questions about care or a legal action, such as a malpractice suit, the medical record is the most important evidence. Consequently, medical records need to be saved. A nurse can say that he or she provided certain care, but if it was not documented, then it is as if that care did not occur.

Iyer and Camp (1999, p. 5) listed the following standard critical concerns that pertain to documentation and still apply today, whether a record is paper or electronic:

- The medical record reflects the nursing process.
- The medical record describes the patient's ongoing status from shift to shift (inpatient care) or from patient visit to patient visit (ambulatory care).
- The plan of care and the medical record complement each other.

Exhibit 13-1 ANA's Principles for Nursing Documentation

Nursing Documentation Principles

Principle 1. Documentation characteristics
Principle 2. Education and training
Principle 3. Policies and procedures
Principle 4. Protection systems
Principle 5. Documentation entries
Principle 6. Standardized terminologies

Principle 1. Documentation Characteristics

High-quality documentation is:
- Accessible
- Accurate, relevant, and consistent
- Auditable
- Clear, concise, and complete
- Legible/readable (particularly in terms of the resolution and related qualities of EHR content as it is displayed on the screens of various devices)
- Thoughtful
- Timely, contemporaneous, and sequential
- Reflective of the nursing process
- Retrievable on a permanent basis in a nursing-specific manner

Principle 2. Education and Training

Nurses, in all settings and at all levels of service, must be provided with comprehensive education and training in the technical elements of documentation and the organization's policies and procedures that are related to documentation. This education and training should include staffing issues that take into account the time needed for documentation work to ensure that each nurse is capable of the following:
- Functional and skillful use of the global documentation system
- Competence in the use of the computer and its supporting hardware
- Proficiency in the use of the software systems in which documentation or other relevant patient, nursing and health care reports, documents, and data are captured

Principle 3. Policies and Procedures

The nurse must be familiar with all organizational policies and procedures related to documentation and apply these as part of nursing practice. Of particular importance are those policies or procedures on maintaining efficiency in the use of the down time system for documentation when the available electronic systems do not function.

Principle 4. Protection Systems

Protection systems must be designed and built into documentation systems, paper-based or electronic, to provide the following as prescribed by industry standards, governmental mandates, accrediting agencies, and organizational policies and procedures:
- Security of data
- Protection of patient identification
- Confidentiality of patient information
- Confidentiality of clinical professionals' information
- Confidentiality of organizational information

Principle 5. Documentation Entries

Entries into organization documents or the health record (including but not limited to provider orders) must be:
- Accurate, valid, and complete
- Authenticated; that is, the information is truthful, the author is identified, and nothing has been added or inserted
- Dated and time stamped by the persons who created the entry
- Legible/readable
- Made using standardized terminology, including acronyms and symbols

Principle 6. Standardized Terminologies

Because standardized terminologies permit data to be aggregated and analyzed, these terminologies should include the terms that are used to describe the planning, delivery, and evaluation of the nursing care of the patient or client in diverse settings.

Source: From American Nurses Association. (2010). *Principles for nursing documentation.* Silver Spring, MD: Author.

- The documentation system is designed to facilitate retrieval of information for quality improvement activities and for research.
- The documentation system supports the staffing mix and acuity levels in the current healthcare environment.

The following guidelines (Iyer & Camp, 1999) continue to be important for all who document:

- Do not include opinion, but only objective information in documentation. The nurse does not make subjective comments (e.g., comments about the patient being uncooperative, lazy, or impolite). Nurses document only what they have done and objective data. A nurse would not document another staff member's actions. Supervision of care, however, can be documented.
- Write neatly and legibly. Many HCOs now use computerized documentation, although not all HCOs have moved to an EMR system. If a computerized system is used, typos (typographical errors) may be a problem. Other issues may arise in electronic systems that use a checklist for a particular section of the EMR but do not allow for narrative notes. Nurses and others may be frustrated when they cannot add a narrative note.
- Use correct spelling, grammar, and medical terminology.
- Use authorized abbreviations. Using unapproved abbreviations increases the risk of errors.
- Use graphic records to record specified patient data, such as vital signs and medication administration.
- Record the patient's name on every page (for hard-copy medical records); this should be part of the EMR.
- Follow HCO rules about verbal and telephone orders.
- Transcribe orders carefully; double-check and ask questions if an order is not clear. In

computerized systems, orders do not need to be transcribed; however, this does not mean that there is no risk of an error in an order. All orders need careful review, and if they are not clear, they may require follow-up.

- Document omitted care.
- Document medications and outcomes.
- Document patient noncompliance/nonadherence and the reason(s) for it.
- Document allergies, and use this information to prevent errors and complications.
- Document sites of injections.
- Record all information about intravenous therapy and blood administration.
- Report abnormal laboratory results.
- Document as soon as possible after care is delivered. If documentation is done late, note this in the record. The nurse should not leave blank areas to come back to for later documentation.
- When quoting, use quotation marks and note the person who made the statement.
- When documentation is corrected because of a mistake, follow the HCO policies regarding corrections as per a hard-copy record or electronic record. Medical records are never rewritten.
- Document patient status change.
- When contacting the physician, document the time, date, name of physician, reason for the call, content, physician response, and steps taken after the call. This note should not include subjective analysis of the response such as the physician was rude.

The Joint Commission does not provide details as to what must be in a medical record (the term used by The Joint Commission for this document is *record of care/treatment and services*), but it does provide some guidelines that are required for accreditation (Clark, 2011; The Joint Commission, 2011):

- Content noted by The Joint Commission that needs to be included consists of the patient's name, address, date of birth, name of any legally authorized representative, assessment, diagnosis, clinician notes and actions, signatures and countersignatures as required, dates, details of procedures performed, laboratory reports, medications administered, and treatment plans. This does not mean that other data cannot be included, and other data are typically included. The content listed here is simply the minimum requirement.

- The record should be clear and understandable.
- The record must create a system of communication and an audit trail.
- Storage of documents must be secure and reasonable. For example, the system would consider who has access to records and prevent casual viewing by non-staff. All Medicare storage rules must be followed.
- HIPAA requirements must be followed.

This list applies to hospital medical records. The content is somewhat different for medical records in other types of settings, such as ambulatory care, long-term care, and home care, although some information would be the same. Nurses are not involved in documenting in all these categories because other staff members also have documentation responsibilities.

In 2010, the Joint Commission standard for record of care/treatment and services was one of the top 10 standards with which HCOs were in noncompliance (Clark, 2011). The three major areas where hospitals often did not meet compliance were as follows:

1. Complete and accurate medical record
2. Verbal orders received and recorded by qualified staff
3. Patient assessed and reassessed per defined time frame

Nurses are involved in all three aspects of these documentation standards.

MEANINGFUL USE

The American Recovery and Reinvestment Act of 2009 specifies the following three components of *meaningful use* (HHS, Centers for Medicare and Medicaid Services [CMS], 2014):

- Use of certified EHR in a meaningful manner (e.g., e-prescribing)
- Use of certified EHR technology for electronic exchange of health information to improve quality of health care
- Use of certified EHR technology to submit clinical quality measures (CQM) and other such measures selected by the Secretary of HHS

Meaningful use involves using certified electronic health record technology for the following purposes (HHS, HealthIT.gov, 2014):

- Improve quality, safety, efficiency, and reduce health disparities
- Engage patients and family
- Improve care coordination, and population and public health
- Maintain privacy and security of patient health information

Ultimately, it is hoped that the meaningful use compliance will result in the following benefits:

- Better clinical outcomes
- Improved population health outcomes
- Increased transparency and efficiency
- Empowered individuals
- More robust research data on health systems

Meaningful use identifies specific objectives that eligible professionals and hospitals must achieve to qualify for CMS reimbursement. Given that most hospitals receive CMS reimbursement, there is obviously a strong incentive to follow these requirements. Nurses are also required to consider meaningful use, particularly if they are in leadership positions where decisions about informatics are made.

In response to the legislation passed in July 2010, the Office of the National Coordinator for Health Information Technology and CMS issued new rules identifying criteria that hospitals and eligible providers must meet to be considered meaningful users of health IT (HHS, 2010). Hospitals and eligible providers are not able to receive federal funding related to the EMR initiative unless they meet these requirements; thus a significant amount of funding depends directly on satisfaction of the meaningful use criteria. There are five purposes for establishing these rules:

1. To improve quality, safety, efficiency, and reduce health disparities
2. To engage patients and their families (through electronic communication)
3. To improve care coordination
4. To ensure adequate privacy and security protection for personal health information
5. To improve the health of the population as well as public health—through data collection and analysis of data

All of these purposes are in line with the IOM *Quality Chasm* reports.

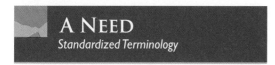

A NEED
Standardized Terminology

Health care has expanded in multiple directions and includes the services of many different healthcare providers. Ensuring effective communication among these myriad providers is not always easy. Certainly, there are issues regarding willingness to communicate, lack of time to communicate, and so on, but a critical problem is the lack of a common professional language. For those entering health care, such as nursing students, this is probably a surprising comment. Each healthcare professional area has its own language; there are some common medical terms, but each profession has a specific language that is often not known or understood by other healthcare professionals. "Creating a common

language is no small task. Developing and adhering to distinct profession-specific terms may be a manifestation of professionals' desire to preserve identity, status or control" (IOM, 2003, p. 123). This problem affects all the core competencies and the ability to develop educational experiences that meet the competencies across healthcare professions, such as nursing, medicine, pharmacy, and allied health. It does not just relate to informatics; however, because informatics is dependent on language, the issue of shared language is even more important in NI.

The IOM has recommended that an interprofessional group created by the Department of Health and Human Services develop a common language across health disciplines "on a core set of competencies that includes patient-centered care, interprofessional teams, evidence-based practice, quality improvement, and informatics" (IOM, 2003, p. 124). Accomplishing this feat will require that healthcare professionals be willing to actively work together to achieve this goal. The next major step will then be getting different healthcare professionals to accept a universal language. This will require compromises.

> The data element sets and terminologies are foundational to standardization of nursing documentation and verbal communication that will lead to a reduction in errors and an increase in the quality and continuity of care. It is through standardization of nurse documentation and communication of a patient's care that the many nurses caring for a patient develop a shared understanding of that care. Moreover, the process generates the nursing data needed to develop increasingly more sophisticated decision support tools in the electronic record and to identify and disseminate best nursing practices. (ANA, 2006)

These statements are an example of why developing and accepting a universal language is difficult but necessary. The statements are nursing focused. How to move from this approach and blend with others, such as medicine, is the challenge.

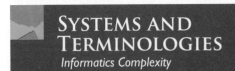

SYSTEMS AND TERMINOLOGIES
Informatics Complexity

Informatics is not as simple as e-mail and Internet. There are many database systems, terms, and other factors that make this a complex area. The following provides examples to illustrate informatics complexity.

Examples of Systematic Collection of Nursing Care Data or Data Element Sets

- *Nursing Minimum Data Set*: This data set describes patient problems across healthcare settings, different populations, geographic areas, and time. These clinical data also assist in identifying nursing diagnoses, nursing interventions, and nursing-sensitive patient outcomes. In addition, the Nursing Minimum Data Set is useful in assessing resources used in the provision of nursing care. The goal is the ability to link data between HCOs and providers. Data can also be used for research and healthcare policy.
- *Nursing Management Minimum Data Set*: This data set focuses on nursing administrative data elements in all types of settings.

Interface Terminologies

- *Clinical Care Classification*: The clinical classifications software for the *International Classification of Diseases*, 10th revision, Clinical Modification (ICD-10-CM) is a diagnosis and procedure categorization scheme that can be used in many types of projects that analyze data on diagnoses and procedures. The software is based on ICD-10-CM, a uniform and standardized coding system. ICD-10-CM includes more than 13,600

diagnosis codes and 3700 procedure codes (Centers for Disease Control and Prevention [CDC], 2011). Clinical care classification focuses on home care and includes diagnoses, interventions, and outcomes.

- *International Classification of Nursing Practice*: This classification system is a unified nursing language system that applies to all types of nursing care. It is a compositional terminology for nursing practice that facilitates the development of and cross-mapping among local terms and existing terminologies. It includes nursing diagnoses, nursing interventions, and nursing outcomes (International Council of Nurses, 2008).
- *Nursing Intervention Classification and Nursing Outcome Classification*: The North American Nursing Diagnosis Association (NANDA) focuses on nursing diagnoses, Nursing Intervention Classification (NIC) on nursing interventions, and Nursing Outcome Classification (NOC) on nursing outcomes.
- *Omaha System*: The Omaha system is a comprehensive, standardized taxonomy designed to improve practice, documentation, and information management. It includes three components: the problem classification scheme, the intervention scheme, and the problem rating scale for outcomes. When the three components are used together, the Omaha system offers a way to link clinical data to demographic, financial, administrative, and staffing data (Omaha System, 2011). The Omaha system is used in home health care, community health, and public health services.
- *Perioperative Nursing Data Set*: The Perioperative Nursing Data Set is a standardized nursing vocabulary that addresses the perioperative patient experience from preadmission until discharge, including nursing diagnoses, interventions, and outcomes. The Perioperative Nursing Data Set was developed by a specialty organization, the members of

the Association of periOperative Registered Nurses, and has been recognized by the ANA as a data set useful for perioperative nursing practice (Association of periOperative Registered Nurses, 2008).

Examples of Multiprofessional Terminologies

- *Logical Observation Identifiers Names and Codes*: This clinical terminology classification is used for laboratory test orders and results. It is one system designated for use in U.S. federal government systems for the electronic exchange of clinical health information (National Library of Medicine, 2008a). This system can be used to collect data about assessments and outcomes for nursing and other healthcare services.
- *Current Procedural Terminology*: This code is used for reimbursement (Larkin, 2008).
- *Systematized Nomenclature of Medicine—Clinical Terms*: This comprehensive clinical terminology is one of several standards approved for use in U.S. federal government systems for the electronic exchange of clinical health information (National Library of Medicine, 2008b). This system is applicable to nursing and other healthcare services and focuses on diagnoses, interventions, and outcomes.

With the increased use of technology for documentation, nursing has been more concerned about two issues (Schwiran & Thede, 2011):

- How to differentiate nursing's contributions to patient care from those of medicine
- How to incorporate descriptions of nursing care into the health record in a manner that is commensurate with its importance to patients' welfare

In a study conducted by Schwiran and Thede (2011), the researchers examined nurses' knowledge of and experience with standardized nursing technologies. The results indicate that most nurses do not have much knowledge of or experience with standardized nursing technologies, such the Nursing

Interventions Classification, Nursing Outcomes Classification, and North American Nursing Diagnosis Association. Given the increasing use of informatics in healthcare settings, such a lack of knowledge and experience can hamper nurses' ability to participate actively in informatics.

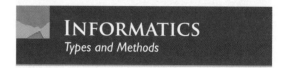

INFORMATICS
Types and Methods

For informatics to be effective, three concerns must be addressed. First, the HCO must have effective and easily accessible IT support services. Staff must be able to pick up the telephone and get this support. Failure of the information system has major implications for patient care, so backup systems are critical.

The second critical concern is staff training. This requires resources: financial resources, trainers, and time. Staff need time to attend training, and there must be recognition that it takes time for staff to learn how to use a system.

Incorporation of informatics with any of the methods described next (and others that are not included here) requires a major change in care delivery. Change is stressful for staff, and it needs to be planned, representing the third concern. Trying to implement too many changes at one time can increase staff stress, impact the success of using more informatics in the future, decrease staff motivation to participate, and increase the risk of errors that might impact patient outcomes.

It is not difficult to find nurses who will complain about a hospital's attempt to increase the use of informatics, particularly if it has been badly planned. Often, in these complaints, staff note that the system selected was not effective and that they had no part in the process. Equipment and software can be very costly, and decisions regarding them are critical. Time must be taken to evaluate equipment and software to make sure they meet the needs and demands of the organization and users such as nurses. Examples of current activities in this area are automated dispensing of medications and bar coding; computerized monitoring of adverse events; the use of electronic medical/health records, provider order entry systems, clinical decision support systems, tablets, smartphones, computer-based and reminder systems; accessing patient records at the point of care; prescribing via the Internet; and using nurse call systems, voice mail, the telephone for advice and other services, online support groups for patients and families, the Internet or virtual appointments, and smartphones. These methods are discussed on the following pages.

Automated Dispensing of Medications and Bar Coding

Pharmacies in all types of HCOs are using or moving toward using automatic medication dispensing systems with bar coding. These systems select the medication based on the order and prepare it in single doses for the patient. The bar code is on the packaged dose. This code can then be compared with the bar code on the patient's identification band using a handheld device. Such a system can decrease errors, and it supports all five rights of medication administration:

1. Right drug
2. Right patient
3. Right amount
4. Right route
5. Right time

Bar coding can also be used to collect data about prescribed and administered drugs. Data can then be used for quality improvement and for research. Bar coding systems are expensive to install and maintain, but they can make a difference in reducing errors.

Computerized Monitoring of Adverse Events

Computerized systems that monitor adverse events assist in identifying and monitoring adverse events.

Developing and using a database of these events facilitates analysis of data and the development of interventions to decrease adverse events.

Electronic Medical/Health Records

The EMR/EHR is slowly replacing the written medical record for an individual patient while the patient receives care within a specific healthcare system. A second type of electronic documentation system is the **personal health record (PHR)**. The PHR is less common than the EMR, but there is hope that it will become standard in the future. The PHR is a computer-based health record for which data are collected over the long term—for a lifetime. With the patient's permission, the healthcare provider can access this record easily to obtain information. To reach this point, there must be agreement on a minimum data set—uniform definitions of data (i.e., standardized language) that would enable all healthcare providers to understand and use the information. There is still much to be done to make this a reality in every HCO, including clinics and medical offices, but the technology is already available.

The **electronic medical record (EMR)** is a record of the patient's history and assessment, orders, laboratory results, description of medical tests and procedures, and documentation of care provided and outcomes. Care plans are included. Information can be easily input, searched, and reviewed, and reports can be printed. Data can be stored over the long term, which is harder to do with written records: Written records require significant storage space, and they may not be easy to find once archived. In addition, written records can be less readable over time. The hard-copy record is also not always easy to access in a hospital unit. If one person is using the record, others cannot use it. With the EMR, this is not a problem as long as staff can access the computerized record system. EMR systems do require security and backup systems to ensure that data are not lost in the event of a power outage or natural disaster.

The following list developed by Iyer and Camp (1999, pp. 129–130) identifies the projected and current advantages of using EMRs:

- Legible records
- Readily available records
- Improved nursing productivity
- Reduction in record tampering
- Support of nursing process in the system
- Reduction in redundant documentation
- Clinical prompts, reminders, and warnings
- Categorized nursing notes
- Automatically printed reports
- Documentation according to standards of care
- Improved knowledge of outcomes
- Availability of data
- Prevention of medication errors
- Facilitation of cost-defining efforts
- Printed discharge information

EMR documentation may take place at the unit workstation, at a hallway computer station, at the bedside in the hospital, or an examining room in a clinic. Bedside systems are better; they are easy to access when the nurse or other healthcare professional needs information, and point-of-care documentation is enhanced.

The ANA believes that the public has a right to expect that health data and healthcare information will be centered on patient safety and improved outcomes throughout all segments of the healthcare system and the data and information will be accurately and efficiently collected, recorded, protected, stored, utilized, analyzed, and reported. Principles of privacy, confidentiality, and security cannot be compromised as the industry creates and implements interoperable and integrated healthcare information technology systems and solutions to convert from paper-based media for documentation and healthcare records to the newer format of EHRs, including individual personal health record (PHR) products. The ANA strongly supports efforts to further refine the concept and requirements of the patient-centric EHR, including the creation of standards-based electronic health records and supporting infrastructures that promote efficient and effective interprofessional and patient communications and decision-making wherever care is provided. Similar attention must address the secondary uses of data and information to generate knowledge that leads to improved and effective decision tools. All stakeholders, including nurses and patients, must be integral participants in the design, development, implementation, and evaluation phases of the electronic health record. This effort requires the attention and action of nurses, the professional and specialty nursing organizations, and the nursing profession to ensure the EHRs are designed to facilitate and support critical thinking and decision making, such as in the nursing process, and the associated documentation activities. It is ANA's position that the registered nurse must also be involved in the product selection, design, development, implementation, evaluation and improvement of information systems and electronic patient care devices used in patient care setting. (ANA, 2009)

Provider Order Entry System

The **provider order entry system** (POES) is included in the EMR, although it can also be a stand-alone system. The healthcare provider inputs orders into this system rather than writing them. One clear advantage of the POES is legibility; written orders are often very difficult to read because handwriting varies, and this has led to many errors. It also takes time to transcribe written physician/provider orders into a form in which the orders can be used. During this process, risk of transcription errors is increased. Typing orders into a computer can also lead to typos, but this is less of a problem than errors with handwritten orders. Clinical decision support systems can be included with the POES. This combination enhances the provider order entry system and can lead to improved care and a decrease in errors.

Clinical Decision Support Systems

Clinical decision support systems have led to major changes in healthcare delivery. These systems provide immediate information that can influence clinical decisions. Some of the systems actually intervene when an error is about to be made. For example, when an order for a medication is put into a patient's EMR, the computerized system can indicate that the patient is allergic to that medication by immediately sending an alert, stopping the order. The nurse can also get alerts that the patient is at risk for falls or decubiti. In the past, nurses depended on textbooks or journals that the unit might have to find information, and such searches were not done effectively. Easy electronic access to current information eliminates many problems related to obtaining information when needed. This, too, can improve the quality of care. Evidence-based practice relies heavily on access to evidence-based practice literature, which is most easily accessible via the Internet and databases. As is true for all electronic methods, healthcare professional critical thinking, as well as clinical reasoning and judgment, must still be applied. Errors can still be made with technology. When HIT is used, staff may go on "automatic pilot," assuming that the electronic system will catch errors, which is not always the case.

More research is needed to fully understand the impact of clinical decision support systems on patient outcomes. A study published in 2011 indicated that there was no consistent association between such systems and the quality of care in an investigation that included 3 billion patient visits (Romano & Stafford, 2011). Only one of 20 indicators—diet counseling for high-risk adults—demonstrated significantly better performance when clinical decision support systems were utilized. In contrast, earlier studies had shown that use of the clinical decision support systems improved outcomes. A critique of the 2011 study questions whether its results were influenced by the following factors: (1) Clinical decision support systems rules may have been different in the systems studied; (2) the study focused on medication management, whereas earlier studies were broader; and (3) the study looked at the outcome of a single visit rather than the cumulative effect. More research is needed to better determine the effectiveness of using clinical decision support systems.

Tablets and Smartphones

Tablet computers such as iPads have become hugely popular with the general public. Most mobile telephones now have Internet capability, such as access to the Internet and storage of information; such devices are referred to as smartphones. These phones give users access to information, Internet, e-mail, and text messaging, and, of course, telephone service. Such handheld devices can hold a significant amount of information, serve as a calendar, keep contact information, and are an effective method for transmission of information.

Nurses who use tablets carry information with them and can look up side effects of a medication or any other type of medical information necessary as they provide care. In some cases, the nurse can access EMRs to get to patient information through the tablet. Some textbooks can now be uploaded into tablets, such as pharmacology and clinical laboratory resources. This is useful information for the nurse to have available—it is accessible in seconds at the point of care with this type of HIT. Nurses working outside a structured setting, such as in public health or in home care, may also find this type of system useful for support information and documentation needs (patient information, visit data, and so on); however, they must be very careful to maintain HIPAA regulations. Tablets are used in public health to collect data such as health assessments; these data are stored locally on the tablet and then uploaded to a secure cloud server (i.e., a server that is encrypted to protect personal health information) when the user is back in network/wireless range. Anytime such technology is used, the data must be protected to keep information secure and confidential.

Computer-Based Reminder Systems

Computer-based reminder systems are used to communicate with patients via e-mail to remind them of appointments and screenings and to discuss other health issues. In the future, this method will most likely take the place of telephone calls to remind patients of appointments. This system also must maintain HIPAA regulations. For example, the healthcare provider must ensure that only authorized parties have access to the computer and e-mail data. More narrowly defined, only the patient should have access to the information unless the patient wants the information shared.

Access to Patient Records at the Point of Care

Many hospitals are moving toward providing access to the patient records either in the patient's room or in the hallway via computers. In the future, more nurses will carry small laptops or tablets that allow access to the EMR when needed. This reduces time spent returning to the workstation to get information. Documentation can be completed as soon as care is provided; this reduces errors and improves quality because all care providers know when care

has been provided. Point-of-care access decreases the chance that details may be forgotten, documented incorrectly, or not documented at all. In addition, it saves nurses time and eliminates the need to delay documentation. For example, if they do not have this type of immediate access, nurses may document at certain times during the shift such as midmorning or near the end of a shift—a system that can lead to errors, incomplete data in the record if the nurse forgets information, and situations in which other providers need current patient information that has not yet been documented.

Internet Prescriptions

There has been rapid growth in access to prescriptions via the Internet. The medications are then mailed to the patient. The consumer does have to be careful and check the legitimacy of the source to prevent errors.

Nurse Call Systems

Nurse call systems are a form of informatics that is very important in communication within a healthcare system. They allow for improved and efficient communication and are a great improvement on the old method of yelling out for a staff member. Many types of nurse call systems exist, such as pagers, light signals, buzzers, methods that allow patients to talk directly to nurses through a direct audio system that the nurse can easily access, smartphones, miniature label microphones, and locator badges. The goal is to get a message to the right person as soon as possible while maintaining privacy and confidentiality. Doing so can improve care, improve patient satisfaction, reduce errors, and make staff more efficient, preventing the unnecessary work of trying to obtain and share information.

Voice Mail and Texting

Computer-based messaging systems are found in all healthcare settings today so that staff can leave and receive voice messages. Staff and patients can use these systems, often reducing the need for callbacks. Complicated systems can annoy consumers, however, and there is an impersonal quality to this form of communication, though it is part of everyday life today. One has to be very careful about leaving voice mails. Clearly, others can listen to messages, and this can lead to a HIPAA violation.

Telephone for Advice and Other Services

Patient advice systems are used mostly by insurers, although some HCOs and providers provide these services as well. In such systems, nurses use their assessment skills and provide advice to patients who call in with questions. Typically, insurers develop standard protocols that the nurses use for common questions, but nurses must still use professional judgment when providing advice. This type of service should not become "cookbook" care in which there is no consideration of assessment and individual patient needs. Assessment is the key to successful telephone nursing, as it enables providers to identify the interventions required that may or may not be found in the guidelines. Some physician offices have telephone advice services that are manned by a physician in the practice or by a nurse. Pediatric practices are the most common type of practice using this system. Patient advice systems via telephone require clear documentation policies and guidelines that include content related to who is called, when, and for what reason, and the required assessment data and interventions. Telephone advice systems are typically used to answer questions, remind patients of appointments or follow-up needs, and check in on how a patient is doing.

Hospitals are using the telephone to begin the admission process for patients with scheduled admissions. Patients are called before the admission date, asked questions related to required admission information, and told what to expect on admission. Pretesting may be scheduled prior to admission. This saves the hospital time and is more cost-effective,

and pretesting can be more convenient for the patient. This method can also identify problems that may impact the needed patient care so that they can be addressed early on.

Online Support Groups for Patients and Families

Online support groups can focus on any problem or disease. Patients and their families can use chat rooms, e-mail, and websites for information sharing. Consumers gain information, education about their health and health needs, and support from others with similar problems. A healthcare provider may or may not be involved. Privacy issues must be discussed with participants, along with the risk of lack of privacy.

Internet or Virtual Appointments

Use of the Internet as a means of increasing accessibility to a physician or advanced practice nurse or to make appointments is increasing. Members of younger generations, as well as some senior citizens, are using the Internet to obtain advice from health professionals. Portable family histories can be maintained in this fashion and passed on to a new primary care provider. Those patients and families who have limited resources—financial, transportation, or insurance—can more affordably receive medical advice in this format. It also keeps some employees from missing work to take a child or other family member to an appointment. Many of these sites link to cellular devices to send an alert of high importance to whoever is on call for virtual hours. This ensures that high-priority questions and requests for advice reach the health professional quickly (Larkin, 2008). These types of services will most likely increase in the future.

As is true with all documentation methods, patient confidentiality must be maintained. Notably, the risk of confidentiality problems increases with use of such technology.

THE FUTURE OF INFORMATICS AND MEDICAL TECHNOLOGY

The future is likely to see major expansion in the use of technology. Some of the possible technological approaches are already being used in some areas. One area that is growing is the use of embodied conversation agents to provide reinforcement of discharge teaching, particularly when there is low health literacy (Paasche-Orlow, 2010). Cutting-edge technology is sometimes hard to believe. Some of the possibilities will be discussed next.

Nanotechnology

Nanotechnology—microscopic technology on the order of one billionth of a meter—will likely impact the diagnosis and treatment of many diseases and conditions (Gordon, Lutz, Boninger, & Cooper, 2007). Some of the pending technologies are highlighted here:

- Sensing patients' internal drug levels with miniature medical diagnostic tools that circulate in the bloodstreams
- Chemotherapy delivered directly to a tumor site, reducing systemic side effects
- New monitoring devices for the home: a talking pill bottle that lets patients push a button to hear prescription information; bathroom counters that announce whether it is safe to mix two medications; a shower with built-in scales to calculate body mass index; measuring devices in the bathroom to track urine frequency and output and upload these data to a system or care manager; non-invasive blood glucose monitors to eliminate sticks; and sensors to compute blood sugar levels using a multi-wavelength reflective dispersion photometer.

Wearable Computing

A computer can be worn, much as eyeglasses or clothing is worn, and interactions with the user are based on the context of the situation (ANA, 2008). With heads-up displays, embedded sensors in fabrics, unobtrusive input devices, personal wireless local area networks, and a host of other context sensing and communication tools, wearable computers can act as intelligent assistants or data collection and analysis devices. Many of these devices are available now using smart fabrics. Such wearable computer and remote monitoring systems are intertwined with the user's activity so that the technology becomes transparent. Sensors and devices can gather data during the patient's daily routine, providing healthcare providers or researchers with periodic or continuous data on the person's health while he or she is at work, at school, exercising, or sleeping, rather than the current snapshot captured during a typical hospital or clinic visit. A few applications for wearable computing devices include sudden infant death syndrome monitoring for infants; ambulatory cardiac and respiratory monitoring; monitoring of ventilation during exercise; monitoring the activity level of post-stroke patients; monitoring patterns of breathing in asthma; assessment of stress in individuals; arrhythmia detection and control of selected cardiac conditions; and daily activity monitors (Offray Specialty Narrow Fabrics, 2007).

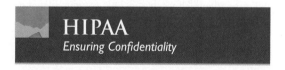

HIPAA
Ensuring Confidentiality

The **Health Insurance Portability and Accountability Act of 1996 (HIPAA)** has had a major impact on healthcare delivery systems and how they communicate. Privacy and confidentiality have long been problematic issues in health care. Because HIPAA focuses on the issue of information and confidentiality, it applies to IT. The law also requires data security and electronic transaction standards. This law was necessary because with the growth of information sharing, it became increasingly evident that existing means of transactions and systems were not ensuring privacy and confidentiality—key elements that had long been part of the healthcare delivery system.

Privacy is the right of a person to have personal information kept private. As discussed, this relates to professional ethics. Privacy restrictions even apply to family members unless the adult patient specifically communicates that it is acceptable for family members to be given information. This cannot be assumed. HIPAA requires that only necessary information be shared among providers, including insurers. Patients may also access their medical records.

Health information cannot be openly shared by healthcare providers—for example, discussing patient information in public places, calling a patient's work or home and leaving a message that reveals information about health or health services, and so on, must not be done. Carrying documents outside an HCO with patient identifier information is prohibited; this constraint has implications for students who may take notes or have written assignments that include this information. How information is carried in tablets, laptops, or smartphones is also of concern. For example, taking pictures on smartphones in clinical settings is a privacy violation. Many institutions have implemented strict policies about the taking of patient photos even if they are de-identified. As a nurse, you should make sure you know your institution's policy on smartphone use in a clinical setting and follow it.

Development of new technology has been moving so fast that critical prior issues have not always been addressed effectively. The 1996 law, however, requires that staff know the key elements of HIPAA and apply them. As a result, HCOs and healthcare profession schools, such as nursing programs, are required to provide information and training about HIPAA. There are large fines if the law is broken. Patients are informed about HIPAA when they enter the health system; they are given written information and asked to sign documents to indicate that they have been informed. Ensuring that the requirements are met must be incorporated into IT, which has become a major method for communicating health information. With the Internet, it is easy for patients to report HIPAA violations. Violations will be examined, and the provider may have to pay a fee for not following HIPAA regulations.

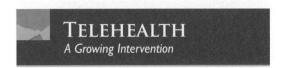

TELEHEALTH
A Growing Intervention

Telehealth, or telemedicine, is the use of telecommunications equipment and communications networks for transferring healthcare information between participants at different locations. Telehealth applies telecommunication and computer technologies to the broad spectrum of public health and medicine. This technology offers opportunities to provide care when face-to-face interaction is impossible (such as in home care, in school-based care, and in rural areas) and can be used in a variety of settings and situations as long as the equipment is available. Two-way interactive video is the most effective telehealth method.

> **Telenursing** refers to the use of telecommunications technology in nursing to enhance patient care. It involves the use of electromagnetic channels (e.g., wire, radio and optical) to transmit voice, data and video communications signals. It is also defined as distance communications, using electrical or optical transmissions, between humans and/or computers. (Skiba, 1998, p. 40)

Issues that arise with telehealth include the cost of equipment and its use; training for staff and for patients if they need to actively use equipment; limited or no insurance coverage for telehealth services; the need for clear policies, procedures, and protocols; privacy and confidentiality of information; and regulatory issues (e.g., a nurse who is located and licensed in one state providing telenursing for a patient in another state where the nurse is not licensed). Telehealth also has implications for international health care because it provides a method for connecting expertise to patients who may need care that is not accessible in their home country.

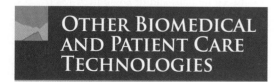

USE OF THE INTERNET

Nurses use the Internet to obtain information and for communication through e-mail. Patients/consumers are also using the Internet for increasingly more health-related purposes. It can be an excellent source for all types of information, including health and medical information.

When the Internet is used as a source of health information, it is important that nurses evaluate the websites, because they are not all of the same quality. A nurse needs to consider the following factors when evaluating a website:

- The source or sponsor of the website: The most reliable sites are sponsored by the government, academic institutions, healthcare professional organizations, and HCOs.
- Current status of the information: When was it posted or revised?
- Accessibility of the information on the site: Can one find what one needs?
- References provided for content when appropriate.

OTHER BIOMEDICAL AND PATIENT CARE TECHNOLOGIES

Examples of other biomedical and patient care technologies are briefly described in this section.

Remote Telemetry Monitoring

Remote telemetry monitoring technology informs staff when a patient's condition has changed. The patient is placed on a monitor, and signals are sent to staff through a page system. Staff may be informed, for example, of the patient's identity, heart rate, and readout of rhythm without being right next to the patient.

Robotics

The use of robotics in patient care is expected to expand in the future (ANA, 2008). Robots have been used for many years to deliver supplies to patient care areas. Robotics enables remote surgeries and virtual reality surgical procedures. Hand-assist devices help patients regain strength after a stroke ("Robotic Brace," 2007). Robots may provide a remote presence to allow physicians to virtually examine patients by manipulating remote cameras ("Telemedicine Pioneer Helps Physicians," 2007). They are also used for microscopic, minimally invasive surgical procedures. For example, the da Vinci surgical system helps surgeons perform such procedures as mitral valve repairs, hysterectomies, and prostate surgeries (da Vinci Surgery, 2008). In the future, robots may also be used in direct patient care—for instance, to help lift morbidly obese patients.

Genetics and Genomics

Advances in mapping the human genome (genetics), understanding individual DNA, and examining the impact of external factors such as the environment (genomics) will have a dramatic impact on patient care (ANA, 2008). These data, especially once they are integrated into EMRs or PHRs, will lead to advances in customized patient care and medications targeted to individual responses to medications. Care and medication can be precisely customized to patients based on their unique DNA profile and how they have responded to medications and other interventions in the past; this will dramatically change how patients are managed for specific diseases and conditions and extend into the prevention of some diseases. The inherent complexity of customized patient care will demand computerized clinical decision support that reflects individual needs and health history. Predictive disease models based on patients' DNA profiles will emerge as clinicians better understand DNA mapping. These advances have implications for a new model of care and for the informatics nurse's participation in the development of genomic IT solutions. More than ever, patients will need to be partners in this development as part of patient-centered care. Nurses are beginning to collaborate more with bioengineers and informatics experts to develop new products, participate in research using these products, and help to develop implementation and evaluation plans to use with these products.

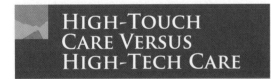

HIGH-TOUCH CARE VERSUS HIGH-TECH CARE

High-touch care is what most people go into nursing for, but nursing is much more than this today. This chapter describes the growing influence of technology on all segments of health care. This influence will not decrease, but rather will increase in the future. Nurses do need to understand and know how to use technology that is applied to their practice areas. They need to be involved in the development of this technology when possible, and they must be involved in the implementation of the technology. But there are concerns. When we talk through machines, do we lose information and the personal relationship? How can this be prevented so that we are not disconnected from our patients? How can we ensure that the information we are getting is correct and complete? Are people able to communicate fully through some of these other means? It is clear that over time, the public has become increasingly comfortable with informatics, which they are using more and more in their everyday lives. As nursing

adopts informatics to an ever greater extent, nurses need to keep in mind the potential for isolation and the need for effective communication, and they must not forget the need for touch and face-to-face communication. When a nurse uses a computer or some type of handheld device asking patient questions and does not look at the patient, this does not engage the patient in the process.

The future will include many more new uses of technology, and change is ongoing. For example, the eICU (e-intensive care unit) is used to monitor patients from afar to improve patient outcomes (Kowalczyk, 2007). In this example a system is attached to four hospitals in Iowa and their ICUs. This system allows intensivists at a remote monitoring center to view patients' vital statistics, electrocardiograms, ventilators, and X-ray and lab results. The eICU includes two-way conference video capability so that patients and staff can interact when required. This type of system has advantages: For example, experts can be located in one place and then consult with multiple locations and staff. This is particularly useful in providing expert medical care for residents in rural and remote areas. There is no reason that this type of system would be limited to physician consultation; it could be used by nurses. For example, a nurse clinical specialist could view data and consult on patient care with nurses in various ICUs. The potential is there for increased access to information and expertise. The other side of this innovation coin is the effect on the touch side of care when the provider is not actually in the room with the patient. It is not clear how this might impact care because these types of systems are very new.

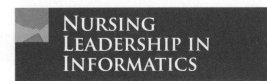

NURSING LEADERSHIP IN INFORMATICS

We are currently at a critical junction for nurses and the IOM informatics competency, with all nurses being called upon to assume more of a leadership role in the expansion of informatics in healthcare.

This call to action corresponds to the recommendations in the IOM's *Future of Nursing* report (2011). Ongoing implementation of the Affordable Care Act will lead to further changes in healthcare delivery and more dependence on informatics, and nurse informaticists should be part of the structure that develops and implements greater use of informatics (HIMSS, 2011).

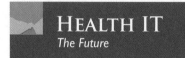

HEALTH IT
The Future

The IOM report titled *Health IT and Patient Safety: Building Safer Systems for Better Care* (2012) makes a strong statement that health IT is not something separated from care delivery or the providers of care.

> We are at a unique time in health care. Technology—which has the potential

to improve quality and safety of care as well as reduce costs—is rapidly evolving, changing the way we deliver health care. At the same time, health care reform is reshaping the health care landscape. As Sir Cyril Chantler of the Kings Fund said, "Medicine used to be simple, ineffective, and relatively safe. Now it is complex, effective, and potentially dangerous." More and more cognitive overload requires a symbiotic relationship between human cognition and computer support. It is this very difficult transition we are facing in ensuring safety in health care. (IOM, 2012, p. ix)

The IOM report highlights patient and family concerns about safety and shared responsibility. These same themes have also been emphasized throughout this text.

CONCLUSION

This chapter has explored the current and future world of healthcare informatics and some aspects of biotechnology. There is much more to this subject than use of e-mail, as the many diverse examples presented in this chapter suggest. The core competency of using informatics is critical for nurses' success in the 21st century. If graduates of the healthcare profession schools cannot understand and use informatics, the safety and quality of the care they provide will be diminished. Communication, coordination, documentation, and care provision (including monitoring and decision making) are linked to informatics. However, each nurse must not get so involved in informatics and technology that the patient as a person is lost—the patient–nurse relationship is an important component of patient-centered care.

CHAPTER HIGHLIGHTS

1. The IOM describes the fifth healthcare profession core competency as "communicate, manage knowledge, mitigate error, and support decision making using information technology" (IOM, 2003, p. 4).

2. Informatics is more than just looking at IT; it also involves understanding how that technology is used to prevent errors and improve care.

3. Informatics is used for evaluating the performance of HCOs and individual healthcare

CHAPTER HIGHLIGHTS (CONTINUED)

providers and has a major impact on quality improvement. Today, it is much easier to collect, store, and analyze large amounts of data that in the past were collected by hand.

4. Insurers rely heavily on informatics to provide insurance coverage, manage data, and analyze performance, which has a direct impact on whether care is covered for reimbursement.

5. Informatics provides opportunities for government at all levels—local, state, national, and international—to collect data and use them for policy decision making and evaluation.

6. A clinical information system is a method of data storage that is generally used at the point of care. It includes such elements as clinical guidelines, patient information, and pharmacopeias to check for drug interactions.

7. A coding system is a mechanism for identifying treatments and procedures with specific labels so as to bill for those services.

8. Computer literacy is knowledge of basic computer technology.

9. Data mining is the ability to drill down and search through databases—for example, to determine trends in a patient or a system. Examining the data for relationships between treatment and patient outcomes is another example.

10. Decision support systems are computerized systems that assist the health professional in making clinical treatment plans.

11. Information literacy is the ability to recognize and retrieve needed data.

12. A minimum data set is the minimum group of categories of data with uniform definitions and categories concerning a specific aspect or dimension of the healthcare system that meets the basic needs of multiple data users. An example is the Nursing Minimum Data Set.

13. Standardized language is a collection of terms with definitions for use in informational systems databases. It enables comparisons to be made when the same term is used by everyone to denote the same condition. Standardized language is necessary for documentation in EHRs.

14. Nursing informatics is a nursing specialty that integrates nursing science, computer science, and information science to manage and communicate data, information, knowledge, and wisdom in nursing practice. This specialty has its own sets of standards, scope of practice, and national certification.

15. Informatics can directly impact care by providing data in a retrievable form for the purpose of assisting with clinical decision making. However, the data are only as reliable as the information entered in the computer.

16. In today's healthcare organizations, documentation is often implemented in an electronic format.

17. Standardized terminology assists in promoting clearer communication across disciplines.

18. Interface terminologies include, but are not limited to, the Clinical Care Classification, the International Classification of Nursing Practice, NANDA, NIC, NOC, the Omaha System, and the Perioperative Nursing Data Set.

19. Multidisciplinary terminologies include, but are not limited to, the Logical Observation Identifiers Names and Codes and the Systematized Nomenclature of Medicine—Clinical Terms.

20. Effective informatics is dependent on accessible IT support and adequate staff training. Change related to informatics, which is inevitable, must be well planned if it is to be successful.

(continues)

CHAPTER HIGHLIGHTS (CONTINUED)

21. Examples of use of informatics in healthcare delivery include the automated dispensing of medications and bar coding for identification; computerized monitoring of adverse events; use of EMRs, provider order entry systems, and clinical decision support systems; use of tablets and smartphones; access to patient records at the point of care; and Internet prescriptions, nurse call systems, voice mail, telephone for advice and other services, online support groups for patients, and Internet or virtual appointments.

22. HIPAA requires that patient data are kept secure and private.

23. Telehealth (telemedicine) is the use of telecommunications equipment and communications networks for transferring healthcare information between participants at different locations.

24. Robotics is the use of robots for the purposes of retrieving supplies, carrying lab specimens from one location to another, or even assisting in surgical procedures.

25. There has been expansion in the area of genomics, or the mapping of the human gene locations, as well as in understanding of its environmental impact.

26. As health informatics expands, nursing must be proactive in increasing its role in informatics and assume more leadership to improve healthcare through better informatics.

DISCUSSION QUESTIONS

1. Explain how the core competency "utilize informatics" relates to the other four IOM core competencies.

2. What is informatics, and why is it important in health care and nursing?

3. Describe the certification requirements for an informatics nurse and the role filled by this nurse.

4. Describe four examples of healthcare informatics and implications for nursing.

5. Why is documentation important?

6. Explain how the EMR and PHR can increase quality of care and decrease errors. Provide examples.

7. Discuss issues related to confidentiality and informatics.

CRITICAL THINKING ACTIVITIES

1. Divide into small teams. Identify an HCO in your local community and try to find out how it uses informatics and applies meaningful use. You can focus on the entire organization or select a department or a unit. Are there any future plans to increase the use of informatics?

Landscape © f9photos/Shutterstock, Inc.

CRITICAL THINKING ACTIVITIES (CONTINUED)

2. In a team of classmates, develop six questions to ask a nurse who works in a hospital that uses an EMR to gather data about staff responses to use of EMRs. Each student on the team will then interview one registered nurse. After the interviews, combine your data and analyze the results.

3. Speak to a registered nurse who works in staff development/education in an HCO. Discuss the training that staff members receive for using

informatics (e.g., type of content, cost and time commitment, challenges).

4. If you have used an EMR in clinical practice, what was it like for you? If you have not yet done this, interview a senior student and ask about the experience.

5. Which biomedical equipment have you used or seen used? How does the use of this equipment impact care?

Circuit Board: ©Photos.com

ELECTRONIC *Reflective Journal*

What is your opinion of the potential conflict between high-touch care and high-tech care? Describe some examples where you thought technology interfered with patient care, either for you or for something you observed. What could have been done to prevent this?

Landscape © f9photos/Shutterstock, Inc.

LINKING TO THE INTERNET

- Alliance for Nursing Informatics: http://www.allianceni.org
- American Nursing Informatics Association: http://www.ania-caring.org/mc/page.do?sitePageId=101757&orgId=car
- American Telemedicine Association: http://www.americantelemed.org
- Ending the Document Game: http://endingthedocumentgame.gov/medicationRecord.html
- Healthcare Information and Management Systems Society: http://www.himss.org/asp/topics_nursingInformatics.asp
- Technology Informatics Guiding Educational Reform (TIGER Initiative): http://www.thetigerinitiative.org/

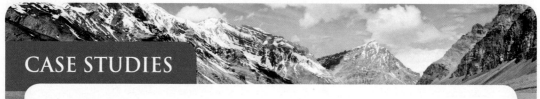

CASE STUDIES

Case Study 1

A 6-year-old has come to the attention of the child welfare department as a possible victim of sexual abuse. The child lives in a very rural part of a western state. Rather than have the child travel a distance to experts, she was taken to the nearest clinic with sexual assault nurse examiners and a knowledgeable pediatrician skilled in sexual abuse examinations. At the time of the examination, pictures were taken of the child's body, including the genital area. These pictures are crucial if charges are filed. To ensure that an accurate diagnosis is made, local experts wish to have a second opinion because the results of the physical examination were not believed to be completely definitive. The experts for the second opinion were linked via the Internet and Internet videoconferencing equipment so that the two teams could talk and view de-identified (because the information was going across unsecure Internet channels) photos. Within 15 minutes, it was determined that the hymen was intact and no penetration had occurred. Other markers indicated that there was evidence of child abuse, but none that supported a claim of sexual assault. This case used an EMR, digitized photos, and Internet consultation to arrive at a diagnosis that had both medical and legal implications.

Case Questions

1. Discuss the impact of the use of these methods in the case on the nurse–patient relationship and on patient confidentiality including HIPAA requirements.
2. How else might this technology be used?
3. What is your opinion of the human, caring part of the care process in relation to this case description?

Case Study 2

The hospital where you work is assessing its electronic medical record (EMR), which has been in use for 1 year. You have volunteered to be on the task force to lead the review. The team meets to discuss critical issues that need to be addressed. Some of the issues are staff acceptance of the new system, errors, and information that is not easy to access in the EMR. The representative from the hospital finance team asks, "What about meaningful use?"

Case Questions

1. What is meaningful use?
2. Why is the team member's question important?
3. How might meaningful use affect what the task force does?

Words of Wisdom

© Roobcio/Shutterstock, Inc.

Marion J. Ball, EdD

Professor Emerita, Johns Hopkins University School of Nursing, Fellow, Center for Healthcare Management IBM Research

Nursing professionals are the foot soldiers of the healthcare delivery system and therefore must be well equipped to carry out the best possible care for our patients. Having a solid understanding of the use of technologic enabling tools is essential to be able to give the best possible patient care. The Technology Informatics Guiding Education Reform (TIGER) initiative is working on bringing the most essential skills for the profession to the table (http://thetigerinitiative.org/). The eight areas TIGER is addressing are:

1. Standards and interoperability
2. Healthcare IT national agenda/healthcare IT policy
3. Informatics competencies
4. Education and faculty development
5. Staff development/continuing education
6. Usability/clinical application design
7. Virtual demonstration center
8. Leadership development

For more information, go to http://www.thetigerinitiative.org/.

In fighting the battle of disease and suffering, nurses are the ones who can win the battle if they are well prepared. This means a good grasp of informatics is an essential ingredient.

Landscape © f9photos/Shutterstock, Inc.

REFERENCES

American Nurses Association (ANA). (2006). Nursing practice information infrastructure: Glossary. Retrieved from http://www.nursingworld.org/npii/glossary.htm

American Nurses Association (ANA). (2008). *Nursing informatics: Scope and standards of practice*. Washington, DC: Author.

American Nurses Association (ANA). (2009). *Electronic health record (Position statement)*. Silver Spring, MD: Author. Retrieved from http://nursingworld.org/MainMenuCategories/Policy-Advocacy/Positions-and-Resolutions/ANA-PositionStatements/Position-Statements-Alphabetically/Electronic-Health-Record.html

American Nurses Association (ANA). (2010). *ANA's principles for nursing documentation*. Silver Spring, MD: Author.

American Nurses Credentialing Center (ANCC). (2014). Informatics nurse certification exam. Retrieved from http://www.nursecredentialing.org/InformaticsNursing

Appleton, C. (1998). Nursing research: Moving into the clinical setting. *Nursing Management, 29*(6), 43–45.

Association of periOperative Registered Nurses. (2008). Perioperative data set. Retrieved from http://www.aorn.org/Secondary.aspx?id=21100&terms=Perioperative%20data%20set

Bodenheimer, T. (2008). Coordinating care: A perilous journey through the healthcare system. *New England Journal of Medicine, 358*, 1065–1071.

Centers for Disease Control and Prevention (CDC). (2011). International classification of diseases (ICD-10). Retrieved from http://www.cdc.gov/nchs/icd/icd10.htm

Clark, S. (2011). Medical record documentation makes top 10 non-compliance list for first half of 2010. *HIM Connection*. Retrieved from http://www.hcpro.com/CCP-258429-237/Medical-record-documentation-makes-Joint-Commission-top-10-noncompliance-list-for-first-half-of-2010.html

da Vinci Surgery. (2008). Surgery enabled by da Vinci®. Retrieved from http://www.davincisurgery.com/davinci-surgery/

Dykes, P., & Collins, S. (2013). Building linkages between nursing care and improved patient outcomes: The role of health information technology. *Online Journal of Issues in Nursing, 18*(3). Retrieved from http://www.nursingworld.org/MainMenuCategories/ANAMarketplace/ANAPeriodicals/OJIN/TableofContents/Vol-18-2013/No3-Sept-2013/Nursing-Care-and-Improved-Outcomes.html

Englebardt, S., & Nelson, R. (2002). *Healthcare informatics: An interdisciplinary approach.* St. Louis, MO: Mosby-Year Book.

Finkelman, A., & Kenner, C. (2012). *Teaching IOM* (3rd ed.). Silver Spring, MD: American Nurses Association.

Gordon, A., Lutz, G., Boninger, M., & Cooper, R. (2007). Introduction to nanotechnology: Potential applications in physical medicine and rehabilitation. *American Journal of Physical Medicine and Rehabilitation, 86*, 225–241.

Healthcare Information and Management Systems Society (HIMSS). (2011, June 17). Position statement on transforming nursing practice through technology and informatics. Retrieved from http://www.himss.org/ASP/index.asp

Institute of Medicine (IOM). (2003). *Health professions education.* Washington, DC: National Academies Press.

Institute of Medicine (IOM). (2011). *The future of nursing: Leading change, advancing health.* Washington, DC: National Academies Press.

Institute of Medicine (IOM). (2012). *Health IT and patient safety: Building safer systems for better care.* Washington, DC: National Academies Press.

International Council of Nurses (ICN). (2008). International classification for nursing practice (ICNP). Retrieved from http://www.icn.ch/icnp_def.htm

Iyer, P., & Camp, N. (1999). *Nursing documentation.* St. Louis, MO: Mosby.

The Joint Commission. (2011). *Comprehensive accreditation manual for hospitals.* Chicago, IL: Author.

Kowalczyk, L. (2007, November 19). Teletreatment. Monitoring from afar, "eICUs" fill the gap. Retrieved from http://www.boston.com/business/globe/articles/2007/11/19/tele_treatment/

Larkin, H. (2008). Your future chief of staff? *H&HN: Hospitals & Healthcare Networks, 82*(3), 30–34.

National Center for Health Statistics. (2010). More physicians switch to electronic medical record. Retrieved from http://nchspressroom.wordpress.com/2010/04/02/more-physicians-switch-to-electronic-medical-record-use/

National Library of Medicine (NLM). (2008a). Logical observation identifiers names and codes. Retrieved from http://www.nlm.nih.gov/research/umls/loinc_main.html

National Library of Medicine (NLM). (2008b). Unified medical language system: SNOMED clinical terms. Retrieved from http://www.nlm.nih.gov/research/umls/Snomed/snomed_main.html

National Quality Forum (NQF). (2013). Electronic quality measures. Retrieved from http://www.qualityforum.org/Projects/e-g/eMeasures/Electronic_Quality_Measures.aspx

Nelson, R., & Joos, I. (1989, Fall). On language in nursing; from data to wisdom. *PLN Vision*, p. 6.

Offray Specialty Narrow Fabrics. (2007). Smart textiles. Retrieved from http://www.osnf.com/p_smart.html

Omaha System. (2011). The Omaha system: Solving the clinical data-information puzzle. Retrieved from http://www.omahasystem.org/

Paasche-Orlow, M. (2010). Usability of conversational agents by patients with inadequate health literacy: Evidence from two clinical trials. *Journal of Health Communication, 15*(suppl 2, special issue), *Health Literacy Research: Current Status and Future Directions*, 197–210.

Richards, J. (2001). Nursing in a digital age. *Nursing Economics, 19*(1), 6–10, 34.

Robotic brace aids stroke recovery. (2007). *Science Daily.* Retrieved from http://www.sciencedaily.com/releases/2007/03/070321105223.htm

Romano, M., & Stafford, R. (2011). Electronic health records and clinical decision support systems: Impact on national ambulatory care quality. *Archives of Internal Medicine, 171*, 897–903.

Schwiran, P., & Thede, L. (2011). Informatics: The standardized nursing terminologies: A national survey of nurses' experiences and attitudes. *Online Journal of Issues in Nursing, 16*(2). Retrieved from http://nursingworld.org/MainMenuCategories/ANAMarketplace/ANAPeriodicals/OJIN/Columns/Informatics/Informatics-Participants-Perception-of-Comfort-in-the-Use.html

Skiba, D. J. (1998). Health-oriented telecommunications. In M. J. Ball, K. J. Hannah, S. K. Newbold, & J. V. Douglas (Eds.), *Nursing informatics: Where caring and technology meet* (pp. 40–53). New York, NY: Springer.

Telemedicine pioneer helps physicians on the move stay close to patients. (2007). Retrieved from http://www.cisco.com/?POSITION=SEM&COUNTRY_SITE=us&CAMPAIGN=tomorrowstartshere&CREATIVE=Brand_Cisco+Systems&REFERRING_SITE=Bing&KEYWORD=what+is+cisco+systems_e|mkwid_6dahF5kH|dc_3648159597_0v0xx7y7d0http://www.hhs.gov/news/press/2013pres/05/20130522a.html

Thompson, D. (2013). U.S. hospitals triple use of electronic health records: Report. Retrieved from http://health.usnews.com/health-news/news/articles/2013/07/08/us-hospitals-triple-use-of-electronic-health-records-report

U.S. Department of Health and Human Services (HHS). (2010). Meaningful use. Retrieved from http://www.hhs.gov/news/imagelibrary/video/2010-07-13_press.html

U.S. Department of Health and Human Services (HHS). (2013). Doctors and hospitals' use of health IT doubles since 2012. Retrieved from http://www.hhs.gov/news/press/2013pres/05/20130522a.html

U.S. Department of Health and Human Services (HHS), Centers for Medicare and Medicaid Services (CMS). (2014). Meaningful use. Retrieved from http://www.cms.gov/Regulations-and-Guidance/Legislation/EHRIncentivePrograms/Meaningful_Use.html

U.S. Health and Human Services (HHS). HealthIt.Gov. (2014). Meaningful use definition and objectives. Retrieved from http://www.healthit.gov/providers-professionals/meaningful-use-definition-objectives

SECTION 4

The Practice of Nursing Today and in the Future

Section IV concludes this text. It summarizes key concerns focusing on the future of nursing, and the importance of nursing leadership. Change in the healthcare delivery system provides many opportunities for nursing, if nursing is ready for them.

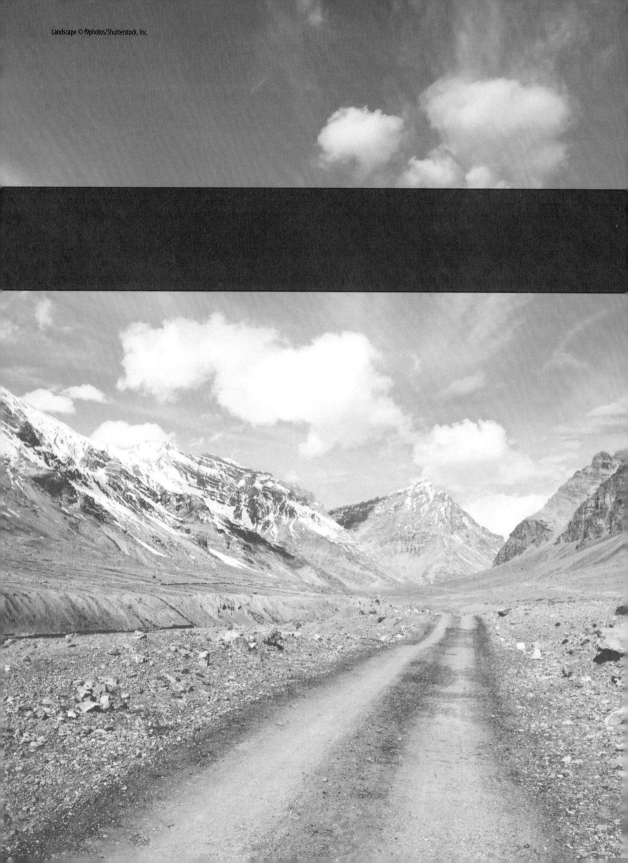

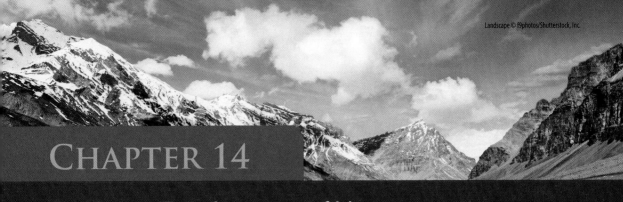

CHAPTER 14

The Future: Transformation of Nursing Practice Through Leadership

CHAPTER OBJECTIVES

At the conclusion of this chapter, the learner will be able to:

- Discuss the relevance of leadership in nursing and differences in management and impact of shared governance
- Examine the factors that influence nursing leadership and management
- Examine the various settings and roles and specialties for nurses and possible future changes in scope of practice
- Critique the various professional practice models
- Discuss the impact of legislation, regulation, and policy on nursing leadership and practice
- Explain the importance of economic value to the nursing profession

- Discuss the impact of the work environment on the nursing profession and the delivery of effective, quality care
- Explain why it is important for nurses to take active leadership roles in quality improvement
- Discuss how the Forces of Magnetism and the Magnet Recognition Program are used to support effective, healthy nursing work environments and nursing leadership
- Examine some of the implications of the Institute of Medicine's report *The Future of Nursing: Leading Change, Advancing Health* and student leadership

CHAPTER OUTLINE

CHAPTER OUTLINE (CONTINUED)

KEY TERMS

Accountability
Accreditation
Advocacy
Assertiveness
Certification
Differentiated practice

Empowerment
Forces of Magnetism
Leadership
Magnet hospital
Management
Power

Practice model
Recognition
Responsibility
Shared governance
Transformational leadership

INTRODUCTION

This is the concluding chapter in this text, but in another sense, it is the beginning of your professional journey. Leadership is key to the success of the profession. Content related to leadership is found throughout this text, such as in discussions about healthcare policy, healthcare organizations (HCOs), coordination and collaboration, communication, interprofessional teams, delegation, conflict resolution, evidence-based practice and research, and the Institute of Medicine (IOM) five healthcare core competencies. The discussion that began here will not end with this text or in a course that introduces the critical elements of the nursing profession. Instead, this chapter marks a new beginning because

it highlights key concerns introduced elsewhere in the text and the content focuses on the future of nursing and the need for greater leadership—both for the profession and for individual nurses. You are the future of nursing. This content explores some of the emerging issues, trends, and initiatives in nursing and leadership, but more change certainly is predicted for the future.

LEADERSHIP AND MANAGEMENT IN NURSING

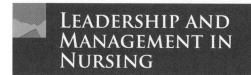

Leadership is important for every nurse, whether the nurse is in a formal administrative/management position or not. Leadership characteristics and skills are required to ensure that patients get the care they need and are important in ensuring that the nursing profession is an active participant in the healthcare delivery system and in the development and implementation of healthcare policy. The topics in this chapter relate to leadership and its importance to nursing, nurses, and patients. The IOM's *Future of Nursing* report (2010) emphasizes the need for nursing to assume more leadership in health care, and to accomplish this nurses need greater leadership competency.

Leadership Models and Theories

To better understand leadership in nursing, a good place to begin is with an overview of leadership models and theories, critical issues, and a comparison of **leadership** and **management**. Leadership and management are not the same, although effective managers need to demonstrate leadership. In general, earlier leadership models and theories emphasized control and getting the job done with little, if any, emphasis on creativity and innovation and staff participation in decision making. The following is a brief summary of some of the key models and theories to illustrate how they have changed over time.

- *Autocratic*: The formal leader (manager/administrator) makes the decisions for the staff; the model assumes staff are not able and not interested in participating in decision making.
- *Bureaucratic*: The focus is on structure, rules, and policies, with decision making placed in the hands of the formal leader (manager/administrator). Staff receive directions. This approach is also related to the autocratic approach.
- *Laissez-faire*: The formal leader (manager/administrator) turns over decision making to the staff, steps back from participation, and lets things happen with little, if any, direction. This can lead to problems because it often means the organization or process may be leaderless.

These approaches have long been used in health care. Indeed, some HCOs still use them or some adaptation of them. Nevertheless, these approaches are not effective in today's rapidly changing environment where staff want to participate more and seeks recognition for their performance and expertise. Over time, new models and theories that built on one another were developed. Often these changes began in other industries and then were adopted by HCOs. Some of these newer theories are highlighted here:

- *Deming's theory*: Effective organizations are dependent on group or team interaction.
- *Drucker's theory*: This theory, which is referred to as modern management, builds on Deming's recognition of the importance of staff group/team participation in the organization and yet also maintains the importance of individual autonomy.
- *Contingency theory*: Multiple variables impact situations, which in turn affects leader–member relationships, tasks, and position power.
- *Connective leadership theory*: The focus is on caring and connecting to others—individuals, groups, and organizations.
- *Emotional intelligence theory*: The focus is on leader–follower relationships, feelings, and self-awareness.
- *Chaos or quantum theory*: A more current theory, this model emphasizes interdependency, sensitivity to change, avoidance of predicting too far into the future, and accountability in the hands of those who do the work.
- *Knowledge management theory*: This theory turns attention to knowledge—the knowledge worker, knowledge-intense organizations, interprofessional collaboration, and accountability. It recognizes the importance of technology and information today. Although this is a new theory, it, too, has historical roots. For example, Drucker used the term *knowledge worker* to describe a person

who works with his or her hands and with theoretical knowledge. Knowledge workers are assets for HCOs—for example, nurses who focus on knowledge rather than titles.

As changes were made in leadership models and theories in the last 20 years, there has been a movement toward greater staff participation, recognition of staff, relationships, and collaboration. This is very different from autocratic, bureaucratic, or even laissez-faire leadership approaches.

As a result of these changes, a newer leadership theory stands out today—a theory that has connections to the theories previously described. This so-called **transformational leadership** is recommended by the IOM (2003b) as the best approach in health care today. This approach emphasizes a positive work environment; recognition of the importance of change and using change effectively; rewarding staff for expertise and performance; and development of staff awareness. Transformational leaders create vision and mission statements with the staff to guide the work of the organization. This leader is described as honest, energetic, loyal, confident, self-directed, flexible, and committed. Staff are able to see these characteristics in a transformational leader and want to work for and with this leader.

Leadership Versus Management

It is easy to confuse leadership and management. A leader can be a leader and not a manager, just as a manager can be a manager and not be a leader. A manager holds a formal administrative position and focuses on four major functions in that position: planning, organizing, leading, and controlling. Today, effective nurse managers need to be able to collaborate, communicate, coordinate, delegate, recognize importance of data and outcomes, manage resources (budget, staff, equipment, supplies, and so on), improve staff performance, build teams, and evaluate effectiveness and efficiency. They use critical thinking and clinical reasoning and judgment,

and they need to be flexible and able to adjust to change, using the planning process.

Leaders gain the position of leadership by their ability to influence others; in contrast, a manager has power because of a formal management position such as team leader, nurse manager, or chief nursing officer. One viewpoint on the difference between leaders and managers is described by Bennis and Goldsmith (1997, p. 4): "There is a profound difference—a chasm—between leaders and managers. A good manager does things right. A leader does the right thing."

With the major changes in management requirements, the following aspects of leadership have become more important (Porter-O'Grady, 1999, p. 40).

- Change focus from process to outcomes
- Align role to the information infrastructure rather than to functional performance
- Focus on team results rather than individual performance
- Manage data complexes rather than individual events
- Facilitate resources that then direct work
- Transfer skill sets rather than make decisions for staff
- Develop staff self-direction rather than giving direction
- Focus on obtaining value rather than simply finding costs
- Focus on consumer-driven structure rather than provider-based system
- Construct horizontal relationships rather than maintain vertical control mechanisms
- Facilitate equity-based partnerships rather than control individual behaviors

Consideration of these factors provides greater opportunity to develop and implement transformational leadership.

There are many myths about leadership that are important to address, and three of them are key to nursing leaders (Goffee & Jones, 2000):

- *Everyone can be a leader.* This is not true. Everyone may have potential to be a leader;

however, it is important to recognize that leadership competencies can and must be developed for a person to actually be a leader.

- *People who get to the top are leaders.* This is not true. There are many people in top administrative positions who would not be described as leaders; in some cases, they cannot even be described as managers.
- *Leaders deliver business results.* This is not true. Leaders do not always meet expected outcomes.

Other authors have echoed the sentiment that *authority* and *leadership* are not interchangeable terms.

> In today's increasingly less hierarchical and more lateral organization structures, leadership is not about position of authority, as much as it is a role of influence. Staff nurses can and must lead through teamwork, through the development of better practices, through the development of centrality in communication networks, and in contributing to the strategic management of units and departments. The leadership role and tasks are pivotal, not peripheral, to the success of the healthcare facilities. (Ferguson & Brindle, 2000, p. 5)

Effective nurse leaders require all the competencies and characteristics mentioned, and it is important that nursing managers are also leaders.

Nursing Management Positions

Nurse managers today carry much more responsibility than in the past. The main purpose of management is to get the job done or to make sure the job is done effectively.

There are three common levels of management. The first level includes managers who work with staff to get the daily work done. The typical title at this level for nursing is nurse manager; this person guides and supervises a unit's staff, both professional and nonprofessional, to ensure that quality patient care is delivered. **Exhibit 14-1** describes nurse manager role characteristics. The second level in an organization consists of middle managers who supervise multiple first-level managers. Such managers might include a nursing director who supervises all the unit nurse managers in the medical division or all the nurse managers in ambulatory care clinics and the emergency department. The upper level is the chief nursing officer. This nurse manager is responsible for the overall work of the nursing service and in some cases may be responsible for other services. Middle-level managers report to the upper-level managers.

What is described here is the most common organization for nursing; however, there are variations from organization to organization. In addition, there are usually some staff who may hold nonmanagerial positions but also need to be effective leaders. These individuals do not have supervisory responsibilities and do not always direct staff, but they must influence staff. For example, a clinical nurse specialist (CNS), advanced practice nurse (APRN), or clinical nurse leader (CNL) may hold this type of position. Another specialist role that has become more important today as health care increases its use of informatics is the nurse informaticist. The nurse informaticist needs leadership competency to guide staff effectively.

Shared Governance: Empowering Nursing Staff

"**Shared governance** can be viewed as a management philosophy, a professional practice model, and an accountability model that focuses on staff involvement in decision making, particularly in decisions that affect their practice" (Finkelman, 2012, p. 126). Through shared governance, nurses in an organization can (Hess, 2004):

1. Control their professional practice
2. Influence organizational resources that support practice

Exhibit 14-1	Role Characteristics of the Nurse with Unit-Based or Service Line–Based Authority

- Promoting care delivery with respect for individuals' rights and preferences
- Participating in nursing and organizational policy formulation and decision making involving staff, such as in shared governance
- Accepting organizational accountability for services provided to recipients
- Evaluating the quality and appropriateness of health care
- Coordinating nursing care with other healthcare disciplines and assisting integrating services across the continuum of health care
- Participating in the recruitment, selection, and retention of personnel, including staff representative of the population diversity
- Assessing the impact of plans and strategies to address such issues as ethnic, cultural, and diversity changes in the population, political and social influences, financial and economic issues, the aging of society and demographic trends, and ethical issues related to health care
- Assuming oversight for staffing and scheduling personnel considering scope of practice, competencies, patient needs, and complexity of care
- Providing appropriate orientation for new staff and individual feedback on staff development and progress

- Encouraging staff members to attain education, credentialing, and continuing professional development
- Evaluating performance of personnel in a fair and transparent manner
- Developing, implementing, and monitoring the budget for defined area(s) of responsibility
- Participating in and involving the nursing staff in evaluative research activities to promote evidence-based practice
- Facilitating educational experience for nursing and other students
- Encouraging shared accountability for professional practice
- Advocating for a work environment that minimizes work-related illness and injury
- Reporting any injuries or safety hazards and taking corrective action as quickly as possible
- Providing an open forum of communication with staff, allowing them ample opportunities to discuss issues and seek guidance
- Understanding and complying with state and federal laws concerning the healthcare services and practice they manage and complying with all the facility regulations and policies

Source: From American Nurses Association. (2009). *Nursing administration: Scope and standards of practice* (pp. 16–18). Silver Springs, MD. Reprinted with permission.

3. Gain formal authority, which is granted by the organization
4. Participate in decision making through committee structure
5. Access information about the organization
6. Set goals and negotiate conflict

In this type of organization, nurses assume an active role in the management of the patient care services. Shared governance is a management model, but it also emphasizes the need for nurses to share accountability and responsibility. Nurses have the authority to make sure the right decisions

are made about the work that they do. **Accountability** means that the nurse accepts responsibility for outcomes or is answerable for what is done. **Responsibility** is to be "entrusted with a particular function" (Ritter-Teitel, 2002, p. 34). These aspects of management are connected to autonomy, or the right to make decisions and control actions. The best situation occurs when the nurse who provides care is also the staff member who works to resolve issues and ensure that patient outcomes are achieved at the point of care, limiting the number or layers of staff who must be involved. Shared governance is dependent on effective collaboration, communication, and teamwork and spreads departmental and organizational decision making over a large number of staff. This approach, however, does not mean that managers can ignore their managerial and leadership responsibilities or that all decisions are made by the staff. If the process blocks decision making—by taking too long to make a decision, for example—this model will not be effective.

Shared governance is not easy to develop, and it can become a barrier to delivery of efficient, high-quality care. It takes time to be effective. Neither staff nor leaders/managers should assume that the approach relieves leaders and managers of their responsibility to do their jobs. Decision making is more decentralized and takes place through a designated committee or council structure, but both staff and managers have responsibilities and accountability. Typically, hospitals that use a shared governance model find that staff are more satisfied and turnover is lower. Staff like working in the organization. Not all hospitals use shared governance, and how it is implemented and its effectiveness can vary widely.

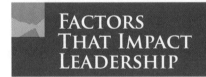

FACTORS THAT IMPACT LEADERSHIP

Generational Issues in Nursing: Impact on Image

Nursing today is composed of three active generations: (1) baby boomers, (2) Generation X, and (3) Generation Y. The so-called traditional generation is no longer in practice, but it had a significant impact on the nursing profession and current practice. **Box 14-1** identifies the time frames for these nursing generations.

Generational issues are important because the generations are part of the image of nursing and have an impact on nursing leadership. When a person thinks of a nurse, which generation or age

Box 14-1	Current Generations in Nursing
Traditional generation	Born 1930–1940
Baby boomers	Born 1941–1964
Generation X	Born 1965–1980
Generation Y (also called millennials)	Born 1981–present

groups are considered? Most people probably do not realize that there is not one age group, but rather several represented in nursing. Nurses in these four generations are different from one another. How does this affect the image of nursing? It means that the image of nursing is one of multiple age groups with different historical backgrounds. How nurses from each generation view nursing can be quite different, and their educational backgrounds vary a great deal, from nurses who entered nursing through diploma programs to nurses who entered through baccalaureate programs. Some of these nurses have seen great changes in health care, and others see the current status as the way it always has been. Technology, for example, is frequently taken for granted by some nurses, whereas others are overwhelmed with technological advances. Some nurses have seen great changes in the roles of nurses, whereas other nurses now take the roles for granted—for example, the advanced practice nurse. If one asked a nurse in each generation for the nurse's view of nursing, the answers might be quite different. If these nurses then tried to explain their views to the public, the perception of nursing would most likely consist of multiple images.

The situation of multiple generations in one profession provides opportunities to enhance the profession through the diversity of the age groups and their experiences, but it has also caused problems in the workplace. What are the characteristics of the various groups? How well do they mesh with the healthcare environment? How well do they work together? The following list summarizes some of the characteristics of each generation, including the traditional generation and its impact (American Hospital Association [AHA], 2002; Bertholf & Loveless, 2001; Finkelman, 2012; Gerke, 2001; Santos & Cox, 2002; Ulrich, 2001; Wieck, Prydun, & Walsh, 2002):

- *The traditional, silent, or mature generation, born 1930–1940*: This generation is important now because of its historical impact on nursing, but members of this group are no longer in practice. This group of nurses was hard working, loyal, and family focused, and they felt that the duty to work was important. Many served in the military in World War II and the Korean War. This period occurred prior to the women's liberation movement. The characteristics of the traditional generation had a major impact on how nursing services were organized and what the expectations of management of nurses were. Some of this impact has been negative, such as the emphasis on bureaucratic structure, and it has been difficult to change in some healthcare organizations.

- *Baby boomers, born 1940–1964*: This generation, which is currently the largest in the work arena, is also the group moving toward retirement. This trend is predicted to lead to greater nursing shortage problems in the future. The baby boomer generation grew up in a time of major changes, including the women's liberation movement, the civil rights movement, and the Vietnam War. They had fewer professional opportunities than are available to nurses today because the typical career choices for women were either teaching or nursing. This began to change as the women's liberation movement grew. Within this generation, fewer men went into nursing, as was true of the previous generation. This group's characteristics include independence, acceptance of authority, loyalty to the employer, workaholic tendencies, and less experience

with technology, although many in this group have led the drive for adoption of more technology in nursing. This generation is often more materialistic and competitive and appreciates consensus leadership. It is a generation whose members chose a career and then stuck to it, even if they were not very happy with that choice.

- *Generation X (Gen-X), born 1965–1980*: The presence of Generation X, along with Generation Y, is growing in nursing. Members of this group will assume more nursing leadership roles as the baby boomers retire. Gen-Xers are more accomplished in technology and very much involved with computers and other advances in communication and information; they have experienced much change in these areas in their lifetimes. These nurses want to be led, not managed, and they have not yet developed high levels of self-confidence and empowerment. What do they want in leaders? They look for leaders who are motivational, who demonstrate positive communication, who appreciate team players, and who exhibit good people skills—leaders who are approachable and supportive. Baby boomers, in contrast, would not look for these characteristics in a leader. Gen-Xers typically do not join organizations (which has implications for nursing organizations that need more members and active members), do not feel that they must stay in the same job for a long time (which has implications for employers that experience staff turnover and related costs), and feel that they want a good balance between work and personal life (which means that they are not willing to bring work home). Compared to earlier generations of nurses, members of Generation X are more informal, pragmatic, technoliterate, independent, creative, intimidated by authority, and loyal to those they know; they also appreciate diversity more. By contrast, the baby boomers with whom the Gen-Xers are working often see things very differently: Baby boomers are more loyal to their employer, stay in the job longer, are more willing to work overtime (although they are not happy about it), and have greater long-term commitment. These differences can cause problems between the two generations, with baby boomers often occupying supervisory positions or senior faculty positions and Gen-Xers found in staff positions or beginning faculty positions, but moving into more leadership positions.

- *Generation Y (nexters, millennials, Generation Next, myPod generation, Gen-Y), born 1980–present*: The millennials are the generation primarily entering nursing now, although second-career students and older students are also entering the profession, representing earlier generations. Key characteristics of this generation are optimism, civic duty, confidence, achievement, social ability, morality, and diversity. In work situations, they demonstrate collective action, optimism, tenacity, multitasking, and a high level of technology skill, and they are also more trusting of centralized authority than Generation X. Typically, they handle change better, take risks, and want to be challenged. This generation is connected to cell phones, personal tablets, and various methods for social networking. They are tech savvy and expect to multitask. Sometimes, however, this makes it difficult for them to focus on one task.

In a profession that includes representatives from multiple generations, it is necessary to recognize that age diversity means great variations in positive and negative characteristics among staff. Some will pull the profession backward if allowed, and some will push the profession forward. "In the workplace, differing work ethics, communication preferences, manners, and attitudes toward authority are key areas of conflict" (Siela, 2006, p. 47).

This also has an impact on the nursing profession's image; it is not a profession that encompasses just one type of person or one age group. People in different age groups are now entering nursing. As one generation moves toward retirement, the next generation will undoubtedly have an impact on the image of nursing. It is critical to avoid gender role stereotyping and to increase the strength of nurses as one group of professionals, while still recognizing that these differences exist and appreciating how they might impact the profession.

Power and Empowerment

Power and empowerment are connected to the image of nursing and the ability to assume leadership. How one is viewed can impact whether the person is viewed as having **power**—power to influence, to say what the profession is or is not, and to influence decision making. Nurses typically do not like to talk about power; they find it to be philosophically different from their view of nursing (Malone, 2001). This belief—that is, viewing power only in the negative—acts as a barrier to success as a healthcare professional. But what are power, powerlessness, and empowerment?

To feel as if one is not listened to or not viewed positively can make a person feel powerless. Many nurses believe that they cannot make an impact in clinical settings, and they are not listened to or sought out for their opinions. This powerlessness can result in nurses feeling like victims. The result may be resentment that is expressed as incivility. Such a feeling of powerlessness can act against nurses when they do not actively address issues such as the image of nurses and when they allow others to describe what a nurse is or to make decisions for nurses. This failure to be proactive merely worsens their image.

What nurses want and need is power—to be able to influence decisions and have an impact on issues that matter. It is clear that power can be used constructively or destructively, but the concern here with the nursing profession is using power constructively. Power and influence are related. Power is about control to reach a goal. "Power means you can influence others and influence decisions" (Finkelman, 2012, p. 341). There is more than one type of power, as described in **Box 14-2**. The type of power a person possesses has an impact on how it can be used to reach goals or outcomes.

Empowerment is also an important issue with nurses today (Finkelman, 2012). To empower is to enable to act—a critical need in the nursing profession. Basically, empowerment is more than just saying you can participate in decision making; staff need more than words. Empowerment is needed in day-to-day practice as nurses meet the needs of patients in hospitals, in the community,

and in home settings. Empowerment also implies that some individuals may lose their power while others gain power.

Staff who experience empowerment feel that they are respected and trusted to be active participants. Staff who feel empowered also demonstrate a positive image to other healthcare team members, patients and their families, and the public. Nurses who do not feel empowered will not be effective in conveying a positive image, because they will not be able to communicate that nurses are professionals with much to offer. Empowerment that is not clear to staff is just as problematic as no staff empowerment. Empowered teams feel a responsibility for the team's performance and activities, which in turn can improve care and reduce errors.

Control over the nursing profession is a critical issue that is also related to the profession's image. Who should control the nursing profession, and who does? This is related to independence and autonomy—key characteristics of any profession. But a key question persists: *What should be the image of nursing?* As a profession, nursing does not appear to have a consensus about its image, given that the types of advertising and responses to these initiatives vary. Nursing needs to control the image and visibility of the profession, and in doing so, may exert more control over the solutions for the following four issues:

1. If nurses had a more realistic image, it would be easier to support the types of services that nurses offer to the public.
2. If nurses had a more realistic image, it would be easier to support an entry-level baccalaureate degree to provide the type of education needed.
3. If nurses had a more realistic image, it would be easier to support the need for reimbursement for nursing services, which involve much more than hand holding.
4. If nurses had a more realistic image, it would be easier to participate in the healthcare dialogue on the local, state, national, and international levels to influence policy.

> ## Box 14-2 Types of Power
>
> - *Informational power:* Power that arises from the ability to access information and share information.
> - *Referent power:* A type of informal power that exists when others recognize that a person has special qualities and is admired; others are willing to follow that person.
> - *Expert power:* Power that exists when a person is respected for his or her expertise, and others will follow. The person may or may not be in a management position; staff may follow another staff member because they feel that person has expertise.
> - *Coercive power:* Power that is based on punishment when someone does not do what is desired. For example, the result might be loss of a raise or promotion, which is a decision made by a supervisor who has formal power.
> - *Reward power:* Power that comes from the ability to reward others when they do as expected. In this case, the person would have to be in a position of authority—for example, a manager.
> - *Persuasive power:* Power that occurs when a person uses persuasion to influence others.

Assertiveness

Assertiveness is demonstrated in how a person communicates—direct, open, and appropriate in respect to others. When a person communicates in an assertive manner, verbal and nonverbal communication become congruent, making the message clearer. Assertive and aggressive communications are not the same. Assertive persons are better able to confront problems in a constructive manner and do not remain silent; they frequently use *I* statements. The problems that the nursing profession has with its image have been influenced by nursing's silence—the inability to be assertive, which is also a critical leadership competency.

Smith (1975) identified some critical rules related to assertive behavior that can easily be applied to the difficulties that nursing has experienced with changing its image, increasing its visibility, and developing leadership—areas that continue to need improvement.

- Avoid over-apologizing.
- Avoid defensive, adverse reactions, such as aggression, temper tantrums, backbiting, revenge, slander, sarcasm, and threats.
- Use body language—such as eye contact, body posture, gestures, and facial expressions—that is appropriate to and that matches the verbal message.
- Accept manipulative criticism while maintaining responsibility for your decision.
- Calmly repeat a negative reply without justifying it.
- Be honest about feelings, needs, and ideas.
- Accept and/or acknowledge your faults calmly and without apology.

Other examples of assertive behavior were identified by Katz (2001, p. 267):

- Express feelings without being nasty or overbearing.
- Acknowledge emotions but remain open to discussion.

- Express self and give others the chance to express themselves equally.
- Use *I* statements to defuse arguments.
- Ask for and give reasons.

Advocacy

Advocacy is speaking on behalf of something important, and it is one of the major roles of a nurse. Leaders are advocates. Typically, one thinks of advocacy for the patient and family, populations, and communities; however, nurses also need to be advocates for themselves and for the profession as a whole. To do this successfully, nurses need to feel empowered and be assertive. All nurses represent nursing—acting as advocates in their daily work and in their personal lives. When someone asks a nurse, "What do you do?", the nurse's response is a form of advocacy. The goal is to have a positive, informative, and accurate response.

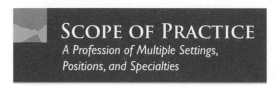

SCOPE OF PRACTICE
A Profession of Multiple Settings, Positions, and Specialties

Multiple Settings and Positions

The practice of nursing takes place in multiple settings, thus offering multiple job possibilities for an individual over the career span. Many nurses change their settings and specialties based on interest and jobs that they want to pursue. Some examples of the many different nursing settings and positions are provided here:

- *Hospital-based or acute care nursing*: This is the area that most students think of first when considering jobs in nursing. It is what is most frequently illustrated in the media (films, television, and so on). Within this setting are multiple specialty opportunities and both clinical and administrative/management/education positions.

- *Ambulatory care*: This is a growing area for nurses, and these venues are considered to be community-based settings. Many types of ambulatory care settings exist, such as clinics, private practice offices, ambulatory surgical centers (both freestanding and associated with hospitals), and diagnostic centers (both freestanding and associated with hospitals). Nurses hold both clinical and administrative/management positions in ambulatory care facilities.

- *Public/community health*: This area, which is growing rapidly, is an important clinical site for nursing students, and within this setting are multiple opportunities. Examples include clinical and administrative/management/education positions in public/community health departments, clinics, school health facilities, tuberculosis control centers, immunization clinics, home health, substance abuse treatment, mental health, and more.

- *Home care*: This setting is very broad, in that numerous home health agencies exist across the United States. Some are owned and managed by government agencies, such as city health departments. Some agencies are owned and managed by other HCOs, such as a hospital. Home health agencies may also be part of national healthcare corporations, for-profit HCOs, or not-for-profit HCOs. Nurses in home care practice in the patient's home. They may also hold administrative/management positions, and some may even own home health agencies.

- *Hospice and palliative care*: This type of setting may be partnered with home care, or it may be a freestanding service. Hospice or palliative care can also be associated with an inpatient unit that is either part of a hospital system or a freestanding facility. Hospice or palliative care has a special mission: to include patients, families, and significant others in the dying process and to make the patient as comfortable as possible while meeting the patient's wishes. Palliative care or comfort care is also used when a life-threatening condition is present that may or may not result in death. Many acute care hospitals now have palliative care teams that provide support to the patient, family, and the staff for a dying patient or a family, for example, who have experienced a fetal demise or neonatal death.

- *Nurse-managed health centers (NMHCs)*: NMHCs are expected to proliferate due to the increased healthcare insurance coverage provided through the Affordable Care Act of 2010. These centers are community-based primary healthcare services that operate under the leadership of an advanced practice nurse, and that focus on health education, health promotion, and disease prevention. The population targeted by the NMHC is usually the underserved. NMHCs are not-for-profit organizations, typically use a sliding scale for payments, and may be Federally Qualified Health Centers (Kovner & Walani, 2010). Since 2010, the number of these centers has grown. In 2012, the National Nursing Centers Consortium (NNCC), a nonprofit member association representing more than 200 nurse-managed centers throughout the United States, was formed. (See "Linking to the Internet" at the end of this chapter.)

- *School nursing*: This setting was also mentioned as an example of public/community health nursing. The focus is on the provision of healthcare services within schools. The role of the school nurse is changing dramatically. Some schools have very active clinics where nurses provide a broad range of healthcare services to students.

- *Occupational health*: This is a unique setting for nursing practice. Nurses who work in this area provide healthcare services in occupational or work settings. Occupational health nurses provide emergency care; direct care including assessment, screenings, and preventive care; and health and safety education. They also initiate referrals for additional care. Some schools of nursing offer graduate degrees in this area.

- *Telehealth/telemedicine*: Nurses work in telehealth by monitoring patients, providing patient and family education, and directing care changes. Home health may also use this method, although it is not common.
- *Parish nursing*: Parish nursing takes place in a faith-based setting, such as a church or synagogue. The nurse is often a member of the organization. Services might include screenings and prevention, health education, and referral services. The members of the faith-based organization are the population whom the nurse serves.
- *Office-based nursing*: Nurses work in physician practices. APRNs may have their own practices or be part of a physician practice. These nurses provide assessment and direct services, assist the physician, monitor and follow up with patients, and teach patients and families. APRNs provide more advanced nursing care.
- *Extended care and long-term care:* Many nurses work in this area, and with the aging population needs will increase in this area of care. Nurses provide assessment, direct care, and support to patients and support and education to families.
- *Management positions*: Nurse managers are found in all HCOs. The key responsibilities of this functional position are staffing, recruitment, and retention of staff, planning, budgeting, staffing, supervising, quality improvement (QI), staff education, and ensuring overall functioning of the nurse manager's assigned unit, division, or department.
- *Nursing education (academic and staff education)*: This is a functional position. Academic

faculty teach in a nursing education program. Nurses may also hold positions in staff development or staff education within HCOs, focusing on staff orientation, ongoing staff education, and the maintenance of continued competencies.

- *Nursing research*: Nurses are involved in nursing research and research conducted by other healthcare providers. They fill many research roles, including serving as the primary investigator leading a research study, collecting data, and analyzing data. Some healthcare institutions refer to this role as a nurse scientist. These nurses are not just doing nursing research; they are also responsible for helping other interdisciplinary team members conduct research.
- *Informatics*: Nurses are active in the area of informatics as a specialty and as a part of their other responsibilities. A nurse might serve on the informatics committee or participate in planning for an electronic medical record; or if the nurse has advanced informatics expertise, the nurse may lead or help with major organizational informatics planning, implementation, and evaluation.
- *Nurse entrepreneurship*: Nurses may serve as consultants or own a healthcare-related business. This is an area that most nursing students do not know much about, as it is a less common role for nurses; however, it is likely that this area will expand in the future.
- *Nurse navigator*: This nurse helps a patient and family navigate the healthcare system. The nurse may coordinate care among several disciplines or provide a bridge between transitional care settings. For example, the patient who has cancer and is discharged home will need care coordination between the acute care facility and the oncology and radiology services. The patient may also need home visits. The nurse navigator helps find services and coordinates the care.

- *Nurse coach*: A nurse coach is a registered nurse who integrates coaching competencies into any setting or specialty area of practice to facilitate a process of change or development that assists individuals or groups to realize their potential (Hess, Dossey, Southard, Luck, Schaub, and Bark, 2013, p. 1). For example, a nurse coach may work with clients to promote health and wellness, help clients cope with chronic illness such as diabetes, or provide education, cardiac rehabilitation, or end-of-life care. Some nurse coaches focus on managerial coaching. The Affordable Care Act of 2010 refers to coaches (Section 4001, 2010): "Partnerships include practitioners of integrative health, preventive medicine, health coaching, public education and more" (Hess et al., 2013, p. 22).
- *Legal nurse consultant*: This nurse usually has completed additional coursework related to legal issues and health care, and the nurse may even be certified in this area. The legal nurse consultant works with attorneys and provides advice about health issues, reviews medical records and other documents, and assists with planning responses to cases. Nurses may be expert witnesses providing expert testimony for cases. Such a nurse should be an expert in the area addressed in the legal case—for example, a psychiatric–mental health nurse would act as the expert witness in a case involving a patient who was injured in a mental health unit.

It is unknown what the future holds for new healthcare settings or new roles, but nursing history has demonstrated that the likelihood of new roles emerging is highly. In an interview with nursing leaders, Porter-O'Grady commented that mobility and portability will become very important in technotherapeutic interventions (Saver, 2006). Technology will extend into patients' lives, and the settings in which care is received will be less connected to hospitals. Others suggest that as patients demand more control

as consumers, there will be more self-diagnostic tests (Saver, 2006). Examples might be apps that are used to monitor and identify medical problems, or monitor diet or exercise. New roles for nurses, in turn, will emerge. For example, nurses will assume more active roles in positions concerned with healthcare quality, in pharmaceutical companies, as nurse practitioners in clinics located in retail stores, managing research and development departments of equipment or biomedical companies, working in or leading medical homes, and in counseling (Saver, 2006). All of this change is occurring now and requires greater nursing leadership competency.

Nursing Specialties

Nursing specialties are part of the profession and expand professionalism. There are numerous general specialties in nursing, such as maternal–child (obstetrics)/women's health, neonatal, pediatrics, emergency, critical care, ambulatory care, public/community health, home health, hospice, surgical/perioperative, psychiatric/mental health/behavioral health, nurse–midwifery, management, legal nurse consulting, nursing consulting, and many more. There are also subspecialties such as diabetic care, wound care, and dialysis. The most important reason why specialties develop is to meet the need for focused practice experience and to ensure that nurses receive the necessary education to provide specialized nursing. Nurses may also become interested in a type of patient or care setting and want to learn more about it, gain more experience, and work in that area. All specialty nursing is based on the core general nursing knowledge and competencies. The same specialty might be offered in multiple settings—for example, a certified nurse–midwife might work in a hospital in labor and delivery, in a private practice with obstetricians, in a clinic, in a freestanding delivery center, in patients' homes, or in his or her own private practice.

There are two ways to view a specialty. One view is based on the nurse who works in a specialty area and thus claims it as his or her specialty (e.g., the nurse works in a behavioral health unit and is considered a psychiatric nurse). A second view, combined with the first, is that the nurse has additional education and possibly certification in a specialty. For example, the psychiatric nurse may have a master's degree in psychiatric–mental health nursing and may be certified in this specialty. The key to truly functioning as a specialty nurse is making a commitment to gain additional education in the specialty. This also includes continuing education.

There are many titles in nursing, but they all do not necessarily indicate a nurse's specialty. These titles are advanced practice nurse/nurse practitioner (APRN), clinical nurse specialist (CNS), and clinical nurse leader (CNL). For certified nurse–midwives (CNM) and certified registered nurse anesthetists (CRNA), their specialties are clear from their titles (midwifery and anesthesia, respectively). An APRN may focus on one or more multiple specialties, such as families, pediatric acute care, adult–gerontology primary care or acute care, pediatric primary care, neonatal nurse practitioner, and psychiatric–mental health. A CNL does not focus on a specific clinical group in the degree program; instead, this is a functional role that may be used in any type of specialty area. For example, a CNL may serve in a medical unit, a pediatric unit, or a women's health unit. The clinical nurse specialist title is also a broader term, but the CNS master's degree does focus on a specific clinical area. Specialty education at the graduate level and certification support professionalism in nursing and help to ensure that nursing remains a profession.

Nurse leaders must continually support staff and the need for professionalism within the work setting. They do this by recognizing education and degrees through differentiated practice, encouraging ongoing staff education (continuing education and academic), ensuring that standards are maintained, working to increase staff participation in decision making, helping staff who want to move into a management position accomplish this goal

(e.g., by directing staff to administration-focused education to prepare for the role), and mentoring staff who want to pursue the administrative track. Nurse leaders also need to encourage staff to participate in professional organizations, publish in professional journals, attend professional conferences, submit abstracts for presentations, and then need to recognize these staff accomplishments throughout the organization.

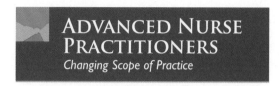

ADVANCED NURSE PRACTITIONERS
Changing Scope of Practice

There has been increasing development in the role of the advanced nurse practitioner. Part of this is the result of Affordable Care Act, but there are other reasons for this trend as well.

> Nurses' role in primary care has recently received substantial scrutiny, as demand for primary care has increased and nurse practitioners have gained traction with the public. Evidence from many studies indicates that primary care services, such as wellness and prevention services, diagnosis and management of many common uncomplicated acute illnesses, and management of chronic diseases such as diabetes can be provided by nurse practitioners at least as safely and effectively as by physicians. (Laurent, Reeves, Hermens, Braspenning, Grol, & Sibbald, 2005, as cited in Fairman, Rowe, Hassmiller, & Shalala, 2010, p. 280)

In its 2010 report on the future of nursing, the IOM recommended expansion of nurses' scope of practice in primary care focused on advanced practice. The critical factor that limits nurse practitioners' scope of practice is state-based regulations. The website for the Center to Champion Nursing in

America (see "Linking to the Internet" at the end of this chapter) provides resources about nursing and about nurse practitioners and their scope of practice. Data are provided describing how specific states regulate nurse practitioner practice.

Other changes are occurring as the result of legislation that are important to the APRN scope of practice. One example is the movement to allow APRNs to sign home health plans of care and certify Medicare patients for home health benefits. Recognizing that to make this change there would need to be legislation, in 2013 bills were introduced in both the U.S. House of Representatives (H.R. 2504) and the Senate (S. 1332 Home Healthcare Planning Improvement Act) and endorsed by the American Nurses Association and others. These bills would allow payment for home health services to Medicare beneficiaries when those services were delivered by (1) a nurse practitioner, (2) a clinical nurse specialist working in collaboration with a physician in accordance with state law, (3) a certified nurse–midwife, or (4) a physician assistant under a physician's supervision. This change would facilitate providing greater home care services to the rural and underserved areas. Because this is federal legislation, it must be passed by both the House and the Senate and signed by the president to become law; however, both bills were referred to committee in 2013, and both now sit waiting in their respective committees for further action. It is not unusual for bills to get frozen in committee and never to move forward. The IOM report of 2011 highlights many new position opportunities for APRNs such as in community health centers, nurse-managed health centers, medical/health homes, and accountable care organizations, but just because they are listed in legislation does not mean they will be implemented or implemented as described.

A number of barriers exist to expanding the role of nurse practitioners in primary care, particularly state laws that limit scope of practice, payment policies, and professional tensions between nurse practitioners, physicians, and physician assistants.

Policy solutions need to (1) remove unwarranted restrictions on scope of practice, (2) equalize payment and recognize nurse practitioners as eligible providers, (3) increase nurses' accountability, (4) expand nurse-managed centers, (5) address professional tensions and focus more on interprofessional teams, (6) fund education for the primary care workforce, and (7) fund research to examine outcomes (Naylor & Kurtzman, 2010).

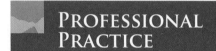

PROFESSIONAL PRACTICE

Today, professional **practice models** are described as having an impact both on the nursing profession and on quality care. Some HCOs are developing, or have developed, their own professional practice models. Differentiated practice, shared governance, and collaboration are important elements of a successful professional practice model, all discussed elsewhere in this text.

Differentiated Practice

Differentiated practice is part of developing a professional practice model. The subject of the level of entry into nursing practice continues to be an issue in the nursing profession. In 1965, a decision was made to establish the bachelor of science in nursing (BSN) as the nursing entry-level degree. This has not yet fully occurred, although several current reports continue to recommend that the BSN should be the entry-level degree (Benner, Sutphen, Leonard, & Day, 2010; IOM, 2010). Associate degree in nursing programs are growing faster than the BSN programs; there are more associate nursing degree graduates, and more associate degree graduates than BSN graduates are practicing today. Despite the emphasis on the BSN in **Magnet hospitals**, data published in 2014 indicated that in these hospitals, regardless of hospital size, staff degrees were broken down in this way: 35.86%, associate degree; 8.46%, diploma; 51.78%, BSN; and 3.78%, master/graduate degree in nursing. The data are somewhat better for pediatric Magnet hospitals: 24.06%, associate degree; 5.58%, diploma; 65.78%, BSN; and 4.50%, master/graduate degree. The number of nursing staff with BSN degrees is a critical factor achieving Magnet status, yet even in Magnet-designated hospitals the percentage of BSN graduates is not high. Clearly, there is still a long way to go before the BSN becomes the entry-level degree (Magnet Program, 2014).

Graduates from all types of nursing programs take the same licensure exam, and this complicates the issue. Registered nurse (RN) licensure is the same for all the graduates regardless of the type of degree earned. Boston (1990) defined differentiated nursing practice as "a philosophy that focuses on the structuring of roles and functions of nurses according to education, experience, and competence" (p. 1). This does not mean that a graduate from one program is necessarily better than another, because many individual factors would determine this. Rather, it indicates that graduates from each program enter practice with different competencies.

Differentiated practice needs to be more evident in nursing. Most employers do not recognize an RN's degree. It is rarely noted on employee identification badges, and if noted, the degree designation is difficult to read on the small name badges. Salaries are most likely not based on the education level of the nurse, although they should be. Much needs to be done by the profession to address this area of concern, and this requires professional leadership.

Examples of Professional Practice Models

Examples of some professional practice models are found in **Figures 14-1, 14-2, 14-3, 14-4**, and **14-5**. Some of these models are not used today, but it is important to understand the evolution of models because sometimes they return or are revised and used as a new model. Notably, the functional model is used less today. Total care is often used in areas such as critical care. Primary care was very popular in the 1980s, but it is less so now because it requires a greater number of RNs. However, some HCOs still use the primary care model today, usually as an adaptation of the original model. The Forces of Magnetism for Magnet hospitals emphasizes the need for HCOs to implement a professional practice model.

TEAM NURSING STRUCTURE

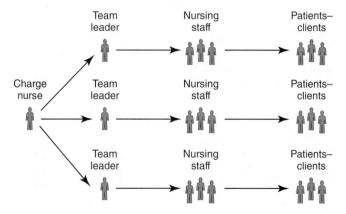

Figure 14-1 Team Nursing Model

Source: From Hansten, R. I., & Jackson, M. (2004). *Clinical delegation skills: A handbook for professional practice.* Sudbury, MA: Jones and Bartlett.

FUNCTIONAL NURSING STRUCTURE

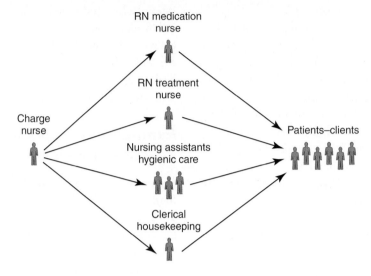

Figure 14-2 Functional Nursing Model

Source: From Hansten, R. I., & Jackson, M. (2004). *Clinical delegation skills: A handbook for professional practice.* Sudbury, MA: Jones and Bartlett.

Why does an HCO need a professional practice model for nursing? The description of the Magnet forces provides some reasons for the need: "Conceptual models provide an infrastructure that decreases variation among nurses, the interventions they will choose, and, ultimately, patient outcomes. Conceptual frameworks also differentiate forward thinking organizations from those where nursing has less of

TOTAL CARE NURSING STRUCTURE

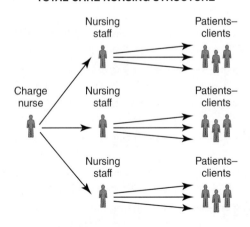

Figure 14-3 Total Patient Care Model

Source: From Hansten, R. I., & Jackson, M. (2004). *Clinical delegation skills: A handbook for professional practice.* Sudbury, MA: Jones and Bartlett.

PRIMARY NURSING STRUCTURE

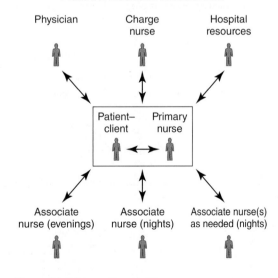

Figure 14-4 Primary Care Model

Source: From Hansten, R. I., & Jackson, M. (2004). *Clinical delegation skills: A handbook for professional practice.* Sudbury, MA: Jones and Bartlett.

CASE MANAGEMENT MODEL

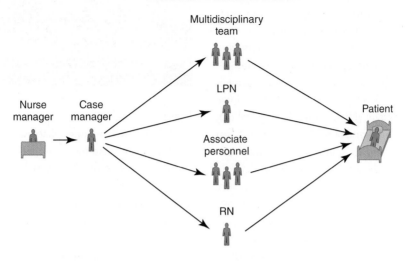

Figure 14-5 Case Management Model

Source: From Hansten, R. I., & Jackson, M. (2004). *Clinical delegation skills: A handbook for professional practice.* Sudbury, MA: Jones and Bartlett.

a voice" (Kerfoot, Lavandero, Cox, Triola, Pacini, & Hanson, 2006, p. 20). These forward-thinking organizations also tend to have a professional rather than technical view of nursing. A model offers nurses "a consistent way of framing the care they deliver to patients and their families" (p. 21).

The American Association of Critical-Care Nurses' Synergy Model for Patient Care is one example (Kerfoot et al., 2006). This model's core premise is closely related to the IOM's five core competencies, particularly patient-centered care. It states that the needs of patients and families drive the characteristics and competencies of the nurse (Kerfoot et al., 2006). The Synergy Model for Patient Care identifies eight important competencies: clinical judgment, clinical inquiry (innovator/evaluator; evidence-based practice, quality improvement, and innovative solutions), caring practices, response to diversity, advocacy and moral agency (ethics), facilitation of learning, collaboration, and systems thinking (American Association of Critical-Care Nurses, 2010). This model can be applied to all types of units, not just critical care. In fact, many hospitals use this model in critical care units

as well as in other units. The Synergy Model for Patient Care identifies standards that are a part of the model. Within this model, patient characteristics are resiliency, vulnerability, stability, complexity, resource availability, participation in care, participation in decision making, and predictability. This is a good fit with the IOM core competencies.

There are other examples of new innovative models (Kimball, Cherner, Joynt, & O'Neil, 2007, pp. 393–394):

- Designing a model that provides the feel of a 12-bed hospital within a large hospital (Baptist Hospital of Miami, Miami, Florida) led to a model for a primary care team led by a patient care facilitator who monitors the nursing team. The team covers 12–16 beds. Key elements in this model are as follows: (1) Every patient deserves an experienced RN. (2) Every novice nurse deserves mentoring. (3) Every patient should have the opportunity to participate in care. (4) Every team member is committed to the needs of the patients. (5) Each team member functions within a defined professional scope of practice.

(6) Work intensity decreases with improved work distribution processes and team support. (7) The model of nursing care is an important element in patient safety and patient, staff, and physician satisfaction.

- The collaborative patient care management model was developed by High Point Regional Health System (High Point, North Carolina). It is a multidisciplinary, population-based case management model. In this model, high-volume, high-risk, and high-cost patients in disease-specific or population-based groups are targeted to reduce length-of-stay and costs and improve patient outcomes.

- The transitional care model focuses on comprehensive hospital planning, care coordination, and home follow-up of high-risk elders (University of Pennsylvania Medical Center). APRNs play a major role in this model of care, working with the elders and guiding their transition to home; in addition, the APRN may implement the plan of care in the elder's home. Dr. Mary Naylor's work in this area has become a national model for examining the cost-effectiveness of managing the transition from hospital to home and between care settings. Her work is an example of comparative effectiveness research that examines the best practice or the effectiveness of a type care—in this case, the transition model (Naylor, Hirschman, O'Connor, Barg, & Pauly, 2013).

Innovative new professional practice models have common elements (Kimball et al., 2007). Specifically, they include an elevated RN role; greater focus on the patient; efforts to smooth patient transitions and handoff to decrease errors and make the patient more comfortable; leveraging of technology to enable care model design, such as electronic medical records, robots, bar coding, cell phone communication, and more; and being driven by results or outcomes. The IOM core competencies also provide an effective start for a professional practice model.

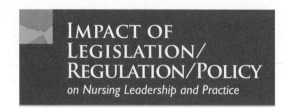

IMPACT OF LEGISLATION/ REGULATION/POLICY

on Nursing Leadership and Practice

Legislation, regulations, and policies emphasize the need for nurses to work collaboratively with other stakeholders in shaping health policy through legislation and regulation. Nurses are involved and will continue to be involved at the local, state, national, and international levels. The current critical health policy issue is the healthcare reform passed in 2010, that is, the Patient Protection and Affordable Care Act. The increasing cost of health care, the increasing number of uninsured and underinsured individuals, and the growing aging population (along with concerns about the ability of Medicare funds to cover all of their care) are all forces that have helped to propel healthcare reform forward, though it has been an intense political battle. The 2010 legislation, which focuses primarily on reimbursement/insurance, impacts nurses and nursing care, and now the implementation phase requires active nursing participation to further develop this important policy. The initiative to enroll currently uninsured people in health insurance met the goal of more than 8 million in early 2014, though this does not mean everyone in the United States has health insurance. It will take time to evaluate the results of this initiative with regard to individual consumer satisfaction, access to care, and quality of care—and, of course, cost of care.

Related to legislation and regulation at the state level, over the last decade many agencies, including state workforce centers, have examined the issue of the nursing shortage. State workforce centers focus on maintaining an adequate supply of qualified nurses within a state to meet healthcare needs, providing analysis and strategies to address unmet needs (National Forum of State Nursing Workforce Centers, 2014). The American Academy of Nursing recently held a technology conference to examine work redesign and the use of technology as a means to transform nursing care. As this initiative evolved, a commission on the workforce was formed, led by representatives from both practice and education. It was quickly recognized that responses to the nursing shortage problem must address the pipeline issue—that is, the faculty shortage, which in turn reflects on educational preparation of the workforce. A subcommittee addressing this issue included regulators from the National Council of Boards of Nursing, accreditation groups such as the National League for Nursing and the American Association of Colleges of Nursing, and officials from higher education and practice. The focus of their work is to identify barriers to increasing enrollments and redesigning education at all levels. To make sweeping changes in this area, regulatory bodies will also need to be included in the conversations to shape the new nursing educational models of the future. The need to produce more nurses does not necessarily mean a compromise on quality of education, but it does mean consideration of differences (Scott & Cleary, 2007).

At the national level, a provision in the Patient Protection and Affordable Care Act (U.S. Public Law 111-148, 2010) established the National Health Care Workforce Commission. Its purposes are fivefold: (1) serve as a resource for Congress, the president, and localities; (2) coordinate activities of the Departments of Health and Human Services, Labor, Veterans Affairs, Homeland Security, and Education; (3) develop and evaluate education and training activities; (4) identify barriers to improved federal, state, and local coordination and recommend ways to address barriers; and (5) encourage innovation. The commission is composed of 15 members (each serving a 3-year term), and the commission as a whole reports to Congress. Membership must include no less than one representative from the following categories:

- Healthcare workforce and health professions
- Employers
- Third-party payers

- Experts in healthcare services and health economics research
- Consumer representatives
- Labor unions
- State or local workforce investment boards
- Educational institutions

The first chairperson of the National Health Care Workforce Commission was a nurse, and other nurses serve on the commission. Though this commission was established is not yet functioning due to lack of fund allocation. This is an example of how legislation can initiate change, but if there is limited or no funding the initiative can be blocked.

There is no doubt that quality care is a major issue being addressed by healthcare legislation. Nurses need to be involved in these initiatives because they directly impact patient care every day in multiple settings. Healthcare legislation at the state level is also important to nurses. For example, many states are trying to pass legislation related to mandatory overtime and staff–patient ratios—and some states have already enacted these types of laws.

There is a nurses' caucus in Congress made up of nurses who serve in Congress. It serves as an important resource for nursing. More nurses are needed to run for office at the local, state, and national levels. Nurses who have an interest in politics and health policy have to plan for this activity, particularly if they want to run for office eventually. This requires a career plan with a time frame and experience in political activities.

Regulation is also an important issue today as change occurs both within the healthcare system and within nursing. One example is the initiative to change regulations related to advanced practice nurses, focusing on changes to allow APRNs to practice independently of physicians, when appropriate. This has not yet occurred in all states. Much of this change is occurring at the state level; however, there is often greater emphasis on the need for changes related to such issues as expansion of reimbursement for APRNs on the federal level. This represents a major change, and it will not be easy to accomplish.

ECONOMIC VALUE AND THE NURSING PROFESSION

Salaries and benefits have long been a concern of nurses. Salaries and benefits vary across the United States. Some nurses have unionized to get better salaries and benefits and to have more say in the decision-making process in the work setting. The nursing profession as a whole has yet to develop effective methods for determining their value in the reimbursement process, and it is important to solve this problem. How does nursing describe the value of nursing services? How does nursing identify costs of nursing services? Some efforts have been made to accomplish this, but there is much more to do. The IOM (2010) comments on this problem by saying that within the fragmented healthcare system, nursing contributions are even more difficult to identify. Most HCOs' accounting systems are not able to capture or differentiate economic value provided by nurses (IOM, 2010, pp. 3–26).

APRNs have brought the issue of payment for nursing services to the forefront. Some examples of issues that have arisen relate to reimbursement. The Federal Employee Compensation Act—a law provides healthcare services to federal employees who are injured on the job—has become very important to APRNs. It is one of the last major federal healthcare programs to deny patient access to advanced practice nurses. APRNs are covered medical providers in Medicare, Medicaid, Tri-Care, and some private insurance plans, and they serve as medical providers in the Veterans Administration, the Department of Defense, and the Indian Health Service. If they choose, most federal employees have access to APRNs through their federal employee health benefit plan.

Because greater emphasis has been placed on healthcare quality, there is now more focus on a pay-for-performance model—third-party payers and government paying for quality care (Saver, 2006). This change is exemplified by the Centers for Medicare and Medicaid Services' and other insurers' refusal to pay for certain complications experienced by patients. In turn, this policy has had an impact on nursing care and on budgetary decisions related to nursing. Because nurses are involved in most of the care that would relate to these complications, nurses have an opportunity to exhibit leadership in this area and demonstrate that they can have a major impact on the quality of care and cost of care by developing effective interventions to assess risk and to prevent these complications. Nurses also need to demonstrate leadership in data collection, analysis of data, and discussion of interventions to resolve problems at all levels throughout hospitals.

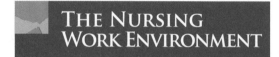

THE NURSING WORK ENVIRONMENT

The Work Environment and Leadership

Quality care is best provided in a healthy, functional work environment. Key issues are staff safety; communication; collaborative, positive work relationships; work design (space/facility); work processes; infrastructures that support staff participation in decision making; and an emphasis on positive work environments that support (reduce staff stress/burnout and high turnover rates) and seek to develop staff. The IOM (2010) report on nursing highlights the unique needs of new graduates and recommends nurse residency programs as a means to increase retention of staff and ensure quality of care. The nursing profession is currently focusing much of its attention on APRNs; however, most nurses are not APRNs but rather staff nurses who have complex needs and work in a complex environment. If these needs are not addressed, the omission will have a major negative impact on patient care—more significantly, it will affect quality as well as nursing practice. We need to know more about the problems, but more importantly nursing needs, to actively address the problems for all nurses and not just focus on APRNs.

Interprofessional Teams and the Work Environment

Interprofessional teams are critical in today's healthcare workplace. The IOM identifies the ability to use interprofessional teams effectively as one of the core healthcare professions competencies, and teams have a major impact on the work environment. Despite this well-known need, an effective approach to preparing nursing students and other healthcare profession students to work on teams is still lacking. The assumption is these individuals will be able to work on teams after they graduate—but that outcome does not necessarily happen. Newhouse and Mills (2002, pp. 64–69) identified key points related to nurse–physician relationships that are important in the development of effective interprofessional teams:

- All teams are not created equal, but careful development of working relationships and clear goals can make all the difference.
- Successful groups are composed of competent team members with the necessary skills, abilities, and personalities to achieve the desired objectives.
- Teams composed of many professions/disciplines are able to expand the number and quality of actions to improve healthcare systems.
- Interprofessional teams work collaboratively to set and achieve goals directed toward innovative and effective care and efficient organizational systems.
- Nurses on the team represent the voice of nursing as a discipline responsible for the holistic care of patients.
- Positive relationships with physicians benefit the patient and enhance the work environment for nurses.
- Nurses must develop the skills to work collaboratively as professional members of the interprofessional team.

Improving the Work Environment

Nurses need to take the lead in HCOs to improve the work environment—by identifying concerns, helping to identify supporting data and analyzing the data, understanding retention of staff, assisting in the development of strategies to resolve problems, and tracking outcomes to improve care. It has been noted that staff are using work-arounds more, and this increases risk of errors in a work environment. A work-around is a "rushed, improvised response to a breakdown in a work process, without pausing to analyze and correct the underlying problem" (Finkelman & Kenner, 2012, p. 222). Efforts to improve and to develop an effective, healthy work environment need to consider the IOM five core competencies and critical elements in the work culture. **Exhibits 14-2** and **14-3** describe examples of improvement strategies.

The March 2014 issue of *Charting Nursing's Future*, a newsletter that was created following the publication of the IOM's *Future of Nursing* report, describes an emerging blueprint for change to transform the nurses' work environment that recommends providers, policy makers, and educators use the following strategies ("An Emerging Blueprint for Change," 2014, p. 8):

- Monitor nurse staffing and ensure that all healthcare settings are adequately staffed with appropriately educated, licensed, and certified personnel
- Create institutional cultures that foster professionalism and curb disruptions
- Harness nurse leadership at all levels of administration and governance
- Educate the current and future workforce to work in teams and communicate better across the health professions

All of these strategies relate directly to the healthcare professions core competencies discussed throughout this text.

Exhibit 14-2   Transition Policy and Strategies

Goal: Anticipate and prepare the nurse labor market for impending shortages, thereby reducing their duration and impact and lowering the economic and noneconomic costs to patients, nurses, and hospitals.

Strategies	Transition Policy
Demand strategies	Speed up development and adoption of technology and use nonprofessional nursing personnel more effectively
	Remove barriers to efficiency and redesign the work content and organization of nursing care
	Strengthen management decision making
	Avoid regulating nurse staffing
Supply strategies	Accommodate an older RN workforce
	Accelerate improvements in working conditions
	Expand the capacity of nursing education programs
	Continue to inform the public about opportunities in nursing
Wage strategies	Assist hospitals and other healthcare employers in financing needed RN wage increases
	Avoid imposing controls on RN wages

Source: From Buerhaus, P. I., Staiger, D. O., & Auerbach, D. I. (2009). *The future of the nursing workforce in the United States: Data, trends, and implications.* Sudbury, MA: Jones and Bartlett.

Finding the Right Workplace for You

Students really begin the process of finding the right work environment for themselves when their clinical courses begin. You as a student nurse begin to consciously or unconsciously assess each work environment you encounter, asking, "Would I want to work here?" In doing so, you also begin to integrate the ideas, "What is a nurse?" and "Is this profession

---

Exhibit 14-3   Long-Run Policy and Strategies

Goal: Expand employment of RNs in the long run by eliminating barriers that lead to an inadequate supply of RNs and by appropriately valuing the contributions of RNs.

Strategies	Long-Run Policy
Supply strategies	Remove barriers to hiring foreign-educated RNs
	Remove stigmas and barriers facing men and Hispanics
Demand strategies	Reinforce development of pay-for-performance systems
	Increase the number of nursing-sensitive outcomes included in pay-for-performance systems

Source: From Buerhaus, P. I., Staiger, D. O., & Auerbach, D. I. (2009). *The future of the nursing workforce in the United States: Data, trends and implications.* Sudbury, MA: Jones and Bartlett.

right for me?" Socialization into the profession begins. By the time senior year arrives, of course, nursing students are actively beginning to consider positions after graduation. Review Appendix B to have a better understanding of staffing, which is a critical issue to consider when assessing positions, and Appendix C, which provides tips related to finding the right workplace for you

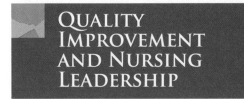

QUALITY IMPROVEMENT AND NURSING LEADERSHIP

There is no question that nurses need to be more active in QI on multiple levels. Staff nurses are critical in preventing quality-related problems, identifying QI concerns on a daily basis, and participating in QI programs at the clinical team level. They should also participate in organization-wide QI activities at all levels. Nurse managers and administrators need to be leaders in the organization in setting QI direction and determining strategies to improve care at all levels. Some nurses should serve in key QI positions. At the health policy level, nurses should be active at the local, state, and federal levels in the development of QI health policy; they can take on many roles to provide leadership in the health policy-making process. Nursing faculty provide QI leadership by ensuring that students, both undergraduate and graduate, are prepared to practice and utilize evidence-based practice and evidence-based management. The following sections discuss examples of some new initiatives that relate to QI and nursing leadership in the need to improve care.

Transforming Care at the Bedside

The creation of Transforming Care at the Bedside (TCAB) is a result of the IOM quality reports.

The development of this initiative began in 2003 through the Institute for Healthcare Improvement (IHI) in conjunction with the Robert Wood Johnson Foundation (Martin, Greenhouse, Merryman, Shovel, Liberi, & Konzier, 2007). The IHI is an effective initiative that provides multiple strategies for improving health care. "The goal is to make fundamental improvements in the healthcare delivery system that will result in safe and reliable care, vitality and teamwork, patient-centered care, and value-added care processes" (p. 445). In 2008, the TCAB program was implemented in 10 hospitals, starting locally (such as in a hospital unit) and then spreading throughout a hospital. The approach that was taken established pilots in hospitals at the level of direct care, which could then have a greater impact.

TCAB looks not only at innovative change, but also at the outcomes from the change. Did care improve? Was care monitored using indicators such as injury from falls, adverse events, readmission, voluntary turnover of RNs, patient satisfaction, and percentage of nurses' time in direct patient care? Examples of some of the innovative ideas that have been tested follow (IHI, 2008):

- Use of rapid response teams to rescue patients before a crisis occurs
- Specific communication models that support consistent and clear communication among caregivers
- Professional support programs such as preceptorships and educational opportunities
- Liberalized diet plans and meal schedules for patients
- Redesigned workspace that enhances efficiency and reduces waste

TCAB has had an impact by introducing effective, innovative changes that can be used in many hospitals. This initiative provides many opportunities for nurses to assume leadership in improving healthcare delivery—leadership can occur at the level of the staff nurse, the nurse manager, or other nurse administrative positions. The TCAB website (listed in the "Linking to the Internet" section of this chapter) provides information on the TCAB framework and current TCAB projects.

Magnet Nursing Services Recognition Program

It is important that nurses take active roles in determining the quality of care and the nurse's role in the process. Nurses run the risk of taking the blame for some of the problems that are found in acute care today. "Politics in healthcare may not end at the bedside, but it certainly begins there. It would be a tragedy if patients and family members blamed nurses for system failures. But the more nurses detach from their patients, the easier it becomes for the rest of us (consumers) to lose sympathy" (Kaplan, 2000, p. 25). The Magnet program is one way to address this issue.

In 1981, researchers conducted a study that explored the issue of attracting and retaining nurses (McClure, Poulin, Sovie, & Wandelt, 1983). This investigation was undertaken before the beginning of the major nursing shortage over the last 8 years; however, the study has played a significant role in attempts to address the shortage because it identified some methods for improving recruitment and retention of nurses. The researchers sought to identify factors or variables that led some acute care hospitals to be more successful in recruitment and retention than other hospitals. The objectives of the Magnet program respond to these needs (American Nurses Credentialing Center [ANCC], 2008):

- Promote quality in a setting that supports professional practice
- Identify excellence in the delivery of nursing services to patients/residents
- Disseminate best practices in nursing services

The Magnet recognition program was established in 1993 and is administered by the ANCC's Commission on the Magnet Recognition Program. Recognition is awarded to acute care hospitals and long-term care facilities. Any size hospital that meets the standards may apply for Magnet status. It is not an easy process to get Magnet status.

The ANCC defines **accreditation** as a voluntary process used to validate that an organization and an approval body meet established continuing education standards. **Certification** focuses on the individual and is a process used to validate that an individual RN possesses the requisite knowledge, skills, and abilities to practice in a defined practice specialty. **Recognition** is a process used to evaluate an organization's adherence to excellence-focused standards (Urden & Monarch, 2002, pp. 102–103). The Magnet program is a recognition program, not an accreditation program.

The first step for an organization that wants to apply for Magnet status recognition is to complete a self-assessment using materials provided by the program. The organization then has a better idea about where it stands and what needs to be improved before completing the application to achieve recognition. The recognition process does not focus solely on management; staff nurses must be involved in all steps in the process. After extensive sharing of information, an on-site survey is completed by the Magnet Recognition Program surveyors. After recognition is obtained—and not all organizations that apply receive Magnet status—the organization must maintain the standards; participate in the American Nurses Association's quality indicator study coordinated by the National Center for Nursing Quality; and provide certain annual monitoring reports to ensure that the requirements for Magnet recognition continue to be met over time. Studies do indicate that achieving recognition has a positive impact on Magnet HCOs, such as improving professional practice, clinical competence, and job experience—all of which influence staff retention rates (Aiken, Clarke, Sloane, Lake, & Cheney, 2008; Havens, 2001; Stone, Larson, Mooney-Kane, Smolowitz, Lin, & Dick, 2006; Ulrich, Buerhaus, Donelan, Norman, & Dittus, 2007). Recognition is not permanent, however, and the HCO must apply for renewal. A website is maintained with current information about the program, and the link is found in the "Linking to the Internet" section of this chapter.

A hospital that has Magnet status also demonstrates a different form of management, focusing more on participative management in which staff have input into decisions, with managers listening to staff, and typically using a decentralized structure, such as shared governance. This difference in management is evident in the role of the nurse executive and throughout all levels of nursing management, as well as in the overall organizational leadership's support of nursing. Effective leadership is present. Staff feel that nursing leaders in the organization understand their needs and provide resources and support for the work that staff do daily. Nurse managers and their roles are also critical to the success of these hospitals. These hospitals have more nurses with BSN degrees because this is a Magnet requirement. Nurses are very active in committees, projects, and so on. Evidence-based practice is actively pursued, and the hospitals are involved in nursing research. Clearly, staffing is of critical concern, and Magnet hospitals use innovative methods to respond to recruitment and retention issues and to provide appropriate levels of staffing per shift. Staff education is valued; there are opportunities for quality staff development, and staff who want to pursue additional academic degrees are encouraged to do so. Promotion can occur through the management track, which is the most common method, but it also should occur through the clinical track. Magnet HCOs offer both opportunities. These HCOs demonstrate higher levels of quality of care, autonomy, a nursing model, mentoring, professional recognition, and respect, and they enable staff to practice nursing as it should be practiced (McClure et al., 1983).

Research in this area did not stop with the original 1981 study. Multiple studies that support the positive impact of Magnet recognition have been conducted. These HCOs have better outcomes—lower burnout rates, higher levels of job satisfaction, and higher quality of care—than non-Magnet HCOs (Laschinger, Shamian, & Thomson, 2001). Another study (Kramer & Schmalenberg, 2002) re-examined 14 Magnet hospitals and identified eight variables that are important in providing quality care. These variables relate to nursing leadership demonstrated by formal leaders in management positions and by staff leaders, emphasizing transformational leadership (pp. 53–55):

1. Working with other nurses who are clinically competent
2. Good nurse–physician relationships
3. Nurse autonomy and accountability
4. Supportive nurse manager-supervisor
5. Control over nursing practice and practice environment
6. Support for education
7. Adequacy of nurse staffing
8. Paramount concern for patients

There are now significant research results that indicate that Magnet HCOs tend to provide quality care that leads to positive outcomes for patients and better work environments for nurses (Aiken, 2002).

As a result of the research on the Magnet program, 14 **Forces of Magnetism** were identified. These forces are organized into five components—structural empowerment; exemplary professional practice; transformational leadership; new knowledge, innovations, and improvements; and empirical quality results (ANCC, 2014). These variables are used to evaluate an HCO and determine whether it can be designated as a Magnet HCO. Nurses who are considering new positions can use these variables to guide their job search, as the variables assist nurses to learn more about the HCO and to assess whether it would be a positive workplace. If the HCO already has Magnet status, the forces should be present, but if not, the nurse applicant can still use the forces as a personal checklist. **Exhibit 14-4** describes the current Magnet forces, which represent the organizational elements of excellence in nursing care.

Exhibit 14-4   Forces of Magnetism

Transformational Leadership

Today's healthcare environment is experiencing unprecedented, intense reform. In a break from yesterday's leadership requirement for stabilization and growth, today's leaders are required to transform their organization's values, beliefs, and behaviors. It is relatively easy to lead people where they want to go; the transformational leader must lead people to where they need to be to meet the demands of the future. This requires vision, influence, clinical knowledge, and a strong expertise relating to professional nursing practice. It also acknowledges that transformation may create turbulence and involve atypical approaches to solutions.

The organization's senior leadership team creates the vision for the future and the systems and environment necessary to achieve that vision. They must enlighten the organization as to why change is necessary and communicate each department's part in achieving that change. They must listen, challenge, influence, and affirm as the organization makes its way into the future. Gradually, this transformational way of thinking should take root in the organization and become even stronger as other leaders adapt to this way of thinking.

The intent of this model component is no longer just to solve problems, fix broken systems, and empower staff, but to actually transform the organizations to meet the future. Magnet-recognized organizations today strive for stabilization; however, healthcare reformation calls for a type of controlled destabilization that births new ideas and innovations.

Forces of Magnetism Represented:

- Quality of Nursing Leadership (Force No. 1)
- Management Style (Force No. 3)

Structural Empowerment

Solid structures and processes developed by influential leadership provide an innovative environment where strong professional practice flourishes and where the mission, vision, and values come to life to achieve the outcomes believed to be important for the organization. Further strengthening practice are the strong relationships and partnerships developed among all types of community organizations to improve patient outcomes and the health of the communities they serve. This is accomplished through the organization's strategic plan, structure, systems, policies, and programs. Staff need to be developed, directed, and empowered to find the best way to accomplish the organizational goals and achieve desired outcomes. This may be accomplished through a variety of structures and programs; one size does not fit all.

Forces of Magnetism Represented:

- Organizational Structure (Force No. 2)
- Personnel Policies and Programs (Force No. 4)
- Community and the Healthcare Organization (Force No. 10)
- Image of Nursing (Force No. 12)
- Professional Development (Force No. 14)

Exemplary Professional Practice

The true essence of a Magnet organization stems from exemplary professional practice within nursing. This entails a comprehensive understanding of the role of nursing; the application of that role with patients, families, communities, and the interdisciplinary team; and the application of new knowledge and evidence. The goal of this component is more than the establishment of strong professional practice; it is what that professional practice can achieve.

Forces of Magnetism Represented:

- Professional Models of Care (Force No. 5)
- Consultation and Resources (Force No. 8)
- Autonomy (Force No. 9)
- Nurses as Teachers (Force No. 11)
- Interdisciplinary Relationships (Force No. 13)

New Knowledge, Innovation, and Improvements

Strong leadership, empowered professionals, and exemplary practice are essential building blocks for Magnet-recognized organizations, but they are not the final goals. Magnet organizations have an ethical and professional responsibility to contribute to patient care, the organization, and the profession in terms of new knowledge, innovations, and improvements. Our current systems and practices need to be redesigned and redefined if we are to be successful in the future. This component includes new models of care, application of existing evidence, new evidence, and visible contributions to the science of nursing.

Force of Magnetism Represented:

- Quality Improvement (Force No. 7)

Empirical Quality Results

Today's Magnet recognition process primarily focuses on structure and processes, with an assumption that good outcomes will follow. Currently, outcomes are not specified and are minimally weighted. There are no quantitative outcome requirements for American Nurses Credentialing Center Magnet Recognition. Recently lacking were benchmark data that would allow comparisons with best practices. This area is where the greatest changes need to occur. Data of this caliber will spur needed changes.

In the future, having a strong structure and processes are the first steps. In other words, the question for the future is not "What do you do?" or "How do you do it?" but rather "What difference have you made?" Magnet-recognized organizations are in a unique position to become pioneers of the future and to demonstrate solutions to numerous problems inherent in our healthcare systems today. They may do this in a variety of ways through innovative structure and various processes, and they ought to be recognized—not penalized—for their inventiveness.

Outcomes need to be categorized in terms of clinical outcomes related to nursing; workforce outcomes; patient and consumer outcomes; and organizational outcomes. When possible, outcomes data that the organization already collects should be utilized. Quantitative benchmarks should be established. These outcomes will represent the report card of a Magnet-recognized organization, and a simple way of demonstrating excellence.

Force of Magnetism Represented:

- Quality of Care (Force No. 6)

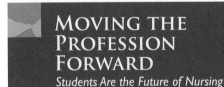

MOVING THE PROFESSION FORWARD
Students Are the Future of Nursing

The Future of Nursing: Leading Change, Advancing Health

The Future of Nursing: Leading Change, Advancing Health (IOM, 2010) is a landmark report from the IOM that addresses the need for nursing leadership. By virtue of its numbers and adaptive capacity, the nursing profession has the potential to effect wide-ranging changes in the healthcare system. Nurses' regular, close proximity to patients and scientific understanding of care processes across the continuum of care give them a unique ability to act as partners with other health professionals and to lead in the improvement and redesign of the health care system and its many practice environments (IOM, 2011, p. S-3).

Related to the 2010 IOM report, the Robert Wood Johnson Foundation conducted a Gallup poll in 2010 entitled "Nursing Leadership from Bedside to Boardroom" (Blizzard, Khoury, & McMurray, 2010). The purpose of the poll was to ask opinion leaders about their views of nursing leadership, particularly nurses' role in the future and potential barriers. Past Gallup Polls typically indicated that the public rated nurses as highly ethical and honest; however, the question was why nurses continued to lag behind as leaders in the healthcare delivery system. The following were the key findings of this opinion poll about healthcare leadership and nursing:

- Respondents rated doctors and nurses first and second out of a list of options for *trusted* information about health and health care.
- Government and insurance executives will have a great deal of influence in health reform in the next 5 to 10 years.
- Respondents perceived patients and nurses as having the least amount of influence in health reform in the next 5 to 10 years.
- Reducing medical errors and increasing the quality of care are two areas where nurses now have a great deal of influence in policy and management.
- Relatively few opinion leaders say nurses currently have a great deal of influence in increasing access to care, including primary care.
- Reducing medical errors, increasing quality of care, and promoting wellness top the list of areas in which large majorities of opinion leaders would like nurses to have more influence.
- Major barriers to nurses' increased influence and leadership were identified as not being perceived as important decision makers or revenue generators compared with doctors; nurses' focus on primary care rather than preventive care, and nursing not having a single voice in speaking on national issues.
- Suggestions for nurses to take on more of a leadership role included making their voices heard and having higher expectations.

These results, which were identified in 2010 just as the Affordable Care Act became law and the *Future of Nursing* report was published, do not paint a positive picture of nursing, but do identify some areas that require active nursing strategies to improve and develop leadership. Some of these elements have improved since 2010, but much more work by nurses is needed.

The *Future of Nursing* report focuses on three nursing areas that need transformation: practice, education, and leadership. The leadership approach discussed is transformational leadership, with its emphasis on collaborative management. The report supports the leadership competencies discussed throughout this text. In particular, it supports interprofessional collaboration and quality improvement by noting that it is important to learn "to be a full partner in a health team in which members from various professions hold each other accountable for improving quality and decreasing preventable adverse events and medication errors" (IOM, 2010, pp. 5–4). Leadership is needed among nurses who hold any position, and this need even extends to nurses who assume more entrepreneurial and business approaches.

In 2014, Sigma Theta Tau International (STTI) joined the effort to improve nursing leadership, albeit from a global perspective. It formed the Global Advisory Panel on the Future of Nursing (GAPFON), whose purpose is to serve as a catalyst to stimulate partnerships and collaborations to advance global health outcomes (STTI, 2014b). This initiative is directly related to the STTI theme, "Serve Locally, Transform Regionally, Lead Globally" (STTI, 2014a).

Susan Hassmiller, a nursing advisor to the Robert Wood Johnson Foundation, identified her vision for a 21st-century nursing workforce, which is related to the recommendations in the IOM's *Future of Nursing* report (2010). This vision includes the following interconnected processes (Hassmiller, 2011):

- Develop nurse-led innovations
- Generate evidence
- Redesign education
- Embrace technology
- Diversify our workforce
- Expand scope of practice
- Foster interprofessional Relationships
- Develop leadership at every level
- Be at the table

Student Leadership

Students need to begin developing their leadership skills while in their nursing educational program.

This can be done by participation in student organizations, such as the National Student Nurses Association (NSNA); working to be invited into Sigma Theta Tau International; or taking on leadership roles in courses and in other on-campus and off-campus activities. The NSNA also offers a leadership academy for student nurses (see the link in the "Linking to the Internet" section at the end of this chapter). Developing leadership takes time, and every nurse needs leadership skills to practice in today's complex healthcare system.

Moving forward implies change. Many people do not like change or do not feel comfortable with it. During an interview, the nurse leader Porter-O'Grady stated, "'Our work isn't changing. Change is our work.' He tells nurses, 'If you looked at change like that, it wouldn't be an enemy'" (Saver, 2006, p. 24). Patton, another nurse leader who served as president of the American Nurses Association, advised, "See opportunities instead of challenges" (Saver, 2006, p. 24). Nurses entering the profession have before them a healthcare delivery system in need of repair, as has been noted by the IOM and reaffirmed in multiple IOM reports. This challenge can be seen as an impossible task or as an opportunity for nurses to step in and assume new roles and expand old roles, if need be. Reforming the U.S. healthcare delivery system requires that nurses are educated, are competent in all five IOM core competencies, provide quality nursing care, are able to communicate and collaborate with others, use political skills, and advocate for patients, families, communities, and the nursing profession. Nurses need to base their decisions on evidence-based practice, whether they are in clinical practice, nursing administration, or nursing education. They need to understand the possibilities that come with technology, participate in determining how technology can be used, and then use it effectively. Change should be based on data and analysis of data. Data will come from QI, another area in which nurses need to step up and participate so that they are among the healthcare professionals who drive quality improvement, thereby influencing how health care is provided. Last but not least, nurses of the future need to recognize that money drives most decisions. Understanding how money flows and how to communicate the value of nurses and nursing care is an important nursing responsibility.

Linda Burns-Bolton, vice president and chief nursing officer at Cedars-Sinai Medical Center, believes that in the future, "Nurses will get the evidence they need when they need it, get information for patients when they need it, deliver safe care, communicate with team members, engage with family members, and leave work feeling satisfied" (Saver, 2006, p. 25). Her view of the future really covers the key elements found in this text and the five IOM core competencies (IOM, 2003a) but is not yet fully realized.

1. Provide patient-centered care
2. Work in interprofessional/disciplinary teams
3. Employ evidence-based practice
4. Apply quality improvement
5. Utilize informatics

Landscape © f9photos/Shutterstock, Inc.

CONCLUSION

This text's content is an introduction to nursing as a profession, to the healthcare system, and, most importantly, to patients, their families, and communities. Nursing is a dynamic profession with multiple possibilities. A nurse can participate in many different nursing positions throughout a career. Some positions require additional education; others do not. As described in this chapter, there are many different settings in which nurses practice. The future holds more change that will lead to new possibilities. You will have the responsibility as a nurse to participate actively in the profession to advocate for your patients (individuals, families, populations, communities) and demonstrate leadership in your practice.

CHAPTER HIGHLIGHTS

1. There is much change occurring in nursing and in health care today.
2. The IOM (2004) report on nursing suggests that transformational leadership is the most effective leadership style. Transformational leaders are confident, self-directed, honest, loyal, and committed, and they have the ability to develop and implement a vision.
3. A leader may or may not hold a formal management position.
4. Nurses should influence how the healthcare delivery system works and be actively involved in healthcare delivery changes in all the clinical, management, or education positions that they may hold.
5. Nursing practice occurs in multiple settings, positions, and specialties.
6. Differentiated practice, shared governance, and collaboration are important elements of a successful professional practice model.
7. Legislation, regulation, and policy emphasize the need of nurses to work collaboratively with other stakeholders in shaping health policy through legislation and regulation.
8. The economic value of nursing focuses on salaries and benefits, but it also needs to consider the value of nurses themselves and how the healthcare delivery system values nursing care.
9. Quality care requires a work environment focused on the need for a healthy, functional work environment.
10. Nurses need to assume active leadership roles in QI.
11. The Magnet Recognition Program recognizes hospitals that provide quality nursing care or excellence in nursing care.
12. The goal of the Transforming Care at the Bedside program is to make improvements in the healthcare delivery system.
13. The IOM's *Future of Nursing* report has had a major impact on nursing education and practice.
14. Students have responsibility to develop leadership competency.

DISCUSSION QUESTIONS

1. Why is leadership important in nursing? Your response should demonstrate knowledge of the differences between leadership and management.
2. Consider one of the issues in this chapter and conduct a literature review on the issue. Share your critique with classmates. How does the issue apply to leadership?
3. What is the Magnet Recognition Program? Why is it important?
4. Visit the website for the Center to Champion Nursing in America (see "Linking to the Internet"). Why is this type of website important to nursing leadership?
5. Why should you as a student begin to work on your leadership competencies?

Landscape © f9photos/Shutterstock, Inc.

CRITICAL THINKING ACTIVITIES

1. What is a nursing professional practice model? Describe one type of model.
2. Visit YouTube on the Internet, and search for "nursing" or "nurses." What do you find? View one of the selections and critique the image portrayed. Discuss your findings in a team with classmates.
3. Explore the American Association of Critical-Care Nurses Synergy Model for Patient Care website (http://www.aacn.org/wd/certifications/content/synmodel.pcms?menu=certification). What do you think about this model of patient care?
4. Consider how the five core competencies might be used as a framework for a professional practice model. Describe your model in narrative form and graphically on large paper your instructor provides. Post it in the classroom. Each team should then explain its model.
5. After completing Critical Thinking Activity 4, each team should review another team's vision and decide which education, regulatory, and practice issues are involved. What role does leadership play?

ELECTRONIC *Reflection Journal*

Circuit Board: ©Photos.com

What do you think the future holds for nursing? Develop your vision of the future of nursing. Save this vision and review it every 6 months while in school to see if your vision changes; then review it again after graduation as you enter into practice. You may find your vision of the future of nursing changes.

Landscape © f9photos/Shutterstock, Inc.

LINKING TO THE INTERNET

- American Association of Critical-Care Nurses: Synergy Model for Patient Care: http://www.aacn.org/wd/certifications/content/synmodel.pcms?menu=certification
- American Nurses Association: Current Federal Legislation: http://www.nursingworld.org/MainMenuCategories/Policy-Advocacy/Federal
- Center to Champion Nursing in America: http://campaignforaction.org
- Institute for Health Improvement: http://www.ihi.org
- Magnet Recognition Program: http://www.nursecredentialing.org/Magnet.aspx
- National Nursing Centers Consortium: http://www.nncc.us/site/
- National Student Nurses Leadership Academy: http://www.nasn.org/AboutNASN
- Transforming Care at the Bedside (TCAB): http://www.ihi.org/engage/initiatives/completed/tcab/pages/default.aspx

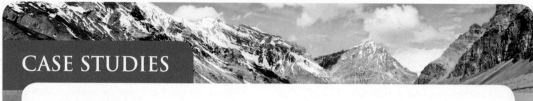

CASE STUDIES

Landscape © f9photos/Shutterstock, Inc.

Case Study 1

The CNL functions as a care coordinator either at the unit level or in a practice. For example, Ms. Apple heads up a busy practice in a cancer institute. As a CNL, she acts as a mentor to novice nurses while coordinating care and helping patients navigate the healthcare maze.

In one patient's case, Ms. Apple identified the need for transportation to and from radiation appointments. She also recognized financial counseling needs because the patient was no longer able to work, and her husband was on disability. Treatment plans needed to be explained, and teaching the patient about medications was necessary. A referral had been made to a radiation interventionist. The family needed knowledge about the problems and explanation about all aspects of care. The CNL pulled the interprofessional team together to ensure clear communication and the creation of an interdisciplinary plan of care.

In some institutions, these positions are called nurse navigators; in others, CNLs, depending on the organization's structure and needs. The CNL, having expertise in interprofessional communication, financial management, and human relations, serves the patient and family to protect and ensure quality patient-focused care and promote safety.

Case Questions

1. Search the Internet to find HCOs that have CNL positions. What can you learn about this new position?
2. Find nursing programs on the Internet that offer the CNL master's degree. Compare and contrast them.
3. How does this new position apply or not apply to the IOM core competencies?

Case Study 2

You have taken a new position as a head nurse for a 30-bed unit. You have been working in the hospital for 7 years—for the first 4 years as a staff nurse and for the last 3 years as the assistant nurse manager on a surgical unit. However, the new position means you have to change units. The chief nursing officer has worked to get you a mentor, another nurse manager, to help you as you transition to the new role and new unit. Before you meet with your mentor for the first time as a mentee, you consider the following questions.

Case Questions

1. What is your personal view of the transformational leadership style? Do you feel competent in applying this style? Why or why not? How might the leadership style of the previous nurse manager impact your transition to the position?
2. What should your unit assessment plan include as you assume your new role?
3. You have been told that the unit has an RN retention problem that has been increasing over the last 2 years. What more do you need to know about the problem?
4. The nursing department uses shared governance. How might this impact you and your new position?

Landscape © f9photos/Shutterstock, Inc.

REFERENCES

Aiken, L. (2002). Superior outcomes for Magnet hospitals: The evidence base. In M. McClure & A. Hinshaw (Eds.), *Magnet hospitals revisited* (pp. 61–81). Washington, DC: American Nurses Publishing.

Aiken, L., Clarke, S., Sloane, D., Lake, E., & Cheney, T. (2008). Effects of hospital care environment on patient mortality and nurse outcomes. *Journal of Nursing Administration, 38*(5), 223–229.

American Association of Critical-Care Nurses. (2010). The AACN synergy model for patient care. Retrieved from http://www.aacn.org/wd/certifications/content/synmodel.pcms?menu=certification

American Hospital Association (AHA). (2002). *In our hands: How hospital leaders can build a thriving workplace.* Chicago, IL: Author.

American Nurses Association (ANA). (2010). *Nursing, scope and standards of practice.* Silver Spring, MD: Author.

American Nurses Credentialing Center (ANCC). (2008). Goals of Magnet program. Retrieved from http://www.nursecredentialing.org/Magnet/ProgramOverview

American Nurses Credentialing Center (ANCC). (2014). Magnet Recognition Program' model. Retrieved from http://www.nursecredentialing.org/magnet/programoverview/new-magnet-model

An emerging blueprint for change. (2014, March). *Charting Nursing's Future, 22*, 8. Robert Wood Johnson Foundation & George Washington University.

Benner, P., Sutphen, M., Leonard, V., & Day, L. (2010). *Educating nurses: A call for radical transformation.* San Francisco, CA: Jossey-Bass.

Bennis, W., & Goldsmith, J. (1997). *Learning to lead: A workbook on becoming a leader.* Reading, MA: Perseus Books.

Bertholf, L., & Loveless, S. (2001). Baby boomers and generation X: Strategies to bridge the gap. *Seminars for Nurse Managers, 9*, 169–172.

Blizzard, R., Khoury, C., & McMurray, C. (2010). Nursing leadership from bedside to boardroom: Opinion leaders' perceptions. Robert Wood Johnson Foundation, *Nursing Research Network.* Retrieved from http://www.rwjf.org; full Gallup Poll report available at http://rwjf.org/files/research/nursinggalluppolltopline.pdf

Boston, C. (1990). Differentiated practice: An introduction. In C. Boston (Ed.), *Current issues and perspectives on differentiated practice* (pp. 1–3). Chicago, IL: American Association of Nurse Executives.

Fairman, J., Rowe, J., Hassmiller, S., & Shalala, D. (2010). Broadening the scope of nursing practice. *New England Journal of Medicine, 364*(3), 280–281.

Ferguson, S. & Brindle, M. (2000). Nursing leadership: Vision and the reality. *Nursing Spectrum, 10*(21DC), 5.

Finkelman, A. (2012). *Leadership and management for nurses: Core competencies for quality care* (2nd ed.). Upper Saddle River, NJ: Pearson Education.

Finkelman, A., & Kenner, C. (2012). *Teaching IOM: Implications of the Institute of Medicine reports for nursing education* (3rd ed.). Silver Spring, MD: American Nurses Association.

Gerke, M. (2001). Understanding and leading the quad matrix: Four generations in the workplace. *Seminars for Nurse Managers, 9*, 173–181.

Goffee, R., & Jones, G. (2000, September–October). Why should anyone be led by you? *Harvard Business Review,* 63–71.

Hassmiller, S. (2011). Vision for 21st century nursing workforce. Retrieved from http://thefutureofnursing.org/21stCenturyNursing

Havens, D. (2001). Comparing nursing infrastructure and outcomes: ANCC Magnet and non-Magnet CNEs report. *Nursing Economics, 19*(6), 258–266.

Hess, D. R., Dossey, B. M., Southard, M. E., Luck, S., Schaub, B. G., & Bark, L. (2013). *The art and science of nurse coaching: The provider's guide to coaching scope and competencies.* Silver Spring, MD: American Nurses Association.

Hess, G. (2004). From bedside to boardroom: Nursing shared governance. *Online Journal of Issues in Nursing, 9*(1). Retrieved from http://www.nursingworld.org/MainMenuCategories/ANAMarketplace/ANAPeriodicals/OJIN/TableofContents/Volume92004/No1Jan04/FromBedsidetoBoardroom.aspx

Institute for Healthcare Improvement (IHI). (2008). Transforming care at the bedside. Retrieved from http://www.ihi.org/engage/initiatives/completed/tcab/pages/default.aspx

Institute of Medicine (IOM). (2003a). *Health professions education.* Washington, DC: National Academies Press.

Institute of Medicine (IOM). (2003b). *Leadership by example.* Washington, DC: National Academies Press.

Institute of Medicine (IOM). (2004). *Keeping patients safe: Transforming the work environment of nurses.* Washington, DC: National Academies Press.

Institute of Medicine (IOM). (2010). *The future of nursing: Leading change, advancing health.* Washington, DC: National Academies Press.

Kaplan, M. (2000). Hospital caregivers are in a bad mood. *American Journal of Nursing, 100*(3), 25.

Katz, J. (2001). *Keys to nursing success.* Upper Saddle River, NJ: Pearson Education.

Kerfoot, K., Lavandero, R., Cox, M., Triola, N., Pacini, C., & Hanson, M. (2006, August). Conceptual models and the nursing organization: Implementing the AACN synergy model for patient care. *Nurse Leader,* 20–26.

Kimball, B., Cherner, D., Joynt, J., & O'Neil, E. (2007). The quest for new innovative care delivery models. *Journal of Nursing Administration, 37*, 392–398.

Kovner, C., & Walni, S. (2010). Nurse managed health centers (NMHCs). Robert Wood Johnson Foundation. *Nursing Research Network*. Retrieved from http://www.rwjf.org

Kramer, M., & Schmalenberg, C. (2002). Staff nurses identify essentials of magnetism. In M. McClure & A. Hinshaw (Eds.), *Magnet hospitals revisited* (pp. 25–59). Washington, DC: American Nurses Publishing.

Laschinger, H., Shamian, J., & Thomson, D. (2001). Impact of Magnet hospital characteristics on nurses' perceptions of trust, burnout, quality of care, and work satisfaction. *Nursing Economics, 19*, 209–219.

Laurent, M., Reeves, D., Hermens, R., Braspenning, J., Grol, R., & Sibbald, B. (2005). Substitution of doctors by nurses in primary care. *Cochrane Database Systematic Reviews, 2*.

Magnet® Program. (2014, February 26). Magnet® program overview. Retrieved from http://www.nursecredentialing.org/Magnet/ProgramOverview

Malone, B. (2001). Nurses in non-nursing leadership positions. In J. Dochterman & H. Grace (Eds.), *Current issues in nursing* (6th ed., pp. 293–298). St. Louis, MO: Mosby.

Martin, S., Greenhouse, P., Merryman, T., Shovel, J., Liberi, C., & Konzier, J. (2007). Transforming care at the bedside. *Journal of Nursing Administration, 37*, 444–451.

McClure, M., Poulin, M., Sovie, M., & Wandelt, M. (1983). *Magnet hospitals: Attraction and retention of professional nurses*. American Academy of Nursing Task Force on Nursing Practice in Hospitals. Kansas City, MO: American Nurses Association.

National Forum of State Nursing Workforce Centers. (2014). About us. Retrieved from http://nursingworkforcecenters.org/AboutUs.aspx

Naylor, M., Hirschman, D. B., O'Connor, M., Barg, R., & Pauly, M. V. (2013). Engaging older adults in their transitional care: What more needs to be done? *Journal of Comparative Effectiveness Research, 2*(5), 1–12.

Naylor, M., & Kurtzman, E. (2010). The role of nurse practitioners in reinventing primary care. *Health Affairs, 29*(5), 893–899.

Newhouse, R., & Mills, M. (2002). *Nursing leadership in the organized delivery system for the acute care setting*. Washington, DC: American Nurses Publishing.

Porter-O'Grady, T. (1999). Quantum leadership: New roles for a new age. *Journal of Nursing Administration, 29*(10), 37–42.

Ritter-Teitel, J. (2002). The impact of restructuring on professional nursing practice. *Journal of Nursing Administration, 32*(1), 31–41.

Santos, S., & Cox, K. (2002). Generational tension among nurses. *American Journal of Nursing, 102*(1), 11.

Saver, C. (2006). Nursing—today and beyond: Leaders discuss current trends and predict future developments. *American Nurse Today, 10*, 18–25.

Scott, E., & Cleary, B. (2007). Professional polarities in nursing. *Nursing Outlook, 55*, 250–256.

Siela, D. (2006, December). Managing multigenerational nursing staff. *American Nurse Today*, 47–49.

Sigma Theta Tau International (STTI). (2014a). About us. Retrieved from http://www.nursingsociety.org/aboutus/Pages/AboutUs.aspx

Sigma Theta Tau International (STTI). (2014b). Global Advisory Panel on the Future of Nursing. Retrieved from http://www.reflectionsonnursingleadership.org/Pages/Vol40_1_STTI_GAPFON.aspx?utm_source=feedburner&utm_medium=feed&utm_campaign=Feed%3A+NursingSocietyRNL+%28Nursing+Society+RNL%29

Smith, M. (1975). *When I say no, I feel guilty*. New York, NY: Bantam

Stone, P., Larson, E., Mooney-Kane, C., Smolowitz, J., Lin, S., & Dick, A. (2006). Organizational climate and intensive care unit nurses' intention to leave. *Critical Care Medicine, 34*(7), 1907–1912.

Ulrich, B. (2001). Successfully managing multigenerational workforces. *Seminars for Nurse Managers, 9*, 147–153.

Ulrich, B., Buerhaus, P., Donelan, K., Norman, L., & Dittus, R. (2007). Magnet status and registered nurse views of the work environment and nursing as a career. *Journal of Nursing Administration, 37*(5), 212–220.

Urden, L., & Monarch, K. (2002). The ANCC Magnet Recognition Program: Converting research findings into action. In M. McClure & A. Hinshaw (Eds.), *Magnet hospitals revisited* (pp. 102–116). Washington, DC: American Nurses Publishing.

Wieck, K., Prydun, M., & Walsh, T. (2002). What the emerging workforce wants in its leaders. *Journal of Nursing Scholarship, 34*, 283–288.

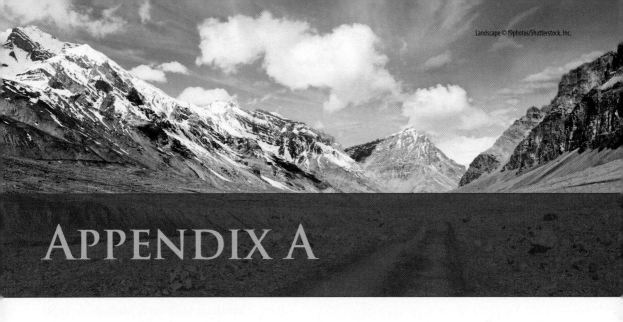

APPENDIX A

Quality Improvement Measurement and Analysis Methods

This appendix presents some examples of QI measurement and analysis methods and information related to quality care. This information is applicable to your clinical experiences throughout your nursing program as you develop QI competency and leadership.

Definitions: Errors

- *Error*: Failure of a planned action to complete as intended or use of the wrong plan to achieve a goal. (Also search for this topic on the Institute for Healthcare Improvement website: http://www.ihi.org.)
- *Adverse Event*: An injury resulting from a medical intervention, not due to the patient's underlying condition. It may or may not be due to an error, and may or may not be preventable. If the adverse event is viewed as result of an error, then it is considered preventable. (Also search for this topic on the Institute for Healthcare Improvement website: http://www.ihi.org.)
- *Misuse*: An avoidable complication that prevents patients from receiving the full potential benefit of services.

- *Overuse*: Potential for harm that exceeds the possible benefit from a service.
- *Underuse*: Failure to provide a service that would have produced a favorable outcome for the patient.
- *Near Miss*: Recognition that an event occurred that might have led to an adverse event. An error almost happened, but staff or the patient/family caught it before it became an error.
- *Active Error*: An error that results from noncompliance with a procedure.
- *Omission*: Missed care should also be considered an error.
- *Common Errors*: Falls, medication errors, development of pressure ulcers due to inadequate skin care, surgical errors such as wrong site, diagnosis (wrong diagnosis, incomplete diagnosis, and so on), wrong patient identification, lack of timely

response, development of nosocomial infections, wound infections, not washing hands, equipment failure, inappropriate use of restraints or used in unsafe manner, documentation errors or inadequate documentation, poor discharge planning or directions.

- *Sentinel Event*: Unexpected events that happen to patients and that result in major negative outcomes such as an unexpected death or critical physical or psychological complication that can lead to major alteration in the patient's health. (Also search for this topic on the Institute for Healthcare Improvement website: http://www.ihi.org.)

Examples of High Risk for Errors and/or Reduced Quality Care

- *Working in Silos*: Not working as a team or using poor communication; individuals or pairs working with little consideration of others who may be working on the same issue, with the same patient, and so on.
- *Joint Commission Annual Safety Goals*: See the annual goals posted on the website: http://www.jointcommission.org/standards_information/npsgs.aspx.
- *Handoffs*: A handoff occurs when a patient experiences a change in provider or setting and there is a transfer of responsibility. (Also search for this topic on the Institute for Healthcare Improvement website at http://www.ihi.org.)
- *Medication Reconciliation*: See the *Apply Quality Improvement* chapter. (Also search for this topic on the Institute for Healthcare Improvement website at http://www.ihi.org.)
- *Workaround*: Occurs when staff use a shortcut to get something done so they do not complete all the steps or substitute different steps in a process. This often happens when staff are behind; rather than figure out the problem they are experiencing, they use a workaround. (Also search for this topic on the Institute for Healthcare Improvement website at http://www.ihi.org.)

- *Health Literacy*: See the *Provide Patient-Centered Care* chapter. Health literacy can impact errors—for example, if the patient does not understand the discharge directions or cannot read them, an error could occur.

Examples of Typical Errors or Concerns of Inadequate Quality Care

- *Hospital-Acquired Complications (HACs):* See the *Healthcare Delivery System: Focus on Acute Care* chapter and the following websites:
  - Centers for Medicare & Medicaid Services, Hospital-Acquired Infections: http://www.cms.gov/Medicare/Medicare-Fee-for-Service-Payment/HospitalAcqCond/Hospital-Acquired_Conditions.html and http://www.cms.gov/Medicare/Medicare-Fee-for-Service-Payment/HospitalAcqCond/index.html.
- *Agency for Healthcare Research and Quality Inpatient Quality Indicators*:
  - *Volume indicators/measures* are proxy, or indirect, measures of quality based on counts of admissions during which certain intensive, high-technology, or highly complex procedures were performed. They are based on evidence, suggesting that hospitals perform more of these procedures may have better outcomes for them.
  - *Mortality indicators/measures for inpatient procedures* include procedures for which mortality has been shown to vary across institutions and for which there is evidence that high mortality may be associated with poorer quality of care.
  - *Mortality indicators/measures for inpatient procedures* include conditions for which mortality has been shown to vary substantially across institutions and for which evidence suggests that high mortality may be associated with deficiencies in the quality of care.

- *Utilization indicators/measures* examine procedures whose use varies significantly across hospitals and for which questions have been raised about overuse, underuse, or misuse.
- *Primary and Secondary Data*: Primary data are data collected from firsthand experience; secondary data are data collected by others.
- *Prevalence and Incidence*: Prevalence is the proportion of the population that has a condition or risk factor. Incidence is the rate of occurrence.
- *Benchmarking*: Measuring quality across healthcare organizations based on same standards.
- *Report Cards*: A published report that provides information about the quality of care for a healthcare organization or provider. (See examples at NCQA's website: http://reportcard.ncqa.org/portal/home.aspx and http://www.ncqa.org/Directories.aspx.)
- *Incident Reports*: Healthcare organizations require that certain incidents, such as medication errors, are reported in written form using a standard form. This provides a record and helps in tracking errors for improvement.
- *Root-Cause Analysis (RCA)*: A method used by many healthcare organizations today to analyze errors, supporting the recognition that most errors are caused by system issues and not individual staff issues. This in-depth analysis is intended to identify causes and then consider changes that might be required to reduce risk of reoccurrence. (Also search for this topic on the Institute for Healthcare Improvement website at http://www.ihi.org.)
- *Failure Mode and Effects Analysis (FMEA):* A tool that "provides a systematic, proactive method for evaluating a process to identify where and how it might fail and to assess the relative impact of different failures in order to identify the parts of the process that are in most need of change" (Institute of Health Improvement, 2011). (Also search for this topic on the Institute for Healthcare Improvement website: http://www.ihi.org.)

- *Plan–Do–Study–Act (PDSA):* A process that is used in planning; four steps are followed to reach effective results. (Also search for this topic on the Institute for Healthcare Improvement website: http://www.ihi.org.)
- *Employee Surveys*: Written questionnaires used to get information from employees on a particular topic—for example, staff safety.
- *Patient/Family Surveys*: Written questionnaires used to get information from patients/families on a particular topic—for example, patient and/or family views of quality care and experience while hospitalized. A common standardized survey that is used by hospitals is offered by Press Ganey. See the website: http://www.pressganey.com/index.aspx.
- *Flow Charts and Decision Trees*: Methods used to describe a process so it can be clearly understood to improve the process or use to help identify when a process is not effective. (Search "decision trees" on Yahoo Images or Google Images.)
- *Patient Safety Indicators (PSI)*: A set of indicators providing information on potential in-hospital complications and adverse events following surgeries, procedures, and childbirth. The PSIs were developed after a comprehensive literature review, analysis of ICD-9-CM codes, review by a clinician panel, implementation of risk adjustment, and empirical analyses. They can be used to help hospitals identify potential adverse events that might need further study; provide the opportunity to assess the incidence of adverse events and in-hospital complications using administrative data found in the typical discharge record; include indicators for complications occurring in hospitals that may represent patient safety events; and design area-level analogs to detect patient safety events on a regional level. (See the Agency for Healthcare Research and Quality [AHRQ] for more information: http://qualityindicators.ahrq.gov/Modules/psi_overview.aspx.)
- *Interviews*: One-on-one collection of data that can be done in person or on telephone.

- *Observation*: Using staff or outside individuals to watch a procedure or work process and collect data on what occurs. This information is then used to track errors, improvement, and so on. An example would be to have observers watching staff to determine compliance with hand washing.
- *Quality Measures*: Tools that help measure or quantify healthcare processes, outcomes, patient perceptions, and organizational structure and/or systems that are associated with the ability to provide high-quality health care and/or that relate to one or more quality goals for health care. These goals include effective, safe, efficient, patient-centered, equitable, and timely care (Centers for Medicare and Medicaid Services [CMS]). (See more information at http://www.cms.gov/Medicare/Quality-Initiatives-Patient-Assessment-Instruments/QualityMeasures/index.html.)
- *Time-out*: During a procedure, the team may use a checklist to confirm the right patient, site, and procedure. If any staff member thinks there may be an error, that staff member can call a stop so that the correct information can be determined—for example, if the wrong site is identified and actions taken to ensure that care provided meets required outcomes.
- *Checklist*: A consistent method for ensuring that what needs to be done is done. The checklist is simple and requires limited if any training to use it. (Also search for this topic on the Institute for Healthcare Improvement website: http://www.ihi.org.)
- *Situation/Background/Assessment/Recommendation (SBAR/ISBAR)*: See the *Work in Interprofessional Teams* chapter. (Also search for this topic on the Institute for Healthcare Improvement website: http://www.ihi.org.)
- *Rapid Response Team (RRT)*: A team of critical care experts who can be called if there is concern about failure to rescue so as to respond quickly to complex and critical needs of patients. (Also search for this topic on the Institute for Healthcare Improvement website: http://www.ihi.org.)

- *Huddle*: A means by which a team gets together periodically during a shift to discuss critical issues. (Also search for this topic on the Institute for Healthcare Improvement website: http://www.ihi.org.)
- *Change of Shift Reports*: Reports that are done routinely, particularly in hospitals units, for bringing new staff coming on up-to-date regarding patient status. Such a report is also an opportunity to discuss quality and safety concerns for individual patients or for the unit or team as a whole.
- *Safety Walk-Arounds*: Staff (usually management but can be other staff) walk through the unit or area of the healthcare organization and identify any safety concerns they may see that would apply to patients, families and visitors, and staff. This information is then used to plan improvement including prevention measures.
- *Crew Resource Management (CRM)*: Communication methodology used in aviation to improve communication and decision making, providing a clear structure for the process. (Also search for this topic on the Institute for Healthcare Improvement website: http://www.ihi.org.)
- *Surveillance*: "Early identification and prevention of potential problems, which requires behavioral and cognitive skills" (Institute of Medicine, 2004, p. 91). Not doing this effectively may result in *Failure to Rescue*.
- *Universal Protocol for Preventing Wrong Site, Wrong Procedure, or Wrong Person Surgery*: The Joint Commission established a procedure to prevent wrong-site, wrong-procedure, and wrong-person surgery errors. This procedure requires staff to utilize the following steps: (1) preprocedure verification, (2) site marking, and (3) use of time-outs. Any staff member may call a time-out if the staff member thinks there is a problem at any point during the procedure.
- *Early Warning System (EWS)*: A "physiological scoring system typically used in general medical–surgical units before patients experience catastrophic medical events" (Duncan & McMullan, 2012, p. 40). This is what triggers

the use of the *Rapid Response Team* to prevent *Failure to Rescue*.

- *Interprofessional Collaborative Teams*: See the *Apply Quality Improvement* chapter.
- *Morbidity and Mortality Conferences*: See the Insitute for Healthcare Improvement age on morbidity and mortality (http://www.ihi.org/resources/Pages/OtherWebsites/AHRQWebMandM.aspx) for additional information on this type of resource, which is used to better understand quality care. Most hospitals hold these conferences regularly to discuss actual patient care and outcomes.
- *Trigger Points*: Clues that there may be an adverse reaction. Standardized lists of trigger points may be used by staff. (Also search for this topic on the Institute for Healthcare Improvement website: http://www.ihi.org.)
- *Electronic Medical/Health Record*: See the *Utilize Informatics* chapter.
- *Computerized Physician/Provider Order System (CPOS)*: See the *Utilize Informatics* chapter.

- *Computerized Decision Support (CDS)*: See the *Utilize Informatics* chapter.
- *Use of Other Technology (e.g., smartphones, handheld computers)*: See the *Utilize Informatics* chapter.
- *Bar Coding*: See the *Utilize Informatics* chapter.
- *Safety Primers (AHRQ)*: See AHRQ's patient safety primers webpage (http://psnet.ahrq.gov/primerHome.aspx) for information a variety of important safety concerns.

References

- Duncan, K., & McMullan, C. (2012, February). Early warning. *Nursing 2012, 38*–44.
- Institute for Health Improvement. (2011). FMEA. Retrieved from http://www.ihi.org/knowledge/Pages/Tools/FailureModesandEffectsAnalysisTool.aspx
- Institute of Medicine. (2004). *Keeping patients safe*. Washington, DC: National Academies Press.

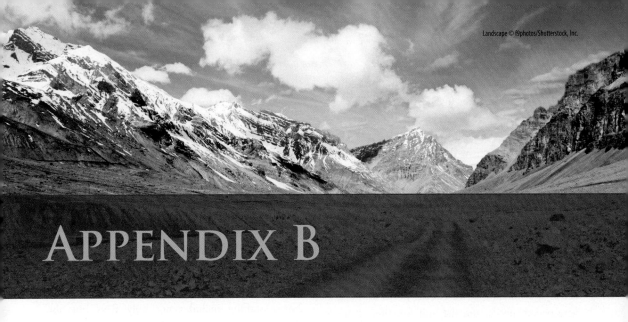

APPENDIX B

Staffing and Healthy Work Environment

Staffing: What a New Nurse Needs to Know

When you search for your first job as a new graduate, it is critical that you inquire about staffing—who does the staffing plan, how far in advance staffing is done, which methods are used, how inadequate staffing areas are covered, and whether overtime is required. Nurses need information about staffing and what input they might have in the staffing pattern.

American Nurses Association Staffing Principles

The American Nurses Association (ANA) staffing principles, which were reissued in 2010, support the need for adequate staffing to delivery of quality patient care. Three underlying assumptions of these principles provide guidance for staffing decisions and are the major ethical concerns related to staffing:

1. Nurse staffing patterns and the level of care provided should not be based on the type of payer.
2. Evaluation of any staffing system should include quality of nurses' work-life outcomes as well as patients' outcomes.

3. Staffing should be based on achieving quality of patient care indices, meeting organizational outcomes, and ensuring that the quality of nurses' work life is appropriate.

"Making nurse staffing decisions is a complex process requiring input from all levels within the nursing structure. Critical to this process are any patient classification and acuity systems currently being used" (ANA, 2010, p. 7). These systems can be useful, but they still lack specificity and reliability for current practice. The critical element is always professional nursing judgment. The following resources may be useful when evaluating staffing (ANA, 2010, p. 11):

- Current *Nursing: Scope and Standards of Nursing* (ANA)
- Appropriate scopes and standards of specialty nursing practice
- Current state nurse practice act and scope of practice information (state board of nursing)
- Current *Code of Ethics with Interpretive Statements* (ANA)

- Copies of relevant facility policies and procedures (e.g., staffing, floating, agency use)
- Copies of the current collective bargaining agreement/contract (if applicable)
- Copies of contracts with outside staffing agencies
- Information on competencies of agency staff
- *Bill of Rights for Registered Nurses* (ANA)
- Principles for delegation

The ANA staffing standards are divided into three categories. First, the principles of the patient care unit focus on the need for appropriate staffing levels at the unit level. These standards reflect both the analysis of individual patient needs and aggregate patient needs, and the unit functions that are important in delivering care. The second category focuses on staff-related principles, such as the type of nurse competencies needed to provide the required care as well as role responsibilities. The third category involves institutional or organizational policies. These policies should indicate that nurses are respected, and they should state a commitment to meeting budget requirements to fill nursing positions. Competencies for all nursing staff (employees, agency, and so on) should be documented. A clear plan should describe how float staff are used and which cross-training is required for these staff so that they are prepared to practice in multiple areas of care. Staff members need to know if they may be switched from one unit to another. There must be a clear designation of the adequate number of staff needed to meet a minimum level of quality care.

The principles identify four critical elements that need to be considered when making staffing decisions (ANA, 2010, p. 23):

1. *Patients:* Patient characteristics and number of patients receiving care.
2. *Intensity of Unit and Care:* Individual patient intensity; across-the-unit intensity (taking into account the heterogeneity of settings); variability of care; admissions, discharges, and transfers; volume.
3. *Context:* Architecture (geographic dispersion of patients, size and layout of individual patient rooms, arrangement of entire patient care units, and so forth); technology (use of beepers, cellular phones, computers); same unit or cluster of patients.
4. *Expertise:* Learning curve for individuals and groups of nurses; staff consistency, continuity, and cohesion; cross-training; control of practice; involvement in quality improvement activities; professional expectations; preparation, and experience.

Staffing Terminology

Nurse staffing includes not only RNs but also licensed practical nurses (LPNs)/licensed vocational nurses and unlicensed assistive personnel (UAPs). All of these staff provide direct care. RNs and LPNs are licensed by the states in which they are employed. The state board of nursing in each state regulates state licensure. RNs assess patient needs, develop patient care plans, and administer medications and treatments, and they must meet the state's nurse practice act requirements. LPNs carry out specified nursing duties under the direction of RNs. Nurses' aides typically provide nonspecialized duties and personal care activities. Some states require that UAPs complete a certification program, at which point they are referred to as certified nurse assistants.

Hospitals and other healthcare organizations (HCOs) have written position descriptions for RNs, LPNs, and UAPs. These descriptions should be followed. They influence staffing because the descriptions identify what staff members may do, which in turn affects the staff mix. Nurse staffing is measured in one of two basic ways:

- Nursing hours per patient per day
- Nurse-to-patient ratio

Nursing hours may refer to RNs only; to RNs and LPNs; or to RNs, LPNs, and UAPs. It is important to know which staff category is identified by the nurse staffing measurement. *Nursing care hours* refers to the number of hours of patient care provided per unit of time or over the course of a specified time. However, it is becoming increasingly clear that, when determining nursing hours of care, one size (or formula) does not fit all. In fact, staffing is most appropriate and meaningful when it is predicated on a measure of unit intensity that takes into consideration the aggregate population of patients and associated roles and responsibilities of nursing staff. (Maguire, 2002, p. 7)

The term *full-time equivalent* is used to describe a position. A full-time equivalent is equal to 40 hours of work per week for 52 weeks, or 2080 hours per year. One full-time equivalent can represent one staff member or several members; that is, a full-time equivalent can be divided (e.g., two staff members each working half a full-time equivalent). Many nursing units employ part-time staff.

The *staffing mix* describes the type of nursing staff needed to provide care. This mix should be determined by considering the type of care needed and patient status, as well as the qualification and competencies needed to provide the care. In some cases, the staff must be RNs; in other situations, a mix of RNs, LPNs, and UAPs is needed, with the RN supervising. This issue is often a concern when the proportion of RNs is compared with other types of nursing staffing. Another factor that needs to be considered is the work level and work flow; for example, the typical time for discharges and admissions or the surgical schedule can make a difference as to when more or fewer staff members are needed (distribution of staff).

Scheduling

The shift, or typical pattern of time worked, is an important factor in scheduling. Some areas of care use multiple types of shifts, whereas others have only one type. Typical shifts are 8, 10, and 12 hours in length. More and more hospitals are using 12-hour shifts, and some schools of nursing are using 12-hour clinical rotations for students. Staff often prefer the 12-hour shift because it allows

for more days off (40 hours can add up quickly). However, there has been concern about 12-hour shifts and the resulting fatigue level that may lead to more errors (Geiger-Brown & Trinkoff, 2010; Institute of Medicine [IOM], 2004; Montgomery & Geiger-Brown, 2010; Trinkoff, Johantgen, Storr, Gurses, Liang, & Han, 2011).

Trinkoff and colleagues (2011) examined the independent effect of work schedules on patient care outcomes. Their study surveyed 633 nurses in 2004 in 71 acute care hospitals in two states. The results indicate that work schedule related significantly to patient mortality when staffing levels and hospital characteristics were controlled. Other concerns are increased risk of infections among staff who are fatigued and ergonomic stressors; accidents that result from driving home tired; and responsibilities at home that further increase nurses' fatigue (Geiger-Brown & Trinkoff, 2010; Worthington, 2001). More research needs to be done to determine the impact of shifts on fatigue and errors.

Split shifts are used to provide more staff at busy times of the day (such as 7:00–11:00 a.m. or later in the day). Part-time staff usually fill in during split shifts, and this has implications for consistency of care and quality with increased risk of errors. "Moving away from 12-hour shifts will require a real change in hospital culture" (Montgomery & Geiger-Brown, 2010, p. 148).

The staffing schedule can contribute to many negative results. Because staff usually do not get off on time, longer shifts can compound the problems associated with 12-hour shifts. For example, when staff work 10- or 12-hour shifts instead of 8-hour shifts, staying 1 hour past the end of their shifts can be very difficult. This is a frequent occurrence because some staff may be arriving late or not coming at all, and temporary coverage is needed until additional staff coverage is found. This makes a 10- or 12-hour shift much longer. In some HCOs, staff are required to rotate shifts so that they may switch back and forth from the day shift to the night shift. This can be hard for many nurses, although some like to work the night shift. **Box B-1** lists some tips for adjusting to the night shift.

Scheduling is not easy and causes a lot of conflict among staff. Nurses invariably want more say in scheduling. Some organizations use computerized request systems so that staff can input their special staffing requests, and others do this in writing or orally. When staffing is posted is also of concern because staff need to make their personal plans. The procedures for schedule changes need to be known by all staff. The trend is for HCOs to develop staffing schedules centrally, although some may do it unit by unit. In addition, a non-nurse scheduler is more common today (Cavouras, 2006). This model has disadvantages because it may leave out or limit important input from nurse managers. However, "one of the most important reasons that people (nurse managers) leave hospital nursing is frustration with schedules and staffing" (Cavouras, 2006, p. 36), so it is important to find

a balance. Scheduling must consider patient needs; staff competencies; individual staff issues such as days off, vacation time, sick leave, and so on; organization needs; legislative requirements; union requirements; shortage concerns; use of external sources for staff (e.g., agencies); standards; and rising labor costs.

Patient classification systems may be used to assist with staffing levels. These computerized systems are used to identify and quantify patient needs, which can then be matched with staffing level and mix. It is thought that these systems are more objective because data related to patients and their needs are used to determine the number and type of staff required per shift.

Some organizations or patient care units use self-scheduling (Hung, 2002). With this system, guidelines are developed for the schedule. Staff are then given a certain amount of time to fill in the schedule based on the guidelines. Individual staff

---

Box B-1	Tips for Working the Night Shift

- Do not exercise before you try to sleep.
- Develop a routine for your time off and sleep time, and maintain it. Set up a plan with family members so that sleep time during the day is not disrupted.
- When you get tired at work, try to do something active. If you are allowed rest time, take it.
- If you feel unusually tired and are administering medications, for example, ask a coworker to double check the dose.
- Drink water instead of snacking. Snack foods at work are not helpful.
- Try to avoid working too many nights in a row. Working more than three nights in a row can cause problems with circadian rhythm.
- Eat lightly before going to sleep.
- Avoid use of sleep medications and alcohol.
- Relax a little before trying to go to sleep.
- Do not think that because you have all day open and do not have to go to work until nighttime that you have extra time for other activities.
- Try wearing sunglasses on the way home from work.
- Keep a diary of your sleep pattern to see if you can find the best time for the longest daytime sleep.
- Avoid excessive use of caffeine.
- Find your own sleep pattern. Each person's sleep pattern is individual.

Source: Summarized information from Pronitis-Ruotolo, D. (2001). Surviving the night shift. *American Journal of Nursing, 101* (7), 63–68.

members do need to consider the schedules that other staff members have already posted. When the designated time period is completed, the nurse manager (or a staff member who is responsible for completing the schedule) reviews it and makes any required changes or additions to ensure that staffing is adequate. This type of scheduling allows staff to feel more in control of the staffing and to work with one another to come up with the most effective arrangement. It also reduces the time that the nurse manager or another scheduler might spend on staffing. More staff input and control over staffing usually result in greater staff satisfaction and less absenteeism, which leads to greater staff empowerment.

The schedule inevitably has holes—positions on the schedule for which there is no staff member. What does the HCO do? One method to fill holes in the schedule is for the HCO to develop a float pool. This is a group of staff (RNs, LPNs, or UAPs) who may be moved from unit to unit based on need. These staff members need to be competent in the relevant area of care and should be flexible and able to adjust quickly to new environments. Float pool staff are HCO employees who are not assigned to a specific unit. Staff who float need orientation and training related to the types of care that they are expected to provide.

When nursing shortages become a serious problem, hospitals increase the number of staff who are not employees of the HCO but rather temporary employees. Agency nurses are nurses hired by a nursing agency; the agency then contracts with an HCO for specific types of staff to fill holes in the schedule. Some hospitals contract with one supplemental staffing agency, whereas others contract with multiple agencies to meet their staffing needs. An agency nurse is paid by the agency (typically more than usual organization staff), must be licensed, and should meet employee competency qualifications or any other criteria required by the HCO. Work assignments can be for one shift, for several days, or for weeks or months.

Another method for responding to incomplete schedules or lack of staff to fill all positions needed is the use of travelers. Travelers are nurses who work for an agency, but not a local agency. They are hired by the agency and then assigned to work at an HCO for a block of time (more than a few days and often several months). The nurse may come from anywhere in the United States. The agency pays the nurse's salary, benefits, and often moving, travel, and housing expenses are covered by the HCOs that use the travelers. Salaries are often very high for these nurses. Nurses can decline a specific assignment, and moving is required. Nurses might even be assigned a management position. Nurses who are employees of the HCO are often concerned about the pay difference; traveling nurses, as well as regular agency nurses, typically earn much more than the full-time employees, which can cause conflict. Travelers must meet the requirements to practice in the state and the HCO requirements.

All these nurses need orientation and should not be expected to just "get to work." It is not easy to change from one HCO to another because HCOs are not all the same. The nurse has to learn quickly to work with a new team. More experienced nurses are better at making this transition, and many of the traveling nurse agencies hire only experienced nurses. Although the fluctuations in the nursing shortage have decreased in some areas, when the shortage begins to increase again, which will occur when more nurses retire, there will be greater need again to use alternative staffing strategies.

Recruitment

Recruitment in nursing involves the recruitment of both nurses and nursing students. Some improvement has occurred in recruitment of nursing students. Notably, the Johnson & Johnson advertising campaign to attract more students to nursing improved enrollment. This multimedia campaign highlighted the value of nursing as a profession and the need for more nurses, sending out a proactive message about nursing. Schools of nursing, states, and the federal government have also increased their efforts to increase scholarship and loan funds for nursing students. Schools of nursing have tried to expand enrollment, and many have been successful.

Unfortunately, there are two major roadblocks to expansion of nursing education programs. The first roadblock is the shortage of nursing faculty, which will only worsen as more faculty reach retirement age. Schools are trying various strategies, such as making collaborative arrangements with hospitals and other HCOs to use their staff as clinical faculty; having nurses with bachelor of science in nursing degrees and sufficient clinical experience assist with clinical teaching; and opening up more master's-level nursing education courses and programs. Offering these programs online and in an accelerated format can help to develop additional faculty.

The second barrier is finding enough clinical sites for clinical experiences. This is a major struggle in some areas that have a lot of schools and only limited healthcare sites. The increased use of simulation laboratories for some of the clinical experiences has decreased some of the need, but it does not solve the problem entirely.

Despite these barriers, nursing schools continue to have more applicants than spots available for them. This imbalance in supply and demand has been impacted by the 21st-century economic conditions as college-age students consider majors that might lead to jobs after graduation. However, the economy has also had a negative impact on nursing overall because there are now fewer job openings. This will change over the next few years as the economy improves and the nursing shortage returns primarily due to expected increase in nursing retirement.

Recruitment of staff is just as challenging. Some HCOs, in an effort to hire new nurses, advertise in local, state, and national newspapers; on radio and television; in professional journals; and on a growing number of Internet sites that offer information about jobs. Many HCOs have offered bonuses to entice new staff when they experience a shortage, although this does not guarantee that a nurse will not then seek a job elsewhere for another bonus. All specialties—not just one specialty or a few—have experienced the shortage. Specialties that usually attract younger nurses because of the fast-paced nature of the work—such as intensive care units, emergency departments, and surgical nursing (operating room and post-anesthesia)—have experienced increasing difficulty attracting nurses with this type of experience; in some areas there simply are not enough nurses to fill these positions. Nurses also listen to other nurses regarding the best places to work.

Disgruntled nurses can do great damage to efforts to attract new staff. HCOs need to recognize all of the many aspects of recruitment that can attract new nurses, yet also push them away. How the nurse is treated from the very beginning of the job application process—on the telephone, responsiveness during the interview, whether a tour is provided, along with the opportunity to talk to staff—is very important. When there are so many openings, the potential employee is in the driver's seat in the recruitment process. With some areas of the United States experiencing a lull in the nursing shortage, some HCOs have moved to requiring baccalaureate degrees for nurses, which has had a major impact on new graduates from other types of programs. The nurse's ability to relocate expands job opportunities. Potential new staff also consider salaries and benefits, scheduling, educational benefits, orientation time, the HCO's reputation and the reputation of its nursing service, and position responsibilities. Magnet status also has become important. In the last few years, new graduates have shown an increasing interest in participating in nurse residency programs.

Retention

After staff are recruited, they need to be retained. There is a great risk of job hopping with so many jobs open. Both new nurses and experienced nurses are leaving nursing. Nurse turnover is very costly (Jones & Gates, 2007). Turnover costs range from $22,000 to more than $64,000 per nurse (Advisory Board Company, 1999; Jones, 2005; O'Brien-Pallas et al., 2006; Stone et al., 2003). It is, however, difficult to define nurse turnover costs (and benefits). What are some of the costs and benefits of turnover (Jones & Gates, 2007)?

Nurse Turnover Costs

- Advertising and recruitment
- Vacancy costs (e.g., paying for agency nurses, overtime, closed beds, and hospital diversions when the emergency department must be closed)
- Hiring (review and processing of applicants)
- Orientation and training
- Decreased productivity (loss of staff who know routines)
- Termination (processing of termination)
- Potential patient errors; compromised quality of care
- Poor work environment and culture; dissatisfaction; distrust
- Loss of organizational knowledge (loss of staff who know the history of the organization and processes)

Nurse Turnover Benefits

- Reductions in salaries and benefits for newly hired nurses versus departing nurses
- Savings from bonuses not paid to outgoing nurses
- Replacement nurses bringing in new ideas, reality, and innovations, as well as knowledge of competitors
- Elimination of poor performers (this is not guaranteed, it is merely hoped)

Focusing on retention is more important than focusing on turnover, but there are benefits and costs related to retention as well (Jones & Gates, 2007). A study that included 229 RNs using a survey on work environments identified some important aspects about the transition to practice from student status (Pellico, Djukic, Kovner, & Brewer,

2009). The survey collected data in two time intervals: (1) the first 6–18 months of practice for RNs and (2) 1 year later. It is critical that HCOs improve retention of new nurses and understand the reasons new nurses leave positions or stay in positions and yet experience frustration that impacts work. Analysis of the survey data indicated the following six themes:

1. *Pressured time:* There was not enough time to get the work done. This is relevant to nursing education, which should provide experiences for students to learn how to better manage time, prioritize, delegate, and make decisions. These types of experiences should be found throughout a nursing curriculum. HCOs also need to improve how work is done in the organization—types of support provided; use of an effective system; ensuring supplies are available and equipment works; considering staffing levels and patient acuity; and so on.

2. *The reality of being a nurse is nothing like the dream:* Nursing programs need to do more to discuss the reality of practice and allow students to discuss their concerns and better understand the healthcare work environment. HCOs need to better understand this type of reaction and provide mentors to help new nurses adjust.

3. *Growing weary:* Critical problems are concern about exhaustion, abuse from colleagues, and other barriers to realizing an effective work environment. Some of these problems can be addressed in nursing education programs rather than waiting for the new nurse to experience them without support. HCOs need to do more in orientation and to provide mentors.

4. *Getting out:* There is no doubt that new nurses are leaving nursing or changing jobs frequently as they try to cope with their response to the work environment. Some may have chosen the wrong profession, but many want to be RNs but do not want to do so if the position comes with many of the issues identified in this study.

5. *Finding one's niche:* For some new graduates, it will take time to find the best specialty, best HCO (employer), and best unit or department for them. Nursing provides many options for positions, and over a lifetime career, many nurses hold a variety of positions.

6. *Upward mobility:* By the second data collection period, some of the nurses were back in school working on master's degrees. The nurses who had remained in nursing positions were more satisfied but saw themselves as changing positions over their careers. They gave suggestions for improving the work environment, such as improving orientation, providing mentoring, increasing pay for work performance, face-to-face annual reviews, and more staff education. This forward-thinking response was not found in all the nurses in the study.

Creating a Healthy Work Environment: Retaining Nurses

Working in a healthcare environment can be a very positive experience, particularly if the environment is one in which staff are respected; communication is open; staff feel empowered and part of the decision-making process; staff safety and health are considered important; and staff feel that they are making a contribution. This, however, is not always the case. Staff experience stress, burnout, and conflict in the workplace. Some signs that students and staff should watch for in themselves, in others, and in organizations follow.

Personal Signs

- Irritability
- Lack of sleep or too much sleep
- Complaining about many aspects of work
- Unwillingness to help others
- Desire to just get the job done and leave
- Less enjoyment during personal time
- Dreading going to work
- High frustration with management

- Angry outbursts
- Gaining or losing weight
- Lack of energy

Attitude and behavior impact others, too—coworkers and family. Burnout is contagious because of this impact. Morale can decrease as staff try to cope with their own stress and burnout. This affects productivity and the quality of care.

Organizational Signs

- Inadequate or confused communication
- Top-down decision making, leaving staff out
- Poorly planned change that is unsuccessful
- Increase in staff complaints
- Staff–management conflict
- Distrust of staff and staff distrust of management

The American Association of Critical-Care Nurses (2005) standards for healthy work environments address the need for improved work environments:

> Each day, thousands of medical errors harm the patients and families served by the American healthcare system. Work environments that tolerate ineffective interpersonal relationships and do not support education to acquire necessary skills perpetuate unacceptable conditions, so do health professionals who experience moral distress over this state of affairs, yet remain silent and overwhelmed with resignation. (p. 11)

Consider again these all-too-familiar situations:

- A nurse chooses not to call a physician known to be verbally abusive. The nurse uses her judgment to clarify a prescribed medication and administers a fatal dose of the wrong drug.
- Additional patients are added to a nurse's assignment during a busy weekend because on-call staff are not available and backup plans do not exist to cover variations in patient census. Patients are placed at risk for errors and injury, and nurses are frustrated and angry.

- Isolated decision making in one department leads to tension, frustration, and a higher risk of errors by all involved. Whether affecting patient care or unit operations, decisions made without including all parties place everyone involved at risk.
- Nurses are placed in leadership positions without adequate preparation and support for their role. The resulting environment creates dissatisfaction and high turnover for nurse leaders and staff as well.
- Contentious relationships between nurses and administrators are heightened when managers are required to stretch their responsibilities without adequate preparation and coaching for success (American Association of Critical-Care Nurses, 2003).
- Only 65% of hospital managers are held accountable for employee satisfaction (University Health System Consortium, 2003).

The standards of the American Association of Critical-Care Nurses (2005) focus on the following areas and can be applied to all nursing specialties:

- *Skilled communication:* Nurses must be as proficient in communication skills as they are in clinical skills. Skilled communication protects and advances collaborative relationships.
- *True collaboration:* Nurses must be relentless in pursuing and fostering true collaboration. True collaboration is an ongoing process built on mutual trust and respect.
- *Effective decision making:* Nurses must be valued and committed partners in making policy, directing and evaluating clinical care, and leading organizational operations. Advocating for patients requires involvement in decisions that affect patient care.
- *Appropriate staffing:* Staffing must ensure the effective match between patient needs and nurse competencies. Remaining focused on matching nurses' competencies to patients' needs points the way to innovative staffing solutions.
- *Meaningful recognition:* Nurses must be recognized and must recognize others for the value each brings to the work of the organization. Meaningful recognition acknowledges the value of a person's contribution to the work of the organization.
- *Authentic leadership:* Nurse leaders must fully embrace the imperative of a healthy work environment, authentically live it, and engage others in its achievement. Nurse leaders create a vision for a healthy work environment and model it in all their actions.

An important part of any nurse's work experience is working with others—relationships—and this affects the healthy work environment. There is even more emphasis on this aspect of the workplace today, with the IOM core competency that focuses on interprofessional teams. Relationships with coworkers can be the deciding factor in how comfortable a nurse feels in the work environment (Trossman, 2005). These relationships take time to develop. With the hectic work environment today and shorter breaks and lunch, staff members have less time to build those relationships. Such relationships can be critical when nurses work together; working together requires communication, trust, mutual respect, and confidence that one will be supported and assisted when needed. "Positive relationships also foster loyalty to each other and to the institutions and the community [an organization] serves" (Trossman, 2005, p. 8). Staff spend a lot of time at work, and it is less stressful when one looks forward to working with the team rather than dreading work or expecting conflict. Healthy work environments are necessary to improve patient safety, staff safety, quality of care, and staff recruitment and retention, and they have an impact on the financial status of the HCO.

References

- Advisory Board Company. (1999). A misplaced focus: Reexamining the recruiting/retention trade-off. *Nursing Watch, 11,* 114.
- American Association of Critical-Care Nurses. (2003). *Strategic market research study.* Aliso Viejo, CA: Author.

- American Association of Critical-Care Nurses. (2005). *AACN standards for establishing and sustaining healthy work environments*. Aliso Viejo, CA: Author.
- American Nurses Association (ANA). (2010). *Utilization guide for the ANA principles for nurse staffing* (reissue). Silver Spring, MD: Author.
- Cavouras, C. (2006). Scheduling and staffing: Innovations from the field. *Nurse Leader, 4*(4), 34–36.
- Geiger-Brown, J., & Trinkoff, A. (2010). Is it time to pull the plug on 12-hour shifts? Part 1. The evidence. *Journal of Nursing Administration, 40*(3), 100–102.
- Hung, R. (2002). A note on nurse self-scheduling. *Nursing Economic$, 20*(1), 37–39.
- Institute of Medicine (IOM). (2004). *Keeping patients safe: Transforming the work environment of nurses*. Washington, DC: National Academies Press.
- Jones, C. (2005). The costs of nursing turnover, Part 2: Application of the nursing turnover cost calculation methodology. *Journal of Nursing Administration, 35*(1), 41–49.
- Jones, C., & Gates, M. (2007). The costs and benefits of nurse turnover: A business case for nurse retention. *Online Journal of Issues in Nursing, 12*(3). Retrieved from http://www.nursingworld.org/MainMenuCategories/ANAMarketplace/ANAPeriodicals/OJIN/TableofContents/Volume122007/No3Sept07/NurseRetention.aspx
- Maguire, P. (2002). Safe staffing and mandatory overtime: Issues of concerns in today's workplace. *Ohio Nurse Review, 77*(10), 4, 7–11.
- Montgomery, K., & Geiger-Brown, J. (2010). Is it time to pull the plug on 12-hour shifts? Part 2. Barriers to change and executive leadership strategies. *Journal of Nursing Administration, 40*(4), 147–149.
- O'Brien-Pallas, L., Griffin, P., Shamian, J., Buchan, J., Duffield, C., Hughes, F., ... Stone, P. W. (2006). The impact of nurse turnover on patient, nurse and system outcomes: A pilot study and focus for multicenter international study. *Policy, Politics, and Nursing Practice, 7*, 169–179.
- Pellico, L., Djukic, M., Kovner, C., & Brewer, C. (2009). Moving on, up, or out: Changing work needs of new RNs at different stages of their beginning nursing practice. *Online Journal of Issues in Nursing, 15*(1). Retrieved from http://www.nursingworld.org/MainMenuCategories/ANAMarketplace/ANA-Periodicals/OJIN/TableofContents/Vol152010/No1Jan2010/Articles-Previous-Topic/Changing-Work-Needs-of-New-RNs.aspx
- Stone, P. W., Duffield, C., Griffin, P., Hinton-Walker, P., Laschinger, H. K. S., O'Brien-Pallas, L. L., & Shamian, J. (2003, November 3). *An international examination of the cost of turnover and its impact on patient safety and outcomes*. Proceedings of the 37th biennial convention, Sigma Theta Tau International, Toronto, ON.
- Trinkoff, A., Johantgen, M., Storr, C., Gurses, A. P., Liang, Y., & Han, K. (2011). Nurses' work schedule characteristics, nurse staffing, and patient mortality. *Nursing Research, 60*(1), 1–8.
- Trossman, S. (2005). Who you work with matters. *American Nurse, 37*(4), 1, 8.
- University Health System Consortium. (2003). *Successful practices for workplace of choice employers*. Oak Brook, IL: Author.
- Worthington, K. (2001). The health risks of mandatory overtime. *American Journal of Nursing, 101*(5), 96.

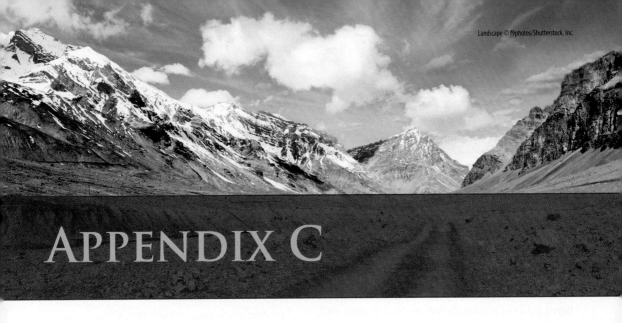

APPENDIX C

Getting the Right Position

Career Development—First Step: First Nursing Position

Career development is a responsibility of every nurse. This process really begins before graduation from a nursing program and licensure.

From Student to Practice: Reality Shock

Reality shock has been identified in nursing as the shock-like reaction that occurs when initial education comes in conflict with work-world values (Kramer, 1974). Another definition is "the incongruency of values and behaviors between the school subculture and the work subculture that leads to role deprivation or reality shock" (Schmalenberg & Kramer, 1979, p. 2). Benner (1984) identified five stages of competence: novice, advanced beginner, competent, proficient, and expert. The first three stages are affected by reality shock. Through the nursing education process, the novice nurse learns the rules for performance but has limited real-life clinical experience during which to apply those rules and to expand clinical reasoning and judgment.

Getting your first job as an RN is a very important step in your career development. Even before graduation, you should take some time to begin a career plan. The plan will change over time, but having a plan provides a guide for personal professional decisions.

Tools and Strategies to Make the Transition Easier

Where to begin? You should begin by developing a résumé, composing a biosketch, and maintaining a professional portfolio. A résumé is a one- or two-page document that describes the person's career. It includes your name, contact information, credentials, education, goals and objectives, and employment and relevant experience (a résumé should be kept current and not be lengthy). The biosketch is a paragraph that provides a short summary of your work history and accomplishments. It should include your name, credentials, and education. It is a narrative rather than a list. Later, curriculum vitae can be developed. This is a more detailed accounting of information found in the résumé and includes publications, presentations, continuing education (CE), honors and awards, community activities, and grants.

503

The portfolio provides evidence of a person's competency. It is not always required for job applications, but sometimes it is, and in some positions, nurses are asked to maintain a portfolio for performance review. A portfolio is a collection of information that demonstrates your experiences and accomplishments, such as committee work, professional organization activities, presentations, development of patient education material, awards, letters of recognition, projects and grants, and so on. The portfolio should include annual goals and objectives and review of outcomes, which should be updated annually.

A professional development plan, which is based on information found in your résumé and portfolio, lays out the direction you want to take with your career over the next year, 2 years, and 5 years. It should include a target time frame and strategies and activities to reach the goals. Self-assessment is a critical activity for any nurse, and this assessment helps you to further develop the career plan.

Interviewing for a New Position

Interviewing for a new position as a nurse should be taken seriously. The first step is setting up the interview. As the potential employee, you should find out the time of the appointment, the location, and the length of the interview. Will there be more than one interview on the same day? Will additional interviews take place later depending on whether the person is considered for the position? Will the interview be with one person or with a group? Do your homework; find out as much as possible about the organization and people who will be at the interview, and think about which types of questions might be asked and how to respond to them. Wear business dress, look neat, and be prepared. Bring a copy of your résumé to all interviews and any other required documents. Make sure you know how to get to the interview, and arrive early to allow yourself time to focus on the interview. Delays can happen when you least expect it, so planning to arrive early helps to prevent lateness.

During the interview, focus on the questions. Look the interviewer in the eye, take a moment to respond, and ask for clarification if you are unsure about the question. Share information about competencies and experiences—successes and challenges, and how you handled them. Ask the interviewer about the organization and the position.

When the interview is completed, thank the interviewer. Follow up to thank him or her (in a letter or via e-mail). Ask about the process—what comes next, when the decision will be made, and so on.

Box C-1 suggests examples of questions to ask at an interview.

Determination of the Best Fit: You and a New Position

How does one choose a position and an organization for employment? It is not easy to know that the fit is a good one. First, know which type of nursing interests you and why. Second, based on what you know about the healthcare organizations (HCOs) in the location where you want to work, focus on those organizations that most interest you. Today, the Internet is a resource for job hunting. Most HCOs, particularly hospitals, have websites. Explore them to learn about their organizations. Talk to people who may know about the organization that interests you.

Students often have clinical experiences in several HCOs, and they can use this opportunity to assess each organization. Do staff seem happy working there? Does the HCO differentiate degrees in nursing and how? What is the quality of care? What are some of the negative aspects of the organization?

Salary and benefits are always an important factor. Potential employees should also consider driving distance, parking, schedules, and general work conditions. Asking about promotions and use of career ladders can yield helpful information, along with how much support is given to staff for education (i.e., orientation, staff development, continuing education, and academic degrees). Regarding education, a new employee would want to know if tuition reimbursement is available, and for whom and at which level. Is it difficult to get release time to attend classes, or is there flexible staffing to allow for this?

Nurses should also ask about staff turnover, use of supplemental staffing (agency, travelers),

Box C-1	Examples of Questions to Ask During an Interview for a Hospital RN Position

- Do you have an opening on one of your _____ units in this hospital? For what shift?
- Would you hire a new BSN-prepared nurse to work in that unit? If no, why not?
- What is the position description for the job? (Ask to see it.)
- Which skills or knowledge (beyond basic preparation) would I need?
- How can I obtain these skills or knowledge?
- What are the opportunities for advancement in the unit?
- What is the culture of the unit?
- Who is the nurse manager and how long has the manager been in the position?
- What is the leadership style of the manager of the unit?
- What is the turnover rate of RNs in the unit?
- What is the relationship of RNs and physicians on the unit?
- Is a team concept practiced on the unit? If so, who are the members of the team?

Source: Modified from Milstead, J., & Furlong, E. (2006). *Handbook of nursing leadership: Creative skills for a culture of safety.* Sudbury, MA: Jones and Bartlett.

mandatory overtime, and change in nurse leaders. Organizations that experience high turnover in staff and nurse managers are organizations that are experiencing problems. Overreliance on supplemental staff indicates that the organization is having problems retaining nurses and developing strategies to cope with the nursing shortage.

Is the organization used for clinical experiences for nursing students? This usually means that the organization is interested in education, but it also means that staff need to be willing to work with students. How is medical staff coverage handled? Are there medical students and residents? It is important to know who covers for medical issues because this has an impact on expectations of nursing staff and collaboration with others. Today hospitals are ranked locally, by state, and nationally. This information can be accessed through the Internet.

The HCO's top leadership, such as the chief executive officer (CEO), is an important person. The CEO signs off on the budget. If the CEO does not recognize the importance of nursing to the organization and to outcomes, this can have a negative impact on how nurses are treated, and it can affect such budget issues as the number of nursing positions, salaries and benefits, and funds for education. The Forces of Magnetism have been used by nurses as criteria for evaluating potential organizations for employment.

Mentoring, Coaching, and Networking

Several methods are used in HCOs to support new staff, and mentoring is one of them. The mentor is more experienced and usually is selected by the staff nurse, but some HCOs assign new staff to mentors. The mentor acts as a role model and serves as a resource. Coaching is another method used for support, encouragement, and career development (e.g., how to go for a promotion or change of career ladder level, or to go back to school for a higher degree).

Networking is a less structured method. All nurses need to learn how to network or make connections with nurses and others who can help them. Professional organizations are good places to network and meet nurses who might provide guidance, support, and/or information. Nurses should keep contact information of potential connections even when they may not have a specific reason to make the contact; one never knows when the information may become important. Networking can also be done in non-healthcare settings that include people who may be helpful to know.

Career Ladder

Many HCOs today have developed career ladder programs for their nurses. The details of these career ladders vary from organization to organization. Typically, there are levels entitled Clinician I, II, III, and so on. The first level is entry level. The levels describe the role and responsibilities, as well as the educational requirements for that position or level. This type of system provides clear criteria for promotion and an increase in salary that does not require moving to a management position, which in the past was the most common path for advancement. The career ladder structure recognizes that clinical work is important and deserves recognition. Nurses have to demonstrate that they meet the criteria for the level that they are requesting. This is the point at which a nurse might use a portfolio and mentor. In some organizations, portfolios are required. Along with identified criteria HCOs need clear procedures for staff who want to apply for a change in level within the career ladder system.

Encouraging staff to participate in the career ladder offers positive outcomes for the organization, such as motivating staff to improve their competencies and increase their education level; increasing efforts to improve care; serving as an attractive recruitment strategy; and increasing retention. Performance improvement should be an active part of any nursing position. Through an active, positive performance improvement program, staff can use self-assessment and assessment from supervisors to further develop their career plans.

Going Back to School, Certification, and Continuing Education

Returning to school for another degree may not be your first thought after graduation and licensure, but when you develop a career plan, additional education should be considered. This decision should be based on

goals and a timeline. You need to consider the best time to begin work on additional education. Competency is an important issue. Do you need more time to achieve competency and to further your development as a professional nurse before entering a graduate program or a specialty? Some specialties may require certain type of practice experience before entering a graduate program—for example, nurse anesthesia programs require practice experience in critical care. Entering into such specialties requires serious thought and planning. Additional education is most productive when you are competent at your current position level and practice effectively as a professional nurse. For many new graduates, achieving this level of competency takes time.

Certification is another way to expand competencies and education; however, it does require that you have a specified amount of experience before taking the examination. Thus you need to plan when to apply and obtain the required experience.

Continuing education (CE) is a professional responsibility. Employers may provide educational experiences that also allow nurses to earn CE contact hours, or they may cover expenses for staff to attend CE programs outside the HCO. Many professional organizations offer CE programs, and some offer web-based programs. Many CE programs are offered via the Internet. Some states require that RNs earn a certain number of contact hours prior to relicensure. Certified nurses must meet CE requirements to continue their certification. CE is more effective if the content relates to the work that the nurse does and is in alignment with the nurse's professional goals. Nurses should keep a file of CE activities and update their records accordingly.

References

- Benner, P. (1984). *From novice to expert, excellence and power in clinical nursing practice.* Menlo Park, CA: Addison-Wesley Publishing Company.
- Kramer, M. (1974). *Reality shock: Why nurses leave nursing.* St. Louis, MO: Mosby.
- Schmalenberg, C., & Kramer, M. (1979). *Coping with reality shock.* Wakefield, MA: Nursing Resources.

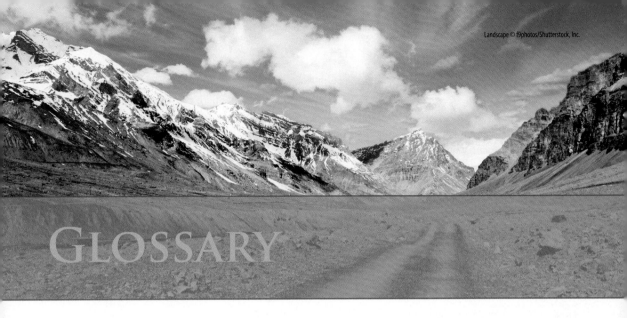

GLOSSARY

accountability An obligation or willingness to accept responsibility.

accreditation The process by which organizations are evaluated on their quality, based on established minimum standards.

acute care Treatment of a severe medical condition that is of short duration or at a crisis level.

advance directive A legal document that allows a person to describe his or her medical care preferences.

advanced practice nurse A registered nurse with advanced education in adult health, pediatrics, family health, women's health, neonatal health, community health, or other specialties.

adverse event An injury resulting from a medical intervention (in other words, an injury that is not caused by the patient's underlying condition).

advocacy Speaking for something important (one of the major roles of a nurse).

advocate A nurse who speaks for the patient but does not take away the patient's independence.

annual limit A defined maximum amount that an employee/policy holder/patient would have to pay, and after that level is reached, he or she no longer has to contribute to the payment for care.

applied research Research designed to find a solution to a practical problem.

apprenticeship A nursing program developed in England that provided on-the-job training and a formal education component.

articulation A formal agreement between two or more institutions that allows specific programs at one institution to be credited toward direct entry or advanced standing at another.

assertiveness Confronting problems in a constructive manner and not remaining silent.

associate degree in nursing A degree offered as culmination of a 2-year program that includes some liberal arts and sciences curriculum but focuses more on nursing.

autonomy The quality or state of being self-governing; the freedom to act on what you know.

baccalaureate degree in nursing A degree from a 4-year nursing program in a higher education institution.

basic research Research designed to broaden the base of knowledge rather than solve an immediate problem.

benchmarking Measurement of progress toward a goal, taken at intervals prior to the program's completion or the anticipated attainment of the final goal.

bias A predisposition to a point of view.

blame-free environment An environment that encourages reporting of errors and focuses more on a systematic view of errors rather than individual causation.

breach of duty The proximate (foreseeable) cause or the cause that is legally sufficient to result in liability for harm to the patient; a breach of due care.

burnout A deterioration of attitude in which a person becomes tired, defensive, frustrated, cynical, bored, and generally pessimistic about the job; exhaustion of physical or emotional strength.

care coordination Establishment and support of a continuous healing relationship, enabled by an integrated clinical environment and characterized by a proactive delivery of evidence-based care and follow-up.

care map An innovative approach to planning and organizing nursing care.

caregiver Someone who provides care to another; not a healthcare professional.

caring Feeling and exhibiting concern and empathy for others.

case management A system of management that facilitates effective care delivery and outcomes for patients through structured care coordination.

certification A process by which a nongovernmental agency validates, based on predetermined standards, an individual nurse's qualification and knowledge for practice in a defined functional or clinical area of nursing.

change agent Someone who engages deliberately in, or whose behavior results in, social, cultural, or behavioral change.

clinical data repository An information warehouse that stores data longitudinally and in multiple forms, such as text, voice, and images.

clinical decision support systems Computerized documentation systems that provide immediate information that can influence clinical decisions.

clinical experience Practicum that occurs when students with faculty supervision provide care to patients for learning experiences.

clinical information system A method of data storage generally used at the point of care.

clinical judgment The process by which nurses come to understand the problems, issues, and concerns of patients; to attend to salient information; and to respond to patient problems in concerned and involved ways. It includes both conscious decision making and intuitive response.

clinical pathways Descriptions of how care is best provided for a specific patient population with specific problem(s).

clinical reasoning The nurse's ability to assess patient problems or needs and analyze data to accurately identify and frame problems within the context of the individual patient's environment. *See also* **clinical judgment.**

code of ethics A list of provisions that makes explicit the primary goals, values, and obligations of the nursing profession; published by the American Nurses Association.

coding system A set of agreed-upon symbols (frequently numeric or alphanumeric) that is used to change information into another form so that it can be better accessed and used.

collaboration Cooperative effort among healthcare providers, staff, and multiple organizations who work together to accomplish a common mission.

communication The exchange of thoughts, messages, or information.

community The people and their relationships that use common services and share specific space environment.

compassion fatigue The feeling of emotion that ensues when a person is moved by the distress or suffering of another, leading to a state of psychic exhaustion.

computer literacy Knowledge of basic computer technology.

confidentiality The responsibility to keep patient information private, except as required to communicate in the care process and with team members.

conflict A state of opposition between persons, ideas, or interests.

conflict resolution A process of resolving a dispute or disagreement.

consumer/customer The ultimate user of a product or service.

continuing education Systematic professional learning designed to augment knowledge, skills, and attitudes.

continuum of care Care services available to assist an individual throughout the course of his or her disease.

coordination Proactive methods to optimize health outcomes.

copayment The fixed amount that a patient may be required to pay per service (doctor's visit, lab test, prescription, etc.).

coping The process of managing taxing circumstances.

corporatization Business; the business of health care.

counselor A person who gives guidance in a specific area of expertise or knowledge.

credentialing A process used to ensure that practitioners are qualified to perform and to monitor continued licensure.

critical thinking Purposeful, informed, outcome-focused (results-oriented) thinking that requires careful identification of key problems, issues, and risks.

culture The knowledge and values shared by a society.

curriculum An integrated course of academic studies that describes the program's philosophy, level, and terminal competencies for students, or what they are expected to be able to accomplish by the end of the program.

data Discrete entities that are described objectively without interpretation.

data analysis software Computer software that can analyze data.

data bank A large store of information, which may include several databases.

data mining Locating and identifying unknown patterns and relationships within data.

database A collection of interrelated data, often with controlled redundancy, organized according to a scheme to serve one or more applications.

deductible The part of the bill that the patient must pay before the insurer begins to pay for services.

delegatee The person to whom someone delegates a task.

delegation The transfer of responsibility to complete a task that is within the scope of the transferee's position.

delegator The person who assigns responsibility or authority.

differentiated practice A philosophy that focuses on the structuring of roles and functions of nurses according to education, experience, and competence.

diploma schools of nursing Nursing programs associated with a hospital that offer a nursing degree that is not offered through a college or university setting; typically 3 years in length.

disease prevention Focuses on interventions to stop the development of disease, but also includes treatment to prevent disease from progressing further and leading to complications. The major levels of prevention are primary, secondary, and tertiary.

disparity An inequality or a difference in some respect.

distance education A set of teaching and/or learning strategies to meet the learning needs of students separate from the traditional classroom and sometimes from traditional roles of faculty; for example, an online course.

diversity All the ways in which people differ, including innate characteristics (e.g., age, race, gender, ethnicity, mental and physical abilities, and sexual orientation) and acquired characteristics (e.g., education, income, religion, work experience, language skills, and geographic location).

do not resuscitate (DNR) A form of advance directive that may be part of an extensive advance directive. This order means that there should be no resuscitation if the patient's condition indicates need for resuscitation.

educator A person who teaches others; typically a professional such as a nurse or teacher.

effective care The provision of services based on scientific knowledge (evidence-based practice) to all who could benefit, and refraining from providing services to those not likely to benefit (avoiding underuse and overuse).

efficient care Care that avoids waste, including waste of equipment, supplies, ideas, and energy.

electronic medical record (EMR) A medical record in a digital format.

e-mail list A list of e-mail addresses that can be used to send one e-mail to all addresses at one time.

e-measurement The secondary use of electronic data to populate standardized performance measures.

empower   To give power to another.

empowerment   Having power or authority.

encryption   Changing written information, especially patient information, into a code that protects the privacy of data for security purposes.

entrepreneur   An innovator who recognizes opportunities to introduce a new process or an improved organization.

equitable care   The provision of care that does not vary in quality because of personal characteristics such as gender, ethnicity, geographic location, and socioeconomic status.

error   The failure of a planned action to be completed as intended or the use of the wrong plan to achieve an aim; errors are directly related to outcomes.

ethical decision making   Ethical dilemmas that occur when a person is forced to choose between two or more alternatives, none of which is ideal.

ethical principles   A standardized code or guide to behaviors for the nursing profession.

ethics   A standardized code or guide to behaviors.

ethnicity   A shared feeling of belonging to a group; peoplehood.

ethnocentrism   The belief that one's group or culture is superior to others.

evidence-based management (EBM)   Use of evidence such as research to support management decisions.

evidence-based practice (EBP)   The integration of the best evidence into clinical practice, which includes research, the patient's values and preferences, the patient's history and exam data, and clinical expertise.

executive branch   The branch of the U.S. government in charge of enforcing and executing the laws.

experimental study   A type of research design in which the conditions of a program or experience (treatment) are controlled by the researcher and in which experimental subjects are randomly assigned to treatment conditions. This design must meet three criteria: manipulation, control, and randomization.

extended care   The provision of inpatient skilled nursing care and related services to patients who require medical, nursing, or rehabilitative services.

failure to rescue   The inability to recognize a patient's negative change in status in a timely manner in order to prevent patient complications and to prevent major disability or death.

family   Two or more individuals who depend on one another for emotional, physical, and/or financial support.

followers   Members of a team.

for-profit   An organization that must provide funds to pay stockholders or owners; this affects the availability of money for other purposes that have an impact on nurses and nursing.

Forces of Magnetism   The identified effective descriptors of healthcare organizations that are designated as Magnet organizations.

handoff   A clinical situation that occurs when the patient is passed from one provider or setting to another; increasing the risk for errors.

health   The state of well-being; free from disease.

Health Insurance Portability and Accountability Act of 1996 (HIPAA)   A law that amended the Internal Revenue Code of 1986 to improve portability and continuity of healthcare information and ensure privacy of patient information.

health literacy   The ability to understand and use health information.

health promotion   Effort to stop the development of disease by emphasizing wellness; includes treatment to prevent a disease from progressing further and causing complications.

healthcare disparity   An inequality or gap in healthcare services that exists between two or more groups.

healthcare report cards   A report that provides specific performance data for an organization at specific intervals, with a focus on quality and safety.

healthy community   A community that embraces the belief that health is more than merely an absence of disease.

Healthy People 2020   A federal initiative to improve the health of all citizens in the United States by establishing goals and leading indicators for communities to strive for; results are monitored and then used to adjust the initiative (goals and indicators).

home care   The provision of healthcare services in the home.

hospice   A philosophy of care for managing symptoms and supporting quality of life as long as possible for the terminally ill.

hypothesis   A formal statement in a research study describing the expected relationship or relationships between two or more variables in a specified population (the sample).

identity   Sense of self as a professional nurse.

illness   A sickness or disease of the mind or body.

informatics   An integration of nursing science, computer science, and information science to manage and communicate data, information, knowledge, and wisdom in nursing practice.

information   Data that are interpreted, organized, or structured.

information literacy   The ability to recognize when information is needed and to locate, evaluate, and effectively use that information.

informed consent   Permission required by law to explain or disclose information about a medical problem and treatment or procedure so that a patient can make an informed choice.

internship/externship   A program that offers nursing students employment (typically during the summer) and includes educational experiences such as seminars, special speakers, and simulation experiences.

interprofessional team-based care   Care delivered by intentionally created, usually relatively small work teams in health care, who are recognized by others and by themselves as having a collective identity and shared responsibility for a patient or a group of patients (e.g., rapid response team, palliative care team, primary care team, operating room team).

interprofessional teamwork   The levels of cooperation, coordination, and collaboration characterizing the relationship between professions in delivering patient-centered care.

intuition   Quick and ready insight.

The Joint Commission   A major nonprofit organization that accredits more than 20,500 healthcare organizations, including hospitals, long-term care organizations, home care agencies, clinical laboratories, ambulatory care organizations, behavioral health organizations, and healthcare networks or managed care organizations.

judicial branch   The branch of the U.S. government that interprets and applies laws in specific cases.

knowledge   An awareness and understanding of facts.

knowledge management   A method for gathering information and making it available to others.

knowledge worker   A person who is effective in acquiring, analyzing, synthesizing, and applying evidence to guide practice decisions.

leader   One who has the ability to influence others; a role that nurses assume, either formally by taking an administrative position or informally as others recognize that they have leadership characteristics.

leadership   The ability to influence others to achieve a common goal or outcome.

legal issues   Questions and problems concerning the protections that make laws (U.S. Congress).

legislative branch   The law-making branch of the U.S. government; made up of the Senate, the House of Representatives, and agencies that support Congress.

living will   A document that describes a person's wishes related to his or her end-of-life care needs.

lobbying   Assembling and petitioning the government for redress of grievances.

lobbyist   An individual paid to represent a special interest group, whose function is to urge support for or opposition to legislative matters.

long-term care   A continuum of broad-ranged maintenance and health services delivered to the chronically ill, disabled, and the elderly.

macro consumer   The major purchasers of care: the government and insurers.

Magnet hospital   A hospital that demonstrates high levels of quality of care, autonomy, primary nursing care, mentoring, professional recognition, respect, and the ability to practice nursing; hospitals awarded this status meet specific standards.

malpractice   An act or continuing conduct of a professional that does not meet the standard of professional competence and results in provable damages to a patient.

management   A formal administrative position that focuses on four major functions: planning, organizing, leading, and controlling.

master's degree in nursing A graduate-level nursing degree of approximately 2 years with specialty focus (e.g., advanced nurse practitioner or clinical specialist).

Medicaid The federal healthcare reimbursement program that covers health and long-term care services for children, the aged, blind persons, the disabled, and people who are eligible to receive federally assisted income maintenance payments.

medical power of attorney The right of a person given by another individual to speak for him or her if he or she cannot do so in matters related to health care. Also known as a durable power of attorney for health care or a healthcare agent or proxy.

Medicare The federal health insurance program for people aged 65 and older, persons with disabilities, and people with end-stage renal disease.

mentor A role model.

mentoring Method used in healthcare organizations to support new staff; the mentor acts as a role model and serves as a resource.

micro consumer The patients, families, and significant others who play a role in patient care and in the decision-making process.

microsystem In healthcare delivery, a small group of people who work together on a regular basis to provide care to discrete subpopulations including the patients.

minimum data set The minimum categories of data with uniform definitions and categories; an example would be the Nursing Minimum Data Set.

misuse An event that leads to avoidable complications that prevent a patient from receiving the full potential benefit of a service.

National Database of Nursing Quality Indicators A system in which nursing data are collected to evaluate outcomes and nursing care.

near miss An event that occurred that could have led to an adverse event but did not.

negligence Failure to exercise the care toward others that a reasonable or prudent person would have under the same circumstances; an unintentional tort.

networking The cultivation of productive relationships for employment or business.

nomenclature A system of designations (terms) elaborated according to preestablished rules; an example would be the International Classification for Nursing Practice.

not-for-profit An incorporated organization whose shareholders or trustees do not benefit financially.

nurse practice act The act that governs nursing practice in the state in which the nurse practices.

nursing The profession of a nurse.

nursing informatics The specialty that integrates nursing science, computer science, and information science to manage and communicate data, information, knowledge, and wisdom in nursing practice.

nursing process A systematic method for thinking about and communicating how nurses provide patient care; this includes assessment, diagnosis, planning, intervention or implementation, and evaluation.

occupational health care Health promotion, disease and illness prevention, and treatment; includes attention to the risks of illness and injury within the work environment.

organizational culture The values, beliefs, traditions, and communication processes that bring a group of people together and characterize the group.

organizational ethics Organizational concerns related to the beliefs, decision making, and behavior of the organization as an entity.

outcomes Measurable benefits of patient care.

outcomes research Research focused on determining the effectiveness of healthcare services and patient outcomes.

overuse The point at which the potential for harm from the provision of a service exceeds the possible benefit.

palliative care Care focused on alleviating symptoms and meeting the special needs of the terminally ill patient and the family.

patient advocacy Respecting patient rights and the patient and ensuring that the patient has the education to understand treatment and care needs.

patient-centered care Identification of, respect, and care for patient differences, values, preferences, and needs; relief of pain; coordination of care; clear communication with and education of the patient; shared decision making; and continuous promotion of disease prevention and wellness.

patient–intervention–comparison–outcome–time (PICOT) To ask a searchable and answerable question. The *P* (patient population) is specific and describes the population in terms such as age, gender, diagnosis, ethnicity, other. The *I* (intervention) relates to prognostic factors, risk behaviors, exposure to disease, clinical intervention or treatment, and so foth. The *C* (comparison intervention) can pertain to another treatment, no treatment, or other. The *O* (outcome) includes factors such as risk of disease, complications or side effects, or adverse outcomes. The *T* is the time, meaning the time involved to demonstrate the outcome.

personal health record (PHR) Computer-based health records that collect data over a lifetime; with permission of the patient, this record can be accessed easily by any provider who needs the information.

plan–do–study–act (PDSA) cycle A systematic approach to planning and decision making.

policy A set course of action that affects a large number of people and is stimulated by a specific need to achieve certain outcomes.

political action committee (PAC) A private group that represents a specific issue or group and works to get someone elected or defeated.

politics The process of influencing the authoritative allocation of scarce resources.

power The ability to influence decisions and have an impact on issues that matter.

practice model A framework used to guide practice.

practicum A course that includes clinical activities and stresses the practical application of theory in a field of study; also referred to as a "clinical."

preceptor An experienced and competent staff member (an RN or, for nurse practitioner students, possibly a nurse practitioner or physician) who has received formal training to function as a preceptor and who serves as a role model to guide student learning, serving as a resource for the nursing student.

prejudice Making assumptions or judgments about the beliefs, behaviors, needs, and expectations of other persons who are of a different cultural background than oneself because of emotional beliefs about the population; involves negative attitudes toward the different group.

prescriptive authority Legal authority granted to advanced practice nurses to prescribe medication.

primary care Initial or entry point of care for patients.

private policy Policy created by nongovernmental organizations.

procedures A definite statement of step-by-step actions required for a specific result.

process Particular course of action intended to achieve a result.

professional ethics Generally accepted standards of conduct and methods in the nursing profession.

professionalism The conduct, aims, or qualities that characterize or mark a profession.

protocols Treatment plans.

provider of care A healthcare staff member who provides care to patients.

provider order entry system A data-entry system that allows healthcare providers to input orders into a computer system rather than writing them.

Public Health Act of 1944 This law consolidated all existing public health legislation into one law.

public policy Policy created by the legislative, executive, and judicial branches of federal, state, and local levels of government that affects individual and institutional behaviors under the government's respective jurisdiction.

qualitative study A systematic, subjective, methodological research approach; analysis of data that does not rely on statistics or mathematical equations.

quality Requirements that maintain high standards.

quality improvement (QI) An organized approach to identify errors and hazards in care, and to improve care overall.

quantitative study A formal, objective, systematic research process that uses statistics for data analysis.

race A biological designation of a group.

randomized controlled trial (RCT) Often referred to as the gold standard in research designs, this is the true experiment in which there is control over variables, randomization of the sample with a control group and an experimental group, and an intervention(s) (independent variable).

reality shock   The reaction of students when they discover that the clinical experience does not always match the values and ideals that they had anticipated.

recognition   A process used to evaluate an organization's adherence to excellence-focused standards.

reflective thinking   Creativity and conscious self-evaluation over a period of time.

regulation   An official rule or order, based on laws, governing processes, practice, and procedures; in nursing, legal regulation governs licensure.

rehabilitation   The restoration of, or improvement of, an individual's health and functionality.

reimbursement   Payment for healthcare services.

research   Investigation or experimentation aimed at the discovery and interpretation of facts about a particular subject.

research analysis   The process of using methods to analyze and summarize results or data.

research design   A specific plan for conducting a study.

research problem statement   A description of the topic or subject for a research study, which provides the context for the research study and typically generates questions that the research aims to answer.

research proposal   A written document that describes recent, relevant literature on the problem area; describes the research topic/problem; and defines the processes or steps that will be followed to answer the research question(s).

research purpose   Identifies the potential uses of research results.

research question   The interrogative statement that directs a research study.

researcher   A person who systematically investigates and studies materials and sources to establish facts and reach conclusions.

residency   A special employment program that helps new RN graduates transition to practice in a structured program that provides content and learning activities, precepted experiences, mentoring, and gradual adjustment to higher levels of responsibility.

resilience   The ability to cope with stress.

responsibility   Moral, legal, or mental accountability.

risk management (RM)   Maintaining a safe and effective healthcare environment and preventing or reducing financial loss to the healthcare organization.

role   Behavior oriented to the patterned expectation of others.

role transition   Gradual development in a new role.

root-cause analysis   An in-depth analysis of an error to assess the event and identify causes and possible solutions.

safety/safe care   Freedom from accidental injury.

scholarship   A fund for knowledge and learning.

scope of practice   A statement that describes the who, what, where, when, why, and how of nursing practice.

secondary caregiver   Assistant who helps home patients with intermittent activities such as shopping, transportation, home repairs, getting bills paid, emergency support, and so forth.

security protections   Methods used to ensure that information is not read or taken by persons not authorized to access it.

self-directed learning   A process in which individuals take the initiative, with or without the help of others, in diagnosing their learning needs, formulating learning goals, identifying human and material resources for learning, choosing and implementing appropriate learning strategies, and evaluating learning outcomes.

self-management of care   The systematic provision of education and supportive interventions to increase patients' skills and confidence in managing their own health problems, including regular assessment of progress and problems, goal-setting, and problem-solving approaches.

sentinel event   An unexpected medical event that results in death or physical or psychological harm, or the risk thereof.

shared governance   A management philosophy, a professional practice model, and an accountability model that focuses on staff involvement in decision making, particularly in decisions that affect their practice.

simulation   Replication of some or nearly all essential aspects of a clinical situation as realistically as possible.

situation–background–assessment–recommendations (SBAR) A systematic communication method that is used to improve communication of critical information about a patient that requires immediate attention and action.

social policy statement A statement that describes the profession of nursing and its professional framework and obligations to society; published by the American Nurses Association.

Social Security Act of 1935 The act that established the U.S. Medicare and Medicaid programs—two major reimbursement programs—and also provided funding for nursing education through amendments added to the law.

software Computer programs and applications.

standard A reference point against which other things can be evaluated and that serve as guides to practice.

standardized language A collection of terms with definitions for use in informational systems databases.

status A position in a social structure with rights and obligations.

stereotype The process by which people use social groups (e.g., gender and race) to gather, process, and recall information about other people; also known as labeling.

stress A complex experience felt internally that makes a person feel a loss or threat of a loss; bodily or mental tension.

stress management Strategies used to cope with stress to alter bodily or mental tension; reducing the negative impact of stress, improving health, and developing health-promoting behaviors.

structure The environment in which services are provided; inputs into the system, such as patients, staff, and environments.

surveillance Purposeful and ongoing acquisition, interpretation, and synthesis of patient data for clinical decision making.

system The coming together of parts, interconnections, and purpose.

systematic review A summary of evidence typically conducted by an expert or a panel of experts on a particular topic; uses a rigorous process to minimize bias for identifying, appraising, and synthesizing studies to answer a specific clinical question and draw conclusions about the data gathered; different methods may be used depending on the type of review such as integrative review or meta-analysis.

team A number of persons associated in work or activity.

team leader The person who leads the team.

teamwork Work done by several associates, with each doing a part but all subordinating personal prominence to the efficiency of the whole.

telehealth The use of telecommunications equipment and communications networks to transfer healthcare information between participants at different locations.

telenursing The use of telecommunications technology in nursing to enhance patient care.

tertiary care Level of care that occurs when there is disability and the need to maintain or, if possible, improve functioning.

theory A body of rules, ideas, principles, and techniques that applies to a particular subject.

therapeutic use of self The nurse's use of his or her personality consciously and in full awareness in an attempt to establish relatedness and to structure a nursing intervention.

time management Strategies used to manage and control time productivity.

timely care Meeting the patient's needs; providing high-quality experiences and improved healthcare outcomes when needed.

training Activities and instruction intended to foster skilled behavior.

types of power Legitimate (formal), referent (informal), informational, expert, reward, and coercive power.

transformational leadership This approach emphasizes a positive work environment, recognition of the importance of change and using change effectively, rewarding staff for expertise and performance, and development of staff awareness. Transformational leaders create vision and mission statements with the staff to guide the work of the organization and are described as honest, energetic, loyal, confident, self-directed, flexible, and committed.

underuse   Failure to provide a service that would have produced a favorable outcome for the patient.

unlicensed assistive personnel   Healthcare workers who are not licensed to perform nursing tasks but are trained and often certified.

utilization review   Evaluating necessity, appropriateness, and efficiency of healthcare services for specific patients or in patient populations.

wisdom   The appropriate use of knowledge to solve human problems; understanding when and how to apply knowledge.

wraparound services   Services that offer social and economic interventions, preferably within the healthcare provider setting to better ensure that full services are provided for complex patient needs.

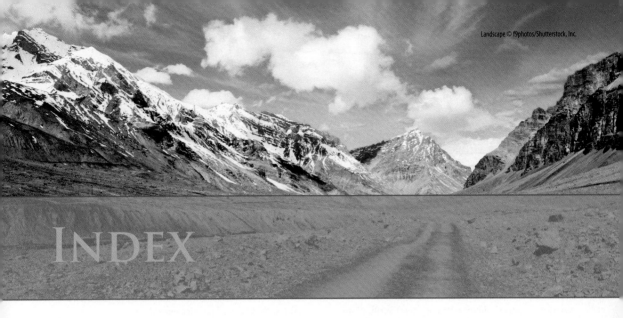

INDEX

Note: Page numbers followed by *b*, *f*, and *t* indicate material in boxes, figures, and tables, respectively.